Physical Rehabilitation in ARTHRITIS

On the cover is a picture of the knees of a 45-year-old woman who has an acute exacerbation of osteoarthritis of the left knee taken with infrared thermography (Agema Thermovision 4000 series). Each color represents a 0.5 °C difference in temperature ranging from the cooler temperatures in the dark blue to warmer temperatures in the light pink. The left knee is clearly hotter than the right. These colors revert towards normal with adequate treatment. (Courtesy R.A. Scudds, PhD, PT.)

Physical Rehabilitation in ARTHRITIS

SECOND EDITION

Joan M. Walker, PhD, MA, Dip TP, BPT, Certifs in PT (NZ)
Professor Emerita
Faculty of Graduate Studies and Faculty of Health Professions
School of Physiotherapy
Dalhousie University
Halifax, Nova Scotia, Canada

Antoine Helewa, MSc(Clin Epid), PT
Professor Emeritus
Department of Physical Therapy
University of Western Ontario
London, Ontario, Canada

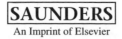

SAUNDERS
An Imprint of Elsevier

SAUNDERS

An Imprint of Elsevier

11830 Westline Industrial Drive
St. Louis, Missouri 63146

PHYSICAL REHABILITATION IN ARTHRITIS SECOND EDITION   ISBN 0-7216-9538-8
Copyright © 2004, Elsevier Inc. All rights reserved.

Previous edition copyrighted 1996

Library of Congress Cataloging-in-Publication Data

Physical rehabilitation in arthritis / [edited by] Joan M. Walker, Antoine Helewa. – 2nd ed.
   p. ; cm.
  Rev. ed. of: Physical therapy in arthritis. c1996.
  Includes bibliographical references and index.
  ISBN 0-7216-9538-8
   1. Arthritis–Physical therapy. 2. Arthritis–patients–Rehabilitation. I. Walker, Joan M. II. Helewa, Antoine. III. Physical theray in arthritis.
  [DNLM: 1. Arthritis–rehabilitation. 2. Physical Therapy Techniques. WE 344 P577 2004]
  RC933.P465 2004
  616.7'22062–dc22

                          2003066832

Acquisitions Editor: Marion Waldman
Developmental Editor: Louise Bierig
Publishing Services Manager: Melissa Lastarria
Project Manager: Joy Moore
Designer: Amy Buxton

Printed in the United States of America

Last digit is the print number: 9 8 7 6 5 4 3 2 1

Author Biography

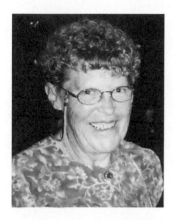

Joan M. Walker qualified as a physiotherapist from the New Zealand School of Physiotherapy in Dunedin, New Zealand. Over the years, she also completed a Teacher's Diploma of Physiotherapy from the Chartered Society of Physiotherapy, England; a Bachelor of Physical Therapy and Master of Arts (Physical Anthropology) from The University of Manitoba, Canada; and a Doctor of Philosophy (Medical Sciences, Growth and Development) from McMaster University, Canada. She has taught on the faculties of the Universities of Toronto, Manitoba, McMaster, Canada; Witwatersrand, South Africa; and Southern California, United States. A former Director at the Dalhousie University School of Physiotherapy, she currently holds the position of Emeritus Professor.

Dr. Walker focused her extensive research on exercise and aging, influences on cartilage and other joint tissues, and lately on post-poliomyelitis. She has written more than 60 peer-reviewed articles, presented more than 50 invited papers and courses, and delivered more than 35 conference presentations. In addition to writing and lecturing, she has served on numerous editorial committees and continues to review for a number of professional journals. Dr. Walker has received the prestigious Mildred Elson Award from the World Confederation of Physical Therapy (1999), the Enid Graham Memorial Lecture Award from the Canadian Physiotherapy Association (2002), The Helen Hislop Award, The Marion Williams Award from the American Physical Therapy Association (1994), and an Honorary Fellowship from the New Zealand Society of Physiotherapists (2003).

With Antoine Helewa she authored the textbook, *Critical Evaluation of Research in Physical Rehabilitation: Towards Evidence-Based Practice* (2000).

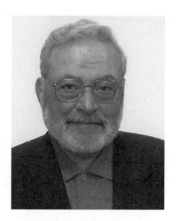

Antoine Helewa is Professor Emeritus at the School of Physical Therapy, University of Western Ontario (UWO), Ontario, Canada.

His professional career in physical therapy spans almost five decades, beginning with undergraduate training in Israel and graduate studies at the University of Toronto and McMaster University, both in Ontario, in physical therapy and clinical epidemiology. He was a lecturer in physical therapy at the universities of Toronto and Manitoba and Director of Professional Services for the Ontario Division of the Arthritis Society. This was followed by an appointment as a tenured Associate Professor and Chair, Department of Physical Therapy at UWO, a post he held for 10 years. In 1990 he was promoted to the rank of full professor.

Professor Helewa has published more than 30 peer-reviewed scientific articles, two textbooks, and numerous monographs. His primary research interests are in the fields of rheumatology, epidemiology, and the development of related outcome measures.

His volunteer activities are extensive; he has served on numerous professional and academic committees, chief among these as President of the Ontario Physiotherapy Association, President of the Canadian Physiotherapy Association (CPA), and founding member of the District Health Council of Metropolitan Toronto. In 1984, he received the Enid Graham Memorial Lecture Award, and in 1995 he became a Life Member of the CPA.

Contributors

Editors

Joan M. Walker, PhD, MA, Dip TP, BPT, Certifs in PT (NZ)
Professor Emeritus
Faculty of Graduate Studies and Faculty of Health Professions
School of Physiotherapy
Dalhousie University
Halifax, Nova Scotia, Canada

Antoine Helewa, MSc(Clin Epid), PT
Professor Emeritus
Department of Physical Therapy
University of Western Ontario
London, Ontario, Canada

Contributors

Priti Flanagan, BSP, PharmD
College of Pharmacy and Division of Geriatric Medicine
Dalhousie University
Halifax, Nova Scotia, Canada

Katherine Harman, PhD, MSc, BSc(PT)
Assistant Professor
School of Physiotherapy
Dalhousie University
Halifax, Nova Scotia, Canada

Donna J. Hawley, RN, EdD
Professor and Director
Institutional Research
Wichita State University
Wichita, Kansas

Mary Ann Keenan, MD
Department of Orthopaedic Surgery
University of Pennsylvania
Philadelphia, Pennsylvania

Peter Lee, MB, ChB, MD (Otago), FRACP, FRCPC
Mount Sinai Hospital
Toronto, Ontario, Canada

Marion A. Minor, PhD, PT
Assistant Professor and Chair
Physical Therapy Department
Faculty of Health Professions
University of Missouri
Columbia, Missouri

Carolee Moncur, PhD, PT
Division of Rheumatology and Bioengineering
University of Utah
Salt Lake City, Utah

Douglas Palma, MD
Albert Einstein Medical Center
Philadelphia, Pennsylvania

Rhonda J. Scudds, PhD, PT
Assistant Professor
Department of Rehabilitation Sciences
The Hong Kong Polytechnic University
Hong Kong, People's Republic of China

Roger A. Scudds, PhD, PT
Associate Professor and Physiotherapy Programme Leader
Department of Rehabilitation Sciences
The Hong Kong Polytechnic University
Hong Kong, People's Republic of China

Elaine Smith, MSW, RSW
MacMillan Bloorview Centre
Toronto, Ontario, Canada

Hugh A. Smythe, MD, FRCP(C)
Professor
Department of Medicine
Faculty of Medicine
University of Toronto
Toronto, Ontario, Canada

Barbara Stokes, Dip, PT
The Arthritis Society
Ottawa, Ontario, Canada

Susan L. Street, MScOT(C), OTRegNS
Doctoral Candidate
Faculty of Graduate Studies
Dalhousie University
Halifax, Nova Scotia, Canada

F. Virginia Wright, MSc(Clin Epid), PT
MacMillan Bloorview Centre
Toronto, Ontario, Canada

Foreword

Arthritis is one of the unique diagnoses in rehabilitation that seems pervasive because of the number of types and subtypes affecting individuals at all ages. Thus, the need to know all aspects of this disease entity, ranging from epidemiology to management, to availability of community resources, can affect the student or practitioner whether they treat clients in pediatric, geriatric, orthopaedic, neurologic, or even cardiopulmonary subspecialties. Given the increasing prevalence of arthritis and the fact that any one type, such as rheumatoid arthritis, can affect more than 1% of the entire U.S. population, offering contemporary knowledge about all aspects of the treatment of clients with arthritis seems invaluable.

This point was made patently clear recently when a physical therapist colleague, specializing in the treatment of older adults with movement limitations precipitated mostly by arthritis, told me of a recent encounter with a client. After performing a comprehensive evaluation, she streamlined what had appeared to be a vast list of exercises into a succinct few, and, in the process, explained to the client why the new sequence was arranged in the prescribed order and had now become self-limited. Furthermore, she instructed the client to take more responsibility for her own exercise program, despite her growing dependence as she approached her 75th year of life. Lastly, my colleague gave the client a list of resources and facilities where she could learn more or engage in activities with peers, some of whom had comparable problems.

The point to be made from this very real occurrence is that, remarkably, this course of action captures the unique attributes contained within the second edition of Walker and Helewa: *Physical Rehabilitation of Arthritis*. Although the first edition could certainly stand alone as a premier text on the subject of management (primarily by physical therapists) of the client with arthritis, this edition has successfully captured contemporary approaches to all aspects of treatment by rehabilitation team members. Each clinically-based chapter is oriented toward evidence-based practice and highlighted by the realities of clinical practice, reduced treatment time, the need for selective and specific prescription of treatment elements, the necessity for both client advocacy and self-responsibility, and the importance of engaging family and community resources. Woven into the fabric of this philosophy is the availability of superb referencing, as well as contemporary tests, measures, and informational bases.

Whereas the entire second edition is a superb clinical and instructional text for any clinician or student who studies or treats clients with arthritis, some chapters hold special appeal. Dr. Walker's update on the historical record of paleopathology in the management of arthritic clients (Chapter 1) preserves the historical perspective of the original contribution while updating contemporary approaches among rehabilitation specialists with a special emphasis on less passive and more progressive interventional approaches. Dr. Peter Lee's treatment of the diagnosis and management of arthritic conditions (Chapter 4) is particularly compelling because he has combined fundamental information with a critical but relevant practice based approach, highlighting clinical features with contemporary referencing.

Priti Flanagan and Joan Walker have added the description of newer medications and specific pharmacologic-client interactions necessary for rehabilitation clinicians to observe (Chapter 6). Also included here are excellent discussions on complementary and alternative medical therapies, an introduction into the developing field of pharmacogenomics, and updated references. F. Virginia Wright and Elaine Smith offer a most comprehensive treatment of the child and adolescent with juvenile rheumatoid arthritis (Chapter 8). Their emphasis is on outcome measures and alternative treatments that can be investigated by family members. The discussion emphasizes adherence to programs, interfacing clients into the community, and the need for clinicians to recognize psychosocial and behavioral problems.

Barbara Stokes also discusses psychosocial issues and the relevance of evidence-based interventions in the management of clients with ankylosing spondylitis (Chapter 10). Roger and Rhonda Scudds with Katherine Harman have revamped the presentation of managing clients with muscle pain syndromes (Chapter 12) and devote considerable effort to targeting discussion to clients with arthritis. This chapter is well-referenced and compact yet comprehensive, while offering treatment and management approaches for fibromyalgia, trigger points, and muscle pain without loss of the need to identify and consider behavioral components for each pain-related problem.

Susan Street has done a marvelous job in revamping the presentation on splinting and orthotics (Chapter 14). Her approach is analytical and speaks to a problem-solving mode that should characterize the thought processes of all good clinicians. The referencing and appendices will be most helpful guides to any rehabilitation professional wishing to order or assist in the fabrication of splints or orthotics for clients with arthritis. Donna Hawley has updated the discussion on psychosocial aspects of client management (Chapter 15), including important discussions on client responsibility, as well as successful mobility and comfort related to sexual activities. Barbara Stokes reminds us that engaging community resources may require an interdisciplinary approach while optimizing available resources (Chapter 16). She also reminds us about the importance of program planning within the context of an evidence-based approach to justify the identification and utilization of resources. The provision of web sites and other resources is invaluable.

Lastly, Antoine Helewa has created essentially a new chapter (Chapter 17) on the importance of critically comprehending and assessing written materials that are actually modeled in the very book he coedited with Joan M. Walker. The information he provides on how to appreciate the strengths and weaknesses of written materials as a necessary precursor to decision making before and during treatment forms the foundation of the growing integration of art and science so necessary to assure optimal care during the rehabilitation of clients with arthritis.

Steven L. Wolf, PhD, PT, FAPTA
Professor, Department of Rehabilitation Medicine
Professor of Geriatrics, Department of Medicine
Associate Professor, Department of Cell Biology
Emory University School of Medicine
Professor of Health and Elder Care
Nell Hodgson Woodruff School of Nursing at Emory University
Director, Program in Restorative Neurology
Emory University Clinic
Atlanta, Georgia

Preface to the First Edition

The need for a textbook focused on physical therapy management in arthritis is derived from the large number of individuals, from children to senior citizens, whose quality of life is impaired by arthritis. The latest survey by the United States Public Health Service listed about 31,000,000 people with these disorders.

Recent years have seen a marked growth of physical therapy in arthritis. Clinical and basic investigations have expanded and more capable people have been attracted to the field. There is now optimism that much can be done to control many of the arthritic disorders through judicious pharmacologic and physical management.

This volume is the first textbook to provide a comprehensive approach to physical therapy management of arthritis, written largely by physical therapists but also including contributions from other health professionals. All of the authors are recognized in North America for their clinical research and educational skills and expertise. We have directed this textbook to the clinician, but also, in recognition of the importance of well-prepared graduates, to physical therapy educators and students. The essential component of rheumatology in the entry-level curriculum has lacked a foundation reference. The editors hope that other health care workers in related fields will find the text a useful resource and addition to their libraries.

Initial chapters examine the historical record of arthritis, physical therapy involvement in the care of patients with arthritis, epidemiology and economics of arthritis. Middle chapters cover pathophysiology of inflammation, immobility and repair, medical and surgical management, psychosocial issues, pharmacology, orthotics and lifestyle factors to establish a firm foundation for physical therapy management. Subsequent chapters then focus on the physical assessment and management of common arthritis disorders, such as pain amplification syndromes, juvenile arthritis, inflammatory arthritis in adults, osteoarthritis, and ankylosing spondylitis.

The editors believe that the textbook presents innovative approaches to the assessment, and to the management of the young and adult patient with arthritis. Uniquely, and we believe appropriately, one chapter focuses on cardiovascular health and physical fitness for the client with multiple joint involvement. The text also addresses the increasingly important area of community-based health care in management of the client with arthritis.

The important area of evaluation of the quality of the growing literature in arthritis, essential to the provision of evidence-based care, is contained in the final chapter. The approach advocated will provide students and graduates with a critical, planned method to review the literature that may be used in fields other than arthritis.

Treatment chapters include case studies, as well as identification of problem issues or research questions. We feel that this textbook will fill a void in the literature, contribute to further research in arthritis by physical therapists, contribute to the delivery of evidence-based care, improve the quality of care, and ultimately improve the quality of the lives of individuals with arthritis.

Many individuals have contributed to this textbook. We have been inspired by patients, students, and colleagues. Particularly, we recognize the valuable contributions of research assistants at our universities, Noreen Delorey, Janice Palmer, Jane Farrell, and Lisa Wilson. We have been assisted by the computer skills of Pat Darling, and by the reference staff of the Kellogg Health Sciences Library, Dalhousie University. We are also grateful for the encouragement of Margaret Biblis, Senior Editor at W.B. Saunders Company, and for the work of Berta Steiner and the staff of Bermedica Production, Ltd.

Joan M. Walker
Antoine Helewa

Preface to the Second Edition

This second edition of *Physical Therapy in Arthritis*, now *Physical Rehabilitation in Arthritis* is truly a revision of all the content, as well as containing new material. The most efficacious approach in the management of any type of arthritis is a multidisciplinary approach, with a multidisciplinary team of varying membership. The new title reflects this approach.

The second edition contains several major changes. Chapter 17 has a new approach with the literature evaluation being replaced by a discussion of specific problems of clinical research in arthritis, as well as measurement properties of common assessment tools. The chapter on fibromyalgia in the previous edition is now a chapter on chronic muscle pain syndromes (Chapter 12) that uses fibromyalgia as one of the examples of those syndromes. Greater attention has been paid to the development of deformities in Chapter 3, and the Glossary has been expanded with the addition of the definitions for more than 15 terms related to deformities.

A content deficiency in the first edition has been corrected in Chapter 5 with a major expansion of detail related to techniques of assessing active joints and isometric muscle testing with a sphygmomanometer. Chapter 6 contains information on new families of drugs in arthritis, such as biologics, and there is a major overhaul of the content on splinting, orthotics, and lifestyle factors in Chapter 14. The resources appendix is expanded, includes some web sites, and lists peer-reviewed journals in rheumatology by ISI impact rating.

Overall, the authors have attempted to provide evidence-based content, and where that is lacking, to provide adequate detail about reported studies that will enable clinicians to have a firmer basis for their therapy choices. All management chapters contain a master plan in the form of an algorithm, covering management from assessment to discharge, and, in addition to a case study, a skeleton case for use in education. Where appropriate, attention has been given to the important personal topic of intimacy and arthritis. Lastly, reflecting that the person with arthritis should be an active, participatory member of the health care team, the term *client* is used, in preference to the more passive term, *patient*.

We welcome several new authors, Peter Lee, (Chapter 4), Priti Flanaghan, (Chapter 6), Roger and Rhonda Scudds and Katherine Harman (Chapter 12), and Susan Street (Chapter 14) and remain very appreciative of our contributing authors, Marian Minor, Carolee Moncur, Virginia Wright and Elaine Smith, Donna Hawley, Mary Ann Keenan, Hugh Smythe, and lastly Barbara Stokes who not only wrote two chapters but also gave other invaluable assistance. The multidisciplinary team of authors has helped us immensely to ensure that the second edition will appeal to a wider range of health care rehabilitative professionals.

Finally, we acknowledge with gratitude the assistance of many who helped make completion of the second edition possible. This edition was prepared working from our homes in northern Ontario and St Margaret's Bay, south of Halifax, a process greatly facilitated by modern electronic mail, and the assistance of James Crouse, MSc, technician at Dalhousie University, School of Physiotherapy. The continued support of the reference staff at the Kellogg Health Sciences Library, Dalhousie University, Halifax, especially Patrick Ellis, librarian, was invaluable. Many colleagues contributed through conversations and discussion, sharing clinical knowledge and experiences, and reading drafts; to them, we are most grateful as their contributions enhance the text revision. We are convinced that this text fills a unique gap in the literature and will be relevant both in educational programs as well as to clinicians caring for clients with arthritis for several years to come.

We appreciate the guidance and input from Andrew Allen, Publishing Director, Health Sciences, Elsevier, and his team, as well as Rondi Ingraham and her staff at Graphic World Publishing Services.

Joan M. Walker
Antoine Helewa

Preface to the Second Edition

Contents

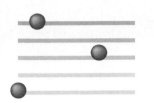

The Historical Record: Paleopathology, Physical Rehabilitation in Management of Arthritis

Joan M. Walker, PhD, PT

Paleopathological Record	Attitudes and Beliefs	Role of Nonmedical Health
Physical Therapy and	Physical Therapy and	Care Professionals in Clinics
Rehabilitation in the	Rehabilitation Today	Education in Rheumatology
Management of Arthritis:		Summary
Past to Present		References

In the United States, self-reported rheumatic diseases are rare in persons younger than 18 years and increasingly common in persons 65 years and older[1] (Table 1-1). In a recent span of 7 years (1990 to 1997), the prevalence of persons in the United States with self-reported arthritis increased substantially to 43 million.[2] For an estimated 8 million persons in the United States, arthritis constitutes a major or contributing cause of activity limitations.[2] Also in 1997, more than 4 million Canadians (1 in 7) were affected by rheumatic disorders.[3]

The increasing prevalence of arthritis, with its associated activity limitations, makes it likely that higher percentages of the workforce will be forced to retire as a result of osteoarthritis (OA) or allied conditions. British studies showed a loss of 4.7 million work days in 1974.[4] At that time, OA was the second leading cause of permanent incapacity in individuals older than 50 years, it affected some 40 million Americans, and it was evident radiologically in more than 80% of individuals 55 years and older.[5] Arthritic conditions constitute a significant, still increasing, social and economic burden in today's societies. Incidence and prevalence are discussed in Chapter 2.

Paleopathological Record

Next to traumatic conditions, arthritis is the oldest and most widespread pathological condition reported in paleopathology (the study of disease and trauma in extinct societies).[6] The fossilized remains of animals and people reveal patterns of injury and disease. These patterns reflect the environment and behavior of the animals and people and are expressions of the stresses and strains to which they were exposed.[7]

First recognized in dinosaurs, arthritis has been seen continuously throughout history. Distinction

PHYSICAL REHABILITATION IN ARTHRITIS, Joan M. Walker, PhD, PT, and Antoine Helewa, MSc(Clin Epid), PT, Elsevier Inc. © 2004.

Table 1-1. Estimated Prevalence Rates per 1000 Persons for Self-Reported Cases of Arthritis by Age and Sex, United States, 1994–1995

AGE (Years)	<24	25–34	35–44	45–54	55–64	65–74	75–84	>85
Male	0.8	5.5	10.5	19.4	29.7	44.5	46.4	42.1
Female	1.5	8.6	15.7	27.7	40.9	52.5	61.1	63.3

Modified from Centers for Disease Control and Prevention: *MMWR Morb Mortal Wkly Rep* 50:335, 2001.
Note: Confidence intervals increased with increasing age.

between rheumatoid arthritis (RA) and OA is not always made or possible; thus reports of "chronic arthritis" are more prevalent in publications. In hominids, chronic arthritis has been observed from the Neanderthal period (e.g., the man of La Chapelle-aux-Saints).[5] Studies of skeletons from the Saxon and Roman period of early England have shown "changes consistent with OA" in at least half the specimens.[8]

Spondylitis (arthritis of the vertebral column) is known to be present in ancient Egyptian populations since 4000 BC. Three of twelve Egyptian royal family mummies from 1570 BC to 324 AD had radiographic evidence of OA in the hips, knees, or spine.[9] Spondylitis also was common in Cro-Magnon and pre-Columbian American populations. In early humans, lumbar involvement was common; dorsal and cervical involvement was rare, with the exception of ancient Egyptians, in whom dorsal involvement was common.[5] By comparison, cervical involvement is common in modern populations, probably related to changing habits and forces. The modern increase in cervical spine involvement may be a reflection of the more sedentary lifestyles, the computer and video game age, and the increased time spent in poor sitting postures.

Hip joint involvement has been observed only in hominids, not in animals. Estimation of the involvement of hand and foot joints is affected by the greater loss of small bones over time. Evidence of arthritis has been observed in all time periods, climates, and locales, as well as in dinosaurs and cave bears, so the paleopathological record offers no support for climate, alcohol, or tobacco as causative factors. Variation in reported frequency of osteophytes (lipping) between early populations (as much as 50% in early Egyptian) is thought to reflect differences in life span. Longer life spans imply a longer exposure to stress.[10]

Systemic population radiography did not reveal evidence of OA in weight-bearing bones of several types of dinosaurs (e.g., tyrannosaurs).[8] OA also is relatively rare in Old World primates.[11] Although an isolated occurrence in dinosaurs, OA affected up to 26% of Pleistocene kangaroos and marsupial oxen.

Colony-raised animals may not constitute an adequate model for the study of "natural" OA.[12] Not only did the frequency of involvement differ significantly (0.8% in free animals compared with 4.8% in colony-raised animals), but the site of involvement differed as well: Shoulder and elbow joints were more affected in colony animals than in free animals, whereas knee joints were more affected in free animals. The longer life spans of colony animals were not considered to give an adequate explanation of these differences.

In the eighteenth century, William Heberden made the first reference to "hard knots, little peas," known now as *Heberden's nodes*. These nodes are frequently seen on digits of patients with OA. Heberden also recognized that these differed from those seen in gout.[5] Of interest is the report that such nodes are visible on ceramic figures made by pre-Columbian Indians (ca. 200 to 650 AD). Although Heberden distinguished between OA and gout, some confusion regarding the relationship between OA and RA remained throughout the nineteenth and early twentieth centuries. Sir William Osler also distinguished between OA and gout, describing at length a chronic disorder of joints termed *arthritis deformans*. Some of the lesions he described now would be termed *RA* (e.g., involvement of synovial membrane); however, he also described new bone formation in spinal ligaments, now termed *ankylosing spondylitis*.[5]

Substantial developments in investigative tools in the fields of radiology, immunology, and genetics have vastly improved our ability to distinguish between the many different types of arthritis. However, we have not advanced much in our ability to prevent or alter the course of many rheumatological conditions.

Hippocrates is credited with "convincing descriptions of gout."[13] The introduction of roentgen rays at the turn of the twentieth century allowed distinction between "atrophic" and "hypertrophic" arthritis, and then between OA and RA. Increasingly, sophisticated laboratory methods of analysis are permitting distinction of many different forms of RA, such as crystal deposition diseases and lupus erythematosus.

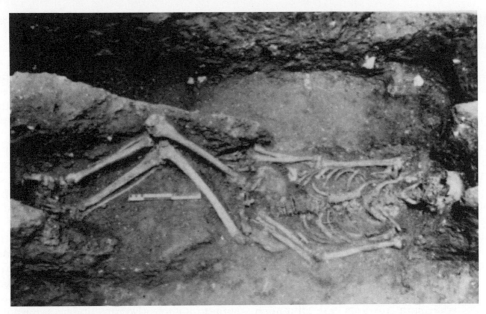

Figure 1-1. Medieval skeleton in situ. Note the flexed knees; this position was not a burial custom and suggests fixed flexion deformities antemortem. Subsequent examination showed extensive, asymmetric sacroiliitis, spondylitis, and peripheral erosive arthropathy with bony proliferation. This picture is cautiously interpreted as a possible example of psoriatic or reactive spondyloarthropathy. (From Dieppe P, Rogers JM: Skeletal paleopathology of rheumatic diseases. In McCarthy DJ, Koopman WJ [eds]: *Arthritis and Allied Conditions*, Vol. 1. Philadelphia, Lea & Febiger, 1993, p 11. With permission.)

Dieppe and Rogers[13] (whose article is recommended to any reader interested in skeletal paleopathology of rheumatoid disorders) cautioned against making a diagnosis of OA solely on evidence of osteophytes, because these alone may reflect only aging changes. Fusion or erosive spondyloarthritis may have been overdiagnosed as ankylosing spondylitis; some cases may be indicative of psoriatic arthropathy or Reiter's disease (Figure 1-1).[13] In contrast to OA, RA has not been convincingly demonstrated in ancient skeletons and RA, of the severity seen today, is "believed to be uncommon, if present at all, in previous centuries."[13] The inability to identify RA clearly, as compared with gout, in old art or literature suggests that it may be a disease of modern origin.[13]

Physical Therapy and Rehabilitation in the Management of Arthritis: Past to Present

Use of massage and exercises for a curative effect dates from prehistoric times. The Chinese used these modalities as early as 3000 BC. Early use also has been recorded by Hindus.[14] Hippocrates (460 to 360 BC) advocated the use of "friction," and Romans, such as Julius Caesar (100 BC) and Galen (131 to 201 AD), apparently valued massage for arthritis. Fuller[15] in 1740 advocated "rubbing and chafing for cutaneous exercise," walking, and riding. He referred to scorbutic rheumatism

in which café, the perfons afflicted are generally ftrong, unable to undergo any sorts of exercifes; and therefore all sorts of exercifes which I shall hereafter mention will agree with them.[15, p 43]

He claimed that moderate exercise augmented the natural heat of the body and increased the velocity of the circulation.

Buchan,[16] writing on domestic medicine in 1803, recommended for obstinate fixed rheumatic pains

a plafter of burgundy pitch worn for some time on the part affected to give great relief in rheumatic joints. The warm baths of Buxton or Matlock in Derbyshire are recommended for chronic or obstinate rheumatism. White mustard, a tablespoonful, taken twice a day. Cold bathing, especially in falt [salt] water often cures rheumatism and also recommend exercife and the wearing of flannel next to the fkin.[16, p 366]

Massage continued to be advocated through the nineteenth century. Roth[17] in 1851 stated that

> rheumatic pains of muscles are cured by pressure on the related nerves. This pressure, such as when given to the nervous accessorius willisii, can cure the most violent rheumatic pains of these parts. Acute rheumatic pains of intercostal muscles may disappear within a couple of hours by a kind of kneeling and rolling of the pectoral and other muscles combined with rotation of the arms. Rheumatic inflammation of the aponeurosis of the nates and left thigh, which occasioned at every movement the greatest pain, was cured in 6 days without medicines or bleedings, save only sawings on the suffering parts and longitudinal frictions of the skin towards the abdomen and back.[17, p 236]

Roth[17] also recognized the value of motion:

> limbs lamed by rheumatism are treated like the stiffness with this difference, that the supra abundant force of the parts adjacent to the diseased one must be diminished by the derivative movements, in order to increase the strength of the parts diseased. Stiffness of the limbs is treated according to the angles corresponding to the articulation in its healthy state, those stiffness that is caused by contractions of muscles and tendons are cured by frictions, combined with slow and extending movements.[17, p 254]

Osler,[18] in 1909, advocated "fresh air," a good diet, hydrotherapy, massage, and range-of-motion exercises; he further stated that salicylates may help and that surgery could correct deformities. Few early medical textbooks, in describing the use of massage, hydrotherapy, and exercise, refer specifically to arthritis but more to "stiffness and lameness of limbs." One of the earliest detailed accounts of physiotherapy in the form of massage for the treatment of chronic rheumatism was given by Goodall-Copestake[19] in 1926:

> Deep massage can be borne and are very beneficial. Careful passive movements gradually increased. Hot air and other baths often beneficial combined with massage. For muscular rheumatism, rest and warmth are essential. Hot applications, hot air or Turkish baths and massage often affords great relief. Time for treatment 15 to 40 minutes daily. For rheumatoid arthritis, massage forms part

of the treatment in every stage of the disease except during acute attacks but it may begin as soon as the pain and swelling have subsided somewhat. Effleurage, frictions, muscle kneadings and passive movements to affected joints. The patient should be encouraged to perform active movements whether painful or not so as to keep up the nutrition of the muscles. Care should be taken not to force movements for fear of rupturing the tendons. If bony changes have occurred in the joints, deep friction should be avoided. The chief objective of treatment, then, is to maintain the strength of muscles. Passive movements must not be given until pain and swelling have subsided.[19, p 169]

Although modern physical therapy (PT) includes only minimal use of massage, it is interesting that if used, it may be in the form of deep transverse frictions. Clients with arthritis obtain relief from general massage; however, there is no scientific evidence to support its use. Also, the modern university-prepared physical therapist is rarely a skilled practitioner in the art of massage.

It is rather remarkable, given the involvement of physical therapists in the management of clients with arthritis, that since the earliest beginnings of the profession there have been so few textbooks devoted to this topic. There are references to treatments for arthritis and nonarticular manifestations that include myalgia, fibrositis, and lumbago. The first major paper in English was written by Forester,[20] a physiotherapist, in 1953. Forester described the conservative treatment of RA, giving special emphasis to changes needed when adrenocorticotropic hormone (ACTH) and cortisone were used.[20] She also emphasized the prevention of deformity, relief of local symptoms, and use of graduated exercise—a change from the earlier emphasis on the use of massage.

Although PT was established as a unique profession at the turn of the twentieth century, even in the 1940s and 1950s, authors of PT texts rarely devoted even a single chapter to the management of patients with arthritis. This state existed despite the recommendation of the British Ministry of Health in 1928 that almost every patient with chronic arthritis at some stage of the disease required physical treatment, usually consisting of the application of heat, either alone or together with massage and movement. It was stated that no scheme of treatment for chronic arthritis could be considered complete unless an extensive range of physical methods of treatment under skilled direction was available. Glover[21] commented that "there appears to be a rapidly increasing demand for such treatment."

Palmer[22] in 1942 continued to advocate the use of effleurage, kneading, and petrissage in the treatment of OA but noted that frictions should be avoided on the articular margins of joints, because they may cause pain and irritation. Movements should be active and performed within the limit of pain. Tidy[23] was one of the few authors to discuss the treatment of different forms of arthritis (e.g., RA, Still's disease, OA, ankylopoietica, infective arthritis). Among the modalities advocated were the use of evaporating lotions such as lead lotion or lead and opium lotion, faradism, radiant heat, and whirlpool baths. Forced movements were not advised; however, manipulation was recommended if stiffness did not respond to traditional therapy. Tidy[23] also recommended massage for all forms of arthritis.

Other modalities in use were histamine ionization or tincture of iodine in chronic cases "for a stronger effect on the circulation," constant current, and surged sinusoidal current to improve blood flow to the limbs.[24] Counterirritants used were galvanic current, ion transfer with vasodilators, high-frequency currents, and ultraviolet rays.[25] It is noteworthy, however, that bed rest was not advised for a patient with RA until swelling and pain had decreased, because it was believed that "irreparable damage would be done."[26]

Generally, the goals of therapy were to increase circulation and metabolism, prevent and relieve local arthritic changes, and correct faulty body mechanisms. The focus in textbooks was on the position of the patient (e.g., wing stoop high-ride sitting) and the movement or technique performed, but not on why the treatment was given. Cyriax[27] was one of the few authors of this time who attempted to identify the structure at fault and define a treatment related to that specific structure. He stated

only when it is realized that arthritis and diffuse capsulitis are synonymous can a masseur understand the theory on which the treatment of nonspecific arthritis is based. The treatment of arthritis is the treatment of the capsule of the joint.[27, p 22]

Cyriax advocated massage to the capsule, mobilization of the joint to strengthen the capsule, exercises, and splinting as required. He considered massage the best treatment for effusion; in addition, he also recommended the use of resisted faradism to obtain full extension of the knee and gait reeducation.[27]

At the middle of the twentieth century the rationale given for PT intervention in arthritis was as follows:

general or systemic physical measures may serve as part of constitutional therapy for increase of circulation and metabolism. Physical measures locally applied serve to prevent and relieve local arthritic changes.[28, p 462]

The practice of massage has been a commonly applied form of therapy in all population groups—ancient and modern. Evidence also exists for the application of orthotic principles across population groups. A report describes an Aleut "midwife" whose fingers had become "crooked and flexed with arthritis; she straightened them by binding them to wooden sticks and thus continued her practice until her death."[29]

Despite the numerous medical textbooks on arthritis and specific forms of arthritis, physical therapists made only a meager contribution to the literature until about the 1970s. Currently there are only two other English-language textbooks about PT in arthritis authored by physical therapists; both were published in the 1980s.[30,31] The establishment of the Association of Rheumatology Health Professionals (ARHP), formerly the Arthritis Health Professions Association, and a section of the American College of Rheumatology (ACR) provided a venue for health professionals interested in this area to interact. Although there has been significant growth in physical therapists' involvement in arthritis, more research that will affect PT and occupational therapy (OT) management and rehabilitation must be done. Only a few physical therapists and occupational therapists are known for research publications in the field of arthritis; noteworthy are Helewa, Jette, Moncur, Minor, Guccione, Krebs, Marks, Stokes, and Banwell. Melvin has contributed to OT arthritis literature, and in nursing Hawley and Lorig are well known. Lorig, a nurse in public health, has made a major contribution to the literature about self-management programs, now used worldwide.

The Arthritis Society in Canada has provided direct physiotherapy, OT, and social work services in most Canadian provinces since the early 1950s. Because physical therapists and occupational therapists received combined training in the early days, only physiotherapy as a service was officially designated. Physical therapists, also provided OT. At present, the two services are distinct in all the provinces where they are provided in Canada. Whereas the initial involvement of occupational therapists focused on splint manufacture and promotion of activity through arts and crafts, modern OT seeks to facilitate clients' independence in the home, and when needed, in the workplace, through the use of adaptive equipment and assistive devices (see Chapter 14) and psychosocial counseling.[32]

With a major focus on fundraising for research and education, the Arthritis Society now provides direct care for clients with arthritis in only three provinces: Ontario, British Columbia, and Nova Scotia. A characteristic of the health service provided by the Society was home care. Physical therapists traveled within about a 50-mile radius of an urban center. In some cases, as in Manitoba, a therapist would spend 2 to 3 days in one away-from-base community. Today, traveling clinics serve as outreach clinics for remote communities. Whereas Ontario's programs are funded by the provincial government, in Nova Scotia a fee is charged for service (Helewa, personal communication). In the United States and Commonwealth countries, arthritis organizations are not known to be involved in direct patient care. Both the Arthritis Society in Canada and the Arthritis Foundation in the United States, as well as similar organizations worldwide, play a significant role in promoting research, public education, and continuing education of therapists involved in arthritis care.

Attitudes and Beliefs

In addition to understanding the pathophysiology of arthritis, a therapist should recognize that clients may differ in their attitudes and beliefs about health and effective health care. Arthritis through the ages has been associated with a rich variety of "folk" remedies, such as the wearing of copper bracelets or the following of a special diet.[33] Today, the terms *alternative* and *complementary* are preferred to the term *folk*. As long as these approaches are not used as substitutes or deterrents to evidence-based care, or the application of "best practice," therapists may be wise to accept some use of alternative or complementary therapy and ensure an environment in which clients feel free to discuss such activities.

Logan[34] suggested that some of the problems encountered when modern health care workers attempt to bring Western-style health care to indigenous groups can be averted if practitioners attempt to understand and appreciate the attitudes and beliefs of different ethnic groups. Health care workers must determine where such beliefs may impede the delivery of care and compliance with prescribed therapy and work out a system of delivery that is sensitive to an individual's philosophy of health. Consideration of such factors is as important in large urban cities of the Western world as it is for the health care worker in third world countries, given the mobility of modern populations.

> Provided the use of alternative or complementary therapies and remedies *does no harm* or does not serve as a substitute to modern evidence-based care, it may be wise not to interfere with such practices.

It can be inappropriate to use a medicine (or therapy) known locally to be hot (or cold).[34] Local beliefs, as in Guatemala, regarding the interplay between beliefs about the natural world and its elements (temperature) may make the therapy not only ineffective but harmful. Logan reported symptoms and diseases recognized by natives and their response to prescribed treatments (acceptance or rejection). Rheumatism is one recognized disease for which natives accept the prescribed treatment of aspirin and Vicks VapoRub (data from Guatemala and New York–based Puerto Rican patients who display similar behavioral patterns in response to treatment of specific disorders). Certain drugs, however, are rejected because they are perceived as being harmful to "the natural order." Because drug therapy is an important component of arthritis management, such behavior can be a serious impediment to the efficacy of planned care.

Therapists working with multicultural populations of clients with arthritis should be cognizant of differences in attitudes and beliefs about health and health care. No study was located that described the impact of such attitudes and beliefs on the delivery of health care by physical or occupational therapists. Therapeutic programs need to be constructed that are sensitive to and compatible with an individual's attitudes and beliefs (i.e., culture-friendly), or adherence is unlikely.

Physical Therapy and Rehabilitation Today

Modern management of the client with arthritis generally requires a client-centered team approach. Members, with varying roles at different stages of the disease, include physicians, rheumatologists, physical and occupational therapists, social workers, nutritionists, orthotists, orthopedic surgeons, hand surgeons, nurses, and most important, the client. Especially in children with arthritis, family members and school teachers should be included. Other team members may include vocational counselors, pharmacists, registered nurses, psychologists, and recreational therapists.

This interdisciplinary team interacts to develop therapy goals and plans. It is part of a multidisciplinary approach to care, in which effort is made to "unify individual treatments into a comprehensive plan."[35] The role of the physical therapist and occupational therapist extends from the client (in the hospital or clinic, at work, or at home) to the family and the public.

Communities have numerous organizations that can assist both the client and the therapy team in the provision of resources (see Appendix I). The community can play a major role in facilitating the independence and mobility of the client with arthritis (e.g., provision of parking spots for the physically challenged, ramp access to buildings, assistance with yard work and snow removal). Employers also have a responsibility and a positive role to play in modifying the workplace as needed and in expanding employment options, such as permitting work pacing and job sharing.

No one health care provider can be expert and knowledgeable regarding all aspects of care; however, knowledge of *who* to contact or refer to, and *when,* is critical to evidence-based management. Banwell[35] has identified the roles and responsibilities of the major health disciplines involved in the management of the client with arthritis, noting that these roles and responsibilities often overlap.

Role of Nonmedical Health Care Professionals in Clinics

Born in part as a result of rising health care costs and long waiting lists resulting from a shortage of rheumatology medical specialists, several projects have been reported in which specially trained health care professionals—nurses[36] and physical and occupational therapists[37-39]—assess clients and manage rheumatic diseases clinics. To date, only three programs involving nurses, physical and/or occupational therapists, and using masked randomized design have been evaluated; more studies with that degree of rigor are needed.[36,40,41]

Education in Rheumatology

The past decade has seen considerable development in the identification of arthritis curricula content for entry-level PT programs. In the early 1980s, 31% of Canadian and U.S. programs had inadequate curricula.[42] Westby[43] surveyed Canadian programs in 1997 and reported a mean of 22 hours of rheumatology instruction but a wide range (8 to 52 hours). Only 3 of the 13 programs had separate courses; most, as in the United States, gave rheumatology instruction in the context of a larger course. In 1997 the ARHP in

the United States updated Moncur's earlier work [44,45] and produced both entry-level and advanced-level PT competencies in rheumatology.[46] No study, however, was located that reported evaluation of the appropriateness and validity of these competencies, in the United States or elsewhere. OT practice guidelines for adults with RA were published in 2000.[47] In Canada, a working group has produced both PT and OT competencies, as yet unpublished.[48]

Summary

The most important advance in the last decade in PT's management, and in rehabilitation of persons with arthritis, is the recognition that passive therapies are of limited use and at best serve only as adjuncts to active therapies. It also is recognized that a major consequence of arthritis is poor cardiopulmonary performance, often leading to serious endurance deficits and serious pathological sequelae, and that physical fitness programs that respect the integrity of joints improve therapeutic outcomes. Occupational therapists play a critical role in facilitating independence and continued activity both in the home and in the workplace. Therapists who function well in a team and use referrals as appropriate will facilitate the health and well-being of clients of all ages with arthritis.

References

1. Lawrence RC, Hochberg MC, Kelsey JL et al: Estimates of the prevalence of selected arthritic and musculoskeletal diseases in the United States. *J Rheumatol* 16:427–441, 1989.
2. Centers for Disease Control and Prevention: Prevalence of arthritis—United States. 1997, *MMWR Morb Mortal Wkly Rep* 50:334–336, 2001.
3. The Arthritis Society: Summary report of Arthritis 2000: the National Arthritis Forum. Ottawa, April 11–13, 1997.
4. Peyron JG, Altman RD: The epidemiology of osteoarthritis. In Moskowitz RW, Howell DS, Goldberg VM et al (eds): *Osteoarthritis: Diagnosis and Medical/Surgical Management.* Philadelphia, WB Saunders, 1992, pp 15–37.
5. Fife RS: A short history of osteoarthritis. In Moskowitz RW, Howell DS, Goldberg VM et al (eds): *Osteoarthritis: Diagnosis and Medical/Surgical Management.* Philadelphia, WB Saunders, 1992, pp 11–14.
6. Ackerknecht EH: Paleopathology. In Landy D (ed): *Culture, Disease, and Healing: Studies in Medical Anthropology.* New York, Macmillan, 1977, pp 71–77.
7. Wells C: *Bones, Bodies, and Disease: Evidence of Disease and Abnormality in Early Man.* London, Thomas & Hudson, 1964, p 17.
8. Rothschild BM: Skeletal paleopathology of rheumatic diseases: the subhomo connection. In McCarty DJ,

Koopman WJ (eds): *Arthritis and Allied conditions,* ed 12. Philadelphia, Lea & Febiger, 1993, pp 3–8.

9. Braunstein EM, White SJ, Russell W et al: Paleoradiographic evaluation of Egyptian royal mummies. *Skeletal Radiol* 17:348–351, 1988.

10. Armelagos GL: Disease in ancient Nubia. In Landy D (ed): *Culture, Disease, and Healing: Studies in Medical Anthropology.* New York, Macmillan, 1977, pp 77–83.

11. Jurmain R: Trauma, degenerative disease, and other pathologies among Gombe chimpanzees. *Am J Phys Anthropol* 80:229–237, 1989.

12. Rothschild BM, Wood RJ: Osteoarthritis, calcium pyrophosphate deposition disease and osseous infection in Old World primates. *Am J Phys Anthropol* 87:341–347, 1992.

13. Dieppe P, Rogers JM: Skeletal paleopathology of rheumatic diseases. In McCarthy DJ, Koopman WJ (eds): *Arthritis and Allied Conditions,* ed 12. Philadelphia, Lea & Febiger, 1993, pp 9–16.

14. Tod EM: *Massage and Medical Gymnastics,* ed 4. London, JMA Churchill, 1951, p 1.

15. Fuller F: *Medicina Gymnaftica: or, every man his own phyfician. A treatise concerning the power of exercise with refpect to the animal oeconomy, and the great neceffity of it in the cure of several diftempers,* ed 7. London, E Curll, 1740.

16. Buchan W: *Domestic Medicine,* ed 18. London, A Strahan, 1803.

17. Roth M: *The Prevention and Cure of Many Chronic Diseases by Movements.* London, John Churchill, 1851, p 254.

18. Osler W: *The Principles and Practice of Medicine,* ed 7. New York, D Appleton, 1909.

19. Goodall-Copestake BM: *The Theory and Practice of Massage,* ed 4. London, AK Lewis, 1926, p 169.

20. Forester AL: The use of physiotherapy in the treatment of rheumatoid arthritis with special reference to its use combined with A.C.T.H. and cortisone. Fellowship Thesis for the Chartered Society of Physiotherapy. London, England, 1953.

21. Glover JA: *A report on chronic arthritis with special reference to the provision of treatment.* London, Ministry of Health, His Majesty's Stationery Office 1928.

22. Palmer MD: *Lessons on Massage,* ed 6. London, Bailliere, Tindall & Cox, 1942, p 42.

23. Tidy NM: *Massage and Remedial Exercise,* ed 7. Bristol, Wright, 1947, p 112.

24. Clayton EB: *Electrotherapy with Direct and Low Frequency Currents.* London, Bailliere, Tindall & Cox, 1947, pp 137–139.

25. The treatment of arthritis. *JAMA* 135:288–289, 1947 (editorial).

26. Solomon WM: Physical treatment of arthritis. *JAMA* 137:128–130, 1948.

27. Cyriax J: *Massage, Manipulation and Local Anaesthesia.* London, Hamish Hamilton Medical Books 1943.

28. Kovacs R: *Electrotherapy and Light Therapy with Essentials of Hydrotherapy and Mechanotherapy,* ed 6. London, Henry Kimpton 1949.

29. Laughlin WS: Acquisition of anatomical knowledge. In Landy D (ed): *Culture, Disease, and Healing: Studies in Medical Anthropology.* New York, Macmillan, 1977, p 258.

30. Banwell BF, Gall V (eds): *Physical Therapy Management of Arthritis.* New York, Churchill Livingstone, 1988.

31. Hyde S: *Physiotherapy in Rheumatology.* London, Blackwell Scientific, 1980.

32. Trombly CA (ed): *Occupational Therapy for Physical Dysfunction,* ed 4. Baltimore, Williams & Wilkins 1995.

33. Jarvis DC: *Arthritis and Folk Medicine.* New York, Holt, Rhinehart & Winston, 1960.

34. Logan MH: Humoral medicine in Guatemala. In Landy D (ed): *Culture, Disease, and Healing: Studies in Medical Anthropology.* New York, Macmillan, 1977, pp 487–495.

35. Banwell BF: Comprehensive care. In Banwell BF, Gall V (eds): *Physical Therapy Management of Arthritis.* New York, Churchill Livingstone, 1988, pp 17–28.

36. Hill J, Bird HA, Harmer R et al: An evaluation of the effectiveness, safety and acceptability of a nurse practitioner in a rheumatology outpatient clinic. *Br J Rheumatol* 33:283–288, 1994.

37. Stokes B, Helewa A, Lineker S: Total assessment of rheumatic polyarthritis: a post-graduate training program for physical therapists and occupational therapists—a twenty year success story. *J Rheumatol* 24:1634–1638, 1997.

38. Hockin J, Bannister G: The extended role of a physiotherapist in an outpatient orthopaedic clinic. *Physiotherapy* 80:281–284, 1994.

39. Campos AA, Graveline C, Ferguson JM et al: The physical therapy practitioner (PTP) in pediatric rheumatology: high level of patient and parent satisfaction with services. *Physiother Can* 54:32–36, 2002.

40. Helewa A, Goldsmith CH, Lee P et al: Effects of occupational therapy home service on patients with rheumatoid arthritis. Lancet 337:1453–1456, 1991.

41. Bell MJ, Lineker SC, Wulkins AL et al: A randomized controlled trial to evaluate the efficacy of community-based physical therapy in the treatment of people with rheumatoid arthritis. *J Rheumatol* 25:231–237, 1998.

42. Jette AM, Becker MJ: Nursing, occupational therapy and physical therapy preparation in rheumatology in the United States and Canada. *J Allied Health* 9:268–275, 1980.

43. Westby MD: Rheumatology instruction in physical therapy undergraduate programs: a survey of Canadian universities. *Physiother Can* 51:264–267, 272, 1999.

44. Moncur C: Physical therapy competencies in rheumatology. *Phys Ther* 65:1365–1372, 1985.

45. Moncur C: Perceptions of physical therapy competencies in rheumatology: physical therapists versus rheumatologists. *Phys Ther* 67:331–339, 1987.

46. Association of Rheumatology Health Professionals: *Standards of practice: physical therapy competencies in rheumatology.* Atlanta, ARHP, 1997.

47. Yasuda YL: *Occupational therapy practice guidelines for adults with rheumatoid arthritis.* Bethesda, Md, American Occupational Therapy Association, 2000.

48. Cyr L, Busby C, Davidson I et al: *Competencies Working Group Final Report: competency in physical and occupational therapy practice in rheumatology.* Vancouver, BC, April 2002 (unpublished).

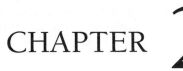

CHAPTER 2

Epidemiology and Economics of Arthritis

Antoine Helewa, MSc(Clin Epid), PT
Joan M. Walker, PhD, PT

Epidemiology is the study of the distribution and determinants of health-related states and events in populations and the application of this study to the control of health problems.[1] Epidemiology has a broad mandate: it is interdisciplinary and involves a variety of topics within each discipline, including clinical, public health, laboratory science, and medical technologies. Most epidemiological applications in arthritis have focused on the more elementary descriptions of disease occurrence; however, increasingly, clinical epidemiological methods are being used as a strategy to evaluate health delivery programs under the rubric of "health services research," using experimental investigative techniques. In this chapter the focus will be on the frequency and distribution of

the various forms of arthritis and their socioeconomic impact. The chapter will end with a discussion of the politics of arthritis.

Is There an Epidemic of Arthritis?

In the past three decades the field of arthritis has received more attention than in previous decades. This can be attributed to a change in the perception of arthritis and people with arthritis—from an affliction of old age with psychosomatic overtones to a group of diseases that respect no age, sex, or geographic boundaries. Even though arthritis affects older individuals more than those in any other age-groups, the politicization of young elderly and not-so-young elderly persons has helped focus attention on this group of diseases as a major health problem. Furthermore, the overall costs of physical and mental disabilities are receiving greater attention from

PHYSICAL REHABILITATION IN ARTHRITIS, Joan M. Walker, PhD, PT, and Antoine Helewa, MSc(Clin Epid), PT, Elsevier Inc. © 2004.

legislators and health insurers. Because of the high prevalence of people with arthritis among the disabled, the field of arthritis has not escaped this scrutiny.

> **Political activity by older adults has helped to focus attention on arthritis as a major health problem.**

The 1994 ground breaking study by the National Arthritis Data Workgroup (NADW) outlined the scope of arthritis in the United States.[2] This group estimated that 38 million Americans—15% of the population, or one in seven people—were affected by arthritis in 1990. More significant is the projection by the NADW that by the year 2020 the number of Americans with arthritis will increase by more than 57% (to 59.4 million Americans) from the 1990 estimate, affecting about 18.2% of the population, or one in five persons.

Is there a looming epidemic of arthritis? Where will these additional people with arthritis come from? Because osteoarthritis affects older adults more than those in any other age-group, the overall increase in the number of older adults contributes to that increase. More significantly, by the year 2020, a large number of older adults will be from the baby boom generation, further swelling the number of those affected. Can a similar case be made for inflammatory arthritis?

> **With aging of the baby boom generation, by the year 2020 more older adults will have arthritis**

Several studies have suggested that the incidence of rheumatoid arthritis (RA) is decreasing, probably as a result of the increased use of oral contraceptives among women. However, true cause-and-effect associations have not been shown.[3-5] Another report indicates that RA is becoming less severe in successive generations of patients, who are less likely to become seropositive, develop subcutaneous nodules, or develop erosive forms of arthritis.[6] Further, the *early* aggressive use of disease-modifying antirheumatic drugs (DMARDs), has had a major impact in the control of joint inflammation as well as the systemic and extra-articular manifestations of the disease. Consequently fewer people than in past years use mobility aids or are bed-bound as a result of the disease or its treatment. Patients with suboptimal response to disease-

modifying antirheumatic drugs who become disabled are helped by increasingly successful reconstructive surgical interventions.

Prevalence and Incidence of Arthritis

Prevalence is the proportion of cases of a disease identified in a population at a given point (*point prevalence*) or during a specified interval (*period prevalence*). Point prevalence is determined in a single survey, and period prevalence is determined in one or more surveys.[7] Incidence is defined as the rate of occurrence of new cases of a disease during a given period in a defined population at risk. Incidence is a more specific and sensitive indicator of disease risk acquisition than is prevalence. Studies of incidence, however, are more demanding than prevalence studies because larger populations are required, and definitions of disease on first diagnosis may be difficult.[7]

In a report by Statistics Canada, based on a 1981 self-report survey of the health of Canadians, 16% (3.5 million) of the population of Canada was estimated to have arthritis; rheumatism; or back, limb, and joint disorders.[8,9] In 85%, the duration of the disorder was longer than 1 year. More women (18.8%) than men (13.2%) reported these complaints. The prevalence among those 65 years of age and older was almost 50%, whereas among those 15 to 64 years of age, it was 17%. In the pediatric age group, the prevalence was 1.3%; however, this still represented a total of 74,000 children with arthritis or rheumatism. The Centers for Disease Control and Prevention analyzed a variety of data for 1997, using International Classifications of Diseases definitions. One analysis, derived from the National Health Interview Survey, showed that prevalence of arthritis has increased by 750,000 per year in the United States between 1990 and 1997.[10] Related analyses documented 744,000 hospitalizations and 44 million ambulatory care visits for arthritis in 1997.[10]

A 1990 Ontario Health Survey based on household interviews showed that musculoskeletal disorders (MSDs) are a leading cause of morbidity in the population. MSDs ranked first in prevalence as the cause of chronic health problems, long-term disabilities, and consultations with a health professional and ranked second for restricted activity days and use of medications.[11] The overall rate of MSDs reported in this study (22%) and that for arthritis and rheumatism (15%) were remarkably similar to rates reported elsewhere, based on self-reported conditions.[9]

In a random sample of 3605 patients aged 25 years and older with chronic pain in general practices in the United Kingdom, 1817 (50.4%) self-reported chronic pain, equivalent to 46.5% of the general population.

Table 2-1. The 1987 Revised Criteria for the Classification of Rheumatoid Arthritis (RA)*

Criterion	Definition
1. Morning stiffness	Morning stiffness in and around the joints, lasting at least 1 hour before maximal improvement.
2. Arthritis of three or more joint areas	At least three joint areas simultaneously have had soft tissue swelling or fluid (not bony overgrowth alone) observed by a physician. The 14 possible areas are right or left PIP, MCP, wrist, elbow, knee, ankle, and MTP joints.
3. Arthritis of hand joints	At least one area swollen (as defined above) in a wrist, MCP, or PIP joint.
4. Symmetric arthritis	Simultaneous involvement of the same joint areas (as defined in 2) on both sides of the body (bilateral involvement of PIP, MCP, or MTP joints is acceptable without absolute symmetry).
5. Rheumatoid nodules	Subcutaneous nodules, over bony prominences, or extensor surfaces, or in juxta-articular regions, observed by a physician.
6. Serum rheumatoid factor	Demonstration of abnormal amounts of serum rheumatoid factor by any method for which the result has been positive in <5% of normal control subjects.
7. Radiographic changes	Radiographic changes typical of rheumatoid arthritis on posteroanterior hand and wrist radiographs, which must include erosions or unequivocal bony decalcification localized in or most marked adjacent to the involved joints (osteoarthritis changes alone do not qualify).

Adapted from Arnett FC, Edworthy SM, Bloch DA et al: The American Rheumatism Association 1987 revised criteria for the classification of rheumatoid arthritis. *Arthritis Rheum* 31:315–324, 1988. With permission.
*For classification purposes, a patient shall be said to have rheumatoid arthritis if he/she has satisfied at least four of these seven criteria. Criteria 1 through 4 must have been present for at least 6 weeks. Patients with two clinical diagnoses are not excluded. Designation as classic, definite, or probable rheumatoid arthritis is not to be made.
PIP = proximal interphalangeal; MCP = metacarpophalangeal; MTP = metatarsophalangeal.

Of these 576 (16.0%) reported that their chronic pain was due to arthritis.[12] A 1996 National Population Health Survey in Canada estimated the overall prevalence of arthritis and rheumatism to be 13.2 % with modal age of 35 to 39 years.[13] Because the population of Canadians aged 15 and older is expected to grow from 23.9 million in 1996 to 30.9 million in 2016—this growth compounded with the aging population—means modal age will rise to 50 to 54 years, with the overall prevalence of people with arthritis and rheumatism increasing to 16.1%.

Seasonal symptom severity in patients with rheumatic diseases is commonly reported. In a U.S. study, about 50% of patients reported seasonal exacerbation of rheumatic symptoms, such as pain and fatigue.[14] Worse symptoms were common in December and January and least symptoms in July.

These variations appear to reflect perception rather than reality, because changes in perceived symptoms do not agree with measured clinical scores.

Inflammatory Arthritis

Epidemiologists have great difficulty in assessing the frequency or natural history of the conditions classified as inflammatory arthritis. Differences in reported incidence and prevalence arise from differences in the interpretation of existing criteria for diagnosis or severity. Whereas classic advanced RA can be reliably diagnosed, recognition of RA during its earliest stages is difficult, because there is no established etiological agent or unique laboratory feature that can be used to define the disease. Furthermore, the disease may follow a variable course for months or years before

Table 2-2. Diagnostic Criteria for the Classification of Juvenile Rheumatoid Arthritis*

Age of onset younger than 16 years
Arthritis in one or more joints defined as swelling or effusion or the presence of two or more of the
    following signs: limitation of range of motion, tenderness or pain on motion, or increased heat
Duration of disease longer than 6 weeks
Type of disease onset during the first 6 months classified as:
Polyarthritis: 5 or more joints
Pauciarticular disease (oligoarthritis): 4 or fewer joints
Systemic disease: arthritis with intermittent fever
Exclusion of other forms of juvenile arthritis

From Cassidy JT, Levinson JE, Brewer EJ Jr: The development of classification criteria for children with juvenile rheumatoid arthritis. *Bull Rheum Dis* 38:1–7, 1989. With permission.

---

becoming typical.[7] For example, using American Rheumatism Association (ARA) criteria for definite RA, rheumatologists achieved a sensitivity (true positives) of 71% and a specificity (true negatives) of 91%.[15] These criteria were revised in 1987,[16] published in 1988, and are still in use. They have a 91% to 94% sensitivity and an 89% specificity (Table 2-1). Therefore to obtain reliable estimates of disease patterns, the diagnosis must be established accurately, and the population studied must be representative.

Several epidemiological studies of RA and related connective tissue diseases[7,17] showed that similarities in the patterns of occurrence are more striking than the discrepancies. On the whole, these diseases tend to be disorders of women with onset most often during the child-bearing ages and tend to affect blacks more often than whites.[18] The sex ratio seems to vary with age. In persons younger than age 60, women predominate by a ratio of 5:1. In persons older than age 60, the sex ratio is approximately equal, suggesting that men may have a protective factor that may be lost at older ages.

Persons of all races develop RA.[7] Prevalence estimates for ARA criteria of definite RA are remarkably constant at 1% in white populations.[19] With use of the same criteria, another report showed that the prevalence of RA in major reported surveys for the average adult (aged 15 and older) ranged from a low of 0.1% in a rural South African black community[20] to 3.0% among Finnish whites.[21] Climate itself does not seem to be a factor.[7]

RA has been associated with lower income and lower educational levels.[22] Overall, the familial aggregation of RA is weak, and a putative susceptibility gene must have a low penetrance.[23]

The natural history of RA varies. Essentially, investigators agree that a high serum level of rheumatoid factor and early bony erosions indicate a poor prognosis.[19] Other factors associated with worse disease are female, white race, two or more swollen upper extremity joints, Raynaud-like phenomena, and malaise or weakness.[24] Because of the systemic nature of RA, reported mortality tends to be high. Factors that are strongly associated with early mortality are a high rheumatoid factor titer, high joint counts, and a worse ARA functional class[25] (see Chapter 5).

> **Connective tissue diseases are usually diagnosed more in women than in men, with onset most often during the child-bearing years. These diseases affect all ethnic groups, and climate does not seem to be a factor.**

Juvenile Arthritis

Juvenile arthritis or juvenile rheumatoid arthritis (JRA) is one of a large group of connective tissue disorders that occur in children and adolescents. By arbitrary definition JRA begins at or before age 16. Incidence and prevalence estimates for JRA vary considerably, due in part to use of two different sets of criteria, ARA criteria[26] (Table 2-2)[27] versus more rigid European criteria; heterogeneity of JRA subtypes; and lengthy periods of remission that complicate inclusion decisions in prevalence studies.[19] The International League against Rheumatism has recently proposed a

Table 2-3. Modified New York Criteria for Diagnosing Ankylosing Spondylitis (AS)

Low back pain of at least 3 months' duration improved by exercise and not relieved by rest
Limitation of lumbar spine in sagittal and frontal planes
Chest expansion decreased relative to normal values for age and sex
Bilateral sacroiliitis, grade 2–4
Unilateral sacroiliitis, grade 3–4
Definite AS if unilateral grade 3 or 4 or bilateral grade 2–4 sacroiliitis and any clinical criteria

From Van der Linden S, Valkenburg HA, Cats A: Modified New York criteria for diagnosing ankylosing spondylitis. Evaluation of diagnostic criteria for ankylosing spondylitis. *Arthritis Rheum* 27:361, 1984. With permission

multiclinic evaluation of new classification criteria.[28] Annual incidence estimates from European-, American-, and Canadian-based studies vary from 2.6 to 12.0 per 100,000 children.[27] Prevalence estimates vary from 0.16 per 1,000 children[29] to 1.13 per 1,000 children.[30] Estimates of distribution of the three JRA subtypes are 50% pauciarticular, 40% polyarticular, and 10% systemic onset types.[27] In the pauciarticular and polyarticular subtypes the female-to-male ratio is 3:1; however incidence is equal in the sexes for the systemic subtype.[27]

Spondyloarthropathies

The spondyloarthropathies are a group of inflammatory joint diseases that have their main effect on the axial skeleton. The primary disorder in this group is ankylosing spondylitis (AS). Other conditions in this group include reactive arthritis and psoriatic arthritis. AS, representing the spectrum of the seronegative forms of arthritis, has a variable prevalence, ranging from virtual absence in Australian aborigines[31] or black Africans[32] to a 10% diagnosed occurrence of sacroiliitis in adult male Haida Indians.[33] The most commonly reported prevalence is 1 per 1000 population, based on surveys of hospital and clinical records, with a sex ratio of three males to one female.[34,35] Criteria for diagnosis of AS were proposed at the Rome symposium[36] and later revised at a New York symposium.[37] A fair degree of variation can be seen in the interpretation of symptoms of pain and stiffness in the dorsal and lumbar spine.[38] A high degree of variation also was seen in the interpretations of radiographic sacroiliitis,[39] especially unilateral and milder bilateral changes in films of persons aged 50 or younger. However, certain manifestations of back pain may be more characteristic of AS than of osteoarthritis[40] (e.g., insidious development, symptoms persisting longer than 3 months, morning stiffness, relief with mild exercise). Subsequently the New York criteria were

further modified by Van der Linden et al,[41] relying on clinical and radiological features only (Table 2-3).

Reiter's syndrome, the most common example of reactive arthritis, has a close clinical relationship to AS, with spinal involvement being seen in nearly one half of patients.[18] Although once considered rare, it is perhaps the leading cause of arthritis among young adult men, especially those in the military. It is sometimes reported in epidemic occurrences, such as after bacillary dysentery. Development of the disease may be triggered by the encounter of a genetically susceptible (HLA-B27) host with some triggering environmental insult, such as an infectious agent.[18] Estimates of prevalence and incidence are limited because of a lack of consensus regarding diagnostic criteria, the nomadic nature of a young target population, and under-reporting of venereal diseases.[42]

Older epidemiological studies showed that 20% of patients with seronegative polyarthritis had psoriasis, but only 1.2% of patients with seropositive arthritis also had psoriasis.[43,44] The prevalence of polyarthritis among individuals with psoriasis was about 7%.[45] Various population studies of this syndrome show conflicting results. A statistical analysis of radiographic changes showed that erosions and mutilation of the distal and proximal interphalangeal joints were the best criteria to distinguish patients with seronegative arthritis and psoriasis from those with seronegative arthritis without psoriasis.[46] This strong association between seronegativity and psoriasis suggests that the presence of psoriasis leads to a more severe form of arthritis.

Osteoarthritis

Population studies of osteoarthritis (OA) show that its occurrence, as expected, increases steadily with age, especially as observed in roentgenographic surveys, in which articular alterations are found in many asymptomatic individuals.[18] However, only 30% of those with radiographic evidence complain of pain in affected sites.

Epidemiological surveys show a strong association between OA and wear and tear, prolonged immobilization, continuous pressure, impact loading, anatomic abnormalities, and previous joint injury.[47–49] Repetitive use of the hands in industry was associated with radiographic evidence of OA in certain joints.[50] Although running does not appear to increase the risk of OA when done as a recreational sport activity, in competitive sport the risk is elevated[51]; this risk also is seen with soccer and basketball. The clear difference between recreational and competitive sport is lessened if degenerative changes are present.[51] Studies suggest that prior trauma and sports participation with high impact loading, especially with torsional forces, predisposes persons to OA.

There is general agreement that obesity is an important risk factor for OA of the knee, is a lesser risk factor for OA of the hip,[52–54] and is also a risk factor for OA of the hand.[50,55] The relationship between weight and OA appears to involve both local and systemic factors.[56,57] Women with body mass index (BMI) of 30 to 35 kg/m^2 had a risk of OA of the knee 4 times that of women with body mass index of <25 kg/m^2; in men the risk of OA of the knee was 4.8 times higher.[56] Interestingly, the risk of development of symptomatic OA was reduced by 50% in over-weight women who lost an average of 11 pounds.[57] Weight management must be part of the overall management of clients with OA, and in populations with growing numbers of overweight children and adults, it should be a strategy to prevent future development of arthritis.

Fibromyalgia

Fibromyalgia (FM) is one of several musculoskeletal pain syndromes or chronic generalized pain syndromes. Signs and symptoms of FM such as tenderness occurs as a continuum in the population and American College of Rheumatology (ACR) criteria for FM merely identify the upper reaches of that continuum.[58] According to ACR criteria, a diagnosis of FM is reached when a subject has a history of widespread pain involving all four quadrants of the body and pain in 11 of 18 tender point sites on digital palpation.[59] Two North American studies of FM, using ACR criteria, found that it was more common in women than in men and that it tended to affect young adults and have serious economic and familial consequences. The Wichita study showed a prevalence for women of 3.4% compared with 0.5% for men,[60] and the London, Ontario, study showed a prevalence of 4.9% versus

1.6%.[61] FM also appears to coexist commonly with certain illnesses such as systemic lupus erythematosus, rheumatoid arthritis, and osteoarthritis.

Socioeconomic Impact of Arthritis

Chronic diseases produce significant economic, social, and psychological problems as a result of their biological effects. It seems reasonable to turn our attention to these problems as we seek ways to improve the overall well-being of clients with these conditions.[62] As the mean age of the population increases in the next decades, the prevalence of these chronic diseases also will increase.

Most studies that attempt to measure the socioeconomic impact of arthritis have been concerned with the costs of RA. A Canadian study showed that the average cost of hospitalization in a rheumatic disease unit for a patient with RA, in 1985 dollars, was about $3,000 Canadian (about $2,200 U.S.) for an average stay of 16 days. This is considerably less than the average per diem cost of $6,600 for hospitalization at that hospital in 1985.[63]

Job-related injuries due to acute repetitive trauma to joints such as the knees, hips, and hands can produce OA years after the initial injury. The costs associated with OA caused by these injuries were estimated in the United States to be between $3.4 billion and $13.23 billion, with a point estimate of $8.32 billion. These costs are on a par with the costs of job-related chronic obstructive pulmonary disease and all asthmas whether job related or not.[64]

Reduced access to tertiary health care services can be another contribution to long-term disability, especially for women with arthritis. Compared with men, women had a higher prevalence of arthritis of the hip or knee and had more severe symptoms and a greater level of disability.[65] However, women were less likely to have undergone hip or knee joint replacements. Despite equal willingness to have the surgery, fewer women than men discussed this treatment option with their physician. The potential need for this surgery was 45 per 1000 among women compared with 21 per 1000 among men.

Apart from sex, the sociodemographic risk factors are similar for musculoskeletal disability and non-musculoskeletal causes of disability.[66] Musculoskeletal disability is independently associated with increasing age, not being married, fewer years of schooling, lower income, and not being employed. Noteworthy in this study is the association between disability and an educational level of grade 8 or less and lower income.[66] Other studies also have shown a strong association between these factors and reported joint symptoms in the population.[67,68]

> The psychosocial impact of RA often results in changes in marital status, employment status, and leisure activities. All may have an impact on response to therapy.

Overall in 1994, the economic impact of musculoskeletal disability in the United States represented about 1% of the gross national product. Even in Canada, according to StatsCan data, arthritis was responsible for the loss of more than $1.4 billion in wages annually and nearly $150 million in tax revenues.[69]

Politics of Arthritis

Compared with heart disease, cancer, or acquired immunodeficiency syndrome, arthritis and politics have not mixed. Generally, people with arthritis are not among the movers and shakers in society, especially because arthritis seems to affect those who are socioeconomically disadvantaged.[66] However, this situation is changing because of the changing demographics of people with arthritis.

> The increase in the number of older adults in our society who are politically active will help empower people with arthritis ("gray power").

Although those with arthritis are largely older adults, they also are well represented in all age-groups. Another factor that may contribute to this change is the high cost of disability. Political and community leaders are becoming more aware of the burden of chronic illness on society, especially the burden resulting from musculoskeletal disability. This increased awareness manifests itself in many ways. Chief among these is the impact of musculoskeletal disabilities on the workplace in terms of absenteeism and therefore compensation costs; low back pain and repetitive injury syndromes are the disorders most commonly seen.

Although older adults have not been vocal in this arena to date, activists and fund raisers for arthritis research are becoming more determined in recruiting these persons, as well as young celebrities to their cause, and these celebrities are more forthright in joining fund-raising campaigns or in lobbying politicians. Tina Wesson of *Survivor* fame, Kathleen Turner, and Ted Brookers, among others, have been very effective in the fight against arthritis in the United States and Canada.

On balance, individuals of all ages are striving for a better quality of life. Those with arthritis are striving for improved services, increased accountability, and cost-effectiveness. Health service providers will no longer be absolute masters of their own turf. Public representation on health service agencies will increase to ensure that care providers are more sensitive and responsive to the needs of their clients. These societal trends have been evolving for at least two decades, and the demand for improved services and quality of life will accelerate, sweeping in its path care providers, politicians, and society's leaders alike.

> Celebrities can be very effective in promoting arthritis as a worthy funding cause and important health problem in today's societies.

Effects on the Practice of Physical Therapy and Rehabilitation

These developments are already having an impact on how physical and occupational therapy are generally practiced. On the one hand, individualized management will no longer be cost-effective as the ranks of people with arthritis swell. On the other hand, the voicing of requests for greater accountability and improved communications will place even heavier demands on overburdened services. All therapists must become innovative in the manner with which their services are delivered to satisfy these opposing challenges. Recent health care reports in North America have highlighted the importance of community rehabilitation delivery systems for patients with chronic disabilities to enhance their integration in their own homes or place of work. This will require all therapists in the field of rehabilitation to introduce innovative service delivery mechanisms that provide for periodic monitoring or follow-up of these unrelenting diseases. Greater reliance on information technology through computer-aided management, and the creation of other support systems such as self-help groups will greatly enhance the effectiveness of physical and occupational therapy and possibly reduce health care costs.

References

1. Thomas CL (ed): *Taber's Cyclopedic Medical Dictionary.* ed 15. Philadelphia, FA Davis 1993.
2. National Arthritis Data Workgroup: Arthritis prevalence and activity limitations. *MMWR Morb Mortal Wkly Rep* 4:433–438, 1994.
3. Linos A, Worthing JW, O'Fallon WM et al: The epidemiology of rheumatoid arthritis in Rochester, Minnesota: a study of incidence, prevalence, and mortality. *Am J Epidemiol* 111:87–98, 1980.
4. Del Junco DJ, Annegers JF, Luthra HS et al: Do oral contraceptives prevent rheumatoid arthritis? *JAMA* 254:1938–1941, 1985.
5. Vandenbroucke JP, Witteman JCM, Valkenburg HA et al: Noncontraceptive hormones and rheumatoid arthritis in perimenopausal and postmenopausal women. *JAMA* 255:1299–1303, 1986.
6. Silman A, Davies P, Currey HLF et al: Is rheumatoid arthritis becoming less severe? *J Chronic Dis* 36:891–897, 1983.
7. Masi AT, Medsger TA: Epidemiology of the rheumatic diseases. In McCarty DJ (ed): *Arthritis and Allied Conditions*, ed 11. Philadelphia, Lea & Febiger, 1989, pp 16-54.
8. Health and Welfare Canada, Statistics Canada: *The Health of Canadians: Report of the Canada Health Survey.* Ottawa, Ministry of Supply and Services, 1981.
9. Lee P, Helewa A, Smythe HA et al: Epidemiology of musculoskeletal disorders (complaints) and related disability in Canada. *J Rheumatol* 12:1169–1173, 1985.
10. Centers for Disease Control: Impact of arthritis and other rheumatic conditions on the health care system: United States 1997. *MMWR Morb Mortal Wkly Rep* 48:349–353, 1999.
11. Badley EM, Rasooly I, Webster GK: Relative importance of musculoskeletal disorders as a cause of chronic health problems, disability and health care utilization: findings from the 1990 Ontario Health Survey. *J Rheumatol* 21:505–514, 1994.
12. Elliott AM, Smith BH, Penny KI et al: The epidemiology of chronic pain in the community. *Lancet* 354:1248–1252, 1999.
13. Badley EM, Wang PP: Arthritis and the aging population: projection of arthritis prevalence in Canada 1991 to 2031. *J Rheumatol* 25:138–144, 1998.
14. Hawley DJ, Wolfe F, Franklin A et al: Seasonal symptom severity in patients with rheumatic diseases: a study of 1224 patients. *J Rheumatol* 28:1900–1909, 2001.
15. Ropes MW, Bennett GA, Cobb S: 1958 revision of diagnostic criteria for rheumatoid arthritis. *Arthritis Rheum* 2:16–20, 1959.
16. Arnett FC, Edworthy SM, Bloch DA et al: The American Rheumatism Association 1987 revised criteria for the classification of rheumatoid arthritis. *Arthritis Rheum* 31:315–324, 1988.
17. Lawrence JS: *Rheumatism in Populations.* London, William Heinemann Medical Books, 1977.
18. Rodnan GP, Schumacher HR: *Primer on the Rheumatic Diseases.* Atlanta, Arthritis Foundation 1983.
19. Hochberg MC: Adult and juvenile rheumatoid arthritis: current epidemiologic concepts. *Epidemiol Rev* 3:27–44, 1981.
20. Beighton P, Solomon L, Valkenburg HA: Rheumatoid arthritis in a rural South African Negro population. *Ann Rheum Dis* 34:136–141, 1975.
21. Laine VAI: Rheumatic complaints in an urban population in Finland. *Acta Rheum Scand* 8:81–88, 1962.
22. Pincus T, Callahan LF: Taking mortality in rheumatoid arthritis seriously: predictive markers, socioeconomic status and comorbidity. *J Rheumatol* 13:841–845, 1986.
23. Del Junco DJ, Luthra HS, Annegers JF et al: The familial aggregation of rheumatoid arthritis and its relationship to the HLA-DR4 association. *Am J Epidemiol* 119:813–829, 1984.
24. Josipovic D: Prognostic indicators in early rheumatoid arthritis. *Clin Exp Rheumatol* 5:26, 1987.
25. Mitchell DM, Spitz PW, Young DY et al: Survival, prognosis and causes of death in rheumatoid arthritis. *Arthritis Rheum* 29:706–714, 1986.
26. Cassidy JT, Levinson JE, Brewer EJ Jr: The development of classification for children with juvenile rheumatoid arthritis. *Bull Rheum Dis* 38:1, 1989.
27. Cassidy JT, Petty RE: Juvenile rheumatoid arthritis. In Cassidy JT (ed): *Textbook of Rheumatology.* New York, Churchill Livingstone, 1990, pp 113–219.
28. Petty RE, Southwood TR, Baum J et al: Revision of the proposed classification criteria of juvenile idiopathic arthritis: Durban, 1997. *J Rheumatol* 25:1991, 1998.
29. Gewanter L, Roghmann KJ, Baum J: The prevalence of juvenile arthritis. *Arthritis Rheum* 26:599–603, 1983.
30. Towner SR, Michet CJ, O'Fallon WM et al: The epidemiology of juvenile arthritis in Rochester, Minnesota 1960–1979. *Arthritis Rheum* 26:1208–1213, 1983.
31. Cleland LG, Hay JAR, Milazzo SC: Absence of HL-A 27 and of ankylosing spondylitis in central Australian aboriginals. *Scand J Rheumatol* 8:30, 1975.
32. Solomon L, Beighton P, Valkenburg HA et al: Rheumatic disorders in South African Negro: part 1—rheumatoid arthritis and ankylosing spondylitis. *S Afr Med J* 49:1292-1296, 1975.
33. Gofton JP, Chalmers A, Price GE et al: HL-A27 and ankylosing spondylitis in B.C. Indians. *J Rheumatol* 2:314–318, 1975.
34. Carter ET, McKenna CH, Brian DD et al: Epidemiology of ankylosing spondylitis in Rochester, Minnesota: 1935–1973. *Arthritis Rheum* 22:365–370, 1979.
35. Masi AT: Epidemiology of B-27 associated diseases. *Ann Rheum Dis* 38:131–134, 1979.
36. Kellgren JH, Jeffrey MR, Ball J: *The Epidemiology of Chronic Rheumatism.* Oxford, Blackwell Scientific Publications, 1963.
37. Bennett PH, Wood PH: *Proceedings of the Third International Symposium on Population Studies of the Rheumatic Diseases.* Amsterdam, Excerpta Medica, 1968.

38. Moll JMH, Wright V: New York clinical criteria for ankylosing spondylitis: a statistical evaluation. *Ann Rheum Dis* 32:354–363, 1973.

39. Hollingsworth PN, Cheah PS, Dawkins RL et al: Observer variation in grading sacroiliac radiographs in HLA-B27 positive individuals. *J Rheumatol* 10:247–254, 1973.

40. Calin A, Porta J, Fries JF et al: Clinical history as a screening test for ankylosing spondylitis. *JAMA* 237:2613–2614, 1977.

41. Van der Linden S, Valkenburg HA, Cats A: Evaluation of diagnostic criteria for ankylosing spondylitis. *Arthritis Rheum* 27:361–368, 1984.

42. Cush JJ, Lipskey PE: Reiter's syndrome and reactive arthritis. In Koopman WJ (ed): *Arthritis and Allied Conditions,* ed 13. Philadelphia, Williams & Wilkins, 1997, pp 1209–1227.

43. Taylor KB, Truelove SC: Immunological reactions in gastrointestinal disease. *Gut* 3:277–288, 1962.

44. Palumbo PJ, Ward KE, Sauer WG et al: Musculoskeletal manifestations of inflammatory bowel disease-ulcerative and granulomatous colitis and ulcerative proctitis. *Mayo Clin Proc* 48:411–416, 1973.

45. Dekker-Saeys BJ, Meuwissen SGM, Van Den Berg-Loonen EM et al: Ankylosing spondylitis and inflammatory bowel disease. II. Prevalence of peripheral arthritis, sacroiliitis and ankylosing spondylitis in patients suffering from inflammatory bowel disease. *Ann Rheum Dis* 37:33–35, 1978.

46. Strober W, James SP: The immunologic basis of inflammatory bowel disease. *J Clin Immunol* 6:415–432, 1986.

47. Peyron JG: Osteoarthritis: the epidemiologic viewpoint. *Clin Orthop* 213:13–19, 1986.

48. Sahlstrom A, Montgomery F: Risk analysis of occupational factors influencing the development of arthrosis of the knee. *Eur J Epidemiol* 13:675–679, 1997.

49. Felson DT, Hannan MT, Nairmark A et al: Occupational physical demands, knee bending and knee osteoarthritis: results from the Framingham study. *J Rheumatol* 18:1587–1592, 1991.

50. Carman WJ, Sowers MF, Hawthorne VM et al: Obesity as a risk factor of osteoarthritis of the hand and wrist: a prospective study. *Am J Epidemiol* 139:119–129, 1994.

51. Lane NE: Exercise: a cause of osteoarthritis. *J Rheumatol* 22:3–6, 1995.

52. Coggon D, Kellingray S, Inkip H et al: Osteoarthritis and the hip and occupational lifting. *Am J Epidemiol* 147:523–528, 1998.

53. Cooper C, Inkip H, Croft P et al: Individual risk factors for hip osteoarthritis: obesity, hip injury and physical activity. *Am J Epidemiol* 147:516–522, 1998.

54. Cooper C: Occupational activity and the risk of osteoarthritis. *J Rheumatol* 22:10–12, 1995.

55. Klippel JH, Crofford LJ, Stone JH et al: *Primer on the Rheumatic Diseases,* ed 12. Arthritis Foundation, 2001.

56. Andersen J, Felson DT: Factors associated with osteoarthritis of the knee in the first National Health and Nutrition Examination Survey (HANES I). *Am J Epidemiol* 128:179–189, 1988.

57. Felson DT, Ahange Y, Anthony JM et al: Weight loss reduces the risk for symptomatic knee osteoarthritis in women. *Ann Intern Med* 116:5353–5359, 1992.

58. Clauw DJ: Musculoskeletal pain and evaluation. In Ruddy S, Harris ED, Sledge CB et al (eds): *Kelly's Textbook of Rheumatology.* Philadelphia, WB Saunders, 2001, pp 417–427.

59. Wolfe F, Smythe HA, Yunus MB et al: The American College of Rheumatology 1990 criteria for the classification of fibromyalgia: report of the Multicentre Criteria Committee. *Arthritis Rheum* 33:160–172, 1990.

60. Wolfe F, Ross K, Anderson J et al: The prevalence and characteristics of fibromyalgia in the general population. *Arthritis Rheum* 38.19–28, 1995.

61. White KP, Speechley M, Harth M et al: The London Fibromyalgia Epidemiology Study: the prevalence of fibromyalgia syndrome in London Ontario. *J Rheumatol* 19:1570–1576, 1999.

62. Meenan RF, Yelin EH, Nevitt M et al: The impact of chronic disease: a socio medical profile of rheumatoid arthritis. *Arthritis Rheum* 24:544–549, 1981.

63. Helewa A, Bombardier C, Goldsmith CH et al: Cost-effectiveness of inpatient and intensive outpatient treatment of rheumatoid arthritis: a randomized, controlled trial. *Arthritis Rheum* 32:1505–1514, 1989.

64. Leigh JP, Seavey W, Leistikow B: Estimating the cost of job-related arthritis. *J Rheumatol* 28:1647–1654, 2001.

65. Hawker GA, Wright JG, Coyte PC et al: Differences between men and women in the rate of use of hip or knee arthroplasty. *N Engl J Med* 342:1016–1022, 2000.

66. Badley EM, Ibanez D: Socioeconomic risk factors and musculoskeletal disability. *J Rheumatol* 21:515–522, 1994.

67. Pincus T, Callahan LF, Burkhauser RV: Most chronic diseases are reported more frequently by individuals with fewer than 12 years of formal education in the age 18–61 United States population. *J Chronic Dis* 40.865–874, 1987.

68. La Vecchia C, Negri E, Pagano R et al: Education prevalence of disease, and frequency of health care utilisation: the 1983 Italian National Health Survey. *J Epidemiol Community Health* 41:161–165, 1987.

69. Gordon DA, Inman RD: Musculoskeletal disability and rheumatology. *J Rheumatol* 21:387, 1994.

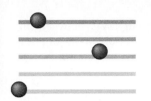

CHAPTER 3

Pathophysiology of Inflammation, Repair, and Immobility

Joan M. Walker, PhD, PT

There are many forms of arthritis in humans; most forms involve joints and often other body tissues. All tissues within a joint may be involved in the pathological process (Figure 3-1).

In most forms of arthritis, the involvement of freely movable joints (diarthroses) produces the greatest dysfunction. Because some joints lack sliding surfaces, they also lack distinct motion. In this chapter, after a brief overview of the different types of joints and their tissues, the following topics are reviewed: pathophysiology of inflammation, aspects of common forms of arthritis, immobilization, loading, and repair mechanisms.

Types of Joints

Joints may be classified by their degree of motion as being fibrous (fixed, synarthroses), cartilaginous

PHYSICAL REHABILITATION IN ARTHRITIS, Joan M. Walker, PhD, PT, and Antoine Helewa, MSc(Clin Epid), PT, Elsevier Inc. © 2004.

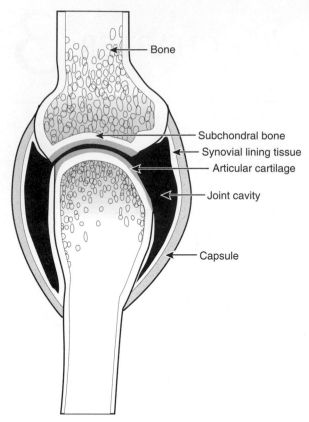

Bone

Subchondral bone
Synovial lining tissue
Articular cartilage

Joint cavity

Capsule

Figure 3-1. Features of a typical synovial joint. The extent of the synovial joint cavity is exaggerated to show features more clearly.

ligament. The intravertebral joint (IVJ) between an intravertebral disk and the inferior and superior surfaces of adjacent vertebrae is classified as an amphiarthrosis; it does not possess a synovial lining tissue. Although each IVJ unit permits only minimal motion, thus fitting the slightly movable classification, collectively IVJs contribute to a considerable range of motion in all planes.

The type and amount of motion, as well as the static and dynamic stability, depend on the shape of the articulating surfaces and the supporting connective tissue structures, that is, ligaments, fibrous capsule, and the bulk of adjacent limb muscles. Inflammatory or degenerative processes may affect all joint tissues. In fact, joints can be viewed as organs for which the health and destruction of individual joint tissues are interrelated, so that pathological changes in one affect the others.

Components of a Diarthrodial Joint

A diarthrodial joint is a load-bearing unit that consists of two or more skeletal surfaces and the subchondral bone covered with hyaline (articular) cartilage (HAC), united by a fibrous capsule. The fibrous capsule is lined by synovial tissue that covers all intra-articular structures except for the central load-bearing portion of disks, menisci, and articular cartilage.

Fibrous ligaments reinforce the capsule and may blend with the capsule or be separate from it. Some ligaments are intra-articular but are extrasynovial (e.g., cruciate ligaments of the knee joint). Joint surfaces are lubricated by synovial fluid (SF). Surface adaptation may be enhanced by intra-articular structures, such as menisci (knee), labra (hip, glenohumeral), or disks (radiocarpal).

Subchondral Bone

HAC overlies and is intimately bound to the subchondral bone plate (SBP), a specialized layer at the articulating surface. The SBP in long bones covers the expanded articular end or epiphysis, which is separated in growth from the bone shaft (diaphysis) by the growth plate (physis). The SBP may have considerable influence on cartilage in health and disease. Its blood supply may be important in HAC nutrition, and the cells may produce peptides that regulate chondrocyte function.[1] Bone is a highly vascular, constantly changing connective tissue. Cells (osteophytes, osteoclasts, osteoblasts) are embedded in the fibrous and the amorphous organic matrix permeated by bone salts.

(slightly movable, amphiarthroses), or synovial (movable, diarthroses). Fibrous joints include fixed joints (sutures), as well as those allowing minimal movement (between tibia and fibula, syndesmosis) and the junction between teeth and their sockets (gomphoses). Cartilaginous joints include symphyses and primary cartilaginous joints (synchondroarthroses). Mechanically, joints are perhaps better described as belonging to one of two major groups: (1) none or minimal motion, fibrous, and cartilaginous, nonsynovial; or (2) movable, synovial.

Synovial joints are distinguished by hyaline cartilage–covered surfaces that are in contact but not intimately bound together. There is a potential joint space for the lubricating fluid (synovial). Some joints are a mixture of types; for example, the sacroiliac joint is synovial in its anterior half, complete with fibrous capsule and lined by a synovial lining tissue, but it is an amphiarthrosis in its posterior half where the two surfaces are united by a strong interosseous

Whereas the exterior bone shaft shell is compact bone, the articulating ends are characterized by cancellous or trabecular bone (spongy) that is more deformable than cortical bone. The organization of SBP differs from that of the underlying bone in that the haversian systems "appear to run parallel to the joint rather than the long axis of the bone."[2] In the knee, SBP is formed by a meshwork of fine trabeculae (<0.2 mm in diameter) with a density of fewer than 2 trabeculae per millimeter of bone. Although SBP is stiffer than HAC, it is more resilient than the underlying bone—about 10 times that of the bone shaft.

The greater resilience of SBP assists in load transmission and is also a factor in the health of HAC. SBP undergoes significant deformation when a load is imposed on the joint surfaces and is the major site of deformation under loading. Thickening or increased stiffness limits the ability of SBP to disperse loads, leading to load concentration and cumulative damage, such as microfractures. Radin[3,4] theorized that either the calcified layer of HAC or SBP is the initial locus of pathological changes leading to osteoarthritis (OA); however, not all workers share this view.

In mature bone, organic material forms about 30% to 50% of its weight, water about 10% to 20% of its weight, and mineral salts (mainly carbonate apatite) about 60% to 70% of the dry weight. Collagen (type I and traces of type V) forms 90% to 95% of the organic matrix.[5] Branches of epiphyseal nutrient arteries pass toward the subchondral bone plate where they anastomose to form a series of arcades, off which a series of end-arterial loops occur. These loops may enter the calcified layer of HAC before returning to connect with venous sinusoids of the epiphyses. Nutrient vessels are accompanied by fine medullated and nonmedullated nerve fibers. The articular surfaces (when small, they are termed *articular facets*) of dry bone are smooth and lack the small vascular foramina typical of bone surfaces. The calcification of the zone of HAC in contact with SBP means that no effective interchange of nutrients occurs between the two layers. In abnormal cartilage, as seen in OA in which there may be vertical splitting of HAC extending into the SBP, the vascular SBP is a source of blood vessels and new cells, thus providing the avascular HAC a means to attempt repair.

It is important to note that, throughout life, bone is constantly remodeling itself. Osteoblasts make new bone, and osteoclasts remove old bone. A potent stimulus for remodeling is a change in the individual's level of physical activity. Radin et al[6] demonstrated a 150% increase in the number of labeled secondary osteons in the tibial SBP of rabbits compared with that in control animals when it was subjected to repetitive impulse loading.

Table 3-1. Components of Articular Cartilage, a Summary*

Component	Wet weight (%)
Major	
Water	60%–85%
Collagen, type II	15%–20%
Aggrecan (and versican)	4%–7%
(50%–85% all proteoglycans)	
Minor	
Link protein	
Hyluronan	
FACIT collagens IX, XII, XIV, XVI	
Interstitial (fiber forming) collagen: types I, V, VI, XI	
Small proteoglycans*	

Data from Poole[10], and Heingard et al.[11]
*See Table 3-3.

Hyaline Articular Cartilage

The HAC covering the subchondral bone plate distributes and transmits loads and shear forces to the underlying bone, protects the underlying bone, and permits synovial joints to have a wide range of almost frictionless movement. HAC is aneural, largely avascular, and only sparsely cellular; it is composed of up to 80% water (Table 3-1).[7]

Because healthy adult articular cartilage contains no blood vessels, the chondrocyte normally exists in a hypoxic acidic environment. HAC may be nourished either from subchondral blood vessels or SF. Because load bearing would imperil blood flow, chondrocytes synthesize specific inhibitors of angiogenesis (formation of new blood vessels) to maintain HAC's avascular state.[8] Anaerobic glycolysis is used for energy production.

Chondrocytes exist in relative isolation, either singly or in small clusters. They synthesize matrix components (collagen, proteoglycan) and the enzymes capable of destroying chondrocytes. Cartilage cells are embedded in the finely textured matrix in small zones that conform to cell shape. A *chondron* refers to the cell surrounded by a thin pericellular matrix. The

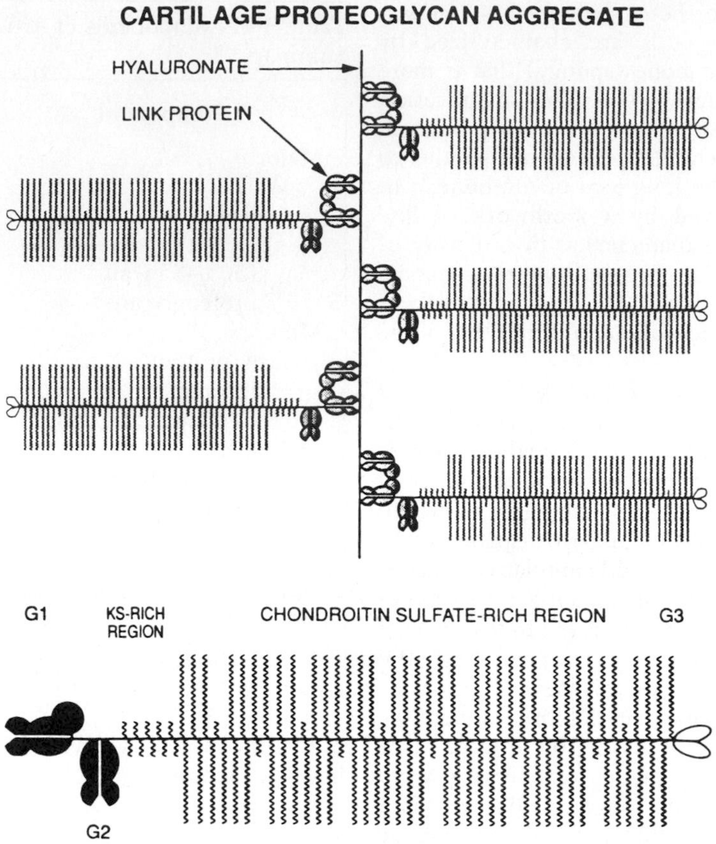

CARTILAGE PROTEOGLYCAN AGGREGATE

Figure 3-2. Cartilage proteoglycan aggregate, several monomers *(bottom)* bound by link proteins to a central hyaluronate core. KS = keratin sulfate. (From Rosenburg L: Structure and function of cartilage proteoglycans. In McCarty DJ, Koopman WJ [eds]: *Arthritis and Allied Conditions,* ed 12, vol 1. Philadelphia, Lea & Febiger, 1993, p. 305. With permission.)

mature chondrocyte has small rounded surface projections and round or oval nuclei. Multinucleated cells are common. The cell cytoplasm contains Golgi apparatus, mitochondria, granular endoplasmic reticulum, a few fat goblets, pigment granules, and glycogen deposits. In immature cartilage, both Golgi apparatus and granular reticulum are particularly prominent, indicative of their ability to synthesize matrix components.[5]

Chondrocytes are exposed to repeated changes in pressure and to deforming forces that have the ability to modify their synthetic function. Proteoglycan synthesis may be stimulated by cartilage compression.[9] A potent stimulus for remodeling is change in an individual's level of physical activity. Chondrocytes in the superficial layers are flattened, whereas those in the deeper layers are more rounded. There is a higher cell density at the articular surface that progressively decreases to be about one half to one third of the superficial layer in the mid to deep zones.[10] HAC is characterized by having relatively sparsely distributed cells and abundant extracellular matrix. This matrix confers to the tissue its specialized loading and mechanical properties. The elastic modulus of the matrix allows some deformation under loading that assists in gradual load distribution. The creep characteristic prevents instantaneous compression on load application. The extracellular matrix is composed of collagens (mainly type II), proteoglycans (in large groups called *aggregates*), nonprotein proteoglycans, and between 60% and 80% water (see Tables 3-1 and 3-2).

The collagen fibers give tensile strength and provide the framework in which cells and proteoglycans are embedded. Water content is greater in the superficial layers.

Proteoglycans

The proteoglycans and glycosaminoglycans (GAGs) are hydrophilic (water-loving) and play an important role in regulating the movement of water within the matrix, thereby influencing the mechanical and lubricant properties of cartilage.[11] Large protein aggregates are groupings of collagen protein monomers and are termed *aggrecans* (Figure 3-2).

Reduced levels of aggrecans are an important feature of joint disease. An aggrecan is bound at intervals with a single central filament of hyaluronate, is stabilized by link proteins, and has three globular domains with chondroitin sulfate (CS-4, CS-6) and keratin sulfate (KS) regions. CS and KS are polysaccharides that consist of sugar residues. Aggrecans have more than 100 negatively charged CS side chains, each with about 50 carboxyl and 50 sulfate groups.

A feature of CS and KS is that their repeating units of GAGs contain closely packed, negatively charged groups so that when these chains are linked to the aggrecan core protein they stand out like bristles on a brush. Protein aggregates occupy a greater volume of solution in vivo because of the strongly repellant forces of thousands of negatively charged groups. In vivo, the protein aggregates are constrained by the collagen network. It is this feature that gives articular cartilage its elastic properties; the tensile forces of the collagen network balance the elastic forces. When cartilage is compressed, interstitial fluid will be extruded from unloaded regions of the cartilage. With relief of pressure, the aggregate will expand (like a sponge) until it is limited by the collagen fiber network; simultaneously, cartilage will imbibe water and the volume of cartilage will be increased.

The other two proteoglycans are dermatan sulfate proteoglycans (DSPG, DSPG-1, biglycan; DSPG-2, decorin). These are multifunctional micromolecules that tend to be most concentrated near the articular surface.[10] They are bound to extracellular matrix macromolecules and regulate or modulate their biological properties.[12] DSPGs inhibit processes involved in tissue development and repair. They may bind to the surface of collagen fibers and inhibit the formation of new collagen fibrils or bind to fibronectin and inhibit cell adhesion, thrombin activity, and clot formation. Their activity could explain why lesions of articular cartilage do not heal well or repair spontaneously.

Figure 3-3 *left* shows the typical two-layered arrangement of HAC. There is an uncalcified superficial layer and a deeper calcified cartilage layer that is bound and merges with the subchondral bone. The junction between the uncalcified and calcified layers is called the tidemark. Within the uncalcified cartilage, there is a superficial or gliding zone, a middle transitional zone, and a deep or radial zone. In each zone cell number, cell shape, orientation, collagen fiber arrangement, and nutrition are relatively unique.

Tidemark and Calcified Layer

The tidemark is the boundary of a metabolically active zone between the calcified and noncalcified layers. Variations in the subchondral bone volume are thought to influence the tidemark region and the changes that lead to OA.[13] Because of the calcifying activities in the tidemark region, the tidemark slowly advances in the direction of the noncalcified cartilage during life. The number of tidemarks increases with aging and in pathological conditions such as OA. The calcified zone tends to become thinner with age.[14]

The difference in orientation of cells within the articular cartilage is shown in Figure 3-3. In the calcified zones, the cells are heavily encrusted with hydroxyapatite (crystals of calcium salts) and are surrounded with calcified matrix in mature cartilage. These cells are considered to be relatively metabolically inactive.[15] Different regions can be distinguished within the matrix. A thin layer of pericellular matrix surrounds each cell (Figure 3-3). Outside of that matrix is the life-sustaining interterritorial matrix; adjacent and surrounding that is the territorial matrix. The latter has a high concentration of KS that may enable the interterritorial matrix to better resist compressive deformation.[16] The fibrillar network is a major component of cartilage, consisting of collagen and of attached, cross-bridging and cross-linking noncollagenous matrix proteins.

Bundles of collagen fibers in the superficial zone of the HAC lie in parallel to the joint cavity, whereas in the transitional zone they are larger and more randomly dispersed. In the radial zone, fibers are coarser than those in the superficial zone, are larger, and have an ascending arcade-type pattern with radial rows in the deepest regions. The fibers in the calcified zone are thicker and orientated perpendicular to the surface.[5,17]

The calcified layer also possesses antiangiogenic (blood vessel formation) molecules.[8] These molecules appear to confirm the ability to inhibit vascular invasion and prevent ossification, which occurs in cartilage of the growth plate. Therefore the calcified cartilage persists and is a transitional zone between the softer uncalcified articular cartilage and the harder subchondral bone. Articular cartilage is bathed by SF and it is via SF that cartilage receives nutrients and extrudes its waste products.

It is important to note that in the healthy joint there is no real joint space. The joint space is a potential

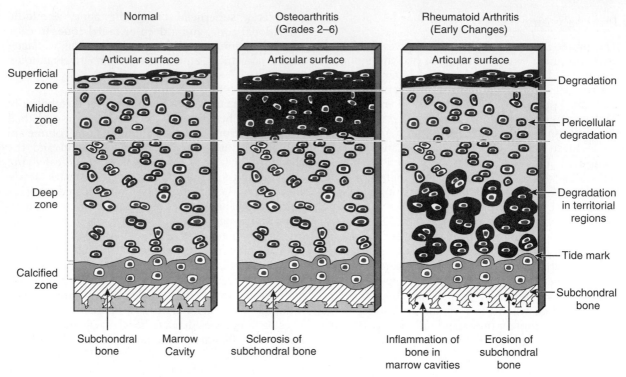

Figure 3-3. Diagrammatic representation of zones of normal cartilage (*left*) and sites of degradation of type II collagen in rheumatoid and osteoarthritic femoral cartilages showing sites of damage. Pericellular degradation is normally seen throughout healthy cartilage. (From Poole AR: Cartilage in health and disease. In McCarty DJ, Koopman WJ [eds]: *Arthritis and Allied Conditions*, ed 12, vol 1. Philadelphia, Lea & Febiger, 1993, p 305. With permission.)

space and the amount of SF present is minimal—about a few drops or milliliters in a healthy joint.

Collagen

As has been stated, articular cartilage, bone, fibrous capsule, tendon, and ligaments are all composed of a high proportion of collagen, which constitutes the extracellular matrix of these tissues. Articular cartilage differs from bone, capsule, tendon, and ligament in that it is composed chiefly of type II collagen rather than type I as in the other tissues (Table 3-2). The collagen superfamily is now recognized to include more than 20 types of collagen, (each with Roman numeral labels) and more than 15 additional collagenous proteins and C-like proteins.[18] The various types of collagen are strands of α-chains that comprise amino acids.

Each collagen is composed of three polypeptides forming a triple helix structure. Type I has two identical polypeptide chains and one that is slightly different; every third amino acid is glycine. Bone matrix is predominantly type I collagen.[19] Type II collagen, in comparison, has three identical helix chains, and contains more hydroxylysine, and is excessively glycosylated.[18,20] The collagen of HAC and fibrocartilage is 50% to 90% type II collagen. Type II is a fibrillar type of collagen found in the tissue as fibrils several thousand molecules in diameter that are packed into bundles to form large fibers. Fibrils are linked together by a number of collagen-binding proteins on the collagen fibril surface.[18] HAC also contains fiber-associated type IX collagen (5% to 20%), two types of short-chained collagen, type VI collagen (also in ligaments), and some type X collagen (principally in the hydrotropic cartilage of the growth plate), as well as a small amount of type XI collagen that may have a role in the regulation of the dimensions of the type II collagen fibril.[18]

The metabolic turnover of collagen is continuous through growth to maturity when the collagen fibers become more metabolically stable and have half-lives

Table 3-2. Location of the Various Types of Collagen in Healthy Human Articular Tissues

Type	Location
I	Fibrous capsule, synovial lining tissues, tendon, menisci, annulus fibrosus, periosteum, perichondrium, bone matrix
II	Hyaline cartilage (primary type), nucleus pulposus, fibrous capsule*
III	Perichondrium, periosteum, synovial lining tissues, tendon, ligament*
IV	Basement membranes (endothelial)
V	Perichondrium, periosteum, endosteal layer bone trabeculae, tendon
VI	Hyaline articular cartilage,* ligaments,* synovium
VIII	Endothelial basement membrane
X	Hypertrophic cartilage (growth plate, within Type II collagen fibers)
XI	Hyaline articular cartilage*
XII	Tendon, hyaline articular cartilage
XIV	Hyaline articular cartilage

Data from Ottani et al,[20] Myllyharju and Kivirikko,[18] and Prockop.[19]
*Small amounts.

of weeks or months.[21] Collagen turnover is increased in some conditions such as malnutrition, starvation, Paget's disease, hypoparathyroidism, and metastatic diseases of bone. The degradation of collagen in these conditions or diseases provides the body with a source of amino acids.

Collagen synthesis is a multistep process with intracellular and extracellular events. Collagen achieves maturity in the extracellular matrix, that is, outside of the cell. Several factors are important in collagen formation. There is increased glucose transport, mediated by a group of glucose-transport proteins that have distinct tissue distributions in HAC and synovial cells. A connective tissue activating protein (CTAP-III) is involved.[11] Amino acids also are transported into the cells. Insulin-like growth factors (IGF-I and IGF-II) stimulate connective tissue replication and extracellular matrix synthesis, that is, the synthesis of proteoglycans. Osteogen, a bone morphogenic protein, is present and can induce the formation of both bone and cartilage. It is theorized that osteogen may be involved in bone and cartilage repair. IGFs also may have a role in cartilage metabolism.[11]

Control of collagen fibril assembly may be a highly regulated process with several molecules participating possibly by binding to the surface of the forming fiber. This assembly also depends upon the exclusion properties of the aggrecan molecule network that may regulate diffusion of collagen precursors.

Collagen-Associated Molecules

A set of small collagen-binding molecules, members of a family of proteins with repeating 25 amino acids, may play an important functional role. These include fibromodulin,[22] decorin,[23] biglycan, and lumican[24] (Table 3-3). Most of these are proteoglycans (decorin, fibromodulin, lumican) that bind to collagen type II fibrillar surface. The nonproteoglycan proteins include proline- and arginine-rich end leucine repeat protein (PRELP),[25,26] chondroadherin,[27] and keratocan.[28] Collagen-associated proteins may function in maintaining the volume of tissue by enforcing the ability of collagen fibrils to resist the swelling pressure exerted by aggrecan.

Fibrous Capsule

The fibrous capsule is a type of regular white connective tissue similar to that of tendons and ligaments. The capsule consists mainly of parallel bundles of collagen (types I and II) with cells sparsely distributed. The fiber diameter varies from 150 to 1,500 mm; a few elastic fibers may be present. Collagen and elastin, fibrous proteins, constitute some 90% of the dry weight tissue, and water content is about 70%. Organic solids are mainly collagen and small proteins; a small portion is proteoglycan. Compared with hyaline cartilage, about 30% is hyaluronic acid, 40% CS, and 20% dermatan sulfate.[2]

The orientation of the fiber bundles reflects the tissue's functional role. This is particularly evident in tendons and ligaments. In the fibrous capsule, the

Table 3-3. Small Proteoglycans of Articular Cartilage*

Biglycan (leucine rich repeat protein in
    extracellular matrix [LRRP-ECM]
Decorin (LRRP-ECM)
Fibromodulin (LRRP-ECM)
Lumican (LRRP-ECM)
Chondroadherin (LRRP-ECM)
Ketatocan (LRRP-ECM)
PRELP Proline- and arginine-rich end leucine
    repeat protein (LRRP-ECM)
Perlican (noncollagenous protein)
Thrombospondin(noncollagenous protein)
COMP (cartilage oligometric matrix protein,
    noncollagenous)
Fibronectin (not cartilage specific)
? Tenascin

*Data from Hocking et al.[25], Neame et al.[27], and Heingard et al.[11]

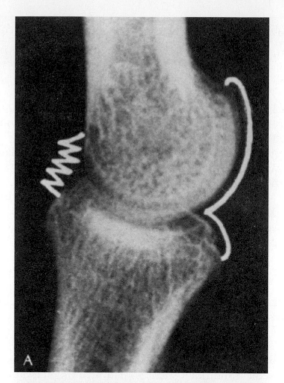

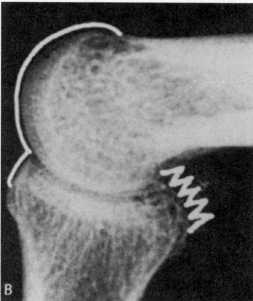

collagen bundles lie both in parallel and as interlacing bundles. The localized thickenings of strongly parallel fibers are the real joint ligaments; those that stand apart from the capsule are often termed *accessory ligaments*. The capsule can be reinforced and/or replaced by tendons and expansions from tendons of the surrounding muscles. The thickness and attachment of the fibrous capsule vary according to the joint. It may be thin and redundant, as in the shoulder joint, or thick and dense, as in the hip and knee joints. The extent of redundancy in the fibrous capsule and its associated synovial tissue or lack thereof has important consequences for the mobility of the joint, especially when it is involved in an inflammatory process. The redundancy permits full range of motion (Figure 3-4).

Ligaments

Ligaments connect bone to bone and provide passive stabilization between bones, limiting joint motion. They may be only hypertrophied extensions of the fibrous joint capsule. Ligaments have a distinct parallel orientation of their fiber bundles with few blood vessels within their substance. Close to where their collagen fibers penetrate the cortical osseous tissue, the tissue becomes mineralized and calcified. This arrangement of progressive stiffening decreases the likelihood of avulsion injuries. As with tendons, the cells (*fibroblasts,* termed *fibrocytes* when old and inactive) are elongated and sparsely distributed. The presence of fibroblasts on the external surface of both

Figure 3-4. Lateral views of an interphalangeal joint in extension (A) and flexion (B). Redundant synovium (shown schematically) gathers above the superior margin in extension and below the inferior margin in flexion. (From Simkin PA: Synovial physiology. In McCarty DJ, Koopman WJ [eds]: *Arthritis and Allied Conditions,* ed 12, vol 1. Philadelphia, Lea & Febiger, 1993, p 200. With permission.)

ligaments and tendons provides a pool of cells from which repair and regeneration can occur.[29] Although tendons are similar to ligaments in constitution, ligaments have a higher ratio of elastin to collagen (4:1) that gives them more extensibility.[1] Polarized light microscopy reveals a sinusoidal wave pattern (crimp) in ligament fibrils. Crimping is thought to give a biomechanical advantage, because with increased tensile deformation more fibrils will be recruited to resist the tensile stress.[30] An alteration in ligament structure may be important in degeneration of articular cartilage.[31]

Tendons

Tendons bridge muscle and bone and function to concentrate the force of a large muscle mass into a small local bone area. They may have a single attachment or multiple attachments. Splitting distributes force to more than one bone. They are formed by longitudinally arranged type I collagen bundles (95%) that are interspersed with a reticular network of types III, V, VI, and IX collagen. Fibrils within a collagen fiber are multidirectional, not longitudinally arranged.[32] Blood vessels tend to be associated with the exterior aspect of the tendon. Some tendons have a specialized insertion into bone (Sharpey's fibers) where fibers run through the periosteum and are continuous with the outer bony lamina. Others become mineralized, blend into fibrocartilage, and merge with bone, as do most ligaments.[1,29] Tendons may be encased in a vascular sheath of discontinuous collagen fibers lined with mesenchymal cells that resemble synovium. This is particularly true of long tendons that traverse multiple joints, as in the wrist and hand and ankle-foot region. Hyaluronic acid secreted by the lining cells may enhance the gliding function of the sheaths. The fibroblasts of both ligaments and tendons are known to synthesize metalloproteinases and cholinase inhibitors, as well as a latent form of cholinase.[1] These have implications in the breakdown and repair of the structures.

Bursae

Bursae are closed sacs lined by mesenchymal cells that are similar to synovial cells. Deep bursae but rarely subcutaneous bursae (e.g., olecranon) may have communications with the joint cavity (e.g., the subacromial bursa at the shoulder joint). Bursae facilitate gliding and provide a low-friction movement of one tissue over another. In life, bursae may develop in response to stress. Similar to that for tendon sheaths, there is a high potential for resolution of bursal inflammation to involve fibrosis, thickening, and adhesions that may seriously impair motion.

Synovial Lining Tissue

Synovial lining tissue (SLT, synovium) borders the joint cavity and covers all intra-articular structures except for the central load-bearing portions of the joint. Because there is no clearly defined membrane, the term *synovial membrane* is considered inappropriate.[33] Immediately adjacent to the joint space is the synovial intima layer. Beneath this layer is the subintimal tissue, which merges on its external surface with the fibrous capsule of the joint or the fibrous outer coating of the tendon sheath or bursae. SLT is a critical tissue in the pathology of arthritis. Because it is vascular, SLT is invariably involved in the inflammatory reaction and release of substances that can degrade articular cartilage. Resolution of inflammation may result in thickening and adhesions that interfere with cartilage nutrition and joint mobility.

The intimal layer consists of cells, one to three deep, that are set in the matrix. This layer is not a continuous layer so that both synoviocytes and the matrix may come in contact with the joint fluid. Between the cells in the intimal layer, there are collagen fibers (type I) and some electron-dense amorphous material that includes hyaluronate. There is no basement membrane, and cell processes (thin branching filaments) appear to provide a supportive membrane for the cells.

The subsynovial layer is a vascular connective tissue framework consisting of fibrous, areolar, and fatty tissues. The predominance of any one of these tissues varies by site and within the joint. Few blood vessels and only nonmedullated nerve fibers penetrate into the SLTs. In the subsynovial layer, there is a rich plexus of blood vessels and lymphatics. The former are believed to be responsible for the transfer of nutrients to the synovial cavity and the formation of SF; the latter are responsible for removal of waste products of HAC. In the intima, capillaries are of the fenestrated variety, which facilitates the movement of solutes and water into the tissues; in subsynovial tissues they are a continuous variety.[34] Vascularity varies both between joints and within the joint. Fibrous synovial surfaces are the least vascular.[35] Blood sacs from the deeper lymphatic plexus penetrate the intima but do not reach the surface, as do capillaries.[36]

Synovial Lining Cells

Although the two main types of synovial lining cells are the macrophage-derived type A and the fibroblast-derived type B, cells with features of both are quite common and are termed *AB lining cells* or *type C transitional cells*. There also are "stellate" cells that do not fit the traditional classification.[36] The two major types of cells do not represent two distinct cell lines but are functional variants of a single cell line.[37] Each cell may be potentially capable, at times, of carrying out either function.

Type A cells with prominent Golgi complexes, many vacuoles and vesicles, filopodia, and small amounts of rough endoplasmic reticulum appear to be equipped for phagocytosis and may be termed *surface macrophages*.[38] These cells have the capacity for endocytosis, are thought to synthesize and secrete hyaluronic acid into the joint fluid, and constitute about 10% to 20% of the lining cells.

Type B cells essentially are the converse of type A cells. They are fibroblast-derived, are concentrated in the deeper parts of the lining, and have prominent nucleoli and long cytoplasmic processes that extend to the surface. They may synthesize a variety of proteins and are hypothesized to be responsible for polypeptide secretion owing to their abundant rough endoplasmic reticulum. They also have the capacity to secrete enzymes that can degrade cartilage and may be primarily involved in synthesizing and releasing neutrophils or neutral proteinases that also can degrade cartilage. Cholinase can digest the collagenous lattice within the articular matrix. Other enzymes produced are gelatinase and strombolycin.[39] Type B cells have a capacity to proliferate and may serve as markers in disease states.[40]

The type A cells are believed to release cytokines, such as interleukin-1 (IL-1) and prostaglandin E_2. IL-1 is an inflammatory mediator that can cause chondrocytes to decrease matrix synthesis and absorb the surrounding matrix. Cytokines may play a major role in perpetuation of synovitis.[39] It is believed that synovial cells also are activated by proteoglycans released from the enzymatically digested cartilage. Synoviocytes may influence the immune response by presenting other targets for immune leukocytes or influence immune leukocytes by expressing cell membrane molecules that affect immune responses.[41]

Tissue cavitation may stimulate fibroblasts and macrophages to differentiate into synovial lining cells, and the environment, composed of SF, cells, and matrix, is necessary to maintain the differentiated state of these cells.[41] Mitotic cells have not been reported in the intima of the synovium. It is believed that intimal cell replacement or regeneration is derived from cells in the subintimal layer.[37,42,43]

SLTs play an important role in the function of the healthy joint and are a significant factor in the patho-

logy of arthritis. SLTs normally function to provide low adherence to the surfaces, a low-friction lining, biological lubricants, deformable packing, and blood supply for the chondrocytes. These tissues also control volume and composition of the SF, transporting nutrients into the joint space and removing metabolic waste; they may have an antimicrobial effect.[36,38] Synovium is heterogeneous, not homogeneous, and SF may poorly represent the tissue fluid composition of any one synovial compartment.[1]

Synovial Fluid

SF is essential for the nutrition and lubrication of the contiguous avascular cartilage surface and tissue. It may help to maintain movement by limiting adhesion formation. SF has a concentration of electrolytes and small molecules similar to that of blood plasma. It is now recognized that although vessel endothelium pore size limits the passage of protein (out of capillaries), the tissue space that must be traversed to reach the synovial cavity (i.e., the synovial interstitium) is a critical control of the passage of small solutes. It is no longer correct to term SF a *dialysate*. Synovial lining cells are responsible for secretion of hyaluronate into SF (Figure 3-5).

A healthy knee joint has about 2.5 ml of SF,[1] sufficient to coat surfaces but not to separate one surface from another. The fluid is usually clear to pale yellow in color of a transparent clarity with high viscosity, and because SF has no clotting factors it does not display spontaneous clotting. Normal synovial fluid is almost acellular. SF contains hyaluronate (GAG chain), a lubricating glycoprotein, and wear-retardant phospholipids.[44] The clearance rates depend upon the molecular size.

The volume of SF depends on conditions in the lining interstitium, the forces acting on it, and the permeability of the tissue surface to water and solutes. The concentration of hyaluronic acid, a nonsulfated GAG, in SF is higher than that in other connective tissue interstitial fluids. Hyaluronic acid is in fluid as a complex with protein and appears to be synthesized by synovial lining cells. About 60% of the protein in SF is albumin, a small molecule that is responsible for the colloid or osmotic pressure of SF.[33]

Hyaluronate is responsible for the high viscosity of SF. Small molecules, such as lactose, carbon dioxide, and inorganic pyrophosphate, are produced by the joint tissues and diffused into the SF; glucose enters SF via a facilitated diffusion. There is little lipid in SF. All plasma proteins can cross the vascular endothelium, traverse the synovial interstitium, and enter SF. The major mechanism is a size-selective

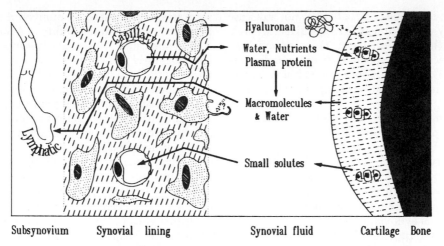

Figure 3-5. Diagram depicting synovial transport pathways (not drawn to scale). (From Levick JR: Synovial fluid determinants of volume turnover and material concentration. In Kuettner K et al [eds]: *Articular Cartilage and Osteoarthritis*. New York, Raven Press, 1992, p 530. With permission.)

process of passive diffusion. In healthy tissue, small molecules, such as albumin, enter easily, whereas large molecules, such as fibrinogen, are mainly excluded.[36] Protein passage from SF to the bloodstream is largely dominated by lymph flow.[45] The interstitial or tissue space of the synovial lining appears to be the important factor in the trans-synovial exchange of small molecules into the SF. Because of capillary infiltration and lymphatic absorption, SF is constantly turning over. Fluid turnover rates and thus the concentration of macromolecules may be increased by 100% to 300% in arthritis.[45]

Lubrication

Because joints exist to provide motion within the constraints of the surrounding soft tissues, an effective lubrication system is vital to protect joint surfaces from shear, stress, and strain that occur when a joint is loaded. Healthy human synovial joints have a remarkable ability to permit reciprocal movements within a wide range of loads and speeds while maintaining stability. Their low frictional resistance gives a remarkable slipperiness to human joints. The type of loading is an important factor in the mechanism of joint lubrication. Human joints may be subject to steady or static as well as dynamic loading; the latter may be very transient, as in jumping. Loading can vary from a very light load, as in the swing phase of gait, to a very high load; for example, heel contact

in gait for which the peak load compression of bone on bone may be 6 times body weight at the hip[46] and as much as 12 times body weight at the ankle joint.[47,48] These high loads tend to occur for only very brief periods (<0.15 second), whereas low loads may occur for longer periods. Joint surfaces can tolerate higher dynamic than static forces.

The body-support interface can play a major role in damping joint forces[49] and can be an important factor in management of clients with arthritis. Radin et al[50] demonstrated negative changes similar to OA in articular cartilage of weight-bearing joints in sheep that walked for long distances on concrete floors. Those that walked on wood chips did not show similar effects. Similarly, Light et al[51] demonstrated that variation in shoe heel construction could decrease the impact of walking on hard surfaces and, by inference, reduce joint loading. Joint forces have an enormous potential to promote degenerative changes in joint tissues that initially are subclinical and may not produce symptoms for years. The repetitive impulsive loading of a variety of activities undertaken in adolescence and young adulthood has potential consequences in later life. Consider the fact that a runner or jogger who runs 20 miles per week over 30 years delivers some 50 million shock waves through his or her body across joint surfaces.[52] Workers in factories or warehouses may spend years standing and moving on unyielding concrete or tiled floors. Some but not all occupations are associated with a higher risk of OA.[53]

Although it is recognized that OA is not a disease just initiated by wear and tear, the typical features of a joint in OA (loss of cartilage, bone remodeling, osteophytes, microfractures, etc.) are strong indicators of remodeling. Damage to tissues results from a variety of causes; repetitive trauma from impulsive loading is one of these.[4,54]

Critical variables in the joint lubrication mechanisms appear to be the following:

- surface compliance or elasticity (adjusts to loading)
- roughness (prevents immediate total contact)
- low coefficient of friction (facilitates lubrication, especially of synovial tissues)
- viscosity and protein lubricants of SF
- velocity of the rolling or sliding motion (maintains a fluid film between surfaces)
- permeability of the surface (blocks large molecules)
- joint surface contour (prevents total contact of surfaces and assists in maintaining a fluid film)

Lubrication of joint surfaces appears optimal when a film of fluid is maintained on the surfaces.

Surface compliance (yielding, conforming) is an important variable because the harder the surface, the higher the friction. If the surface is compliant under loading, more of the joint surface is brought into contact. With higher loads, because of surface compliance, joint surfaces become more congruent and stability of the joint is increased. It is believed that surface roughness produces points of contact between the surfaces, and in unloaded "dips," fluid is trapped when the joint is loaded, thus providing a fluid film between the surfaces.[34] Cartilage surface roughness, detected by electron microscopy, may only represent artifacts.[55] Pathological changes, as seen in rheumatoid arthritis (RA) and OA, alter these factors, limit the ability to maintain a fluid film, and enhance the potential for boundary lubrication and surface wear.

The remarkable slipperiness of human joints is measured by the coefficient of friction (COF). The COF is the shear force needed to make one surface slide on another divided by the normal force pressing them together. The lower the COF, the lower is the resistance to sliding. The theorized COF for cartilage on cartilage is between 0.02 and 0.001,[56,57] and is lower than that of a skate on ice (0.03).

It is believed that *fluid film mechanisms* can operate in healthy joints under most conditions. This means that a very thin layer of incompressible fluid separates joint surfaces. A number of mechanisms are proposed to explain the ability of a fluid film to exist. A fluid film can be generated when high loads compress cartilage; fluid will be extruded, especially on surfaces ahead of the load. Even when the load is high, as long as motion is occurring, a fluid film is still theoretically present to separate the two joint surfaces (hydrostatic mechanism). Elastic deformation of the surfaces (elastohydrodynamic mechanism) can assist in maintaining a small fluid film.

When an individual stands for long periods, as, for instance, on guard duty, a condition is created in which the fluid film would not be maintained; cartilage, however, may weep in the noncontact areas just ahead of the load, providing a fluid film in those areas. *Boundary lubrication* is theorized to operate with surface-to-surface contact. There are roughened dips of the cartilage that are not in full contact as the surfaces are separated by a thin layer of large molecules adsorbed onto the surface. These molecules in the SF are theorized to be hyaluronic acid–protein complexes that, because of their size, cannot penetrate cartilage ("boosted" lubricant mechanism). Although under this condition, friction will increase with a greater contact area of the surface cartilage, these molecules help lower the COF. Hyaluronate is less important in boundary lubrication than glycoproteins, such as lubrican synthesized by synovial cells; however these may act together in certain situations.[58] Dipalmitoyl phosphatidylcholine (DPPC), a phospholipid, may be the active boundary lubricant in SF.[44,59] In boundary lubrication, the coefficient of friction is theorized to be from 0.1 to 0.5, independent of the speed of sliding or the load.[48]

Several theories have been proposed for the lubrication of synovial joints; however difficulties with mathematical models have prevented credible demonstration in synovial joints. The models of boundary, hydrodynamic, and fluid film lubrication are favored, but many variables in theoretical models are poorly defined.[60] Further details on theorized lubrication mechanisms can be found in several articles.[48,61–63]

It is important to recognize that arthritic changes, regardless of the specific name, significantly alter the variables that should ensure the existence of a fluid film to lubricate joint surfaces and slippery structures, such as tendon sheaths and bursae. Such changes promote early contact of a greater area of the load-bearing surfaces and enhance their wear. Disruption of the surfaces then permits ingress and egress of substances that can maintain and enhance the pathological changes.

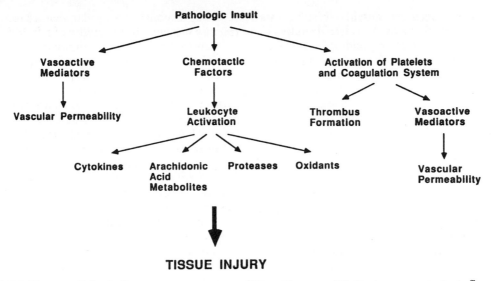

Figure 3-6. Mediators of the inflammatory response. (From Fantone JC: Basic concepts in inflammation. In *Sports-Induced Inflammation: Clinical and Basic Science Concepts*. Park Ridge, Ill, American Academy of Orthopedic Surgeons, 1990, p 26. With permission.)

Inflammation and Repair

The typical protective reaction of most body tissues to injury, pathological insult, and microbes is inflammation. The classic inflammatory process, as seen in wound repair, is characterized by redness, swelling, heat, and pain. The process involves increased vascular permeability, vasodilatation, cell proliferation, neovascularization, and fibroplasia. In this review of inflammation and repair in arthritis, the models will be RA and OA; changes specific to other forms of arthritis will follow.

In RA the inflammatory reaction is initiated, and a variety of molecules and cells are involved. Antigen-antibody complexes are involved and may represent the body's efforts to restore tissue integrity and function—an attempt to heal. The ability of a tissue to exhibit the classic inflammatory response is strongly related to its vascularity. Hence in arthritis, SLTs invariably demonstrate a degree of inflammation, whereas HAC, being avascular, does not demonstrate the typical inflammatory response. Similarly, strongly fibrous, less vascular structures such as tendons and ligaments demonstrate a poor inflammatory response.

Healing with restoration of the original tissue depends on the intrinsic ability of the tissue to regenerate and the complexity of the tissue. When regeneration does not occur, there is replacement by fibrous tissue, which organizes into a firm scar and often lacks the characteristics of the original tissue.

HAC has a very limited and imperfect repair mechanism, particularly if the defect involves only HAC; that is, it does not extend into the subchondral bone plate.[1,64] Mitotic figures have been observed rarely in healthy HAC,[65–67] although hypertrophic cells and cell clusters have been observed in osteoarthritic cartilage.[68] This indicates an attempt by local chondrocytes to reconstitute the extracellular matrix and repair the defect.

In ligaments and tendons, which are poorly vascularized, healing times are long.[69] Healing is complicated by the need to reconstitute the typical compact, precise arrangement of collagen bundles on which their function depends. An inflammatory process involving these structures results in extensive fibrosis due to the action of the fibroblasts laying down scar tissue. Extensibility, tensile strength, and loading characteristics of this scar tissue are compromised by the random organization of fibers and by cross-linking of new fibrils. Scar tissue may stretch over time, lengthening the overall structure and decreasing joint stability.

In comparison, bone retains a high regenerative capacity throughout its life span. The periosteum is a source of stem cells, and most parts of the skeleton are well vascularized. Healing times are long, passing through a collagenous phase (callus) and through differentiation into cartilage and eventually bone. The regenerative capacity of bone means that this tissue also is very responsive to altered loading (stress).

With progressive damage to articular cartilage and exposure of collagen fibers, there is altered loading on the subchondral bone, which responds by remodeling. Remodeling is evident in OA when thickening (sclerosis) of trabeculae occurs and when osteophytes (excess bone formation, i.e., Heberden's nodes in the hand) form at joint margins. These changes in bone, exclusive of osteophytes, eventually occur in RA. Exposure of subchondral bone allows joint debris to be compressed into medullary spaces, forming debris cysts. Such cysts may be "walled off" by sclerosed bone. Bony changes are enhanced by degradation of articular cartilage or by detachment of cartilage due to its splitting.

Tissue damage leads to extravasation of plasma, initiation of intrinsic and extrinsic coagulation (wounds), complement cascade, and release of important mediators of repair (Figure 3-6).[70] Inflammatory mediators include histamine, bradykinin, substance P, prostaglandins, and leukotrienes.[38] A major source of prostaglandins in human tissues is polyunsaturated fatty acids including arachidonic acid. At present, great attention is being focused on arachidonic acid–derived prostaglandins. Therapeutic intervention to inhibit the cyclooxygenase enzyme

(COX-2) responsible for inflammatory prostaglandins recently has been introduced.

Cell membrane phospholipids of injured cells and inflammatory cells may release arachidonic acid. Two enzyme pathways (lipoxygenase and cyclooxygenase) are critical in the conversion (oxygenation and hydrolysis) of arachidonic acid into other acids and metabolites (e.g., prostaglandins, thromboxane) (Figure 3-7 and Table 3-4). Products of the lipoxygenase pathway are much more potent than those of the cyclooxygenase pathway.[71] Varieties of prostaglandins (I_2, E_2) enhance vascular permeability because they produce vasodilation; effusion is increased. Nonsteroidal anti-inflammatory drugs (NSAIDs) act on this pathway to inhibit synthesis of prostaglandins and thromboxane. Prostaglandins of the E series and I_2, however, also inhibit inflammatory cell function (mast cell, neutrophil, macrophage) "secondary to their ability to activate adenylate cyclase and increase intracellular cAMP."[70] Although the main ability of prostaglandins is to influence vascular tone and permeability, prostaglandin E_2, produced by rheumatoid synovia, has been demonstrated to produce tissue injury via stimulation of bone resorption.[36]

Effusion is common when inflammatory processes involve joint tissues. Damaged tissues, particularly SLT, are infiltrated with leukocytes; there is an influx of neutrophils via increased blood flow and time-related chemoattractants. Neutrophils can cause further damage due to release of proteolytic enzymes and oxygen free radicals. Platelets release protease inhibitors that limit tissue damage. Platelets release serotonin and cytokines including transforming growth factors alpha and beta (TGF-α, TGF-β) and platelet-derived growth factor. Cytokines are peptide growth factors secreted by a variety of inflammatory cells and have multiple biological activities that regulate a variety of cell types. Cytokines are believed to be responsible for many features of RA, including systemic effects, as a result of transport from inflamed synovium into the general circulation.[72]

Neutrophils and macrophages arrive to remove cellular and matrix debris. Neutrophils release TGF-β,

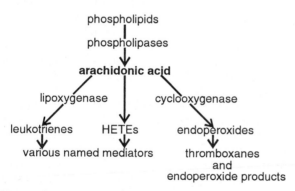

Figure 3-7. Steps in the production of inflammatory mediators, a simplistic version. HETEs = hydroxyeicosatetraenoic acids.[71]

Table 3-4. Sites and Effects of Arachidonic Acid Products

Microvascular	Increase or decrease vessel permeability
Polymorphonuclear leukocytes	
Macrophages	Increase or decrease adherence to surfaces
T-lymphocytes	Alter response to other stimuli
Platelets	

which acts as a monocyte and a fibroblast chemo-attractor and activates fibroblast differentiation from stem mesenchymal cells. Mononuclear cells differentiate into macrophages, produce pro-inflammatory mediators such as IL-1, tumor necrosis factor (TNF), and matrix degrading enzyme (collagenase) and also can express cellular fibronectin, which will contribute to the initial repair of tissue matrix. IL-1 is secreted by synoviocytes.[73] With TGF-α, IL-1 can increase the synthesis of proteases, such as metalloproteases (collagenase, stromelysin, serine proteases) and plasminogen activators. IL-1 also has been shown to favor synthesis of collagen types I and III over that of types II and IX.[33] TGFs are cytokines believed to be linked to the OA disease process and catabolism of HAC. The normal balance between matrix synthesis and degradation is upset in arthritis. The enzymatic processes involve both chondrocytes and synoviocytes; both can produce degradative enzymes. Matrix pH and physical factors, such as temperature, influence the enzymatic activity. Collagenase, for example, is more active at high joint temperatures (36° versus 33° C).[33] If cells are even mildly heated, they synthesize *heat shock proteins,* which are found present in synovia of RA and OA joints. It is believed that the temperature of an inflamed joint can induce synthesis of these proteins.[74] Such data support the use of cold over heat for acutely inflamed joints.

Complement System

The complement system, a group of many plasma proteins, also is involved in the body's defense and immune systems. There are two pathways: the classic complement pathway, which may be activated by inflammatory mediators, immune complexes, and microbial products; and the alternate pathway, which may be activated by cell products, microbial products, and foreign substances, such as x-ray contrast material.[70] The results of activation of either pathway are similar—formation of a membrane attack complex, which can induce cell lysis.

As a result of matrix degradation, basic fibroblast growth factor and TGF-β, normally bound to matrix proteoglycans, are released. Such extracellular messenger proteins (termed *cytokines* or *growth factors*) are involved in both tissue degradation and synthesis. The degradative effects of IL-1 can be controlled by IGF and TGF-β, which can stimulate collagen transcription and induce synthesis by connective tissue cells of tissue-inhibiting metallo-proteases and plasminogen activator 1. IGF-I and IGF-II can stimulate chondrocyte mitotic activity as well as proteoglycan and collagen synthesis. Fibro-blastic growth factors also can stimulate chondrocyte mitotic activity.

In acute inflammation tissues are infiltrated with polymorphonuclear leukocytes. In chronic inflammation, mononuclear cells, macrophages, and lymphocytes dominate the cellular infiltration. Neo-vascularization (angiogenesis) appears necessary to sustain chronic inflammation.[75] Angiogenesis is the primary vascular response in chronic inflammation and provides fresh monocytes and other inflammatory cells. Also seen in chronic inflammatory states is fibrosis and potentially suppuration due to a bacterial infection (septic arthritis). The fibrosis phase may convert the proliferative fibrofatty connective tissue formed in the inflammatory process into adhesions that mature into strong scars, particularly if the part is immobilized. Such scars may result in significant joint contractures with consequent loss of mobility. For further information on the complex cellular, molecular, and immune mechanisms affecting the inflammatory response the reader is referred to Fantone,[70] McCarty and Koopman,[76] and Ruddy et al.[77]

Cartilage Breakdown

Mechanisms of HAC breakdown involve multiple factors and an imbalance between extracellular matrix degradation and synthesis. Radin et al[54] considered *repetitive impulsive loading* (RIL) to be a major factor. Other factors are stress deprivation (immobilization, bed rest, weightlessness), excessive loading (body weight, obesity), developmental etiologies (hip dysplasia, Perthes' disease, coxa valga),[78–80] joint surface incongruity, and joint instability (cruciate ligament trauma, generalized ligamentous laxity). Radin et al[54] stated that the *type of load and manner of loading* are more important than the actual load on joint surfaces. RIL is detrimental to both HAC and subchondral bone. There is a greater potential for damage when loading is more rapid and tensile and shear rates are higher. RIL produces microfractures (subclinical) in subchondral bone, leading to cumulative damage.

Microklutziness is proposed as a mechanism of damage by RIL. This is a type of incoordination—a failure of deceleration at heel strike—that results in a large heel strike transient detectable only with high-speed data collection.[54,81] There may be a relationship between obesity, microklutziness, and OA. Potentially, individuals with these movement characteristics could be identified by gait analysis, and their movement patterns could be altered, decreasing the severity of later OA.

It is thought that RIL activates the secondary ossification center, which gradually thins the articular cartilage layer and increases the shear forces in the deeper layers. The tidemark advances (duplicative tidemarks are seen in HAC in OA), and there is thinning of the noncalcified layer. There is loss of proteoglycans, surface fibrillation, and vertical and horizontal splitting of HAC. Splitting and fibrillation of the cartilage surface produces articular debris in SF, which further irritates the synovial lining tissues and maintains the chronic inflammatory state. Catabolic enzymatic activity, RIL, and other causes produce the excess tissue damage that results in abrasion of cartilage and exposure of the subchondral bone.[54] When collagen and proteoglycans of the extracellular matrix are broken down by the pathological process in arthritis, their proteins or fragments may elicit an inflammatory immune response that triggers an inflammatory reaction.[82] Circulating antibodies to different types of collagens are increased in RA, psoriatic arthritis, and ankylosing spondylitis; in ankylosing spondylosis, this suggests an immune response to cartilage collagens.

Reduced levels of aggrecan are an important feature of joint disease. Although aggrecan levels may be normal early in the course of OA, with progression these levels drop significantly. Aggrecananse, a member of the ADAMTS family of zinc-binding metalloproteinases, is largely responsible for the proteolytic degradation of the aggrecan molecules and the drop in their levels.[83] Although the enzyme aggrecananse is involved in the normal turnover of aggrecan, it also increases turnover with immobilization of joints and shows increased activity in many arthritic inflammatory processes.[84] The loss of aggrecan from cartilage may be extensive, but the process may be reversible with an outcome that looks like repair.[85,86] The relative roles of the different enzymes are unclear and may vary with different joint pathologic conditions. With the loss of aggrecan from cartilage there may be a change in the osmotic environment that impairs water retention, decreases the efficiency of load bearing, and may have an adverse impact on the repair process.

In RA, free radicals, cytokines, neutral proteinase, and catabolic enzymes (derived from synoviocytes, chondrocytes, polymorphonuclear leukocytes) play a major role in articular cartilage breakdown; these substances also are involved in osteoarthritic HAC breakdown.[3,87,88] In osteoarthritic cartilage there is extensive damage to type II collagen fibers, with eventual unwinding of the helix and the appearance of collagen fibrils.[10,21] This process appears to commence in the superficial layers and progresses to the deep layers. Although cartilage proteoglycan loss can be reversed, loss of the structural integrity of cartilage and its collagen framework results in irreversible disintegration of the cartilage.[89] Repair occurs with fibrocartilaginous tissue in which type I collagen, rather than the normal type II, predominates and may facilitate calcification of repair tissue. It should be noted that type II collagen appears to block deposit of hydroxyapatite crystals required for calcification.

Synovial Lining Tissue Changes

It is important to note that synovitis, inflammation of the SLTs, may result from a variety of stimuli and creates an environment that is hostile to articular cartilage. In inflammatory arthritis the HAC may be an innocent bystander, damaged by the inflamed, infiltrated synovium. Stimuli to synovial inflammation in arthritis include substances normally foreign to the joint space, such as cartilage wear particles, matrix molecules, immune complexes, hemosiderin (an iron blood corpuscle pigment), implant wear particles (i.e., from artificial ligaments), hydroxyapatite (released from bone matrix), and surgical chemical agents (ethylene oxide, glutaraldehyde).[90] Synovial intimal cells, absorptive by nature, take up such substances, which have been shown to persist indefinitely in the intimal layer. However, this process may cause the intimal cells to secrete substances that are harmful to articular cartilage and provokes a chronic inflammatory reaction.

Vessels in the subsynovial layer become congested and dilated. Synovial villi proliferate and are larger. There is an increase in intimal cell size (hypertrophy) and number (hyperplasia) and in its matrix. SLTs show fibroblastic proliferation and increased fibrosis. A fibrinous exudate is seen on the surface. This inflammatory infiltrate may progress into a neovascular pannus that invades tendon sheaths and the joint, spreads over the joint surfaces, and destroys the articular cartilage.[75] This pannus is highly vascular and contains several cell types: macrophages, histocytes, mast cells, lymphocytes, and fibroblasts. Inflammatory cells may rarely be directly adjacent to articular cartilage; however, cytokines and other mediators released by nonnuclear cells can affect cartilage from a distance.[91] Pannus is a characteristic feature of RA.

Joint effusion may accompany the synovitis, particularly in RA. The vascular changes allow transit into the joint space of substances not usually found there, such as large plasma proteins (e.g., fibrinogen), cells, enzymes, and inflammatory mediators. Proteinases may overwhelm proteinase inhibitors, permitting enzymes to have a destructive effect, especially on articular cartilage. IL-1 and prostaglandin E_2 may enhance the destructive effect.[90] The enzymatically degraded cartilage releases proteoglycans that also may activate the synovial cells (termed *suicide reaction*, in which cartilage hastens its own destruction). A vicious cycle develops with synovial intimal cells releasing more collagenase and proteinases, cytokines, and IL-1, which further weakens the cartilage and enhances mechanical damage. This process can lead to fibrous ankylosis, particularly in RA-like conditions.

The destruction and loss of articular cartilage occurs particularly in biomechanically vulnerable areas subjected to loading and leads to subluxation or potential dislocation of the joint, seen more often in small joints of the hand and foot. In chronically inflamed SLT of the joint capsule, especially in redundant folds and tendon sheaths, the fibrosis produces adhesions that may significantly limit both the normal gliding of tendons and the total joint range. Because immobilization and rest aggravate adhesion formation, this observation supports use of gentle active assisted movement through range in the acutely inflamed joint.

Specific Joint Involvement

Structural Features of Importance in Arthritis

A sound knowledge of normal anatomy and articular motion is critical to the understanding as well as the prevention and control of deformity so often seen in arthritis. For detailed coverage of this important topic, consult anatomical textbooks. Certain structural features are highlighted here:

- In synovial joints the surrounding connective tissues (capsule, ligaments, tendomuscular units) are taut when the joint is in the close-packed position, usually one of extension. The joint then has maximum stability and minimal motion. An effused joint adopts the loose-packed position, when the surrounding soft tissues are "unwound" and lax, and there is minimal stability and maximal motion. The loose-packed position is one of flexion.[91] An effused joint places more stress on the surrounding soft tissues and is vulnerable to subluxation, dislocation, and deformity.
- Hinge joints, such as the interphalangeal joints, or modified hinge joints, such as the knee, are especially vulnerable because (1) there is a disparity between the proximal convex surface and the poorly adapted slightly concave distal surface and (2) no muscle force provides lateral stability. Collateral ligaments act most efficiently in the close-packed position to provide lateral stability[91]; however, when stretched by effusion these ligaments permit lateral displacement and deformity.
- In both the hand and the foot, flexor (palmar, plantar) muscles, principally interossei and lumbricals, exert greater force than the opposing extensor mechanism. Further, their attachment into the extensor expansion in the region of the middle phalanx, exerts a force that eventually displaces the extensor expansion from the dorsal aspect to between the metacarpal/metatarsal heads. This process, aggravated by joint effusion, produces characteristic deformities, especially in the hand.
- In certain joints, such as the knee, glenohumeral, and carpal/tarsal, there is communication between the joint cavity and adjacent bursa (e.g., subacromial in shoulder) and/or tendon sheaths (biceps). Effusion involving the main joint cavity also will be accompanied by effusion of certain tendon sheaths and bursa.
- In the relaxed state certain joints are predisposed to adhesions, contractures, and loss of mobility because in the typical posture of the joint, redundant folds of the lax synovium-lined joint capsule are in contact. The glenohumeral joint is a good example of this; there are many others.
- Where tendons play over bony surfaces, the tissue is protected by synovium-lined sheaths. These sheaths are prone to inflammation; however, owing to space constraints they are also prone to adhesions, strictures, or nodules that restrict normal tendon play within the sheath and may cause locking. Frictional stress between the tendon and the bony surface may result in fraying and rupture of an inflamed and weakened tendon.
- Certain regions are particularly prone to effusion problems due to the crowding of structures in a narrow space, for example, the carpal tunnel region at the wrist. Effusion of tendon sheaths may exert compression, resulting in paresthesia and/or neuropraxia of the median nerve that traverses the same tight space.

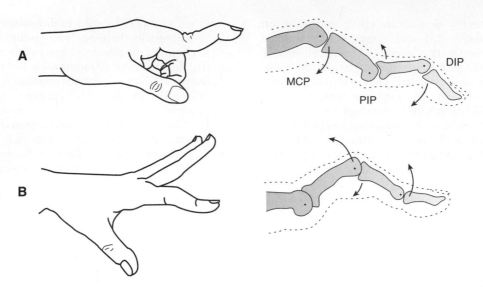

Figure 3-8. Diagrams to show the mechanism of swan-neck deformity (A) and boutonnière deformity (B).

Disease-Specific Changes in Alignment and Function

In RA the primary involvement and changes within synovium of small joints in the hand and foot stretch and weaken periarticular tissues. This produces mechanical imbalances that may progress to subluxation, dislocation, and severe deformity.

> **A 1:1 relationship between dysfunction and deformity has not been demonstrated.**

In RA, along with tenosynovitis, nodules may develop in sheaths producing "trigger fingers." Contracture of intrinsic muscle tendons and/or erosion of the palmar or plantar plates may cause collateral ligaments to "bow string," producing "swan-neck" deformity of the digit(s) (Figure 3-8, A). Erosion of the extensor mechanism over proximal interphalangeal joints may cause a buttonhole (boutonnière) deformity (Figure 3-8, B) and an inability to extend the digit.

In OA, deformity in the hand or foot may be aggravated by the presence of mucous cysts associated with osteophytes (Heberden's nodes, see Figure 4-20) and in gouty arthritis with urate crystal deposits (tophi). Pathological changes involving other tissues, such as calcification of fingertip pulp in scleroderma or in the skin (psoriatic arthritis, systemic lupus erythematosus), contribute to the eventual deformity.

In RA particularly, disease progression with resultant laxity of supporting structures and erosion of joint surfaces may lead to spinal subluxation (atlantoaxial) and neurological symptoms due to excessive pressure on spinal nerves and the spinal cord.[92] Spondylolisthesis (slippage, commonly at L4–L5) may occur in OA with potential stenosis of the spinal canal and neurological symptoms.

The previous chain of events affecting joint tissues in the pathology of arthritis may be arrested at any point by intrinsic and extrinsic (e.g., drug) factors.

Pathological Changes in Specific Conditions

Only certain aspects of the pathophysiology of specific conditions will be covered below. For greater detail see Chapter 4, Diagnosis and Medical Management, as well as Chapters 8 to 12 on specific therapies.

Rheumatoid Arthritis

RA is a destructive chronic synovitis in multiple diarthrodial joints (polyarthritis) with a variety of systemic manifestations. In RA there is persistent immunologic activity with prominent involvement of $CD4^+/CD29^+$ memory T cells.[93] Local production of immunoglobulin (Ig) and autoantibody rheumatoid

> **A sound knowledge of anatomy is essential for understanding and control of deformities common in arthritic conditions.**

factor (RF) plays a role in tissue destruction. Macrophages and lymphocytes have roles in the early synovial inflammatory process. Cytokines, such as TNF-α and IL-1, and the interaction of lymphocytes and macrophages with these cytokines may result in formation of inflammatory mediators (prostaglandins) and release of matrix proteases. There is a chronic cascade of events with inflammatory and immunological components causing cartilage and bone damage as a result of the synovial inflammation. The rheumatoid synovium exhibits variable histopathological characteristics, and infiltration of large numbers of mononuclear cells is characteristic, especially in the chronic phase of RA. It is presumed that small lymphocytes differentiate into Ig- and RF-secreting plasma cells.[93] Lymphoid follicles develop in synovial tissues and are one source of Ig and RF. Hypertrophy and hyperplasia are characteristic features of synovium in RA, as well as microvascular abnormalities, especially of capillaries and postcapillary venules in the acute phase; neovascularization and pannus formation are prominent features. In RA, as with many inflammatory arthritis conditions, pathological changes are not restricted to those of the joint tissues given emphasis in this chapter. Changes are often seen in ocular tissues and in cardiopulmonary, skin, and reticuloendothelial systems.

Psoriatic Arthritis

Synovial changes in psoriatic arthritis (PA) are not distinguishable from those in RA except that there is a greater tendency for bony ankylosis to occur, especially in interphalangeal and carpal joints.[94] There is a marked difference from the pattern of joint involvement in RA. In PA it may be symmetrical, asymmetrical, and sometimes oligoarticular. Cellular infiltration is predominantly lymphocytic. TGF α may be involved in the generalized abnormality of blood vessels and the abnormally fast keratinocyte growth rate (3 days versus 3 weeks).[94] Dystrophy (e.g., pitting) of nails may occur in 60% to 80% of patients with PA.[95] In all studies reported about 20% of patients have joint disease that precedes skin involvement.[96,97]

Ankylosing Spondylitis

This form of arthritis involves specific areas of the body, primarily the spine, and appears to maximally involve the junction of ligaments to bone (enthesis). Enthesopathy involves vertebra in an ascending order with a process that commences around the sacroiliac joint. With inflammation at ligament junctions (enthesitis), bone becomes eroded and cartilage and cortical bone are replaced by fibrous and granulation

tissues. New bone formation (syndesmophytes) causes ascending ossification of the inflamed tissues resulting in ossification of spinal ligaments, intervertebral disks, facet joint capsules, and ankylosis ("bamboo spine"). Typically, there is a "squaring" off of the vertebral bodies. Changes may cause symptoms of cauda equina as well as vertebrobasilar artery insufficiency.[98] Peripheral joints exhibit synovitis similar to that in other forms of inflammatory arthritis, differing only in the distribution of joints affected and, compared with RA, in the absence of RF and usual antigen HLA-B27 positivity.[99]

Infectious Arthritis (Reactive Arthritis)

A number of microorganisms may produce an infectious process at a site distant from the primary infection and cause a suppurative (staphylococcal arthritis) or nonsuppurative inflammatory process (reactive arthritis). One form of nonsuppurative arthritis, Reiter's syndrome, is associated with other pathologic changes (classically a syndrome of arthritis, ureteritis, and conjunctivitis) in less than 33% of patients.[93] About 60% of patients with Reiter's syndrome have subclinical inflammation of the terminal ileum and colon. Pathological changes are similar to those in RA; however, enthesitis is more common. Bony erosions and pannus formation are uncommon, but will be seen with persistent inflammation.

Suppurative infectious arthritis in the absence of direct penetration of the joint by an object, or trauma, reflects failure in the body's extensive defense mechanisms. Under healthy conditions the joint cavity is highly protected from transmission of infectious agents. The initial site of infection is distant to the joint. Joint sepsis may result from agents such as gonococcus, staphylococcus, *Mycobacterium tuberculosis*, *Salmonella* species, and *Haemophilus influenzae* gram-positive bacteria (particularly in young children). (Hence another name is *organism-associated arthritis*.) Septic arthritis is also a grave and costly complication of patients with joint replacements.

The inflammatory process is similar to that of other forms of arthritis. Because of the tamponade (compression) of subsynovial vessels and resultant increase in intra-articular pressure, diffusion of solutes is slowed. This process may allow bacterial cells to remain dormant even in the presence of drugs.[100] Furthermore, although antibiotics may destroy the microorganisms, drug therapy does not remove microbial products. The persistence and retention of these products either within the joint cavity, embedded in joint crevasses, or in the articular cartilage, may cause a persistent chronic inflammatory response (postinfectious synovitis), with further potential for irritation, damage, and dysfunction. Although all joint tissues are vulnerable to damage from the infectious inflammatory process, articular cartilage is particularly vulnerable to the presence of pus, because chondrolysis is irreversible. Rupture of tendon sheaths may occur.

Because the deeper layers of HAC are vascularized in the growing child, the infectious agent may reach the joint space via small capillaries that cross the epiphyseal growth plate. This route is blocked in the older child and adult unless partial defects exist in the osteocartilaginous barrier (tidemark).[1] However, agents may reach the joint via joint anastomoses, via sideways extension into the subperiosteum, and, in certain joints, from dependent synovial fold reflections (i.e., glenohumeral).

Bacterial infections may involve fibrocartilaginous midline joints that lack SLT (symphysis pubis, sternomanubrial, sternoclavicular, posterior sacroiliac). When these joints are involved, osteomyelitis in adjacent bone may occur.[101] Bacteria, ticks (Lyme disease), and other microbial organisms in a joint can activate IL-I, TNF, and the complement, resulting in aggravation of the inflammatory process owing to production of chemotactic factors, mediators of inflammation, and other biologically active substances. The interested reader is referred to reviews for further detail.[76,77]

Hemophilic Arthritis

In hemophilia, repeated joint hemorrhages can produce severe articular cartilage damage, particularly in large peripheral joints such as the knee. The damage can be more severe than that in OA.[102] Large amounts of hemosiderin, an iron-containing pigment, may be deposited as coarse aggregates in the synovium. These aggregates may persist indefinitely and act as an irritant promoting further disintegration of articular cartilage as a result of release of chondrolytic enzymes. The presence of plasmin (fibrinolysin) in SF in acute hemorrhages may enhance enzyme degradation. The contribution of interosseous bleeding to the development of often large cysts or cavities in the subchondral bone has not been established.[103] Accelerated maturation and hypertrophy of adjacent epiphyses may result in stature reduction. (Growth disturbances, local and systemic, and premature closure of growth plates also may cause short stature in patients with juvenile RA.) Repeated hemorrhages cause repetitive acute inflammatory episodes that are often associated with marked atrophy of muscles about the joint.

Crystal-Associated (Gouty) Arthritis

Various crystal deposits, such as monosodium urate monohydrate (MSU) in gout and calcium pyrophosphate dihydrate (CPPD) may cause crystal-induced inflammation with ensuing arthritis. The presence of MSU or CPPD crystals in joint fluid may be both a result of and a cause of joint inflammation,[104] because crystals may be released from enzymatic degradation of cartilage or mechanical disruption of its architecture.

In gout, the common lesion is joint degeneration with deposition of MSU or uric acid crystals from extracellular fluids in and around joint tissues. These tophaceous deposits can cause acute inflammatory episodes with severe destruction of articular structures. Single or multiple joints may be affected. Crystals, the end product of purine metabolism, may be deposited on and in articular cartilage, as well as subchondral bone.[102] Hyperuricemia (supersaturation of urate in serum), a biochemical abnormality, is a characteristic feature, when gout is the disease state.[105]

The tophaceous deposits (solid urate) may form in various soft tissues, such as the helix of the ear, olecranon, prepatellar bursa, and Achilles tendon. Other features of gout may include ulceration of the tense skin overlying the tophi, renal disease, and crystals in the SF during quiescent periods (termed *intercritical*). Except for interphalangeal joints of the hand and foot and carpal region, bony ankylosis is unusual.[106]

Neuropathic Arthritis

In neuropathic joint disease, arthritis, progressive and degenerative, develops as a result of sensory loss in a joint.[107] Sensory loss may result from diabetes mellitus with peripheral neuropathy, neurosyphilis, syringomyelia, paraplegia, and tabes dorsalis. Joint changes are similar to those in OA, but early effusion with later subluxation, para-articular debris, and bony fragmentation are considered diagnostic features. Compared with OA a greater degree of bony sclerosis, osteophytosis, and fragmentation of bone is seen on radiographs.[108]

Effect of Unloading and Immobility

Articular cartilage, ligaments, and tendons are sensitive to abnormal loading. When unloaded, as in immobilization, there is rapid deterioration of biochemical and mechanical properties.

Ligaments

In response to unloading and immobility ligaments show atrophy, decreased strength, and stiffness as well as disorientation of collagen fibers and matrix.[29,69,109] Loss of ligament strength appears exponential over time. Although the loss may be minimal in the first few weeks, if immobilized for 6 to 9 weeks, ligaments are only 50% as strong and stiff as healthy ligaments. Bone resorption at the insertion sites further weakens the ligament.[29,110] Ligaments also tend to be less stiff and more resilient after immobilization.[111] The stiffness in a joint after immobilization is probably due to binding of nonligamentous periarticular tissues. After immobilization, recovery of ligament properties is not homogeneous in all parts; the bony insertion area may recover in a few weeks, whereas recovery of ligament substance may take months.[112,113]

Studies in animal models demonstrate that because the scar tissue formed in ligaments during immobilization is smaller in mass, materially weaker, and less viscous, ligaments are more vulnerable to repeat injury at comparable loads. Bray et al,[114] with a rabbit model of an anterior cruciate ligament–deficient knee, showed that short periods of immobilization may retard osteoarthritic changes associated with joint instability; this result may relate to stability provided by immobilization. If instability is not corrected by immobilization, deterioration will continue. In ligaments, the short-term "benefit" of immobilization may not be worthwhile.[113,115]

Tendons

After immobilization negative changes have been observed in tendon ultrastructure,[116] tensile strength,[117] and biochemistry.[32] A study of repaired Achilles tendons in which functional casting, allowing about 20 degrees of motion, was compared with rigid casting showed improved biomechanical parameters postsurgically.[118]

It is pertinent to note that in arthritis, unlike with isolated ligament injuries in sports, ligaments are not healthy before a period of immobilization. Inflamed joints, however, are subjected more to unloading and temporary immobilization for shorter time periods using removable splints. Because rest is a basic principle of management of acute and chronic arthritis, the negative effects of immobilization on joint tissues produce a dilemma for the clinician, who has to determine the balance between the period of rest to decrease inflammation and the occurrence of further functional loss. Anti-inflammatory drug therapy is an important component of treatment.

More studies are required to establish the most efficacious postsurgical approach with regard to functional casting and use of continuous passive motion equipment.

Articular Cartilage

Synthesis activity by chondrocytes decreases when articular cartilage is unloaded by being deprived of mechanical stimuli (rest, non-weight bearing).[119,120] Unloaded cartilage shows decreased thickness (atrophy), decreased hydration, decreased chondroitin sulfate, and decreased synthesis of GAGs.[121] Collagen synthesis, but not the total amount of collagen, may be enhanced. Effects of unloading on collagen may occur in all collagenous tissues. Fiber-fiber distances and lubrication between fibers is decreased. This hinders fiber-on-fiber gliding and enhances cross-linking and adhesion formation. The collagen arrangement is more random. Fibers may be thicker, because fewer fibers are laid down without regard to the mechanical requirements of the tissue.

When exposed to rigid immobilization, articular cartilage shows changes similar to that of OA; cell necrosis may occur.[120,122,123] These changes presumably are related to interference with the nutrition of the chondrocytes (pressure driven from SF through the cartilage matrix) due to absent or decreased amounts of cyclic compression and expansion of articular cartilage that occurs with intermittent loading.[124] Although immobilization prevents joint motion and is associated with unloading of joint surfaces, some areas of the cartilage joint surface may be subjected to increased loading depending on the position of immobilization.

If cartilage previously exposed to unloading is loaded, there may be "gross functional failure of matrix."[125] This appears to be related to a defect in the ability of proteoglycans to reform the hyaluronic acid–binding region of the aggregates. Cell-matrix interaction probably plays an important role in the response of the chondrocyte to mechanical compression or lack thereof.[126] Unloaded cartilage is less stiff, and the proteoglycan matrix is impaired, which may make articular cartilage more vulnerable to injuries if exposed to sudden, heavy loading. A gently graduated program may reverse such changes; however, restoration of healthy structure and characteristics is uncertain.[127] Therapists should recognize that after immobilization or unloading (rest), articular cartilage is less stiff and less capable of tolerating high loads, loads normally within the physiological capacity of healthy cartilage.

Bone

The response of bone to altered mechanical stimuli is important in arthritis. If mechanical stimuli are reduced by rest or immobilization, bone loss occurs, with a decrease in bone quantity but not in the quality or composition. Adaptive remodeling, the laying down of more bone, is stimulated by altered stress or a change in mechanical stimuli. Frost's "mechanostat" theory[128] postulates that remodeling is stimulated by decreased mechanical usage with concomitant net loss of bone and is inhibited by increased mechanical usage with a net increase in bone mass. Because the internal architecture of subchondral bone influences the load transfer to cortical bone, changes in bone associated with arthritis are important.

The changes in bone as a result of immobilization and decreased loading are significant and clear-cut: increased resorption and decreased trabeculae volume and bone mineral content. This mineral loss can be reversed; however, recovery is not as rapid.[129] The slower rate of reconstitution is more important in progressive arthritic conditions than in fractures occurring in a young adult.

Increased Loading

In OA it is predicted that excessive mechanical loading (repetitive impulse loading) produces fatigue fractures, microscopic cracks in and around osteons that involve individual trabeculae and, over time, reduce the strength and stiffness of bone.[130] As previously noted, there is evidence that faulty deceleration at the heel strike phase of gait, microklutziness, is the mechanism that causes the microdamage associated with RIP and resulting in clinical OA.[54] If the damage is excessive, resorption exceeds deposition and failure occurs at the macroscopic level, such as crush fractures of vertebral bodies and contour changes in joint surfaces. These changes in bone place greater stress on articular cartilage and are postulated to provoke OA. Research has not yet established whether such microcracks can trigger a cellular response that will repair the damaged matrix.

Aging

The pathological changes in bone in arthritis also may encompass changes associated with the natural decline in bone mass due to aging. This decline occurs at a greater rate in women than in men and may lead to osteoporosis. In osteoporosis there is reduced mineral mass, excessive resorption, increased bone porosity, more numerous and larger Haversian canals, and weaker and more brittle bone.[131,132] Moderate to severe arthritis, especially RA, enhances the osteoporotic process owing to limited mobility and activity; the probability of fractures is further enhanced. Although OA is not an inevitable consequence of aging, its incidence and prevalence increases with each decade.[133]

With aging there also is an increased risk of adult-onset diabetes. Insulin-dependent diabetes causes more marked osteopathic changes[134,135] with mechanical weakening of bone.[136,137] Bone mineral loss may be further aggravated by long-term corticosteroid therapy used in RA and juvenile RA, increasing the potential for stress fractures.

With advancing age there is a gradual decrease in the number of chondrocytes in HAC; however, the remaining cells, in an attempt to maintain their extracellular matrix, become more metabolically active. The rate of collagen and proteoglycan synthesis is increased; however, proteoglycan size decreases with age due to increased breakdown by enzymes, and net loss exceeds new synthesis.[138] Another change associated with aging is reduction in the ratio of collagen to proteoglycans. These changes reduce the ability of cartilage to withstand forces to which it is exposed.[139]

Pain Medication and Modulation

The mechanism(s) producing the sensation of pain, common in arthritic conditions, probably is not derived from cartilage damage, because articular cartilage is aneural. Pain sensation may be derived from increased pressure that results from abnormal motion, abnormal geometry, excessive loading, and distention of joint capsule tissues and other soft tissues related to the joint. Articular nerves contain both myelinated and unmyelinated fibers. Pain and vasomotor fibers are small in diameter. Unmyelinated nerve fibers are postganglionic sympathetic fibers that terminate in the walls of the many articular blood vessels found in subsynovial tissues.[140–144]

The articular nociceptive system is inactive in the healthy state but is activated by excessive levels of mechanical stress or deformation and in the presence of inflammation when chemical irritants (prostaglandins, bradykinin, serotonin, histamine) accumulate in the tissues. If vascular permeability is decreased by fibrosis or by acute inflammatory processes, the concentration of these chemical irritants increases.

In the presence of effusion or hemarthrosis, the synovial cavity is no longer a potential space and intra-articular pressures (IAP) normally subatmospheric at rest (0 to 5 mm Hg) becomes supra-atmospheric, up to 20 mm Hg in the resting knee in RA and over 100 mm Hg with isometric exercise.[145] Sustained synovitis with increased SF volume and pressure provokes tension and even pain. When an effusion forms rapidly, pain is more likely.[146] There is a critical effusion pressure, which in turn impairs and reduces synovial blood flow.[147]

The viscoelasticity of synovial cavity tissues influences the relationship between IAP and SF volume (compliance curve). At very small sub-atmospheric pressures the cavity tissues are most stretchable, neither collapsed nor distended. With increase in volume the stiffness of these tissues increases rapidly and linearly so that cavity walls are tense and stretched. If the increase in volume persists, as in chronic synovitis, stress relaxation occurs because of loss of tension in the cavity walls and the pressure, despite constant volume, will decrease. Thus a rapidly forming effusion (traumatic, infective, hemarthrotic) will be associated with more pain (and can be relieved by aspiration) than a slowly forming effusion.[148]

A patient with an effused joint will adopt a position in which the cavity tissues are under the least tension (in the knee about 30 to 40 degrees of flexion) (Figure 3-9).[149] Motion away from this position, in either direction, will increase IAP and potentially pain. Active motion, as displayed in Figure 3-9, is associated with higher IAPs. The greater the effusion (volume), the greater is the sensitivity of pressure to change in the joint angle. Increased IAP in the knee has been shown to excite joint afferents strongly, probably through end organs in the capsule.[141] Firing of these afferents inhibits activation of muscles acting on the joint (quadriceps), contributing reflexly to disuse atrophy. Simultaneously, antagonists (hamstrings) may be stimulated to assist in maintenance of a loose-packed joint position that accommodates the effusion.[140]

Elasticity and viscosity in particular contribute to total stiffness, a common and important symptom in arthritis. Different joint tissues appear to vary in their contribution to total stiffness from joint to joint. This symptom that may be confused with pain has not proven to be easily quantifiable by biomechanical devices. Mechanical perception thresholds in patients with RA are reported to be normal.[150]

Several investigators suggested that a disease-related loss or alteration in joint or muscle proprioception is present in OA.[151–153] Function, such as gait, may be affected by changes in joint position sense that may

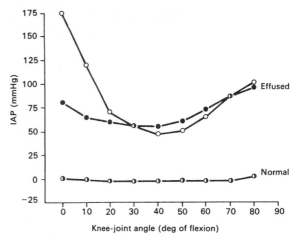

Figure 3-9. Intra-articular pressures (IAPs) recorded at a range of joint angles during active (○) and passive (●) positioning of the knee before and after injection of 10 ml of dextran into the joint (◑). Coincident IAPs are shown for both active and passive positioning. Note that in the effused knee IAPs are lowest at about 30 to 40 degrees. (From Baxendale RH, Ferrell WR, Wood L: Intra-articular pressures during active and passive motion of normal and distended knee joints. *J Physiol* 369:179P, 1985. With permission.)

result from small fluctuations in disease activity (i.e., effusion, intra-articular pressure changes) and may not be due solely to the presence of pain. Merry et al[154] showed high IAP in chronic synovium inflammation with RA but not in acute traumatic effusion during exercise. They theorized that failure of normal reflex muscle inhibition may be the cause in persistent RA involving joints.[154]

Does reflex muscle inhibition precede or follow arthrogenous muscle weakness and atrophy? O'Reilly et al[155] showed in 300 subjects with knee pain a strong association between knee pain, disability, and incomplete muscle activation. Others have suggested, on demonstration of a strong correlation between body weight and extensor strength, that muscle strength may be important in preserving protective muscle reflexes.[156] O'Connor et al[81] theorized that individuals who show large heel strike transients may have differences in their central program generator, with the neural mechanism governing lower limb motion. Although this may increase their susceptibility to OA, this theory remains to be proved.

Kidd et al[157] hypothesized that sensory nerve endings in synovial tissues also may, by releasing neuropeptides, modulate the response of synovial tissues to a variety of noxious stimuli that may result from joint damage. This mechanism may selectively activate preganglionic sympathetic cells, which project to the opposite side, and is reflected in symmetrical joint involvement, common in RA. This projection to the contralateral side leads to recruitment of macrophages in the absence of a full inflammatory response.

In an acute inflammatory state, synovial inflammation is associated with increased blood flow and raised local temperature. In chronic inflammation with capsular fibrosis, however, there is reduced blood flow. A change in synovial plasma flow is correlated with a variation in intra-articular temperature. Theoretically, a swollen but *cool* joint, indicative of reduced blood flow, is metabolically more impaired than a swollen hot joint (increased blood flow). In the knee intra-articular temperature has been shown to be decreased by cold therapy and increased by heat therapy.[158]

Modulation of Pain

Identification and removal of the cause(s) of arthritis are not yet achievable; therefore therapy must be directed at relief of signs and symptoms and prevention or delay of further damage. The interaction of increased IAP, tension, and pain strongly supports the approach that the most efficient modulation of pain is reduction and control of joint effusion.

Many modalities are in use to control pain (drugs, transcutaneous electrical nerve stimulation, thermal agents, acupuncture) and may be effective in accordance with the "gate theory."[159] Stimulation of large-diameter, myelinated fibers blocks the transmission of pain impulses from small-diameter, unmyelinated fibers at the synapse (presynaptic inhibition) and from reaching the dorsal gray column. Some modalities (i.e., cold) act to decrease the firing rate of muscle spindle afferents, thereby decreasing reflex muscle contractions, which decreases the tension on the effused joint tissues and lowers the pain threshold on motion. Management of abnormal mechanical deformation or stress by splinting also serves to decrease awareness of pain by limiting motion into areas of range where IAP is increased. Other mechanisms invoked by drug therapy are given in Chapter 6. The therapist and client, however, must be aware that control and reduction of joint effusion are most likely to give long-lasting relief from pain.

> **Reduce and control effusion to decrease pain.**

Restoration of Joint Surfaces

In considering the potential for restoration of joint surfaces, it is pertinent to distinguish between repair and regeneration. *Repair,* is "the replacement of damaged or lost cells and extracellular matrices with new cells and matrices," and *regeneration* is "a form of repair that produces new tissue that is structurally and functionally identical to the normal tissue."[160]

Bone is characterized by an ability to heal without fibrous tissue (scar) and, when healed, to regain its former strength and functional capabilities. Articular cartilage, however, is notorious for its limited potential for either repair or regeneration. Thus arthritis, regardless of type, tends to be progressive once changes are initiated. Because articular cartilage is avascular, it is incapable of producing an inflammatory reaction, which is the typical tissue response to injury and the initial phase of a repair process. This may explain the failure to heal in partial thickness defects of articular cartilage.[7]

Healing of articular cartilage appears to depend on whether the defect penetrates the subchondral plate. Several studies over the years have amply demonstrated that healing by articular cartilage only occurs in small-thickness defects ($\frac{1}{8}$-inch diameter) and does not occur in large or full-thickness defects, with or without motion.[161,162] Chondrocyte proliferation and matrix remodeling are needed for repair of superficial deficits; mutagens for chondrocytes, such as basic fibroblast growth fiber and bone morphogenic proteins may enhance this process.[163]

Based on unpublished data, Sokoloff[164] suggested that if the pressure on the joint surface can be relieved (i.e., surgically), resurfacing of the OA joint surface can occur. The regenerated surface, however, was fibrocartilaginous but apparently functionally adequate. However, it has not been established that the repair "cartilage" has the typical three-dimensional structure of articular cartilage and therefore will function normally.[165] Drug therapy may arrest or modify the enzymatic degradation of the joint surfaces that occurs in inflammatory arthritis (e.g., RA); however, it cannot reconstitute altered geometry and restoration is unlikely.

The type of training that best improves the ability of articular cartilage to withstand stress and that positively contributes to repair of articular cartilage has not been established. Exercise has been shown to increase blood flow and perfusion of soft tissues in the canine joint; however, effects on cartilage remain unclear.[166] Such data support the use of only minimal activity to preserve range of motion in the acutely inflamed joint and also support the value of vigorous exercise in chronically inflamed joints. An increase in articular cartilage thickness, increased cell size, and improved anabolic processes of articular cartilage all have been demonstrated after exercise training in animal models.[167–169] A species-specific effect may exist, because running exercise in rats has been shown to increase tendon collagen synthesis, but in mice there was a decrease in total collagen and in collagen tensile strength. A type-specific response also may exist, with flexor tendons responding to exercise differently from extensor tendons.[170]

Although cells of healthy articular cartilage appear to have suppression or loss of their ability to replicate their DNA, when degeneration occurs, as in the early stages of OA, chondrocytes appear to recover their ability to divide.[68,171] Chondrocytes may migrate from adjacent areas; however, they have not been shown to proliferate and restore the matrix components.[172] Overall, repair by surviving cells seems absent when a cleft involves only articular cartilage, not subchondral bone. Salter et al,[173] over the past two decades, have demonstrated healing of full-thickness drill hole defects and free intra-articular periosteal grafts with continuous passive motion with hyaline-like tissue. Results have been less impressive in mature animals. How newly synthesized articular cartilage responds to normal loading over time has not been established. The evidence, however, is that physical signals such as motion and load are important in facilitating cartilage repair processes, however imperfect these may be. Data from animal studies also suggest that intermittent rather than continuous mechanical stress induces beneficial metabolic changes in chondrocytes and that absence of motion is detrimental.

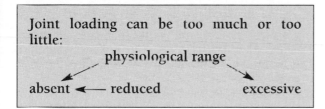

Joint loading can be too much or too little:

physiological range

absent ◄── reduced   excessive

Bone, in comparison with articular cartilage, is a dynamic tissue that retains throughout life the capacity for regeneration. Remodeling is ensured because of penetration of blood vessels from underlying bone; this process, however, enhances further calcification of articular cartilage.[174,175] According to Wolff's law, as loads on bone change, remodeling reorients load-bearing trabeculae so that they are aligned with new trajectories of principal stress.[176] A program of graduated weight bearing/loading is important, because subchondral bone responds to cyclic loading by increased stiffness and strength.[174]

Conclusion

Inflammatory and degenerative pathologic changes affect not only the joint and its tissues but also has influence at a distance. Often systemic effects are often present that may influence the client's response to therapy. Current therapeutic approaches that involve joint replacement, grafting, cell seeding, and genetic manipulations require the clinician to have a sound knowledge of the content in this chapter—articular tissues and their response to injury and disease.

Cartilage and other articular tissues respond positively to loading and negatively to unloading, so that loading may be the most controllable intervention available. There remains a need to define the margins of safety in the application of exercise and loading at different stages of the arthritic process and in different types of arthritis.

Acknowledgment

The contributions of Jerry Tenenbaum, MD, FRCP, to this chapter and of Mike Smit, computer science student at Dalhousie University, to the references are gratefully acknowledged.

References

1. Sledge CB, Reddi AH, Walsh D et al: Biology of the joint. In Ruddy S, Harris ED, Sledge CB (eds): *Kelley's Textbook of Rheumatology*, ed 6. Philadelphia, WB Saunders, 2001, pp 1–21.
2. Mankin HJ, Radin EL: Structure and function of joints. In McCarty DJ, Koopman WJ (eds): *Arthritis and Allied Conditions*, ed 12. Philadelphia, Lea & Febiger, 1993, pp 181–197.
3. Radin EL: Osteoarthrosis. In Wright V, Radin EL (eds): *Mechanics of Human Joints*. New York, Marcel Dekker, 1993, pp 341–354.
4. Radin EL: Mechanically induced periarticular and neuromuscular problems. In Wright V, Radin EL (eds): *Mechanics of Human Joints*. New York, Marcel Dekker, 1993, pp 355–370.
5. Soames RW: Skeletal system. In Williams PL, Bannister LH, Berry MM et al (eds): *Gray's Anatomy*, ed 38. New York, Churchill Livingstone, 1995.
6. Radin EL, Martin RB, Burr DB et al: Effects of mechanical loading on the tissues of the rabbit knee. *J Orthop Res* 2:221–234, 1984.

7. Mankin HJ: The articular cartilages, cartilage healing and osteoarthritis. In Cruess RL, Rennie WRJ (eds): *Adult Orthopaedics,* New York. Churchill Livingstone, 1984, p 207.

8. Moses MA, Sudhalter J, Langer R: Identification of an inhibitor of neovasculization from cartilage. *Science* 248:1408–1410, 1990

9. Urban J: Present perspectives on cartilage and chondrocyte mechanobiology. *Biorheology* 37:185–190, 2000.

10. Poole AR: Cartilage in health and disease. In McCarty DJ, Koopman WJ (eds): *Arthritis and Allied Conditions,* ed 12. Philadelphia, Lea & Febiger, 1993, pp 279–333.

11. Heingard D, Lorenzo P, Saxne T: Matrix glycoproteins, proteoglycans and cartilage. In Ruddy S, Harris ED, Sledge CB (eds): *Kelley's Textbook of Rheumatology,* ed 6. Philadelphia, WB Saunders, 2001, pp 41–53.

12. Rosenberg L: Structure and function of cartilage proteoglycans. In McCarty DJ, Koopman WJ (eds): *Arthritis and Allied Conditions,* ed 12. Philadelphia, Lea & Febiger, 1993, pp 229–243.

13. Oettmeier R, Abendroth K, Oettmeier S: Analysis of the tidemark on human femoral heads. I. Histochemical, ultrastructural and microanalytical characterization of the normal structure of the intercartilaginous junction. *Acta Morphol Hung* 37:155–168, 1989.

14. Lane LB, Bullough PG: Age-related changes in the thickness of the calcified zone and the number of tidemarks in adult human articular cartilage. *J Bone Joint Surg* 62B:372–375, 1980.

15. Kenzora JE, Yosipovitch Z, Glimcher MJ: The calcified cartilage zone of adult articular cartilage: a viable functional entity. *Orthop Trans* 2:120–121, 1978.

16. Poole CA, Flint MH, Beaumont BW: Morphological and functional interrelationships of articular cartilage matrices. *J Anat* 138:113–138, 1984.

17. Jurvelin JS, Arokoski JB, Hunziker EB et al: Topographical variation of the elastic properties of articular cartilage in the canine knee. *J Biomech* 33:669–675, 2000.

18. Myllyharju J, Kivirikko KJ: Collagens and collagen-related diseases. *Ann Med* 33:7–21, 2001.

19. Prockop DJ: What holds us together? Why do some of us fall apart? What can we do about it? *Matrix Biol* 16:519–528, 1998.

20. Ottani V, Raspari M, Ruggeri A: Collagen structure and functional implications. *Micron* 32:251–260, 2001.

21. Prockop DJ, Williams CJ, Vandenburg P: Collagen in normal and diseased connective tissue. In McCarty DJ, Koopman WJ (eds): *Arthritis and Allied Conditions,* ed 12. Philadelphia, Lea & Febiger, 1993, pp 213–227.

22. Ezura Y, Chakravarti S, Oldberg, A et al: Differential expression of lumican and fibromodulin regulate collagen fibrillogenesis in developing mouse tendons. *J Cell Biol* 151:779–788, 2000.

23. Ingram RT, Clarke BL, Fisher LW: Distribution of noncollagenous proteins in the matrix of adult human bone: evidence of anatomic and functional heterogeneity. *J Bone Miner Res* 8:1019–1029, 1993.

24. Blochberger TC, Vergnes JP, Hempel J et al: cDNA to chick lumican (corneal keratan sulfate proteoglycan) reveals homology to the small interstitial proteoglycan gene family and expression in muscle and intestine. *J Biol Chem* 267:347–352, 1992.

25. Hocking AM, Shinomura T, McQuillan DJ: Leucine-rich repeat glycoproteins of the extracellular matrix. *Matrix Biol* 17:1–19, 1998.

26. Bengtsson E, Morgelin M, Sasaki T et al: The leucine rich repeat protein PRELP binds perlecan and collagens and may function as a basement membrane. *J Biol Chem* 277:15061–15068, 2002.

27. Neame P, Tupp H, Azizan N: Noncollagenous, nonproteoglycan macromolecules of cartilage. *Cell Mol Life Sci* 55:1327–1340, 1999.

28. Corpuz LM, Funderburgh JL, Funderburgh ML et al: Molecular cloning and tissue distribution of keratocan. *J Biol Chem* 271:9759–9763, 1996.

29. Woo SLY, Livesay GA, Runco TJ et al: Structure and function of tendons and ligaments. In Mow VC, Hayes WC (eds): *Basic Orthopaedic Biomechanics,* ed 2. Philadelphia, Lippincott-Raven, 1997, pp 209–252.

30. Yahia LH, Drouin G: Microscopical investigation of canine anterior cruciate ligament and patellar tendon: collagen fascicle morphology and architecture. *J Orthop Res* 7:243–251, 1989.

31. Gill MR, Oldberg A, Reinholt FP: Fibromodulin-null murine knee joints display increased incidences of osteoarthritis and alterations in tissue biochemisty. *Osteoarthritis Cartilage* 10:751–757, 2002.

32. Kannus P: Structure of tendon connective tissue. *Scand J Med Sci Sports* 10:312–320, 2000.

33. McCarty DJ: Synovial fluid. In McCarty DJ, Koopman WL (eds): *Arthritis and Allied Conditions,* ed 12. Philadelphia, Lea & Febiger, 1993, pp 63–84.

34. Ghadially FN: Fine structure of joints. In Sokoloff L (ed): *The Joints and Synovial Fluid.* New York, Academic Press, 1978, pp 105–176.

35. Knight AD, Levick JR: The effect of fluid pressure on the hydraulic conductance of the interstitium and fenestrated endothelium in the rabbit knee. *J Physiol* 360:311–332, 1985.

36. Simpkin PE: Biology and function of the synovium. In Finerman GAM, Noyes FR (eds): *Biology and Biomechanics of the Traumatized Synovial Joint: The Knee as a Model.* Rosemont, Ill, American Academy of Orthopedic Surgeons Symposium, 1991, pp 5–16.

37. Ghadially FN: *Fine Structure of Synovial Joints.* London, Butterworth, 1983.

38. Henderson B, Edwards JCW: *The Synovial Lining in Health and Disease.* London, Chapman and Hall, 1987.

39. Chapman WW, Swaim R, Froshsin H Jr et al: Degradation of human articular cartilage by neutrophils and synovial fluid. *Arthritis Rheum* 36:51–58, 1993.

40. Wilkinson L, Pitsillides A, Worrall J et al: Light microscopic characterization of the fibroblast-like

synovial intimal cell synoviocyte. *Arthritis Rheum* 35:1179–1184, 1992.

41. Fox RI, Kang H: Structure and function of synoviocytes. In McCarty DJ, Koopman WL (eds): *Arthritis and Allied Conditions*, ed 12. Philadelphia, Lea & Febiger, 1993, pp 263–278.

42. Barland P, Novikoff AB, Hamerman D: Electron microscopy of the human synovial membrane. *J Cell Biol* 14:207–220, 1962.

43. Ghadially FN, Roy S: *Ultrastructure of Synovial Joints in Health and Disease.* London, Butterworth, 1969.

44. Hills BA, Butler BD: Surfactants identified in synovial fluid and their ability to act as boundary lubricants. *Ann Rheum Dis* 43:641–648, 1984.

45. Levick JR: Synovial fluid determinants of volume turnover and material concentration. In Kuettner K et al (eds): *Articular Cartilage and Osteoarthritis.* New York, Raven Press, 1992, pp 529-541.

46. Simoneau G, Dyhre-Paulsen P, Voigt M et al: Bone-on-bone forces during loaded and unloaded walking. *Acta Anat* 152:133–142, 1995.

47. Scott SH, Winter DA: Internal forces of chronic running injury sites. *Med Sci Sports Exerc* 22:357–367, 1990.

48. Unsworth A: Lubrication of human joints. In Wright V, Radin E (eds): *Mechanics of Human Joints.* New York, Marcel Dekker, 1993, pp 137–162.

49. Bruggemann GP: Biomechanics in gymnastics. *Med Sport Sci* 45:142–176, 1987.

50. Radin EL, Orr RB, Kelman JL et al: Effect of prolonged walking on concrete on the knees of sheep. *J Biomech* 15:487–492, 1982.

51. Light LH, McLellan GE, Klenerman L: Skeletal transients on heel strike in normal walking with different footwear. *J Biomech* 13:477–480, 1980.

52. Dickinson JA, Cook SD, Leinhart TM: The measurement of shockwaves following heel strike while running. *J Biomech* 18:415-422, 1985.

53. Cooper C, Inskip H, Croft P et al: Individual risk factor for hip osteoarthritis: obesity, hip injury and physical activity. *Am J Epidemiol* 147:523–528, 1998.

54. Radin EL, Schaffler M, Gibson G et al: Osteoarthritis as a result of repetitive trauma. In Kuettner KE, Goldberg VM (eds): *Osteoarthritis Disorders.* Rosemont, Ill, American Academy of Orthopaedics Surgeons Symposium, 1995, pp 197–203.

55. Clarke IC, Contini R, Kenedi RN: Friction and wear studies of articular cartilage: a scanning electron microscopy study. *J Lubr Tech* 97:358–368, 1975.

56. Radin EL, Paul IL: A consolidated concept of joint lubrication. *J Bone Joint Surg* 54A:607–616, 1972.

57. Charnley J: How our joints are lubricated. *Basel, Sandoz Pharma AG, Triangle*, 4:175–179, 1960.

58. Swann D, Silver F, Slayter H et al: The molecular structure and lubricating activity of lubricin isolated from bovine and human synovial fluids. *Biochem J* 225:195–201, 1985.

59. Hills BA: Remarkable anti-wear properties of joint surfactant. *Ann Biomed Eng* 23:112–115, 1995.

60. Martin RB, Burr DB, Sharkey NA: *Skeletal Tissue Mechanics.* New York, Springer, 1998, pp 289–305.

61. Unsworth A: Tribology of human and artificial joints. *Proc Inst Mech Eng* 205:163–172, 1991.

62. McCutchen CW: Lubrication of joints. In Sokoloff L (ed): *The Joints and Synovial Fluid.* New York, Academic Press, 1978, pp 437–483.

63. Mow VC, Hayes WC (eds): *Basic Orthopaedic Biomechanics*, ed 2. Philadelphia, Lippincott-Raven, 1997.

64. Bobic V, Noble J: Articular cartilage: to repair or not to repair? *J Bone Joint Surg Br* 82:165–166, 2000.

65. Stockwell RA, Meachim G: The chondrocytes. In Freeman MAR (ed): *Adult Articular Cartilage.* London, Pitman Medical, 1979, pp 69–145.

66. Hulth A, Lindberg L, Telhag H: Mitosis in human osteoarthritic cartilage. *Clin Orthop* 84:197–199, 1972.

67. Havdrup T, Telhag H: Mitosis of chondrocytes in normal adult joint cartilage. *Clin Orthop* 153:248–252, 1980.

68. Havdrup T, Telhag H: Scattered mitosis in adult joint cartilage after partial chondrectomy. *Acta Orthop Scand* 48:424–429, 1978.

69. Woo SLY, Ohland KJ, McMahon PJ: Biology, healing and repair of ligaments. In Fineman GAM, Noyes FR (eds): *Biology and Biomechanics of the Traumatized Synovial Joint: The Knee as a Model.* Rosemont, Ill, American Academy of Orthopaedic Surgeons Symposium, 1991, pp 241–274.

70. Fantone JC: Basic concepts in inflammation. In Leadbeater WB, Buckwalter JA, Gordon SL (eds): *Sports-Induced Inflammation: Clinical and Basic Science Concepts.* Park Ridge, Ill, American Academy of Orthopedic Surgeons, 1990, pp 23–54.

71. Goetzl EJ, Goldstein IM: Arachidonic acid metabolites. In McCarty DJ, Koopman WJ (eds): *Arthritis and Allied Conditions*, ed 12. Philadelphia, Lea & Febiger, 1993, pp 479–494.

72. Szekanecz Z, Koch AE: Cytokines. In Ruddy S, Harris ED, Sledge CB (eds): *Kelley's Textbook of Rheumatology*, ed 6. Philadelphia, WB Saunders, 2001, pp 275–288.

73. Howell DS, Pelletier JP: Etiopathogenesis of osteoarthritis. In McCarty DJ, Koopman WL (eds): *Arthritis and Allied Conditions*, ed 12. Philadelphia, Lea & Febiger, 1993, pp 1723–1734.

74. Evans CH, Brown TD: Role of physical and mechanical agents in degrading the matrix. In Woessner JF, Howell DS (eds): *Joint Cartilage Degradation.* New York, Marcel Dekker, 1993, p 199.

75. Folkman J, Brean H: Angiogenesis and inflammation. In Gallin JI, Goldstein IM, Snyderman R (eds): *Inflammation: Basic Principles and Clinical Correlates*, ed 2. New York, Raven Press, 1992, pp 821–840.

76. McCarty DJ, Koopman WJ (eds): *Arthritis and Allied Conditions*, ed 12. Philadelphia, Lea & Febiger, 1993.

77. Ruddy S, Harris ED, Sledge CB (eds): *Kelley's Textbook of Rheumatology*, ed 6. Philadelphia, WB Saunders, 2001.

78. Salter RB: *Textbook of Disorders and Injuries of the Musculoskeletal System,* ed 3. Baltimore, Williams & Wilkins, 1999.

79. Stulberg SD, Cordell LD, Harris WH et al: Unrecognized childhood hip disease: a major cause of idiopathic osteoarthritis of the hip. In The Hip Society: *The Hip, Proceedings of the Third Open Meeting of the Hip Society.* St Louis, CV Mosby, 1975, pp 212–228.

80. Smith BW: Recognizable patterns of human deformation: identification and management of mechanical effects on morphogenesis. *Major Probl Clin Pediatr* 21:1–21, 1981.

81. O'Connor B, Brandt KD: Neurogenic factors in the etiopathogenesis of osteoarthritis. *Rheum Dis Clin North Am* 19:581–605, 1993.

82. Poole AR: Inflammatory mechanisms in soft tissues. In Leadbeater WB, Buckwalter JA, Gordon SL (eds): *Sports-Induced Inflammation.* Park Ridge, Ill, American Academy of Orthopedic Surgeons, 1990, pp 285-299.

83. Tortorella MD, Burn TC, Pratta MA et al: Purification and cloning of aggrecanase-1: a member of the ADAMTS family of proteins. *Science* 284:1664–1666, 1999.

84. Sandy JD, Flannery CR, Naeme PJ et al: The structure of aggrecan fragments in human synovial fluid: evidence for the involvement in osteoarthritis of a novel proteinase which cleaves the GLU 373-Ala 374 bone of the interglobular domain. *J Clin Invest* 89:1512–1516, 1992.

85. Fosang AJ, Last K, Knauper V et al: Fibroblast and neutrophil collagenases cleave at two sites in the cartilage aggrecan interglobular domain. *Biochem J* 295:273–276, 1993.

86. Arner EC, Pratta MA, Trzaskos JM et al: Generation and characterization of aggrecanase. *J Biol Chem* 274:6594–6601, 1999.

87. Mankin HJ, Brandt KD: Pathogenesis of osteoarthritis. In Ruddy S, Harris ED, Sledge CB (eds): *Kelley's Textbook of Rheumatology,* ed 6. Philadelphia, WB Saunders, 2001, pp 1391–1408.

88. Krane SM: Mechanisms of tissue destruction in rheumatoid arthritis. In McCarty DJ, Koopman WJ (eds): *Arthritis and Allied Conditions,* ed 12. Philadelphia, Lea & Febiger, 1993, pp 763–780.

89. Buckwalter JA, Mankin HJ: Articular cartilage: Part II. Degeneration and osteoarthrosis, repair, regeneration and transplantation. *J Bone Joint Surg* 79-A4:612–632, 1997.

90. Rodosky MW, Fu FH: Induction of synovial inflammation by matrix molecules, implant particles and chemical agents. In Leadbeater WB, Buckwalter JA, Gordon SL (eds): *Sports-Induced Inflammation.* Park Ridge, Ill, American Academy of Orthopedic Surgeons, 1990, pp 357–381.

91. MacConaill MA, Basmajian JV: *Muscles and Movement.* Baltimore, Williams & Wilkins 1969.

92. Lipson SJ: The cervical spine. In Kelley WN et al (eds): *Textbook of Rheumatology,* ed 4. Philadelphia, WB Saunders, 1993, pp 1798–1807.

93. Cush JJ, Lipsky PE: Cellular basis for rheumatoid inflammation. *Clin Orthop* 265:9–22, 1991.

94. Bennett RM: Psoriatic arthritis. In McCarty DJ, Koopman WJ (eds): *Arthritis and Allied Conditions,* ed 12. Philadelphia, Lea & Febiger, 1993, pp 1079–1094.

95. Scarpa R, Oriente P, Pucino A et al: Psoriatic arthritis in psoriatic patients. *Br J Rheumatol* 23:246–250, 1984.

96. Gladman DD, Rahman P: Psoriatic arthritis. In Ruddy S, Harris ED, Sledge CB (eds): *Kelley's Textbook of Rheumatology,* ed 6. Philadelphia, WB Saunders, 2001, pp 1071–1077.

97. Gladman DD, Anhorn KB, Schachter RK et al: HLA antigens in psoriatic arthritis: a follow up study. *J Rheumatol* 13:586–592, 1986.

98. Hunter T: The spinal complications of ankylosing spondylitis. *Semin Arthritis Rheum* 19:172–182, 1989.

99. Van der Linden S, Van der Heihle D: Ankylosing spondylitis. In Ruddy S, Harris ED, Sledge CB (eds): *Kelley's Textbook of Rheumatology,* ed 6. Philadelphia, WB Saunders, 2001, pp 1039–1053.

100. Schmid FR: Principles of diagnosis and treatment of bone and joint infections. In McCarty DJ, Koopman WJ (eds): *Arthritis and Allied Conditions,* ed 12. Philadelphia, Lea & Febiger, 1993, pp 1975–2001.

101. Ho G Jr: Bacterial arthritis. In McCarty DJ, Koopman WJ (eds): *Arthritis and Allied Conditions,* ed 12. Philadelphia, Lea & Febiger, 1993, pp 2003–2023.

102. Hough AJ: Pathology of osteoarthritis. In McCarty DJ, Koopman WJ (eds): *Arthritis and Allied Conditions,* ed 12. Philadelphia, Lea & Febiger, 1993, pp 1699–1722.

103. Weisman MH: Arthritis associated with hematologic disorders, storage diseases, disorders of lipid metabolism and dysproteinemias. In McCarty DJ, Koopman WJ (eds): *Arthritis and Allied Conditions,* ed 12. Philadelphia, Lea & Febiger, 1993, pp 1457–1482.

104. Terkeltaub RA: Pathogenesis and treatment of crystal-induced inflammation. In McCarty DJ, Koopman WJ (eds): *Arthritis and Allied Conditions,* ed 12. Philadelphia, Lea & Febiger, 1993, pp 1819–1834.

105. Levinson DJ, Becker MA: Clinical gout and the pathogenesis of hyperuricemia. In McCarty DJ, Koopman WJ (eds): *Arthritis and Allied Conditions,* ed 12. Philadelphia, Lea & Febiger, 1993, pp 1773–1806.

106. Good AE, Rapp R: Bony ankylosis: a rare manifestation of gout. *J Rheumatol* 5:335–337, 1978.

107. Ellman MH: Neuropathic joint disease (Charcot joints). In McCarty DJ, Koopman WJ (eds): *Arthritis and Allied Conditions,* ed 12. Philadelphia, Lea & Febiger, 1993, pp 1407–1426.

108. Resnik D, Niwayama G: *Diagnosis of Bone and Joint Disorders with Emphasis on Articular Abnormalities.* Philadelphia, WB Saunders 1981.

109. Woo SLY, Matthews V, Akeson WH et al: Connective tissue response to immobility: correlative study of biomechanical and biochemical measurements of normal and immobilized knees. *Arthritis Rheum* 18:257–262, 1974.

110. Noyes FR: Functional properties of knee ligaments and alterations induced by immobilization: the

correlative biomechanical and histological study in primates. *Clin Orthop*; 123:210–242, 1977.

111. Hildebrand KA, Frank CB: Biology of ligament injury and repair. In Johnson R, Lombardo J (eds), *Current Review of Sports Medicine*, ed 2. Philadelphia, Current Medicine, 1998, pp 121–131.

112. Wren TAL, Carter DR: A microstructural model for the tensile constitutive and failure behaviour of soft skeletal connective tissues. *J Biomech Eng* 120:55–61, 1998.

113. Yasuda T, Kinoshita M, Abe M et al: Unfavourable effect of knee immobilization on Achilles tendon healing in rabbits. *Acta Orthop Scand* 71:69–73, 2000.

114. Bray RC, Shrive NG, Frank CB et al: The early effects of joint immobilization on medial collateral ligament healing in an ACL-deficient knee: a gross anatomic and biomechanical investigation in the adult rabbit model. *J Orthop Res* 10:157–166, 1992.

115. Frank CB: Ligament. In Zachazewski J, Magee D, Quillan W (eds): *Athletic Injuries and Rehabilitation*. Philadelphia, WB Saunders, 1996, pp 9–25.

116. Enwemeka CS: Membrane-bound intracytoplasmic collagen fibrils in fibroblasts and myofibroblasts of regenerating rabbit calcaneal tendons. *Tissue Cell* 23:173–190, 1991.

117. Murrell G, Lilly EG 3rd, Goldner RD: Effects of immobilization on Achilles tendon healing in a rat model. *J Orthop Res* 12:582–591, 1994.

118. Stehno-Bittel L, Reddy GK, Gum S et al: Biochemistry and biomechanics of healing tendons: Part I. Effects of rigid plaster casts and functional casts. *Med Sci Sports Exerc* 12:582–591, 1998.

119. Akeson WH, Eichelberger L, Roma N: Biochemical studies of articular cartilage. II. Values following the innervation of an extremity. *J Bone Joint Surg* 40A:153–162, 1958.

120. Akeson WH, Woo SLY, Amiel D et al: The connective tissue response to immobility: biochemical changes in the periarticular connective tissue of immobilized rabbit knee. *Clin Orthop* 93:356–362, 1973.

121. Caterson B, Lowther DA: Changes in the metabolism of the proteoglycans from sheep articular cartilage in response to mechanical forces. *Biochem Biophys Acta* 540:412–422, 1978.

122. Enneking WF, Horowitz M: The intra-articular effects of immobilization of the human knee. *J Bone Joint Surg* 54A:973–985, 1972.

123. Helminen HJ, Jurvelin J, Kuusela T et al: Effects of immobilization for 6 weeks on rabbit knee articular surfaces as assessed by the semi-quantitative stereo-microscopic method. *Acta Anat* 115:327–335, 1983.

124. Stockwell RA: Structure and function of the chondrocyte under mechanical stress. In Helminen HJ et al (eds): *Joint Loading*. Bristol, Wright, 1987, pp 126–148.

125. Palmoski MJ, Perricone E, Brandt KD: Development and reversal of proteoglycan, aggregation defect in normal canine knee cartilage after immobilization. *Arthritis Rheum* 22:508–517, 1979.

126. Quinn TM, Grodzinsky AJ, Buschmann MD et al: Mechanical compression alters PG deposition and matrix deformation around individual cells in cartilage explants. *J Cell Science* 111:573–583, 1998.

127. Tammi M, Paukkonen K, Kiviranta I et al: Joint loading induced alterations in articular cartilage. In Helminen HJ et al (eds): *Joint Loading*. Bristol, Wright, 1987, pp 64–88.

128. Frost HM: Bone "mass" and the "mechanostat": a proposal. *Anat Rec* 219:1–9, 1987.

129. Tuukkanen J, Wallmark B, Jalovaara P et al: Changes induced in growing rat bone by immobilization and reimmobilization. *Bone* 12:113–118, 1991.

130. Imhof H, Breitenseher M, Kainberger F et al: Degenerative joint disease: cartilage or vascular disease? *Skeletal Radiol* 26:398–403, 1999.

131. Martin RB, Burr DB: *Structure, Function and Adaptation of Compact Bone*. New York, Raven Press, 1989.

132. Nilas L, Christiansen C: Bone mass and its relationship to age and in menopause. *J Clin Endocrinol Metab* 65:697–702, 1987.

133. Arthritis prevalence and activity limitations. *MMWR Morb Mortal Wkly Rep* 43:433–438, 1994.

134. Hough FS: Alterations of bone and mineral metabolism in diabetes mellitus. Part II. Clinical studies on 206 patients with type I diabetes mellitus. *S Afr Med J* 72:120–126, 1987.

135. McNair P: Bone and mineral metabolism in human type I (insulin-dependent) diabetes mellitus. *Dan Med Bull* 35:109–121, 1988.

136. Einhorn TA, Boskey AL, Gundberg CM et al: The mineral and mechanical properties of bone in chronic experimental diabetes. *J Orthop Res* 6:317–323, 1988.

137. Dixit PK, Stern AMK: Effect of insulin on the incorporation of citric and calcium into bones of alloxan-diabetic rats. *Calcif Tissue Int* 27:227–232, 1979.

138. McCulloch CAG: Deregulation of collagen phagocytosis in aging human fibroblasts: effects of integrin expression and cell-cycle. *Exp Cell Res* 237:383–393, 1997.

139. Kuettner KE, Aydelotte MB, Thonar E: Articular cartilage matrix and structure: a minireview. *J Rheumatol* 18:46–48, 1991.

140. Dee R: The innervation of joints. In Sokoloff L (ed): *The Joints and Synovial Fluid*, vol 1. New York, Academic Press, 1978, pp 177–204.

141. Johansson H, Sjolander P: Neurophysiology. In Wright V, Radin E (eds): *Mechanics of Human Joints*. Philadelphia, Marcel Dekker, 1993, pp 243–292.

142. Zimny ML: Mechanoreceptors in articular tissues. *Am J Anat* 182:16–32, 1988.

143. Wyke BD: The neurology of joints. *Ann R Coll Surg Engl*, 41:25–50, 1967.

144. Wyke BD: The neurology of low back pain. In Jayson MIV (ed): *The Lumbar Spine and Back Pain*. London, Pitman Medical, 1980, pp 265-321.

145. Gaffney K, Williams R, Jolliffe V et al. Intra-articular pressure changes in rheumatoid and normal peripheral joints. *Ann Rheum Dis* 54:670–673, 1995.

146. Jayson MIV, Dixon A St J: Intra-articular pressure in rheumatoid arthritis of the knee. *Ann Rheum Dis* 29:401–408, 1970.

147. Knight AD, Levick JR: Time-dependence of the pressure-volume relationship in the synovial cavity of the rabbit knee. *J Physiol* 335:139–152, 1983.

148. Levick JR: Synovial fluid and trans-synovial flow in stationary and moving normal joints. In Helminen HJ et al (eds): *Joint Loading*. Bristol, Wright, 1987, pp 149–186.

149. Baxendale RH, Ferrel WR, Wood L: Intra-articular pressures during active and passive motion of normal and distended knee joints. *J Physiol* 369:179P, 1985.

150. Helliwell PS: Joint stiffness. In Wright V, Radin E (eds): *Mechanics of Human Joints*. New York, Marcel Dekker, 1993, pp 203–218.

151. Marks R, Wessel A, Quinney HA: Proprioceptive sensibility in women with normal and osteoarthritic knee joints. *Clin Rheumatol* 12:170–175, 1993.

152. Skinner HB, Barrack RL, Cook SD et al: Joint position sense in total knee arthroplasty. *J Orthop Res* 1:276–283, 1984.

153. Andriacchi TP, Natarajan RN, Hurwitz DE: Musculoskeletal dynamics, locomotion, and clinical applications. In Mow VC, Hayes WC (eds). *Basic Orthopaedic Biomechanics,* ed 2. Philadelphia, Lippincott-Raven, 1997, pp 37–68.

154. Merry P, Williams R, Cox N et al: Comparative study of intra-articular pressure dynamics in joints with acute traumatic and chronic inflammatory effusions: potential implications for hypoxic-reperfusion injury. *Ann Rheum Dis* 50:917–920, 1991.

155. O'Reilly SC, Jones A, Muir KR et al: Quadriceps weakness in knee osteoarthritis: the effect on pain and disability. *Ann Rheum Dis* 57:588–594, 1998.

156. Slemeda C, Brandt KD, Heilman DK et al: Quadriceps weakness and osteoarthritis of the knee. *Ann Intern Med* 127:97–104, 1997.

157. Kidd BL, Gibson SJ, O'Higgins F et al: A neurogenic mechanism for symmetrical arthritis. *Lancet* 11:1128–1129, 1989.

158. Oosterveld FG, Rasker JJ: Effects of local heat and cold treatment on surface and articular temperature of arthritic knees. *Arthritis Rheum* 37:1578–1582, 1994.

159. Melzack R, Wall PD: Pain mechanisms: a new theory. *Science* 150:971–978, 1965.

160. Woo SLY, Buckwalter JD: *Injury and Repair of the Musculoskeletal Tissues: Preface*. Park Ridge, Ill, American Academy of Orthopaedic Surgeons, 1988.

161. Akeson WH, Amiel D, Woo SLY: Physiology and therapeutic value of passive motion. In Helminen HJ et al: *Joint Loading*. Bristol, Wright,1987 pp 375-394.

162. Hasler EM, Herzog W, Wu JZ: Articular cartilage biomechanics: theoretical models, material properties, and biosynthetic response. *Crit Rev Biomed Eng* 27:415–488, 1999.

163. Gimenaz-Gallego G, Cuevas P: Fibroblast growth factors, proteins with a broad spectrum of biological activities. *Neurol Res* 16:313–316, 1994.

164. Sokoloff L: Loading and motion in relation to aging and degeneration of joints: implications for prevention and treatment of osteoarthritis. In Helminen HJ et al: *Joint Loading*. Bristol, Wright, 1987, pp 412–424.

165. Buckwalter JA, Mankin HJ: Articular cartilage. Part II. Degeneration and osteoarthrosis, repair, regeneration and transplantation. *J Bone Joint Surg* 79-A4:612–632, 1997.

166. Simkin PA: Synovial physiology. In McCarty DJ, Koopman WJ (eds): *Arthritis and Allied Conditions*, ed 12, vol 1. Philadelphia, Lea & Febiger, 1993, pp 199–212.

167. Kiviranta I, Tammi M, Jurvelin J et al: Moderate running exercise augments glycosaminoglycans and thickness of articular cartilage in the knee joint of young beagle dogs. *J Orthop Res* 6:188–195, 1988.

168. Tammi M, Saamanen AM, Jauhiainen A et al: Proteoglycan alterations in rabbit knee articular cartilage following physical exercise and immobilization. *Connect Tissue Res* 16:163–175, 1983.

169. Paukkonen K, Selkanaho K, Jurvelin J et al: Cells and nuclei of articular cartilage chondrocytes in young rabbits enlarged after non-strenuous physical exercise. *J Anat* 142:13–20. 1985.

170. Woo SLY, Akeson WH: Response of tendons and ligaments to joint loading and movements. In Helminen HJ et al (eds): *Joint Loading*. Bristol, Wright, 1987, pp 287–315.

171. Telhag H: Mitosis of chondrocytes in experimental osteoarthritis in rabbits. *Clin Orthop* 86:224–229, 1972.

172. Frenkel SR, Di Cesare PE: Degradation and repair of articular cartilage. *Front Biosci* 4:D671–685, 1999.

173. Salter RB: *Continuous Passive Motion (CPM): A Biological Concept for the Healing and the Generation of Articular Cartilage, Ligaments, and Tendons—From its Origination to Research to Clinical Applications*. Baltimore, Williams & Wilkins, 1993.

174. Helminen HJ, Hyttinen MM, Lammi MJ et al: Regular joint loading in youth assists in the establishment and strengthening of the collagen network of articular cartilage and contributes to the prevention of osteoarthrosis later in life: a hypothesis. *J Bone Miner Metab* 18:245–257, 2000.

175. Rubin CT, Rubin JE: Biology, physiology and morphology of bone. In Ruddy S, Harris ED, Sledge CB (eds): *Kelley's Textbook of Rheumatology,* ed 6. Philadelphia, WB Saunders, 2001, pp 1611–1634.

176. Pugh J: Biomechanics of arthritis. In Winter D, Norman R, Wells R et al (eds): *Biomechanics IX-A*. Champaign Ill, Human Kinetics, 1985, pp 135–139.

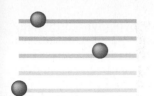

CHAPTER 4

Diagnosis and Medical Management of Conditions with Arthritis

Peter Lee, MB, ChB, MD (Otago), FRACP, FRCPC

What is Arthritis?

The term *arthritis* refers to inflammation within a joint, regardless of the causative process, which results in pain, stiffness, and swelling and which may lead to joint damage. In arthritis joint damage occurs as a result of two main pathologic changes: *inflammation* and *degeneration*. Inflammation may be either acute (typified by acute gouty arthritis or infection) or chronic (as in rheumatoid arthritis). The process of degeneration as the primary cause of joint damage is seen in osteoarthritis. In this chapter the typical clinical presentations of some of the inflammatory and degenerative joint disorders will be described and their pathologic features and some aspects of their medical management will be outlined. Other related conditions, such as systemic lupus erythematosus (SLE) and scleroderma, in which arthritis is not always the dominant feature, but which are often associated with joint problems, also will be considered in this chapter. Definition of unfamiliar terms may be found in Appendix IV (Glossary).

Patient Assessment

Effective treatment of rheumatic disorders depends on an accurate diagnosis based upon the history,

PHYSICAL REHABILITATION IN ARTHRITIS, Joan M. Walker, PhD, PT, and Antoine Helewa, MSc(Clin Epid), PT, Elsevier Inc. © 2004.

physical examination, and relevant laboratory investigations. The following is an overview of assessments normally undertaken in the management of clients with arthritis. Detailed assessment techniques are covered in Chapter 5.

History

A detailed history is an invaluable diagnostic tool. This is particularly important in mild or early disease (as in ankylosing spondylitis [AS]), in diseases in remission, and with disorders (for example, gout and palindromic arthritis) that are only intermittently active. Physical examination in these situations may be entirely normal. A history of definite joint swelling, usually associated with morning and inactivity stiffness, is strongly suggestive of arthritis rather than noninflammatory causes of joint pain, such as fibromyalgia, osteoarthritis, or referred pain from the neck and back. Furthermore, the pattern of joint involvement may point toward a particular diagnosis. In polyarticular diseases, such as rheumatoid arthritis (RA), the number of joints that are painful or swollen and duration of morning stiffness correlate with disease activity. A history of extra-articular manifestations (such as eye inflammation, skin and nail lesions, hair loss, oral ulceration, bloody diarrhea, and urethral discharge) may provide important clues for definitive diagnosis.

Many rheumatic diseases, when active, are associated with constitutional manifestations. Common symptoms include fever, anorexia, weight loss, and fatigue, which may be severe and activity limiting. The occurrence of fevers also may alert the clinician to the possibility of an infectious etiology (as in septic arthritis) or septic complications. Few rheumatic disorders are considered to be hereditary, but a positive family history may be obtained, particularly from patients with AS and gout. A detailed drug history is necessary to ascertain response (or lack of) to previous treatment and to document specific adverse reactions. Information about functional status, especially for activities of daily living and the ability to perform housework or employment-related tasks, is important in assessing the overall impact of the disease on the patient.

Physical Examination

A general physical examination is carried out with the objective of making a specific diagnosis and determining disease severity and activity. Features of extra-articular disease are looked for and documented. Patients are screened for the presence of medical disorders, such as hyper- or hypothyroidism and malignancies, which may present with musculoskeletal manifestations. In the joint examination, the presence of swelling confirms that the patient has active arthritis. The numbers of tender and swollen joints are noted as markers of disease activity. A count of the number of joints with deformities or restricted movement provides an index of joint damage and is a reflection of the aggressiveness of the disease or ineffective treatment. The absence of joint swelling and a predominance of soft tissue tenderness would suggest nonarticular causes of pain, such as fibromyalgia and referred pain from the neck or back. Restricted spinal mobility (and chest expansion), particularly in young persons, suggests a diagnosis of AS. Weakness of the proximal muscles occurs in polymyositis and dermatomyositis, as well as with other connective tissue diseases (SLE and systemic sclerosis).

Laboratory Investigations

In rheumatology, diagnoses are largely clinically based and seldom depend on a laboratory test. The exceptions are osteoarthritis, septic arthritis, and gout. With osteoarthritis a radiograph (or arthroscopic examination) is necessary to confirm the presence of articular cartilage destruction and joint space narrowing. A diagnosis of septic arthritis depends on a positive culture of synovial fluid aspirated from the involved joint. Demonstration of birefringent (splitting a ray of light in two) crystals on polarized microscopy in synovial fluid analysis is diagnostic of gout or pseudogout. In polymyositis and dermatomyositis the diagnostic gold standard is a muscle biopsy showing the presence of an inflammatory cell infiltrate as well as muscle cell necrosis and regeneration.

Most rheumatic diseases are multisystem disorders, and laboratory investigations are necessary to screen for possible involvement of internal organs (especially of the gastrointestinal tract, kidneys, liver, heart, and lungs) and immunological abnormalities. A raised erythrocyte sedimentation rate (ESR) or C-reactive protein (CRP) level usually correlates with the presence of active inflammation, but in the inflammatory arthropathies, such as RA, there is often a poor relationship between laboratory and clinical measures of disease activity.

Rheumatoid Arthritis

RA is a chronic systemic inflammatory disorder of uncertain etiology and is characterized by a symmetrical polyarthritis that invariably affects the small joints of the hands and feet. Although its course is quite variable, if untreated progressive joint damage and functional disability will develop.

Epidemiology

RA affects approximately 1% of the adult population with a female-to-male ratio of 3:1. The disease occurs worldwide but appears less commonly in Asia and Africa compared with Europe and North America. Although RA can affect persons of all ages, the incidence rises with increasing age with a peak between 40 and 50 years.[1] (See also Chapter 2.)

Etiology

The cause of RA remains unknown, but the disease is considered to be genetic on the basis of a genetically related susceptibility and exposure to environmental factors, which activates the immune system. The possibility of a viral or bacterial infection being the triggering factor has been extensively investigated without any definitive findings. Support for a genetic predisposition comes from studies showing a clustering of RA among families and a high concordance rate (30% to 50%) among monozygotic twins.[2] The genetics of RA is complex, and multiple genes appear to be involved. However genes with the greatest impact lie within the HLA-D region of the genome. There is an increased frequency of HLA DR4 and overrepresentation (more often than expected) of a set of HLA-DRB1 alleles among patients with RA. All share a common sequence of amino acids through positions 70 to 74 in the third hypervariable region. This sequence not only appears to confer susceptibility but also may influence the severity of RA.[3]

Pathophysiology

The pathogenesis of RA involves a series of immunological events leading to joint inflammation and destruction. The main pathological feature of RA is the presence of synovitis, characterized by hyperplasia and inflammation of the synovium and an inflammation exudate in the joint cavity. Compared with the lining of a normal joint, rheumatoid synovium is considerably thickened, hypercellular, and hypervascular with markedly increased numbers of small blood vessels (Figure 4-1). An important component of the disease is the recruitment and infiltration of inflammatory cells, mainly macrophages and T cells, into the synovium.[3] These cells are derived from the circulation and have been activated by antigenic exposure before their migration into the perivascular tissues. This complex process is regulated by the up-regulation of adhesion molecules on endothelial cell surfaces. Selected inflammatory cells stick to these molecules and transmigrate through the blood vessel wall into the synovium.

Inflammatory cells mediate the inflammatory process through both cell-to-cell contact and the production of proteins called cytokines, some of which have pro-inflammatory and others anti-inflammatory properties.[3] The important inflammatory cytokines are interleukin (IL)-1, IL-6, IL-8, and tumor necrosis factor-α (TNF-α) produced by activated macrophages. Although IL-1 has been shown to cause both cartilage and bone destruction in RA, it is apparent that TNF-α plays a central and dominant role in regulating IL-1 and other cytokines. Pro-inflammatory cytokines also promote the proliferation of fibroblasts and synoviocytes as well as stimulating the production of matrix metalloproteinase, degradative enzymes, which play an important role in tissue damage. The understanding of these inflammatory pathways has been key to the development of novel therapies for RA in recent years. Such new treatments are being directed against specific cytokines such as TNF-α and IL-1, rather than suppressing the immune system in a nonspecific and blind manner.

Chronic inflammation results in joint damage, leading to deformities, restricted movement, and loss of function. In RA the proliferating synovial tissues (commonly referred to as *pannus*) causes damage to articular cartilage both by direct invasion (Figure 4-2) and through the release of tissue-degrading enzymes (metalloproteinases, stromelysin, collagenases). Adjacent tissues become involved in the destructive

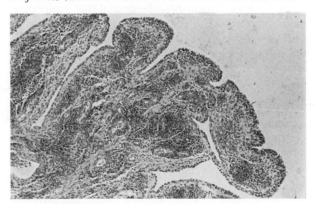

Figure 4-1. An example of chronic rheumatoid synovitis. The surface shows excessive folding and long finger-like processes referred to as villous hyperplasia. Villous hyperplasia is characteristic of chronic rheumatoid synovitis but not diagnostic. (© 1972-1999 American College of Rheumatology Clinical Slide Collection. Used with permission.) See color plate 1.

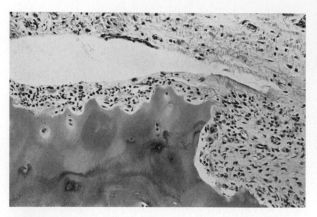

Figure 4-2. A high-power histological view in rheumatoid arthritis that demonstrates an inflammatory membrane (pannus) actively destroying subjacent articular cartilage. (Reprinted from the Clinical Slide Collection on the Rheumatic Diseases, © 1991, by permission from the American College of Rheumatology.) See color plate 1.

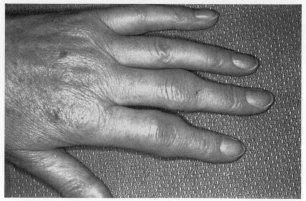

Figure 4-3. Soft tissue swelling occurs as an early finding in rheumatoid arthritis and usually appears as typical fusiform or spindle-shaped enlargement of proximal interphalangeal joints. The second and third fingers of this patient are most involved. (Reprinted from the Clinical Slide Collection on the Rheumatic Diseases, © 1991, used by permission from the American College of Rheumatology.) See color plate 1.

process with bony erosions and rupture of tendons and ligaments. For further details on the pathophysiology of inflammation, see Chapter 3.

Clinical Features

The hallmark of RA is the presence of a symmetrical polyarthritis affecting the small joints of the hands and feet. In the hands the metacarpophalangeal (MCP) and proximal interphalangeal (PIP) joints are predominantly involved with sparing of the distal interphalangeal (DIP) joints (Figure 4-3). Onset of the disease may be insidious or abrupt. A mono-articular presentation is uncommon. Joint stiffness associated with physical inactivity is a consistent feature of active arthritis. This symptom is most prominent on getting out of bed in the morning and referred to as *morning stiffness*. The duration of morning stiffness (time from arising to the time when the stiffness wears off) correlates with active disease and has long been utilized as a measure of disease activity in RA and other inflammatory arthropathies.

Although RA is a disease predominantly of peripheral joints, the apophyseal joints of the spine are also synovial lined and may be affected. Neck pain is common with active disease. In severe cases, atlantoaxial subluxation may occur and rarely results in spinal cord compression. Similarly, bursae and tendon sheaths are synovium-lined structures and can potentially be involved in any polyarthritis. Inflam-

mation of the olecranon bursa will result in a localized swelling at the back of the elbow and heel pain can occur on the basis of a retrocalcaneal bursitis. A tenosynovitis often affects the extensor tendons over the dorsal aspect of the wrist and flexor tendons in the hands. Persistent inflammation may lead to tendon damage and eventual rupture with loss of movement in the involved digits.

> **Duration of morning stiffness gives an indication of the severity of the inflammatory process.**

Uncontrolled RA will eventually lead to joint damage. The deformities occurring in the hands and feet in RA are classic with MCP joint subluxation and ulnar deviation, swan-neck, and boutonnière deformities of the fingers (Figure 4-4), metatarsophalangeal (MTP) joint subluxation with cocked-up or hammer toes (Figure 4-5). Flexion deformities, particularly of the elbows and knees, may occur early and once established are difficult to correct. Chapter 3 gives further detail on the pathomechanics of inflammation and immobility.

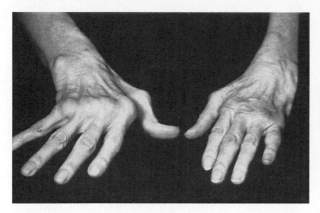

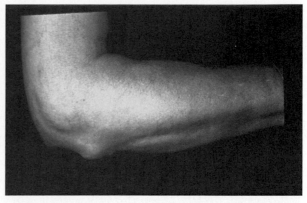

Figure 4-4. Rheumatoid arthritis. Ulnar deviation and subluxation of metacarpophalangeal joints have occurred in the patient's right hand. These joints also appear swollen. Muscle atrophy has developed in the dorsal musculature of both hands. (Reprinted from the Clinical Slide Collection on the Rheumatic Diseases, © 1991, used by permission from the American College of Rheumatology.) See color plate 1.

Figure 4-6. Rheumatoid nodule located on the upper extensor surface of the forearm. (Reprinted from the Clinical Slide Collection on the Rheumatic Diseases, © 1991, by permission of the American College of Rheumatology.) See color plate 2.

Extra-Articular Manifestations

RA is a systemic disorder and with active disease constitutional manifestations including fatigue, anorexia, weight loss, and low-grade fever can occur. Other organs may be involved, resulting in a variety of extra-articular manifestations. Their presence may be helpful in making a diagnosis of RA and are indicative of a more severe form of the disease.

Skin Lesions

Rheumatoid nodules occur in up to 50% of patients with RA during the course of the disease. Their presence is invariably associated with a positive test for rheumatoid factor. The lesions occur most often in the subcutaneous tissues over pressure areas, such as the upper extensor surface of the forearm (Figure 4-6). However rheumatoid nodules can occur at any location including the fingers, over tendons, and within internal organs such as the lungs. Regression of these lesions may occur as the disease goes into remission.

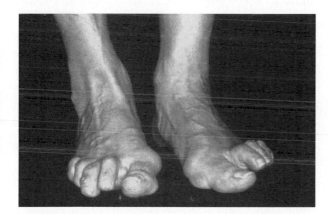

Figure 4-5. The most common foot deformities in rheumatoid arthritis are hallux valgus and hammer toes. The 'cock-up' toe deformities in this patient are associated with subluxation of the metatarso-phalangeal joints. Superimposed painful corns and bunions result primarily from irritation caused by faulty-fitting shoes. (Reprinted from the Clinical Slide Collection on the Rheumatic Diseases, © 1991, used by permission from the American College of Rheumatology.) See color plate 2.

Vascular Lesions

Inflammation of small- to medium-sized blood vessels (vasculitis) may occur in RA, resulting in a variety of manifestations. Leukocytoclastic vasculitis results in palpable purpura whereas necrotizing vasculitis may lead to potentially more serious lesions including skin ulceration, neurological manifestations (such as a mononeuritis), bowel infarction, or gastro-intestinal bleeding.

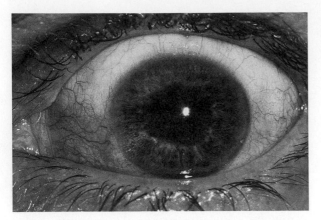

Figure 4-7. Episcleritis in a patient with rheumatoid arthritis. The superficial layers of the nasal portion of the eye are involved. (Reprinted from the Clinical Slide Collection on the Rheumatic Diseases, © 1991, by permission of the American College of Rheumatology.)

Ocular and Oral Manifestations

Patients with RA may present with a painful, red eye due to episcleritis or scleritis (Figure 4-7). Repeated episodes of scleritis may result in thinning of the sclera (scleromalacia) and rarely perforation. Sjögren's syndrome consists of dryness of the eyes and mouth in association with RA or other connective tissue diseases. The condition can occur without a connective tissue disease being present and is referred to as primary Sjögren's syndrome. There is intense infiltration of the lacrimal and salivary glands by inflammatory cells, resulting in tissue damage and decreased secretion of tears and saliva. Involvement of other exocrine glands may result in dryness of the skin, vagina, and respiratory passages. Patients with Sjögren's syndrome have a marked increase risk of developing non-Hodgkin's lymphoma. The use of artificial tears or lubricating ointment provides excellent symptomatic relief in most instances. Cholinomimetic agents such as pilocarpine (Salagen) may stimulate an increase in saliva production.

Respiratory Lesions

Inflammation involving the cricoarytenoid joints results in hoarseness and occasionally dysphagia. A variety of pulmonary manifestations can occur in RA including pleurisy, which causes chest pain and which may be associated with pleural effusion. Intrapulmonary rheumatoid nodules can occur as solitary or multiple lesions. A diagnosis is usually made through the exclusion of other potential causes of lung nodules

such as infections and cancer. The occurrence of pulmonary fibrosis, typically affecting the basal segments of the lungs bilaterally, is characteristic of many connective tissue diseases including RA.

Cardiac Manifestations

Trivial pericardial effusions are frequently seen in up to 50% of patients with RA on echocardiography. Clinical pericarditis with chest pain and an audible friction rub is uncommon. Constrictive pericarditis with tamponade can occur on rare occasions.

Neurological Manifestations

A number of neurological complications can occur in RA. Most common is an entrapment neuropathy at the wrist, resulting in a carpal tunnel syndrome. This is usually seen early in the course of the disease, can be a presenting feature, and is invariably associated with active inflammation in the adjacent wrist. Entrapment of the ulnar nerve at the level of the elbow usually occurs late and is associated with severe joint damage. A tarsal tunnel syndrome is seen less often.

RA may be associated with a peripheral neuropathy. A mononeuritis or mononeuritis multiplex may develop on the basis of a necrotizing vasculitis with manifestations such as a foot or wrist drop. Severe atlantoaxial subluxation can result in spinal cord compression. However such manifestations are more likely to occur with cervical subluxation at a lower level where the spinal canal is narrower.

> **Watch for neurological symptoms when cervical subluxation exists.**

Laboratory Tests

Laboratory tests are not necessary for the diagnosis of RA, but information obtained provides supportive evidence and helps in determining disease severity and prognosis. Serial testing is usually necessary to monitor for potential adverse reactions to disease-modifying antirheumatic drugs (DMARDs).

A mild or moderately severe normochromic, normocytic anemia is often seen in active RA. This is associated with a low serum iron level, but the iron-binding capacity is normal or low. The anemia does not respond to iron supplements because the problem is due to nonutilization of adequate iron stores rather than a true deficiency. A true iron deficiency anemia commonly occurs on the basis of blood loss from nonsteroidal anti-inflammatory drug-induced gastric or duodenal erosions or ulcers. In this situation the serum ferritin level will be very low with a high iron-binding capacity. The ESR and CRP levels are often elevated in RA but often these levels correlate poorly with clinical measures of disease activity.

The use of various DMARDs in RA may result in leukopenia, thrombocytopenia, or pancytopenia. Leukopenia can also be due to Felty's syndrome, originally described as the combination of RA with splenomegaly, leukopenia (due predominantly to a decreased neutrophil count), and leg ulcers. Subsequently lymphadenopathy and thrombocytopenia were included as possible manifestations. The disease mechanism is uncertain, but Felty's syndrome tends to develop in patients with RA who have had longstanding, severe disease.

Rheumatoid factor is an autoantibody directed against immunoglobulin (Ig) G. It is present in the serum of 70% to 80% of patients with RA. The presence of rheumatoid factor supports a diagnosis of RA in a patient presenting with typical clinical features. However the presence of rheumatoid factor is not diagnostic for RA because it can be found in association with other connective tissue diseases (especially SLE and Sjögren's syndrome), chronic infections, and other nonrheumatic conditions. It can also be seen in some normal individuals, particularly in older age-groups. The role of rheumatoid factor in the pathogenesis of RA is uncertain, but its presence (especially in high levels) is usually associated with more severe disease and poorer prognosis. Antinuclear antibodies (ANAs) may be detected in 20% to 40% of patients with RA, usually in those with extra-articular manifestations and severe disease.

Radiology

Radiological manifestations are not helpful in the diagnosis of RA because the abnormalities seen (periarticular erosions and loss of joint space) are nonspecific and are common to all chronic inflammatory arthropathies. However x-ray films are useful in the overall assessment of the patient and staging of the disease. The occurrence of early erosions (within the first year) indicates the presence of more aggressive disease. Serial x-ray films are helpful in assessing disease progression and efficacy of treatment. Increasing numbers of erosions and loss of joint space over time are a consequence of persistently active disease resulting in progressive joint damage. Views of the hands and feet are most useful for this purpose (Figure 4-8). Views of other peripheral joints are usually only necessary to confirm the presence and establish the severity of damage, which has been suspected clinically. Atlantoaxial subluxation can be diagnosed with lateral views of the cervical spine taken in both flexion and extension. Subluxation is considered to be present when the separation between the arch of C1 and the odontoid process (C2) is greater than 2.5 mm with the neck in flexion.

Course and Prognosis

RA is a chronic disease with a variable and unpredictable course. Spontaneous remissions are uncommon, occurring in no more than 10% of patients followed over a 10-year period.[4] Patients having the most severe form of RA present with a persistently active polyarthritis, which does not respond to medical treatment and leads to rapid and progressive joint damage. In most patients, however, the clinical course is up and down with periodic exacerbations, followed by a return of the disease to the baseline condition. Factors predicting more severe disease and poorer outcome include the presence of rheumatoid factor, nodules, other extra-articular manifestations, and the presence of the HLA-DR4 haplotype.[5] Recent epidemiological studies indicate that RA is a more aggressive disease than originally thought. Other studies show that 50% of patients who had been hospitalized in the early stages of their disease were no longer working after 10 years.[6] Radiological evidence of erosions is evident early in the disease course, and 70% of patients with RA exhibit radiological damage within 2 years of disease onset.[7] With this realization, RA is

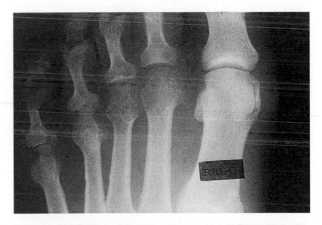

Figure 4-8. X-ray film of a rheumatoid foot showing joint space narrowing and large erosions involving the fourth and fifth metatarsal heads and adjacent phalanges. (Reprinted from the Clinical Slide Collection on the Rheumatic Diseases, © 1991, by permission from the American College of Rheumatology.)

now treated earlier and much more aggressively than has been the practice in the past.

Nevertheless, in most patients, RA is a severe, chronic disorder with progressive joint damage, resulting in major functional limitation and work disability. Furthermore, several studies over the past decade have demonstrated increased mortality rates compared with those in the general population. Patients with severe RA tend to die 10 to 15 years earlier than expected owing to cardiovascular and cerebral vascular disease, infections, gastrointestinal bleeding, and pulmonary and renal involvement.[8]

Treatment

Although there is no cure for RA, treatment is available that can at least control the disease and retard damage. The principle of treatment is to control inflammation to relieve pain and stiffness, restore function, and, in the long term, reduce the rate of damage and preserve joint integrity. The fact that the course of RA is progressively destructive with joint damage occurring early emphasizes the need for prompt diagnosis, identification of prognostic factors, and early aggressive treatment. Poor prognostic factors include the early onset of severe disease with polyarticular involvement, joint erosions, extra-articular manifestations, and the presence of rheumatoid factor. In the past nonsteroidal anti-inflammatory drugs (NSAIDs) were considered the mainstay of treatment for RA. Although NSAIDs produce symptomatic improvement in patients with RA, they do not alter the course of the disease. Therefore treatment with NSAIDs alone is inadequate except for the treatment of very mild disease. In most patients with RA, there is a need for the early introduction of a DMARD.

Education and Physical and Occupational Therapy

Ongoing education of the patient with RA is important in the overall treatment plan. Patients need to be informed and understand the nature of their disease and the principals of treatment. Hopefully proper attention to this area will result in better adherence with treatment and improved outcome.

> **Remember that rheumatoid disease is a systemic disorder in which joints are often the primary target.**

Physical therapy (PT) and occupational therapy (OT) have an important role in the management of the patient with RA both in the early stages and late in the course of the disease. In the presence of active disease, appropriate exercises will help maintain normal range of movement and prevent the development of flexion contractures. In joints that have already been damaged, strengthening of atrophic muscles and restoring range of movement will help improve function. OT plays an important role in educating the patient about joint protection. Splinting promotes rest, reduces joint trauma, and leads to a reduction in inflammation as well as improving alignment. Assessment of function and the provision of assistive devices can improve the quality of life and maintain independence. For detail of PT and OT management, see Chapters 9 and 14.

Drug Therapy

Nonsteroidal Anti-Inflammatory Drugs   NSAIDs are the most commonly used medications in the treatment of RA, especially in early disease. They have both anti-inflammatory and analgesic properties and exert their effect by inhibiting the production of prostaglandins. Prostaglandins occur in two forms, one of which supplies physiological functions such as maintaining the integrity of the gastric mucosa and renal cortical blood flow. Prostaglandins are also produced by inflammatory cells and are important mediators of inflammation. The older NSAIDs unfortunately inhibit the production of both physiological and pro-inflammatory prostaglandins. This can result in potentially serious side effects including gastric and duodenal ulcers and renal toxicity. Endoscopic evidence of gastric ulceration is seen in 15% to 20% of chronic users of NSAIDs, and complications such as perforation and bleeding occur at an annual rate of 1% to 4%.[9] Renal toxicity includes renal failure and sodium and water retention with the precipitation of heart failure and adverse affects on the control of hypertension. NSAIDs therefore need to be used with caution in patients with there is a history of peptic ulceration or major concurrent illnesses and in elderly patients.

In recent years, a new generation of NSAIDs has been developed. These are the cyclooxygenase enzyme (COX-2) inhibitors (such as celecoxib, meloxicam, and rofecoxib) which selectively inhibit pro-inflammatory but spare physiological prostaglandins, resulting in a substantial decrease in the frequency of gastrointestinal side effects.[10,11] Renal toxicity, however, remains a potential problem.

The numerous NSAIDs that are currently available are about equally effective. All have been shown to be more effective than placebo in controlled clinical trials. Because of their better safety profile, the COX-2 inhibitors are now the NSAIDs of choice, but they are substantially more expensive. Although NSAIDs play a useful role in the management of RA, they do not influence the course of the disease or prevent progressive joint damage.

Corticosteroids Corticosteroids are powerful anti-inflammatory drugs. However their role in the treatment of RA is limited by adverse reactions associated with higher doses and long-term use. Complications of treatment include diabetes mellitus, hypertension, weight gain, avascular necrosis, and osteoporosis (which can occur even with low doses given over a prolonged period). Nevertheless corticosteroids are very useful in the management of RA.

The most common use of corticosteroids in RA is in the form of intra-articular injections using long-acting formulations such as methylprednisolone acetate (DepoMedrol). These injections are extremely useful and effective in the management of the patient who just has one or two joints with active disease. Although the effect of this treatment is mainly local, sufficient absorption of the injected material occurs to produce a systemic effect and a general reduction in disease activity. Local corticosteroids, in the form of eye drops and subconjunctival injections, are used to treat the eye manifestations of RA (episcleritis and scleritis).

High-dose systemic corticosteroid therapy is seldom used in RA except in the management of potentially serious extra-articular manifestations such as vasculitis. On the other hand, low doses (prednisone 2.5 to 7.5 mg daily) are often prescribed for patients with severe disease. This may help bridge the gap while one waits for DMARDs to become effective, especially in a patient who has marked limitation of function. In the elderly patient low-dose prednisone may help control disease and preserve independence while avoiding use of potentially toxic DMARDs.

Disease-Modifying Antirheumatic Drugs Often referred to as second-line drugs, DMARDs have become the cornerstone in the treatment of RA because of their ability to favorably alter the course of the disease. The currently available DMARDs are listed in Table 4-1. All are slow-acting drugs because it usually takes several months of therapy before a clinical response occurs. While their precise mechanisms of action are not known, they are thought to reduce disease activity in RA through modulation of the immune system. Although they all have been shown to be more effective than placebos in the treatment of RA, DMARDs seldom induce a complete remission. Some degree of disease activity usually persists and joint damage may continue to progress. Invariably the disease will recur when these drugs are discontinued.

Until about 1980, intramuscular *gold* (sodium aurothiomalate and sodium aurothioglucose) was the DMARD of first choice. Despite its efficacy, toxicity and secondary treatment failure were problems leading to its discontinuation in 75% of patients after 5 years of therapy. The main side effects with intramuscular gold are rash, bone marrow depression, and proteinuria due to a membranous glomerulonephritis.

The antimalarial drugs *chloroquine* and *hydroxychloroquine* are the least effective of the available DMARDs with the exception of auranofin (oral gold). However their use remains popular because of their relatively better safety profile compared with other DMARDs. The antimalarial drugs are therefore often used for the treatment of early and milder cases of RA. Retinopathy with impairment of vision is a potentially serious side effect. Its occurrence can be minimized by the use of maintenance dose guidelines based on lean body weight (chloroquine 3 mg/kg/day, hydroxychloroquine 6 mg/kg/day) and regular (annual or biannual) eye examination by an ophthalmologist. Less eye toxicity has been reported with hydroxychloroquine than with chloroquine.

Sulfasalazine is a combination of a salicylate with a sulfasalazine molecule. The salicylate component is not absorbed, which explains its usefulness in the treatment of inflammatory bowel disease. Developed in 1940, sulfasalazine is one of few drugs specifically formulated for the treatment of RA. The dose range is 2 to 3 g daily. A regular complete blood count is needed to monitor for possible bone marrow suppression.

Methotrexate has become the DMARD of first choice during the past two decades because of its efficacy and favorable safety profile. At least 50% of

---

Table 4-1. Currently Available DMARDs

Gold, intramuscular:
    Sodium aurothiomalate
    Sodium aurothioglucose
Gold, oral: Auranofin
Antimalarial drugs
    Chloroquine
    Hydroxychloroquine
Penicillamine
Sulfasalazine
Cytotoxic drugs
    Azathioprine
    Methotrexate
    Cyclosporine
Leflunomide

patients who start taking methotrexate are still taking it after 5 years. The drug acts by inhibiting folic acid metabolism and a small daily dietary supplement (1 mg) of folic acid has been shown to reduce gastrointestinal and hepatic toxicity without compromising efficacy. The relatively small dose required to achieve disease remission in RA contributes to both the lower cost and reduced toxicity of methotrexate compared with other DMARDs. The starting dose is 7.5 mg once weekly, increasing to up to 25 mg weekly. In more resistant disease, the higher doses are often administered by subcutaneous or intramuscular injection to ensure adequate absorption. Methotrexate is hepatotoxic and may suppress the bone marrow. Regular monitoring of liver function and a complete blood count are necessary on a regular basis to monitor for possible toxicity. For obvious reasons, heavy alcohol consumption and a history of infectious hepatitis are relative contraindications for its use. Of other cytotoxic drugs, azathioprine is less effective than methotrexate, and the use of cyclosporine is limited because of its renal toxicity.

Leflunomide acts by inhibiting pyrimidine metabolism. The dose is 10 to 20 mg once daily. The main side effects are marrow suppression, hepatic toxicity, and diarrhea. It has a very long half-life (about 16 days) and the use of oral cholestyramine will facilitate clearance of the drug through the gastrointestinal tract in patients with serious toxicity. Both leflunomide and methotrexate are potentially teratogenic and should be avoided when pregnancy is a possibility.

Combinations of different DMARDs are often used when single agents alone fail to achieve adequate control of RA. Combinations shown to be more effective than the individual treatments alone include methotrexate plus sulfasalazine (with or without hydroxychloroquine), methotrexate plus cyclosporine, and methotrexate plus leflunomide. This approach cannot only produce better therapeutic results but also may be associated with less toxicity because of the smaller doses of individual drugs used. Of the currently available DMARDs only methotrexate, sulfasalazine, and leflunomide have been shown in serial radiological studies to retard the progression of joint erosions.

Biologic Agents

The use of biologic agents introduces a new and more rational approach to the treatment of RA. The cytokine TNF-α plays a central role in the pathogenesis of RA, initiating events leading to inflammation and joint destruction. Currently two biologic agents that neutralize TNF-α have been approved for the treatment of RA in North America. *Infliximab* is a chimeric (part mouse and part human) antibody to TNF-α that is administered intravenously. It is rapidly effective in controlling inflammation both in RA and Crohn's disease.[12] Coadministration of methotrexate is necessary to prevent the development of antibodies against infliximab and loss of efficacy.

Etanercept is a genetically engineered molecule consisting of two human soluble TNF-α receptors attached to the Fc portion of human IgG. Etanercept is administered by subcutaneous injection twice weekly and acts by absorbing and inactivating TNF-α before it is able to attach to binding sites on inflammatory cells and result in their activation.[13] Both infliximab and etanercept have been shown to be capable of not only controlling inflammation in RA but also retarding significantly the progression of joint erosions. The treatments are generally well tolerated, but the occurrence of demyelinating disorders and serious opportunistic infections (tuberculosis in particular) in some patients is of concern. Biologic agents are extremely expensive (about $20,000 Canadian per year), and their use can have a significant impact on health care costs. For this reason their use is currently limited to patients in whom conventional DMARD therapy has failed.

Other pro-inflammatory cytokines are also being targeted in the treatment of RA, and many new agents are under development. *Anakinra* is an IL-1 receptor antagonist approved for treatment of RA in the United States.[14] Daily subcutaneous injection is necessary. Chapter 6 gives further detail on drug therapy.

Surgery

Orthopaedic surgery in RA is most useful to help restore function in the patient who has sustained severe joint or tendon damage from inadequately controlled inflammation. Surgical synovectomy in the patient with active arthritis is no longer popular because it was realized that the excised synovium rapidly grew back unless the disease was adequately controlled with medical treatment. A tenosynovectomy, however, is a useful procedure when a prolific tenosynovitis, such as that seen at the back of the wrist, is present with threatened or actual damage to the enveloped tendons. This procedure may be combined with repair of the disrupted tendons.

Joint Replacement Hip and knee arthroplasty with replacement of the severely damaged joint surfaces are highly successful procedures. More than 90% of patients undergoing these procedures have a favorable outcome with pain relief and improved function. Apart from the usual operative and perioperative risks, the main long-term complications are infection and loosening of the prosthesis. If the replaced joint becomes infected, removal of the prosthesis may be necessary. Loosening usually occurs after a period of 10 to 15 years resulting in a recurrence of weight-bearing pain that eventually requires revision of the procedure. The indication for hip and knee joint replacement is the presence of severe pain with major functional limitations (such as not being able to climb stairs, difficulty with transfer, being housebound, or inability to walk a distance of 100 m or a city block).

Shoulder and elbow replacements are carried out less often. Compared with hip and knee replacements, these procedures are technically more difficult with respect to fixation of the prosthesis to bone. With shoulder and elbow replacements, the range of movement is usually not greatly improved postoperatively, but the procedures result in excellent pain relief. For this reason alone patients are usually very satisfied. Subluxed MCP joints can be replaced with realignment of the digits and improved function. The best functional results are obtained in hands with intact and functioning interphalangeal joints (without severe deformities).

Patients with fixed subluxation of the MTP joints experience significant weight-bearing pain, which is not relieved with orthotics. Painful callous formation occurs, and the skin underlying the prominent metatarsal heads may breakdown, resulting in local sepsis. Such patients will benefit from forefoot reconstruction, which usually requires resection of the metatarsal heads, base of the proximal phalanges, or both. This shortens the foot, allowing the contracted flexor tendons to relax and the deformed toes to fall back into normal alignment. Satisfactory prostheses have not yet been developed for the replacement of severely damaged wrists and ankles. In both situations, fusion of the joints results in excellent pain relief and improved function. Chapter 7 gives further detail on the surgical management in arthritis.

Spondyloarthropathies

The term *seronegative spondyloarthropathy* refers to a group of related disorders consisting of AS, psoriatic arthritis, Reiter's syndrome (reactive arthritis), and the articular manifestations associated with inflammatory bowel diseases. These disorders are linked together through having a number of characteristic laboratory and clinical features in common. The conditions are referred to as *seronegative* because tests are usually negative for rheumatoid factor, which is more typically positive in RA and other collagen disorders.

Although sacroiliitis and spondylitis (inflammation of the axial skeleton) is characteristic of AS, these manifestations can occur in all of the other seronegative disorders as well. Other clinical manifestations shared by the group include iritis, enthesitis, and dactylitis. Enthesitis is inflammation at sites of tendon attachment to bone (enthesis). Commonly patients will present with heel pain due to inflammation at the attachments of the Achilles tendon or plantar fascia to the calcaneum. Dactylitis is due to active arthritis involving the interphalangeal joints along with a flexor tenosynovitis, resulting in swelling of the whole finger or toe (and hence the commonly used term *sausage digit*).

Epidemiology

Of the spondyloarthropathies, AS has been most extensively studied through epidemiological surveys. The findings indicate that both genetic and environmental factors play a role in the pathogenesis of the disease.[15] AS is seen often among first-degree relatives with the disease with a concordance rate of approximately 60% in monozygotic twins. A strong association has been found between AS and inheritance of the HLA-B27 antigen (identified on the cell surface by tissue typing techniques). The prevalence of the HLA-B27 antigen in the Caucasian population is 7% but is considerably increased in those with AS (90%) and Reiter's syndrome (50% to 80%).[15] In families of patients with AS, 10% to 20% of adult first-degree relatives inheriting the HLA-B27 antigen were found to have the disease.

The presence of the HLA-B27 antigen therefore appears to confer a higher risk of development of AS (and Reiter's syndrome). How this occurs is unknown, but it is likely that the HLA-B27 antigen allows increased susceptibility to the effects of certain infections, especially from the gut. This theory is supported by the fact that spondylitis is increased among patients with inflammatory bowel disease and dysentery due to certain pathogens (*Yersinia, Shigella, Salmonella*) may trigger the onset of reactive arthritis. Reiter's syndrome, on the other hand, is a symptom complex consisting of arthritis, conjunctivitis, and urethritis due to a sexually transmitted *Chlamydia trachomatis* infection. (See also Chapter 2.)

Ankylosing Spondylitis

AS is characterized by the presence of inflammation, resulting in pain and stiffness of the spine. The prevalence of AS varies among ethnic groups, being rare in the Japanese, Australian aborigines, and African

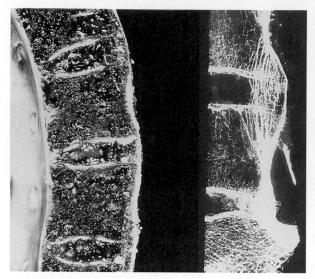

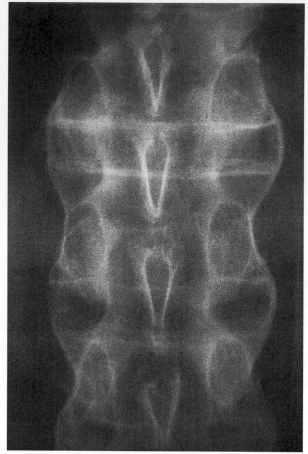

Figure 4-9. Ankylosing spondylitis. Gross sagittal section of the lumbar spine on *left* with accompanying x-ray film on *right* showing bony bridging of adjacent vertebrae due to ossification of the outer layers of the annulus fibrosis. (Reprinted from the Clinical Slide Collection on the Rheumatic Diseases, © 1991, by permission from the American College of Rheumatology.)

Figure 4-10. Ankylosing spondylitis. X-ray film of the lumbar spine showing ossification of the outer layers of the annulus fibrosus, resulting in bony bridging and appearance of a 'bamboo spine.' (Reprinted from the Clinical Slide Collection on the Rheumatic Diseases, © 1991, by permission from the American College of Rheumatology.)

blacks, higher among whites (1 to 2 per 1000), and considerably higher in adult male Haida Indians (4.2 per 1000). AS occurs more often in males with a male-to-female ratio of about 3:1.[15]

Pathology

AS begins with inflammation of the sacroiliac joints and lower spine. Typically, the process spreads slowly up the spine. The inflammation characteristically targets sites where ligaments and tendons attach to bone (enthesis). The latter process may be associated with both localized bone resorption and new bone formation, resulting in squaring of the vertebral bodies and formation of syndesmophytes.[15] Peripheral joints may be involved, but usually the large joints such as the hips, knees and shoulders are affected.

Early in the disease loss of spinal mobility is primarily due to active inflammation. As the disease progresses, ossification of the outer layers of the annulus fibrosus (Figure 4-9) and spinal ligaments occur, resulting in the characteristic "bamboo spine" appearance (Figure 4-10). Fusion of the apophyseal joints adds to the permanent loss of spinal movement.

The rigid spine becomes osteoporotic and subject to fracture, often after mild trauma.

Criteria for Diagnosis

Clinically a diagnosis of AS is based upon a characteristic history of inflammatory type back pain, loss of spinal mobility, and the presence of radiological evidence of sacroiliitis.

Clinical Presentation

The onset of AS is usually insidious, beginning in late adolescence or early adult life and uncommonly after the age of 45 years. The usual presenting symptoms are pain and stiffness in the low back. In common with other inflammatory arthropathies, the symptoms are usually worse during and after periods of immobility. Active AS is therefore characterized by frequent waking during the night and prolonged morning stiffness, which is relieved by physical activity (or a hot shower). As in RA, the duration of morning stiffness is commonly utilized as a measure of disease activity. AS runs a variable course. Some patients experience little loss of spinal mobility, whereas in others the course is relentless, resulting in a completely rigid spine (Figure 4-11). Occasionally, AS may present with extra-articular manifestations, iritis in particular,

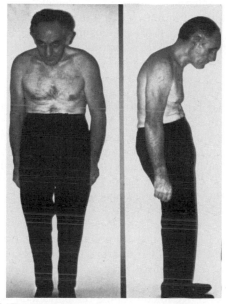

Figure 4-11. On the *left* a frontal view of a patient with ankylosing spondylitis demonstrates the characteristic upward gaze of the eyes when looking straight ahead, necessitated by the flexion deformity of the neck. These postural changes are typical of the more advanced forms of this disease. The lateral view of the same patient on the *right* demonstrates forward protrusion of the head, flattening of the anterior chest wall, thoracic kyphosis, protrusion of the abdomen, and flattening of the lumbar lordotic curvature. The partially fixed thoracic cage is primarily responsible for the muscular atrophy seen in the chest muscles. (Reprinted from the Clinical Slide Collection on the Rheumatic Diseases, © 1991, by permission from the American College of Rheumatology.)

and less often with symptoms of complete heart block or aortic insufficiency.

Physical Examination

The characteristic abnormality on physical examination is loss of spinal mobility in all three planes (flexion-extension, lateral flexion, rotation). The earliest changes have been shown to occur at the level of the thoracolumbar junction, moving upward as the disease progresses. Various methods have been proposed for measuring loss of spinal movement.[16] In practice, measuring the finger-to-floor distance with the thoracolumbar spine fully flexed provides a rapid and reproducible method for comparing spinal mobility between visits.

Postural changes are seen with disease progression. In early AS flattening of the lower spine with loss of the lumbar lordosis is seen. Later in the course a thoracic kyphosis may develop. The latter can be severe with progressive lowering of the horizon and loss of forward gaze. Progression of the kyphosis can be followed by serially measuring the occiput-to-wall distance, carried out with the patient's heels and back against the wall and spine fully extended. (See Chapter 10.)

AS may be associated with a peripheral arthritis typically involving large joints, in particular the hips, knees, and shoulders. Small joint involvement is uncommon. Pain with localized tenderness and swelling may occur on the basis of an enthesitis. Usually this affects the back and sole of the heel where the Achilles tendon and plantar fascia attach, respectively, but it can occur at any tendon-bone junction. (See also Chapter 5.) Patients with AS may exhibit signs of extra-articular manifestations, which includes iritis, complete heart block, aortic insufficiency, prostatitis, and apical pulmonary fibrosis.

Radiological Changes

The earliest radiological change is seen in the sacroiliac joints (sacroiliitis), consisting of blurring of the joint margins, erosions with pseudo-widening of the joint space, and subchondral sclerosis (Figure 4-12). Late in the disease, the sacroiliac joints may fuse completely with obliteration of the joint space (Figure 4-13).

Early changes may be seen in the lumbar spine with squaring of the vertebral bodies. This is due to resorption of the usually prominent corners of the vertebral bodies from enthesitis (Romanus lesions). There may be complete or incomplete bridging of the intervertebral disc spaces by syndesmophytes. These lesions develop through the ossification of the annulus fibrosis and longitudinal ligaments, giving

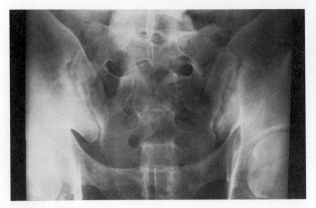

Figure 4-12. X-ray film of the sacroiliac joints in early ankylosing spondylitis showing the presence of bilateral sacroiliitis. There is erosion of the cortical margins (resulting in irregularity and pseudo-widening) and bony sclerosis. (Reprinted from Berens DL: Roentgen features of ankylosing spondylitis. *Clin Orthop* 74:23, 1971. With permission.)

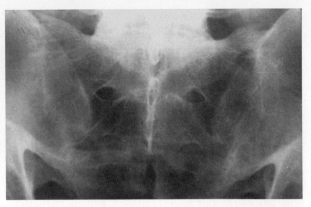

Figure 4-13. There is almost complete obliteration of the sacroiliac joints. Bony trabeculae are noted crossing the residual sacroiliac joint space. There is no gross sclerosis at this time. A moderate degree of osteopenia is present. (Reprinted from Berens DL: Roentgen features of ankylosing spondylitis. *Clin Orthop* 74:23, 1971. With permission.)

rise to the bamboo spine appearance. Fusion of joints may occur, most often affecting the apophyseal joints in the cervical spine.

Laboratory Findings

In the spondyloarthropathies, laboratory tests do not show any consistent or characteristic abnormalities, except for a negative test for rheumatoid factor. The ESR may be raised in the presence of active disease. Testing for the HLA-B27 antigen is not carried out routinely. The test is not diagnostic, but a positive test in a patient with a characteristic history raises the likelihood of a diagnosis of AS.

> **Seronegative inflammatory arthritic conditions have a primary effect on the axial skeleton, and the serological test for *rheumatoid factor* is characteristically negative.**

Management

The management of AS requires close collaboration between physician and physiotherapist. A major long-term disability associated with this disease is the development of a severe and permanent flexion deformity of the spine. If this deformity is allowed to progress, the patient will have great difficulty walking because of the limited field of forward vision. Respiratory capacity may become limited because of

ankylosis of the costovertebral joints, restricting chest expansion. It is essential, therefore, that health professionals be involved in management of AS from the beginning with an educational program promoting the importance of regular active and postural back exercises. The object is to maintain optimal spinal alignment and preserve range of movement. (See also Chapter 10.)

The cornerstone of medical management in AS is the use of NSAIDs. All are potentially effective; none has been shown to be superior over others, although the COX-2 inhibitors have not yet been comprehensively studied. DMARDs such as methotrexate may be effective in controlling the peripheral arthritis but are ineffective in the treatment of spondylitis. Short courses of prednisone (20 to 30 mg daily for 2 to 3 weeks) followed by a rapid taper are often helpful in controlling severe exacerbations of AS.

In the past, radiation was an effective therapy for resistant AS, but use of radiation has been largely abandoned because of concerns about the possible risk of leukemia. Intravenous pamidronate (a bisphosphonate) and use of the TNF-α antagonists have shown promising results. Iritis requires referral to an ophthalmologist. The usual treatment is local administration of corticosteroids. See also Chapter 6 for further details on drug therapy. Severe spinal deformities can be corrected surgically with a spinal osteotomy, but this requires a skilled surgeon familiar with the technique.

Reiter's Syndrome (Reactive Arthritis)

Reiter's syndrome consists of arthritis, urethritis, and conjunctivitis.[17] The disorder is characteristically precipitated by an infectious episode, which may be either genitourinary or gastrointestinal. The genitourinary infection is usually sexually transmitted and is due to *C. trachomatis*. Gastrointestinal infections with *Shigella, Salmonella, Campylobacter,* or *Yersinia* may be also followed by a similar illness. Reiter's syndrome has become synonymous with the term *reactive arthritis*. Although the arthritis has been initiated by an infection, the responsible organisms are not found in the joint. The majority of patients show HLA-B27 antigen positivity, and most patients are young males. Reiter's syndrome also is seen among patients with human immunodeficiency virus infection, often in a more severe form.

Clinical Manifestations

Urethritis, when present, is usually the first manifestation of classic Reiter's syndrome, but it can occur with both postvenereal and postenteric forms of the disease. Conjunctivitis presents with the urethritis or follows it by several days and is usually mild and transient. The arthritis begins acutely 2 to 4 weeks after the venereal infection or gastroenteritis and affects predominantly lower limb joints in an asymmetric distribution. Dactylitis may occur with inflammation of the whole digit. Spinal or sacroiliac involvement resulting in low back pain occurs in approximately 50% of patients. A variety of extra-articular manifestations may be seen including iritis, painless oral ulcers, nail dystrophy, aortic insufficiency, and neurological complications. Most are uncommon except for the iritis, oral ulcers, and nail changes. Two rare but distinct lesions may be seen in Reiter's syndrome. Keratodermia blenorrhagica is a pustular skin rash occurring on the soles or palms that resembles the lesions of psoriasis. Balanitis circinata is a characteristic rash involving the glans or shaft of the penis. Patients with severe disease may experience fevers and profound weight loss.

Course and Management

In the majority of patients, Reiter's syndrome runs a self-limiting course over a 6- to 12-month period. Relapses occur in up to 15% of patients, possibly due to reinfection in some, whereas in 15% of patients the disease has a chronic course, often with a destructive arthritis. NSAIDs are the main treatment for the arthritis. In severe or recurrent disease, the use of DMARDs such as methotrexate, azathioprine, or sulfasalazine may be necessary. When an infection is present, a 10- to 14-day course of antibiotics is usually given. However prolonged antibiotic therapy has not been shown to influence the course of the arthritis.

Enteropathic Arthritis

Ulcerative colitis and Crohn's disease (inflammatory bowel disease, IBD) may be associated with a peripheral arthritis in approximately 10% to 20% of patients. The typical pattern is similar to that seen in Reiter's syndrome with an asymmetrical oligoarthritis, mainly affecting the lower limb joints. Peripheral arthritis usually occurs in the presence of active bowel inflammation and subsides with control of the IBD. In ulcerative colitis, total colectomy will result in a permanent remission of the arthritis. Spondylitis and sacroiliitis occurs in approximately 10% of patients with IBD and are usually associated with the presence of the HLA-B27 antigen. Treatment is similar to that for Reiter's syndrome, but NSAIDs should be used with caution because they may exacerbate the bowel manifestations. In severe disease, systemic corticosteroids are required to control the bowel inflammation.

Psoriatic Arthritis

Psoriasis is a relatively common skin condition with an overall prevalence of about 2%.[18] Between 5% and 7% of patients with psoriasis will have arthritis; it occurs more commonly in those with extensive skin lesions. The etiology of psoriasis and psoriatic arthritis is unknown, but there is strong evidence for a genetic basis. A number of HLA antigens, including HLA-Cw6, have been reported to be associated with psoriasis and psoriatic arthritis.[19] The presence of the HLA-B27 antigen carries a higher risk for the development of psoriatic spondylitis. Although the male-to-female ratio is equal, spondylitis tends to occur more often in men and a symmetrical polyarthritis more often in women. Peak onset is between 30 and 55 years, similar to that for RA.

Clinical Features

Most patients presenting with psoriatic arthritis (70%) will have had the skin lesions for many years. In some (15%) the psoriasis and arthritis will present at about the same time, whereas in a minority the arthritis will precede the skin lesions by many years. The typical psoriatic skin lesion is a well demarcated, erythematous plaque covered with a silvery scale. These lesions vary considerably in size and extent, occurring most commonly on the scalp, umbilicus,

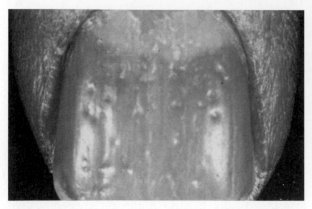

Figure 4-14. Pitting of the nail is a characteristic finding in many patients with psoriasis and is often associated with arthritis of the distal interphalangeal joints. (Reprinted from the Clinical Slide Collection on the Rheumatic Diseases, © 1991, by permission from the American College of Rheumatology.) See color plate 2.

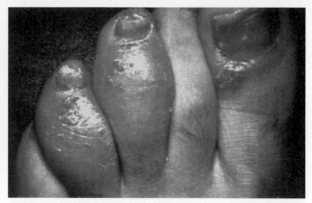

Figure 4-16. Psoriasis can be seen involving the first, third, and fourth toes. This is accompanied by psoriatic arthritis of interphalangeal joints of the third and fourth toes. The sausage shape of these toes is caused by soft tissue swelling more marked than that usually seen in rheumatoid arthritis. (Reprinted from the Clinical Slide Collection on the Rheumatic Diseases, © 1991, by permission from the American College of Rheumatology.) See color plate 3.

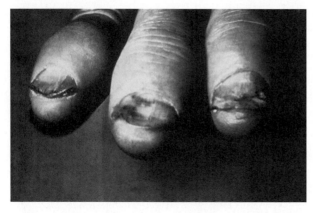

Figure 4-15. Swelling and deformity of the distal interphalangeal joints and uplifting of the distal portion of the nails (onycholysis) are typical of psoriasis. Fragmentation and brown discoloration of the nails are present; total nail destruction may occur. (Reprinted from the Clinical Slide Collection on the Rheumatic Diseases, © 1991, by permission from the American College of Rheumatology.) See color plate 2.

gluteal folds, and extensor surfaces of the elbow and knees. Patients with mild psoriasis are often unaware that they have the disease. Psoriasis may affect the nails with pitting of the surface, onycholysis (lifting of the nail from the nailbed), and dystrophic changes (Figure 4-14 and Figure 4-15). These abnormalities are nonspecific, but multiple pits on a single nail is characteristic of psoriatic arthritis.

Patterns of Presentation
The arthropathy in psoriatic arthritis is quite variable, and different patterns have been recognized:

1. Classic psoriatic arthritis: In this form, there is predominant involvement of the DIP joints of the hands, which are rarely involved in RA (Figure 4-15).
2. Arthritis mutilans: This rare form of psoriatic arthritis results in severe joint destruction in the hands (and occasionally in the feet). The arthritis is associated with osteolysis (bone resorption), resulting in shortening and telescoping of the involved digits.
3. Symmetric polyarthritis: This form resembles RA and may be difficult to differentiate from it clinically.
4. Monoarthritis and oligoarthritis: One to a few joints are involved in an asymmetrical distribution. A dactylitis (sausage finger or toe) may occur with swelling of the whole digit (Figure 4-16).
5. Spondylitis: This is found particularly among patients who have the HLA-B27 antigen.

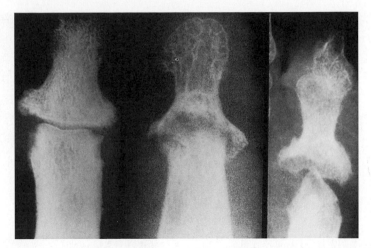

Figure 4-17. Psoriatic arthritis (x-ray film). Progressive destructive changes in the distal interphalangeal joint resulting in a 'pencil-in-cup' appearance (right). (Reprinted from the Clinical Slide Collection on the Rheumatic Diseases, © 1991, by permission from the American College of Rheumatology.)

Radiology

Apart from joint erosions similar to those seen in RA, a number of distinct radiological abnormalities may be seen with psoriatic arthritis including periostitis, bony ankylosis, and the "pencil-in-cup lesion." The latter is a destructive arthropathy involving MCP, MTP, or interphalangeal joints with bone resorption producing the characteristic appearance (Figure 4-17). Spondylitic changes may be seen in the spine with or without sacroiliitis (which can be unilateral).

Management

The treatment of psoriatic arthritis is similar to that for RA with the use of NSAIDs and the early introduction of DMARDs for more severe disease. Methotrexate may help control the skin lesions as well as the arthritis in psoriatic arthritis. Antimalarial drugs need to be prescribed with caution because they can sometimes result in worsening of the skin lesions. The activity of the arthritis often parallels that of the psoriasis, and exacerbations occur more often in the winter when there is less exposure to ultraviolet light. Coordination of treatment between rheumatologist and dermatologist is often necessary for optimal results.

Osteoarthritis

Osteoarthritis (OA, degenerative joint disease) is characterized by progressive destruction of hyaline cartilage followed by remodeling of the affected joint. The term *osteoarthrosis* is preferred by some, in recognition of the fact that the primary pathological process is more degenerative than inflammatory.

OA is separated into primary and secondary forms. The disease is considered to be primary when there is no obvious underlying cause. OA is considered to be secondary when there is an identifiable etiological factor such as an inflammatory arthropathy (for example, RA), infection, fractures with disruption of the articulating surface or malalignment of the limb, avascular necrosis, metabolic conditions (such as hemochromatosis), and leg length discrepancy. Families with early-onset OA due to rare, inherited mutations of collagen have been described.[20]

OA is the most common form of arthritis. Its prevalence increases steadily with age, and radiographic changes of OA are seen in the knees of more than 50% of the population older than the age of 65 years. After the age of 75 years virtually everyone has evidence of OA in at least one joint.[21] Men and women are equally affected before age 45, but after age 45 the prevalence is higher in women.[22] OA has been linked to various occupations and sporting activities. Continuous overuse of a joint may be related to the subsequent development of OA. Long-distance running, however, does not lead to increased OA of the hips or knees if there is no preexisting structural abnormality.

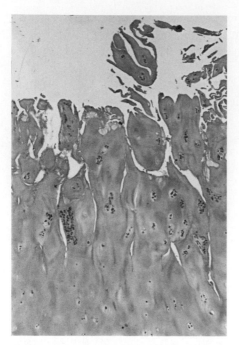

Figure 4-18. A medium-power histological view of the superficial zone of articular cartilage demonstrating characteristic osteoarthritis degeneration including dislodgement of small cartilaginous fragments. (Reprinted from the Clinical Slide Collection on the Rheumatic Diseases, © 1991, by permission from the American College of Rheumatology.) See color plate 3.

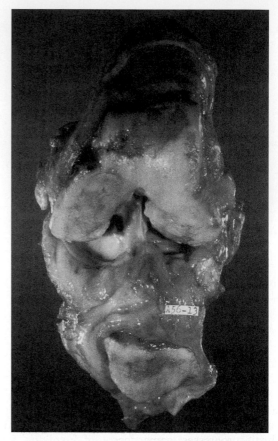

Figure 4-19. Osteoarthritis of the knee. The joint has been opened anteriorly and the patella turned downward. There are large eroded areas of articular cartilage on the intercondylar femoral surfaces and on the patella. (Reprinted from the Clinical Slide Collection on the Rheumatic Diseases, © 1991, by permission from the American College of Rheumatology.)

Pathology

OA begins with abnormalities within the articular (hyaline) cartilage.[23] The normally smooth articular surface becomes disrupted with fibrillation and the formation of deep clefts (Figure 4-18). There is progressive loss of cartilage, eventually resulting in complete exposure of the underlying bone (Figure 4-19). The process is not simply degenerative in nature, because there is evidence of repair occurring at sites of damage, with the proliferation of metabolically active chondrocytes. New bone is laid down with the formation of characteristic osteophytes at joint margins. Abnormalities occur in the subchondral bone with increased density (sclerosis) and the formation of cysts. Mild to moderate synovitis occurs in some patients, but inflammation is not usually a prominent feature of OA unless there is superimposed pseudo-gout or trauma. Thickening and stiffness of the joint capsule contributes to the resulting restricted joint movement.

Pathogenesis

Cartilage consists mainly of water, collagen (mainly type II), and proteoglycans (PGs). The PG consists of a central protein core with glycosaminoglycan side chains. Collagen provides tensile strength, and the PG aggregates confer structural stability to cartilage. In normal cartilage there is a balance between the continuous enzymatic breakdown of collagen and PG and their replacement by the activity of chondrocytes. In OA there is increased enzyme activity and decreased PG, reflecting an up-regulation of the degradative process and a net loss of cartilage.[22]

A number of theories in the causation of OA have evolved. The initial event may be abnormal mechanical stress across a joint, resulting in aberrant chondrocyte metabolism. Chondrocytes produce increased quantities of degradative enzymes (metalloproteinases) including collagenases, gelatinases, and stromelysin, which breakdown collagen and PGs. Chondrocytes also produce increased amounts of cytokines including IL-1 and TNF-α, which further stimulates production of metalloproteinases. Such enzymes are normally neutralized by naturally occurring tissue inhibitors, which obviously become overwhelmed in OA. Calcium pyrophosphate dihydrate crystals are often deposited in degenerating articular cartilage. With cartilage breakdown these crystals can be shed into the joint, become ingested by inflammatory or synovial cells, and result in acute or chronic inflammation (pseudo-gout).

Clinical Features

The joints usually involved in OA are DIP and PIP joints; first carpometacarpal joints of the hands, hips, and knees; first MTP joints in the feet; and apophyseal joints in the midlower cervical and lower lumbar spine. The presenting symptoms are pain, stiffness, and restricted movement of the affected joint. Pain is initially mild, being worse after rest, improving with mobilization, but aggravated by overactivity. As the arthritis progresses, some degree of functional loss becomes inevitable.

OA affecting the hands is usually a benign disease. Although there may be progressive deformity with loss of movement and dexterity, severe crippling does not commonly occur. The involved joints appear enlarged owing to the formation of marginal osteophytes. In the PIP and DIP joints these occur as hard, nodular, nontender lesions, known as Bouchard's and Heberden's nodes, respectively (Figure 4-20). Involvement of the first carpometacarpal joint results in a characteristic deformity with a squared appearance and loss of ability to abduct the first metacarpal. Subsequently there may be a secondary hyperextension deformity of the first MCP joint. Pain is quite variable. It is often aggravated by vigorous physical activity. Some patients have little pain despite the presence of clinically severe disease. Some loss of dexterity is inevitable and in advanced OA there is difficulty with grasp and a tendency to drop things.

The hips and knees are major weight-bearing joints, and for this reason OA at these sites is potentially a more serious problem. With OA of the hip, pain is typically felt in the groin or trochanter. Occasionally referred pain is felt over the medial aspect of the knee. Slow progression is usual with increasing pain, stiffness, and restricted function. With advanced disease pain during rest is often present. Clinically there is reduced range of movement with flexion contractures and stress pain. In the knee, the patellofemoral articulation and medial compartment are most commonly involved. Small effusions may be present, but other signs of active inflammation are characteristically absent unless there is superimposed trauma or pseudo-gout. Crepitus can be felt during passive movement of the joint if complete loss of articular cartilage has occurred.

OA of the first MTP joint occurs often and is often associated with the gradual development of a valgus deformity of the big toe (hallux valgus). Pain arises, either from the degenerative changes within the joint or because of a bursitis, which has developed over a prominent metatarsal head and is aggravated by wearing of tight shoes.

Degenerative disease of the spine is closely associated with increasing age. By the age of 70 years, 90% of the population will show evidence of degeneration of the axial skeleton. Radiological changes are often seen within the fifth decade but are not necessarily symptomatic. The areas most severely affected are the lower cervical, upper thoracic, and lower lumbar spinal segments where the spine has the

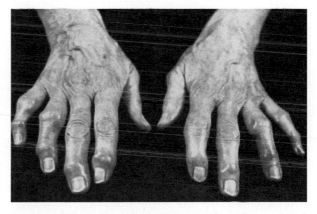

Figure 4-20. Bony enlargement can be seen in distal and proximal interphalangeal joints. The changes in proximal interphalangeal joints (Bouchard's nodes) and distal interphalangeal joints (Heberden's nodes) are common findings in degenerative joint disease of the hands. (Reprinted from the Clinical Slide Collection on the Rheumatic Diseases, © 1991, by permission from the American College of Rheumatology.) See color plate 3.

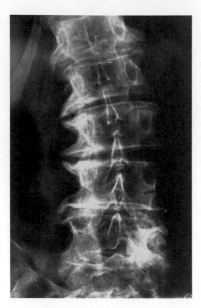

Figure 4-21. This anteroposterior projection of the lumbar spine shows scoliosis and narrowing of the intervertebral spaces on the concave side where extensive osteophyte formation is present. Adjacent bony margins are sclerosed. The zygapophyseal articulations are not well demonstrated, but show narrowing and sclerosis, particularly on the concave aspect of the spine. (Reprinted from the Clinical Slide Collection on the Rheumatic Diseases, © 1991, by permission from the American College of Rheumatology.)

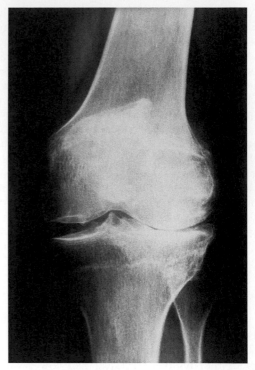

Figure 4-22. Osteoarthritis of the knee (x-ray film). Posterolateral view showing lateral joint space narrowing with sclerosis of the adjacent joint margins. (Reprinted from the Clinical Slide Collection on the Rheumatic Diseases, © 1972, by permission from the American College of Rheumatology.)

greatest curvature and is most mobile. Degenerative changes occur in both the apophyseal joints and intervertebral discs (Figure 4-21). The apophyseal joints are also synovium-lined joints and are subject to development of OA. This is a potential cause of neck or back pain and stiffness. In addition, marginal osteophytes may extend into the adjacent neural foramina, resulting in pressure on the nerve root. These patients present with radicular pain and may have signs of a root lesion with numbness, weakness, and loss of tendon reflexes. Similar manifestations can occur as a result of a lateral disc protrusion. Intervertebral disc degeneration results in loss in height of the disc space, malalignment of the spine, causing increased mechanical stress on the apophyseal joints.

Investigations

Unlike the inflammatory arthropathies, primary OA is not associated with any laboratory abnormalities. In most instances an x-ray film of the involved joint is necessary to confirm the diagnosis and to help assess the stage and severity of the disease. Evidence of loss or narrowing of the joint space is essential for a diagnosis of OA (Figure 4-22). Other characteristic radiological findings are the presence of marginal osteophytes, subchondral cysts, and sclerosis of the subchondral bone. In advanced disease there is complete loss of joint space and remodeling of the bone ends.

> Symptoms of inflammatory disease of the spine are often worse after immobility and are improved by exercise. In contrast, symptoms of degenerative disease are usually directly related to exertion.

General Management

Patient education plays a major role in the management of OA. With hand involvement, it is important to reassure patients that this condition, while progressive, rarely leads to severe disability and handicap. Patients need to be informed of the fact that overuse of a damaged joint will result in more severe pain. They need to pace themselves and avoid overactivity. The use of assistive devices will reduce forces, especially on damaged weight-bearing joints. The difficulty with canes, however, is getting patients to accept them; unfortunately vanity often prevails. For the same reason, weight reduction is strongly advised for obese patients and may help reduce symptoms and improve function in OA of the hip and knee. Referral to a dietitian may be necessary, especially for morbidly obese patients. Physical therapy plays an important role in restoring or maintaining range of movement, muscle bulk and strength, and function (see also Chapter 11).

Medical Management

Analgesic drugs play an important role in the management of pain in OA. Acetaminophen taken intermittently or on a regular basis is often effective and is more desirable than NSAIDs in elderly patients with concurrent illnesses if potential toxicity to the latter is a major concern. However there is evidence that NSAIDs are more effective than acetaminophen in the treatment of OA.[21] Toxicity can be minimized by use of the lowest effective dose, the preferential use of COX-2 inhibitors, or the use of misoprostol or proton pump inhibitors concurrently with older NSAIDs. Nevertheless NSAIDs, including the COX-2 inhibitors, need to be avoided in patients with heart failure, poorly controlled hypertension, renal disease, and history of a bleeding gastric or duodenal ulcer.

The use of over-the-counter medications, such as glucosamine and chondroitin sulfate, has become very popular in the treatment of musculoskeletal pain including that of OA. Although many patients claim benefit from these treatments, there is no convincing evidence, based on controlled clinical trials, that they are more effective than placebo. A sound scientific basis for their use is lacking.

Intra-articular (IA) corticosteroid injections may provide significant relief of symptoms from individual joints for brief periods. The response, however, is quite variable and unpredictable. IA corticosteroid injections may be useful for providing short-term relief for patients waiting for an arthroplasty, for those in whom arthroplasty is contraindicated, and to control acute inflammation such as that caused by pseudo-gout.

The term *viscosupplementation* has been given to a procedure involving the IA injection of sodium hyaluronate (HA). In OA, the concentration of HA in synovial fluid is diminished with a reduction in molecular weight and compromise of its homeostatic properties. HA is used to restore the normal rheological properties of synovial fluid in OA. The use and mode of action of HA remain controversial, but the procedure does appear to be beneficial in temporarily relieving pain in some patients with OA of mild to moderate severity.[25]

Arthroplasty with total joint replacement is indicated in patients with severe OA of the hip and knee. The indication for joint replacement is the presence of severe pain, usually occurring at rest as well as during activity and resulting in marked limitation of function and adverse effects on quality of life. The outcome of total hip and knee replacement is generally excellent with relief of pain and restoration of function. Infection and loosening of the prosthesis are the main long-term complications. See also Chapter 7 for further details on joint replacements.

> **Weight loss is important in reducing pain in weight-bearing joints; a referral to a dietitian is part of management.**

Crystal-Induced Arthritis (Gout)

Gout is an acute inflammatory condition occurring in response to the formation of monosodium urate monohydrate (uric acid) crystals due to hyperuricemia. Uric acid is an end product of purine metabolism and is normally excreted through the kidneys and gastrointestinal tract. Hyperuricemia occurs as a result of either overproduction of uric acid or reduced renal clearance. Secondary causes include renal failure and hematological malignancies, especially after chemotherapy. Rarely, hyperuricemia may be due to inherited abnormalities affecting the enzymes responsible for the breakdown of purines and formation of uric acid.

Not all patients with hyperuricemia develop gout; approximately 10% of the population have asymptomatic hyperuricemia. Gouty arthritis occurs as a result of uric acid crystals forming within a joint. In the long term, deposition of uric acid may also occur in soft tissues to form tophi, in bones resulting in a destructive arthropathy, and in the kidney with the formation of stones and renal damage.

Gout occurs more commonly in males with peak age at 40 to 50 years. It is uncommon in children, unless there is an inherited enzyme abnormality, and in premenopausal women. There is a common association with obesity, hypertension, lipid abnormalities, heavy alcohol intake, and diuretic use.

Gouty arthritis most often affects the first MTP joint, heels, ankles, and knees, usually presenting as a monoarthritis. An attack of gout is quite characteristic with a rapid onset and associated redness and swelling of the joint. The pain is usually excruciating, with the patient being unable to walk or tolerate touching of the involved joint. Fever and chills may occur, raising the possibility of septic arthritis in the differential diagnosis.

A diagnosis of gout is usually made on clinical grounds, but joint aspiration and synovial fluid analysis should be carried out if infection is suspected. The presence in the synovial fluid of negatively birefringent needle-shaped crystals identified on polarized microscopic examination is diagnostic of gout (Figure 4-23). In older patients, a similar arthritis, known as pseudo-gout, is due to the release of calcium pyrophosphate dihydrate or calcium apatite crystals from deposits in articular cartilage.

NSAIDs are the treatment of choice for acute gouty arthritis. An attack will resolve within days to 1 or 2 weeks, depending on how promptly treatment is initiated. Colchicine is now seldom used, except in low doses for prophylactic purposes, because its efficacy in acute gout is less predictable and it is often associated with side effects. An IA corticosteroid injection is very effective and is particularly applicable postoperatively for patients who have not yet resumed eating. Patients having frequent attacks of gout, especially those with a history of renal stones or tophi, should be treated with allopurinol to normalize the serum uric acid level. This will prevent or reduce the occurrence of further attacks of joint inflammation, as well as lead to the gradual resorption of uric acid deposits from various tissues. Allopurinol inhibits the enzyme xanthine oxidase and thereby reducing the production of uric acid.

Rheumatic Diseases in Childhood

Juvenile rheumatoid arthritis (JRA), referred to as juvenile chronic arthritis (or juvenile idiopathic arthritis) in Europe, comprises a heterogeneous group of systemic inflammatory disorders affecting children younger than the age of 16 years. The prevalence of JRA according to population studies in the United States is between 57 and 113 cases per 100,000

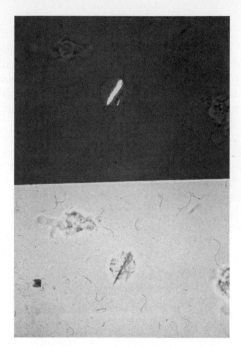

Figure 4-23. This photograph shows monosodium urate crystals that have been phagocytosed by a polymorphonuclear leukocyte in the joint fluid during an acute attack of gout. In the *top section,* compensated polarized light microscopy clearly demonstrates two longer crystals (~13 µm) and one shorter crystal (~9 µm). The *bottom section* shows the same field under ordinary light microscopy. The top section is diagnostic and the bottom section is not. Here only one of the longer crystals is identifiable. (Reprinted from the Clinical Slide Collection on the Rheumatic Diseases, © 1991, by permission from the American College of Rheumatology.) See color plate 3.

children.[26] Although considerably less common than arthritis in adults, JRA is a major cause of childhood disability. Overall, girls are more often affected than boys, but sex and age ratios vary between the different subtypes of JRA. JRA may develop at any age during childhood.

Three major subsets of JRA have been defined on the basis of clinical features at presentation of the disease with prognostic implications. Although family members are seldom affected, JRA is associated with a marked increase in the frequency of HLA-A2 and specifically of the HLA-DR, -DQ and -DP genotypes.[27] These correlate with the type of onset and course, indicating a genetic influence on disease expression.

Classification

Pauciarticular Onset (Oligoarthritis)

In this subset, four or fewer joints are involved. This is the most common form of JRA, accounting for about 60% of all occurrences. Mostly presenting before the age of 5 years, it occurs more often in females. These children seldom complain of pain and usually have a limp. The knee is the joint involved most often, followed by the ankle.

Antinuclear antibodies (ANAs) are found in up to 75% of patients, and there is a strong association with the occurrence of chronic anterior uveitis. This eye manifestation is often asymptomatic and an annual ophthalmological examination is essential because if the uveitis is untreated, it may result in loss of vision. Some patients in this subgroup will develop psoriasis later in life whereas in others (mainly boys) the condition will evolve into ankylosing spondylitis (AS) during or after adolescence. The prognosis for patients with pauciarticular disease is usually excellent. Because of the limited number of joints involved, major functional disability is uncommon. Active joint inflammation however, may continue for many years.

Polyarticular Onset

Approximately 30% of children with JRA have a polyarticular onset with five or more joints involved. This subset is further divided into those who are positive for rheumatoid factor (RF) and those who are negative. The RF-negative subset of the disease occurs throughout childhood and mainly affects the knees, wrists, and ankles in a symmetrical pattern. RF-positive polyarticular onset JRA has a more aggressive course, resembling RA of adult onset. Most patients are females, presenting between the ages 12 and 16 years.

The typical pattern is a symmetrical involvement of the small joints of the hands and feet. Unlike in adult-onset RA, the DIP joints are commonly affected. Flexor tenosynovitis is common. Subcutaneous nodules and other extra-articular manifestations seen in adult RA may occur. Prognosis is less favorable than that for pauciarticular onset disease and nearly one half of these children will still have active disease 10 or more years after onset.

Systemic Onset

About 10% of children with JRA have a systemic onset. This subset is characterized by the occurrence of a high spiking fever, which in combination with a salmon-pink rash over the upper trunk and proximal extremities is virtually diagnostic of the disease. In addition to arthritis, prominent visceral involvement with lymphadenopathy, hepatosplenomegaly and pericarditis may be present. About 50% of these children will recover completely, especially if there is pauciarticular involvement. In the remainder the disease will have a progressive course with variable loss of function.

Radiology

Apart from erosions, joint space narrowing, and atlantoaxial subluxation, other radiological changes are seen with JRA and distinguish it from adult RA. Premature epiphyseal closure results in stunted bone growth, whereas stimulation of the epiphysis by local inflammation leads to bony overgrowth. These changes are commonly seen in the metacarpals and vertebral bodies. Periostitis may result in widening of the phalanges, and joint fusion may be seen, most commonly affecting the upper cervical apophyseal joints.

Management

A coordinated, multidisciplinary team approach involving a pediatric rheumatologist, social worker, physical therapist, occupational therapist, and, if necessary, a specialized orthopedic surgeon is important from the onset of JRA. Education of the child and family plays an extremely important role. The simplest, safest and most conservative measures should be the first applied. Aspirin and other NSAIDs are used initially, together with physical measures to control pain and restore motion and function. Splints are a useful adjunct to prevent or correct joint deformities. Detail of rehabilitation management is given in Chapter 8. See also Chapter 14.

If the disease does not respond adequately to conservative management, DMARDs of the categories used in adult RA are added. Currently methotrexate is the drug of choice because of its efficacy in low doses. As in the management of adult RA, intraarticular (IA) corticosteroid injections may be indicated when one or two joints fail to respond to systemic treatment. Oral corticosteroids are avoided unless there is uncontrolled systemic disease with severe disability because of the risk of growth retardation.

The long-term outcome for patients with JRA is quite variable. A study from Taplow (United Kingdom) showed that after 15 years of follow-up, 83% of children were working or had normal function but 22% had severe functional impairment.[28] In the Cincinnati study, however, 45% still had active disease after 15 to 20 years.[29] For this group, it is important to consider the development of transition clinics to facilitate the passage from a pediatric setting to adult rheumatology care. It is important to keep in mind that residual pain and dysfunction may persist even though the arthritis is no longer active.

Connective Tissue Diseases

Systemic Lupus Erythematosus

SLE is a systemic inflammatory disorder with multiorgan involvement that is associated with the presence of autoantibodies. The etiology of SLE is unknown, but genetic factors play an important role, with a much higher frequency among first-degree relatives of patients with the disease. SLE occurs more often in females, with a female-to-male ratio of 5:1 and a peak incidence between the ages of 15 and 40 years. The prevalence is about 1 per 2000.[30] Recent studies suggest that the prognosis for patients with SLE has improved steadily over the last 30 years. In the earlier studies, 50% of patients died within 6 months of diagnosis. In more recent series, 95% are functioning normally 10 years after diagnosis. It is not certain whether this change is related to improvements in treatment or to the early diagnosis of milder cases of the disease.

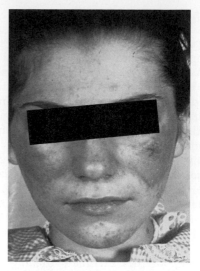

Figure 4-24. Malar rash in a patient with systemic lupus erythematosus. The rash consists primarily of erythema on the malar and chin areas. This type of lesion is suggestive but not diagnostic of systemic lupus erythematosus. (Reprinted from the Clinical Slide Collection on the Rheumatic Diseases, © 1991, by permission from the American College of Rheumatology.) See color plate 4.

Pathology

The pathological abnormalities in SLE are seen throughout the body and consist of inflammation, vasculitis, and immune complex deposition.[31,32] Active skin involvement is characterized by damage in the zone between the epidermis and dermis. Liquefaction or vacuolar necrosis of the basal layer of the epidermis occurs and is associated with the deposition of immune complexes. Other cutaneous changes include epidermal atrophy, hyperkeratosis, perifollicular and perivascular dermal inflammation, dermal edema, fibrosis, and loss of skin appendages.

Renal abnormalities are seen in most patients who have a kidney biopsy. The pathological findings include cellular and matrix proliferation, inflammation, basement membrane thickening, and immune complex deposition. The glomeruli are most prominently affected. Grading schemes have been devised based upon the extent of the proliferative changes within the glomeruli, alterations in the basement membrane, and evidence of disease activity and chronicity (damage). These classifications are useful in the assessment of disease severity and in predicting outcome. Advanced renal disease is characterized by the presence of small, atrophic, and scarred kidneys.

Clinical Presentation

SLE is a systemic disorder, and the clinical presentation varies considerably between patients, depending on which organs are involved. Active disease is often associated with constitutional manifestations such as fever, fatigue, anorexia, and weight loss. A diagnosis of SLE is usually based on evidence of multiorgan involvement, with the presence of antinuclear antibodies (ANAs) in the serum. Although diagnostic criteria have been developed, their application is mainly for research purposes.

Disease Manifestations

Skin and Mucous Membrane The skin rash of SLE is quite varied and is often brought on by exposure to sunlight. The classical skin lesion in SLE is the butterfly rash (Figure 4-24), which is seen on both cheeks and across the bridge of the nose. In some patients, the rash may extend onto sun-exposed areas such as the upper chest (in a V-shaped distribution) and arms. Discoid lesions typically heal with scarring and can occur in the absence of systemic manifestations (discoid lupus). Subacute cutaneous lupus erythematosus is a relatively distinct skin lesion, which does not scar but is exacerbating and remitting. Alopecia is common and can be diffuse or patchy. Mucous membrane lesions include oral, nasal, and vaginal ulcers; along with alopecia they tend to recur with active disease. Lesions due to vasculitis include purpura and ulceration, depending on the size of blood vessels affected.

Musculoskeletal   Arthralgias are common in SLE. A polyarthritis, often resembling RA in appearance, can occur but has a more benign course and does not result in erosions. Rarely, the typical hand deformities of RA develop due to tendon and ligament damage, a condition known as Jaccoud's arthropathy. In contrast to the deformities found in RA, those seen in SLE are usually completely reducible. A myositis resembling polymyositis and resulting in proximal muscle weakness is sometimes seen.

Cardiac and Pulmonary   A number of pulmonary manifestations are seen in SLE including pleurisy, pulmonary emboli, pulmonary hypertension, interstitial lung disease, pneumonitis, and pulmonary hemorrhage. In most instances the presenting symptom is dyspnea or chest pain. In the patient presenting with a fever and pulmonary manifestations, infection should be seriously considered in the differential diagnosis.

Chest pain and dyspnea also can be due to involvement of the heart. Pericarditis is not uncommon. Heart failure and arrhythmias may occur rarely as a result of myocarditis. The endothelium may be involved with the formation of sterile vegetations on heart valves (Libman-Sacks endocarditis). Coronary vasculitis is uncommon, but patients with SLE often have accelerated atherosclerosis and early onset ischemic heart disease.

Vascular   Inflammation of small blood vessels (leukocytoclastic vasculitis) usually results in palpable purpura. Involvement of larger vessels has potentially more serious implications, depending on the location of the lesions. Manifestations include skin ulceration, mononeuritis, bowel infarction, or gastrointestinal bleeding.

Gastrointestinal   Gastrointestinal manifestations are common and patients may present with nausea, vomiting, abdominal pain, or diarrhea. The causes are varied and include diffuse (nonseptic) peritonitis, bowel inflammation (colitis), pancreatitis, and vasculitis. Vasculitic involvement of the mesenteric arteries may result in infarction of the bowel with perforation or hemorrhage. Hepatitis occurs rarely.

Renal   Renal involvement in SLE has important implications in that it is a marker of more severe disease and reduced survival. It is detected by urinalysis, demonstrating the presence of proteinuria, microscopic hematuria, and cellular casts. When involvement is severe, the serum creatinine and urea levels may be elevated, indicating organ failure. Clinical evidence of lupus nephritis rarely occurs unless the patient develops severe nephrotic syndrome with peripheral edema or hypertension. A renal biopsy may be needed to ascertain the type and severity of the nephritis.

Neuropsychiatric   Central nervous system (CNS) involvement in SLE is common and has adverse prognostic implications. The presentation is quite variable, and manifestations include headaches, seizures, strokes, cranial and peripheral neuropathies, depression, organic brain syndrome, and psychosis.

Laboratory Findings

The characteristic laboratory finding in SLE is the presence of ANAs. The ANA test is positive in 95% of patients with SLE, and it is a useful screening test for the disease. However the test is very nonspecific, and results can be positive in numerous other clinical situations. Antibodies may be produced against a number of nuclear proteins (antigens). Some of these, anti-Sm and anti-dsDNA, are highly specific for SLE and their presence can be of diagnostic value. Furthermore the presence of high levels of anti-dsDNA antibodies usually correlates with the presence of active lupus nephritis. In this situation, there is deposition of immune complexes with complement consumption, resulting in decreased C3, C4, and CH50 levels in the serum. Both the elevated anti-dsDNA antibody levels and decreased levels of complement components will return to normal with remission of the disease.

Hematological abnormalities in SLE consist of leukopenia, thrombocytopenia, anemia, or pancytopenia. The anemia may be immune mediated and hemolytic in type with positive Coombs test. Other laboratory abnormalities include hypergammaglobulinemia, a false-positive test for syphilis, and raised ESR.

The presence of a raised activated partial thromboplastin time (APPT) may indicate the presence of a circulating anticoagulant. This, along with the presence of anticardiolipin antibodies in the serum, occurs with the antiphospholipid syndrome. The latter may be associated with SLE and results in recurrent spontaneous abortions and an increased risk of both venous and arterial thrombosis.

Management

Patient education has an important role in the management of SLE. The patient should recognize that the disease often has a fluctuating course and may require treatment continued over many years. The disease often enters periods of remission, sometimes lasting for several years, during which patients may be free of all symptoms.

The drug treatment required for SLE will depend on the activity and severity of the disease. With milder forms of SLE symptomatic treatment may be sufficient. For arthralgias and arthritis, the use of NSAIDs is the primary treatment. The antimalarial drugs (chloroquine and hydroxychloroquine) are very useful for controlling mild disease, especially for arthritis and skin manifestations that are not adequately controlled with more conservative treatment.

Corticosteroids are very effective in the treatment of SLE, but their long-term use is limited by significant side effects. Short-term, low-dose prednisone (10 to 20 mg daily) is used for the control of severe, disabling constitutional manifestations (such as fevers and fatigue), pleuritis, and pericarditis. Severe organ involvement or life-threatening manifestations such as lupus nephritis, CNS disease, and myositis require high-dose corticosteroid therapy (prednisone 1 mg/kg/day) of sufficient duration to control the disease, followed by a slow reduction in dose. An immunosuppressive drug such as azathioprine or methotrexate is added if the maintenance dose of corticosteroids needed to control the disease is unacceptably high. Oral or pulse intravenous administration of cyclophosphamide is indicated when severe renal or CNS disease cannot be controlled with high-dose corticosteroid therapy. (See also Chapter 6.)

Systemic Sclerosis (Scleroderma)

Systemic sclerosis (SSc) is a systemic disorder of uncertain etiology, characterized by the presence of inflammation, fibrosis, and a vasculopathy involving small blood vessels. The main pathological abnormality is excess production of collagen by fibroblasts, resulting in skin thickening and similar fibrotic changes of other organs. Although the cause is unknown, evidence points to an underlying genetic susceptibility with precipitation of the disease by environmental factors. Prolonged exposure to silica dust and industrial solvents such as trichloroethylene is known to induce the disease in predisposed persons. SSc is relatively uncommon with an incidence of between 5 and 15 cases per 1 million population. The female-to-male ratio is about 3:1.[33]

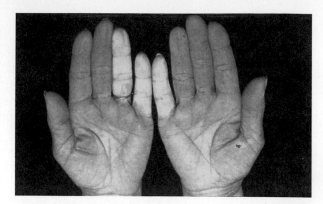

Figure 4-25. The marked pallor of the fourth and fifth digits of the left hand and of the fifth digit of the right hand is characteristic of Raynaud's phenomenon. (Reprinted from the Clinical Slide Collection on the Rheumatic Diseases, © 1991, by permission from the American College of Rheumatology.) See color plate 4.

Clinical Features

Raynaud's phenomenon is the most common presenting symptom, with episodes of pallor or cyanosis involving the fingers and toes after cold exposure (Figure 4-25). On rewarming, the digits often become red or flushed. When severe, Raynaud's phenomenon may lead to painful ischemic ulcers or gangrene.

Skin thickening is the most characteristic feature of SSc and first appears in the hands and feet, spreading proximally as the disease progresses. The involved skin is tight and tethered to the underlying tissues. This results in restricted movement and function. Mouth opening is often reduced and flexion contractures often develop, particularly in the hands, elbows, and knees (Figure 4-26). Other skin manifestations include telangiectasia (damaged, dilated small blood vessels) seen on the face, lips, chest, and hands and calcinosis (deposits of calcium salts in the subcutaneous tissues).

The gastrointestinal tract is invariably involved. Fibrosis is associated with atrophy of the smooth muscle in the gut wall, resulting in dysmotility. Dysphagia and heartburn occur early in the disease and may be followed by constipation, pseudo-obstruction, small bowel bacterial overgrowth, and malabsorption. An erosive arthritis and myositis involving proximal muscles may occur. Involvement of the heart, lungs, and kidneys has important prognostic implications with reduced survival. The main lung manifestations are pulmonary fibrosis and

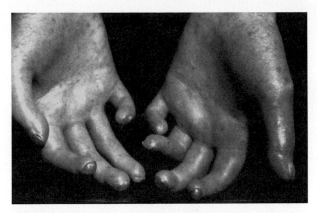

Figure 4-26. The terminal phalanges of both the second and third fingers are shortened and the nails are deformed as a result of bony resorption of the distal phalanges. Flexion contractures and a tightened indurated skin (sclerodactyly) are also shown. (Reprinted from the Clinical Slide Collection on the Rheumatic Diseases, © 1991, by permission from the American College of Rheumatology.) See color plate 4.

primary type pulmonary hypertension. Myocardial fibrosis may result in congestive heart failure and arrhythmias can lead to sudden death. The main renal manifestation is hypertensive renal crisis with malignant level hypertension and rapidly progressive kidney failure.

The extent of skin involvement separates SSc into two distinct subtypes.[34] In limited scleroderma the skin thickening is confined to the face and distal extremities (below the elbows and knees). This subset is associated with the presence of anticentromere antibodies; less severe heart, lung, and renal involvement; and more favorable prognosis. In diffuse scleroderma, the skin thickening spreads proximal to the elbows and knees, often with trunk involvement. These patients have a greater risk of developing severe pulmonary fibrosis, hypertensive renal crisis, and cardiac manifestations. This form of SSc is associated with the presence of antitopoisomerase-1 (anti-Scl 70) antibodies and a poorer prognosis.

Management

The treatment of scleroderma is mainly supportive. In the early stages, active and passive exercises of the fingers and other affected joints are important to maintain range of motion. Splinting has not been found to be helpful.

Patients with Raynaud's phenomenon need to protect themselves from cold exposure. If the manifestation is severe, vasodilators, especially calcium channel blocking agents such as nifedipine and percutaneous nitroglycerin, may help improve peripheral blood flow. Severe heartburn often requires aggressive treatment with proton pump inhibitors, alone or together with motility-enhancing agents such as domperidone.

In most patients with diffuse SSc, the disease will peak after 5 to 6 years, followed by regression and softening of the skin. Any organ damage sustained before this time, however, will be permanent. With severe, diffuse scleroderma, penicillamine and methotrexate have been used in attempts to induce an early remission (and prevent serious internal organ involvement). However these therapies have not been shown by controlled clinical studies to be more effective than placebo.

Polymyositis and Dermatomyositis

Polymyositis is an idiopathic inflammatory disease of skeletal muscle. In dermatomyositis there is involvement of the skin as well. The incidence has been estimated to be between 2 and 10 cases per 1 million persons.[35]

Clinical Features

Polymyositis is characterized by symmetrical weakness of the proximal muscles, affecting particularly the shoulder and pelvic girdles. In severe disease more distal limb muscles and the upper esophagus may be involved. The latter results in dysphagia and increased risk of aspiration. Onset is usually gradual with difficulty raising the arms, climbing stairs, and getting up off a chair. In dermatomyositis, a similar myopathy is seen in association with characteristic skin lesions on the face and hands. Periorbital edema occurs with a violaceous discoloration of the upper eyelids. Slightly raised or flat erythematous plaques over the MCP and PIP joints are known as Gottron's papules. Other disease manifestations include arthritis, Raynaud's phenomenon, calcinosis, pulmonary fibrosis, and myocarditis, which may result in cardiac failure or arrhythmias. Dermatomyositis may be associated with cancer, particularly in older patients,

Laboratory Abnormalities

In active myosis, enzymes including creatine kinase, aldolase, transaminases, and lactic dehydrogenase leak from the damaged muscles, resulting in elevated serum levels. Electromyography demonstrates characteristic abnormalities with insertional irritability and polyphasic motor unit action potentials of low amplitude and short duration.

A muscle biopsy is necessary to confirm a diagnosis of inflammatory myopathy. The characteristic findings are the presence of a chronic inflammatory cell infiltrate, predominantly of lymphocytes, along with evidence of muscle cell necrosis and regeneration. Because of the patchy nature of the disease, muscle biopsy in an otherwise typical patient may sometimes yield normal findings.

Medical Management

High-dose oral corticosteroids (prednisone 40 to 60 mg daily) are given until there is improvement in muscle strength and the serum enzyme levels return to normal. The dose is then slowly reduced while the creatine kinase level and muscle power are closely monitored. Azathioprine or methotrexate may be added as corticosteroid-sparing agents if the dose of prednisone cannot be lowered to a safe maintenance level without flare-up of the disease. Intravenous immune gammaglobulin has been used in the treatment of resistant disease, but definitive proof of its efficacy is lacking. Inclusion body myositis is a variant of the disease with more involvement of distal muscles and is often resistant to treatment.

Fibromyalgia

Although fibromyalgia (FM) is a noninflammatory and nonarticular disorder, it has been included in this chapter because of its importance as the most common rheumatic cause of chronic diffuse musculoskeletal pain. Clinically FM is a syndrome consisting of chronic, diffuse pain with fatigue and the finding of multiple tender points at specific sites.

The etiology of FM is unknown and investigations have not revealed any consistent pathophysiological abnormalities. Some cases appear to have been precipitated by a traumatic event, infection, or surgery. Others occur together with chronic disorders associated with pain or disordered sleep such as RA, SLE, nocturnal myoclonus, and sleep apnea. There is evidence pointing to decreased cerebral blood flow in the area of the thalamus and caudate nucleus. Dysfunction of the hypothalamic-pituitary-adrenal axis, increased levels of substance P in the cerebro-spinal fluid, reduced growth hormone production, and decreased blood levels of serotonin (an important neurotransmitter) have all been described. FM in most patients has no obvious underlying cause. The majority of cases occur between the ages of 30 and 50 years. FM has been found to affect 3.4% of adult women and 0.5% of adult men in the United States.[36]

Clinical Features

Patients with FM complain of diffuse pain and stiffness, which is worse on arising in the morning. Although the pain is diffuse, it is usually most prominent in the neck, low back, and respective girdle areas. FM is characteristically associated with disturbed sleep. Patients with FM sleep very lightly and are easily aroused. Waking often during the night is usual, and patients will invariably waken in the morning feeling nonrefreshed and experience chronic fatigue during the day. Both pain and fatigue are aggravated by physical activity, emotional stress, and changes in the weather. Other problems commonly seen with FM include headaches, poor concentration and memory (cognitive dysfunction), paresthesias in the upper limbs, nocturia (irritable bladder), dry eyes and mouth, and irritable bowel syndrome.

On physical examination patients with FM generally appear healthy. The characteristic finding is the presence of diffuse soft tissue tenderness in a symmetrical distribution. Tenderness is most prominent at defined focal anatomic points (Figure 4-27). These tender points are considered to be positive when pain is elicited by applying pressure either by firm palpation or using a dolorimeter (with 4 kg of force). Classification criteria, proposed by the American College of Rheumatology, consist of widespread pain together with tenderness of at least 11 of the 18 specific tender points.[37] Certain sites such as the heel

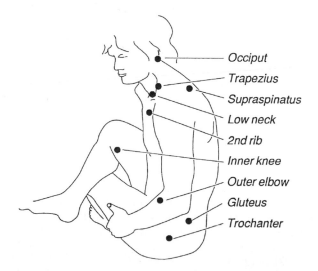

Figure 4-27. The tender points in fibromyalgia (American College of Rheumatology criteria); possible total of 18 points bilaterally. (Courtesy Dr. H.A. Smythe.)

pads and midforehead are usually not tender in FM and are utilized as control points.

Laboratory investigations are normal in primary FM. However, blood tests are usually ordered to help rule out secondary causes. Approximately one third of patients with FM will have an abnormal electro-encephalogram (EEG) with alpha wave intrusion superimposed upon the normal delta wave pattern. These abnormalities are thought to be related to the sleep disturbance, which is a consistent feature of FM. However, the EEG is normal in the majority.

Treatment

Successful treatment of FM depends on a comprehensive program, ideally utilizing the resources of a multidisciplinary team consisting of a rheumatologist, a physiotherapist, a psychologist, and a social worker.

Drug therapy in FM is focused on pain relief and regulation of the sleep disturbance. Unfortunately pharmacotherapy alone has not been successful in the management of FM. NSAIDs and simple analgesics such as acetaminophen have not been shown to be helpful. Narcotic analgesics are to be avoided because of potential addiction. The use of tricyclic anti-depressants such as amitriptyline at a low dose (10 to 25 mg) and muscle relaxants (cyclobenzaprine 10 mg) taken early in the evening may improve sleep but has been shown to be helpful in only about 30% of patients for short periods. Side effects, especially drowsiness, further limit their use. FM is often associated with anxiety and depression, and these problems need to be treated in conjunction.

Several studies have demonstrated the effectiveness of aerobic exercises in reducing pain and improving the level of function in FM.[38,39] The difficulty is in getting patients sufficiently motivated to get involved. The usual excuse is that they are in pain or too tired, and physical activity only makes them feel worse. Much encouragement is needed for them not only to become more active physically but also to learn to pace their activities to avoid exhaustion and aggravation of pain. At the beginning, a little exercise often is more productive than a lot at one time. Walking is an excellent activity as are aquatic exercises in a warm pool. Working out in a group may help induce motivation. Cognitive behavior therapy is becoming popular, and evidence indicates that patients with FM benefit by developing better coping skills and reducing pain behavior (see also Chapter 12 and Chapter 15).

FM is a major cause of physical disability with 30% or more of patients being unable to work and 25% or more receiving disability pensions. FM is a chronic condition, and complete remissions are rare.

However, a 10-year prospective study showed that at the end of the follow-up period, 66% of patients reported that they were "a little" to "a lot" better than when FM was first diagnosed.[40] The most favorable prognosis is for younger women with milder disease and for children.

References

1. Lawrence RC: Rheumatoid arthritis: classification and epidemiology. In Klippel JH, Dieppe PA (eds): Rheumatology. London, Mosby Year-Book, 1994, pp 3.1–4.
2. Winchester R: The molecular basis of susceptibility to rheumatoid arthritis. Adv Immunol 56:389–466, 1994.
3. Firestein GS: Etiology and pathogenesis of rheumatoid arthritis. In Ruddy S, Harris E Jr, Sledge CB (eds): Kelley's Textbook of Rheumatology, ed 6. ch 64, Philadelphia, WB Saunders, 2001.
4. Short CL, Bauer W, Reynolds WE: Rheumatoid Arthritis. Cambridge, Harvard University Press, 1957.
5. Van Zeben D, Hazes JM, Zwinderman AH et al: Association of HLA-DR4 with a more progressive disease course in patients with rheumatoid arthritis: results of a follow-up study. Arthritis Rheum 34:822–830, 1991.
6. Yelin E, Meenan R, Nevitt M et al: Work disability in rheumatoid arthritis: effects of disease, social and work factors. Ann Intern Med 93:551–556, 1980.
7. Brook A, Corbett M: Radiographic changes in early rheumatoid arthritis. Ann Rheum Dis 36:71–73, 1977.
8. Wolfe F, Mitchell DM, Sibley JT et al: The mortality of rheumatoid arthritis. Arthritis Rheum 37:481–494, 1994.
9. Lichtenstein DR, Syngal S, Wolfe MM: Nonsteroidal antiinflammatory drugs and the gastrointestinal tract: the double-edged sword. Arthritis Rheum 38:5–18, 1995.
10. Everts B, Wahrborg P, Hedner T: COX-2 specific inhibitors: the emergence of a new class of analgesic and anti-inflammatory drugs. Clin Rheumatol 19:331–343, 2000.
11. Simon LS: Are the biologic and clinical effects of the COX-2 specific inhibitors an advance compared with the effects of traditional NSAIDs? Curr Opin Rheumatol 12:163–170, 2000.
12. Lipsky PF, van der Heijde DM, St Clair EW et al: Infliximab and methotrexate in the treatment of rheumatoid arthritis. N Engl J Med 343:1594–1602, 2000.
13. Moreland LW, Cohen SB, Baumgartner SW et al: Longterm safety and efficacy of etanercept in patients with rheumatoid arthritis. J Rheumatol 28:1238–1244, 2001.
14. Bresnihan B, Alvaro-Gracia JM, Cobby M et al: Treatment of rheumatoid arthritis with recombinant human interleukin-1 receptor antagonist. Arthritis Rheum 41:2196–2204, 1998.
15. Van der Linden S, Van der Heijde D: Ankylosing spondylitis. In Ruddy S, Harris E Jr, Sledge CB (eds): Kelley's Textbook of Rheumatology, ed 6. ch 69, Philadelphia, WB Saunders, 2001.

16. Miller MH, Lee P, Smythe HA et al: Measurement of spinal mobility in the sagittal plane: new skin contraction technique compared with established methods. *J Rheumatol* 11:507–511, 1984.

17. Yu DTY, Fan PT: Reiter's syndrome and undifferentiated spondyloarthropathy. In Ruddy S, Harris E Jr, Sledge CB (eds): *Kelley's Textbook of Rheumatology*, ed 6, ch 70. Philadelphia, WB Saunders, 2001.

18. O'Neill T, Silman AJ: Historical background and epidemiology. *Bailliere's Clin Rheumatol* 9:245–261, 1995.

19. Eastmond CJ: Psoriatic arthritis, genetics and HLA antigen. *Bailliere's Clin Rheumatol* 8:263–276, 1994.

20. Prockop DJ: Mutations in collagen genes as a cause of connective tissue disorder. *N Engl J Med* 326:540–546, 1992.

21. Peyron JG: Epidemiology and etiology approach to osteoarthritis. *Semin Arthritis Rheum* 8:288–306, 1979.

22. Acheson RM, Collart AB: New Haven survey of joint diseases. *Ann Rheum Dis* 34:379–389, 1975.

23. Mankin HJ, Brandt KD: Pathogenesis of osteoarthritis. In Ruddy S, Harris E Jr, Sledge CB (eds): *Kelley's Textbook of Rheumatology,* ed 6, ch 91. Philadelphia, WB Saunders, 2001.

24. Geba GP, Weaver AL, Polis AB et al: Efficacy of rofecoxib, celecoxib and acetaminophen in osteoarthritis of the knees: a randomized trial. *JAMA* 287:64–71, 2002.

25. Mahen E: Hyaluronan in knee osteoarthritis: a review of the clinical trials with Hyalgan. *Eur J Rheumatol Inflamm* 15:17–24, 1995.

26. Singsen BH: Rheumatic diseases of childhood. *Rheum Dis Clin North Am* 16:581–599, 1990.

27. van Kerckhove C, Luyrink L, Taylor J et al: HLA-DQA1*0101 haplotypes and disease outcome in early onset pauciarticular JRA. *J Rheumatol* 18:874–879, 1991.

28. Allen RC, Ansell BM: Juvenile chronic arthritis: clinical subgroups with particular relationship to the adult pattern of disease. *Postgrad Med J* 62:821–826, 1986.

29. Wallace CA, Levinson JE: Juvenile rheumatoid arthritis: outcome and treatment of the 1990's. *Rheum Dis Clin North Am* 17:891–905, 1991.

30. Ward MM, Pyun E, Studenski S: Long-term survival in systemic lupus erythematosus: patient characteristics associated with poorer outcome. *Arthritis Rheum* 38:274–283, 1995.

31. Boumpas DT, Austin HA, Fessler BJ et al: Systemic lupus erythematosus: emerging concepts. Part 1: Renal, neuro-psychiatric, cardiovascular, pulmonary and hematologic disease. *Ann Intern Med* 122:940–950, 1995.

32. Boumpas DT, Fessler BJ, Barlow JE et al: Systemic lupus erythematosus: emerging concepts. Part 2: Dermatologic and joint disease, the antiphospholipid antibody syndrome, pregnancy and hormonal therapy, morbidity, mortality and pathogenesis. *Ann Intern Med* 123:42–53, 1995.

33. Silman AJ, Black CM, Welsh KI: Epidemiology, demographics, and genetics. In: Clements PJ, Furst DE (eds): *Systemic Sclerosis*. Baltimore, Williams & Wilkins, 1996, pp 23–49.

34. LeRoy EC, Black C, Fleischmajer R et al: Scleroderma (systemic sclerosis): classification, subsets and pathogenesis. *J Rheumatol* 15:202–205, 1988.

35. Medsger TA, Oddis CV: Inflammatory muscle disease. In: Klippel JH, Dieppe PA (eds): *Rheumatology*. London, Mosby Year-Book Europe, 1994, pp 6.12.1–14.

36. Wolfe F, Ross K, Anderson J et al: The prevalence and characteristics of fibromyalgia in the general population. *Arthritis Rheum* 38:19–28, 1995.

37. Wolfe F, Smythe HA, Yunus MB et al: The American College of Rheumatology 1990 criteria for the classification of fibromyalgia: report of the Multicenter Criteria Committee. *Arthritis Rheum* 33:160–172, 1990.

38. Martin L, Nutting A, MacIntosh BR et al: An exercise program in the treatment of fibromyalgia. *J Rheumatol* 23:1050–1053, 1996.

39. Meiworm L, Jakob E, Walker UA et al: Patients with fibromyalgia benefit from aerobic endurance exercise. *Clin Rheumatol* 19:253–257, 2000.

40. Kennedy M, Felson DT: A prospective long-term study of fibromyalgia syndrome. *Arthritis Rheum* 39:682–685, 1996.

Plate 1

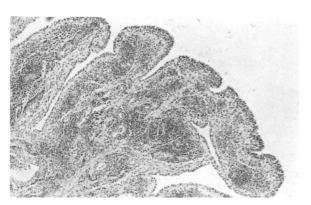

Figure 4-1. See page 51.

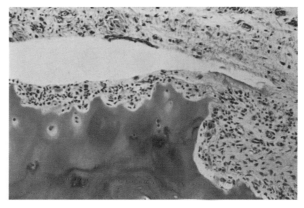

Figure 4-2. See page 52.

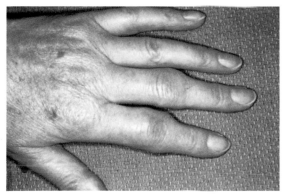

Figure 4-3. See page 52.

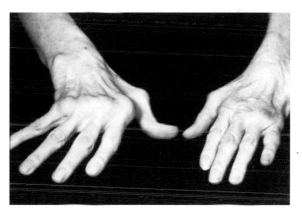

Figure 4-4. See page 53.

Plate 2

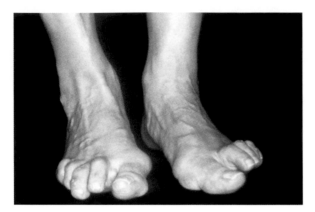

Figure 4-5. See page 53.

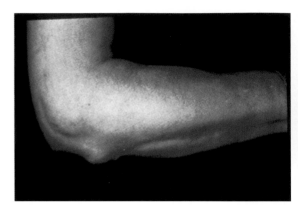

Figure 4-6. See page 53.

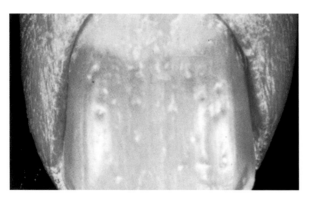

Figure 4-14. See page 64.

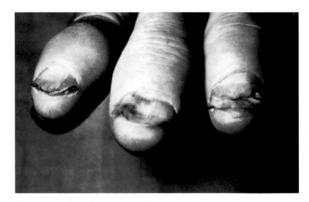

Figure 4-15. See page 64.

Plate 3

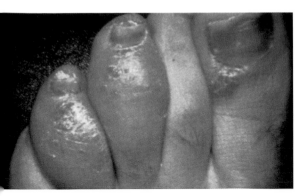

Figure 4-16. See page 64.

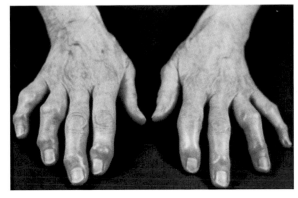

Figure 4-20. See page 67.

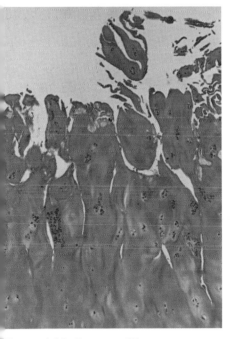

Figure 4-18. See page 66.

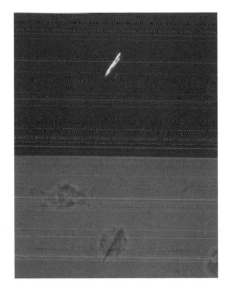

Figure 4-23. See page 70.

Plate 4

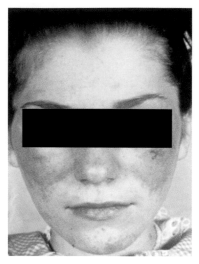

Figure 4-24. See page 72.

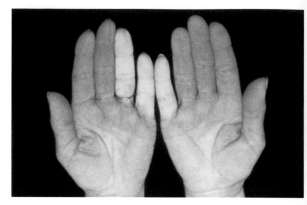

Figure 4-25. See page 74.

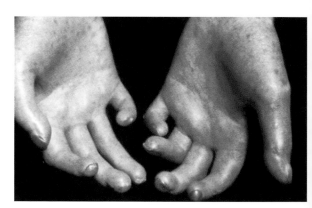

Figure 4-26. See page 75.

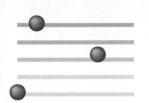

CHAPTER 5

Assessment of Joint Disease

Hugh A. Smythe, MD, FRCP(C)
Antoine Helewa, MSc(Clin Epid), PT

In this chapter a general approach to musculoskeletal diagnosis and assessment, using specific clinical skills that are not described in standard texts, is emphasized. In the rheumatic diseases the musculoskeletal assessment focuses on the evaluation of *inflammation, damage, and function.*

In the section on peripheral joint problems, the techniques needed to assess inflammation separately

from damage are discussed in detail, because anti-inflammatory and reconstructive therapies are so different. Damage is discussed in a general approach rather than a joint-by-joint description of the many possible patterns. Function is reviewed separately, because restoration of function is an important part of the treatment plan. Laboratory investigations, radiographic changes and other disease features are discussed in Chapter 4.

The section on pain amplification syndromes is important, not only because the entities are common

PHYSICAL REHABILITATION IN ARTHRITIS, Joan M. Walker, PhD, PT, and Antoine Helewa, MSc(Clin Epid), PT, Elsevier Inc. © 2004.

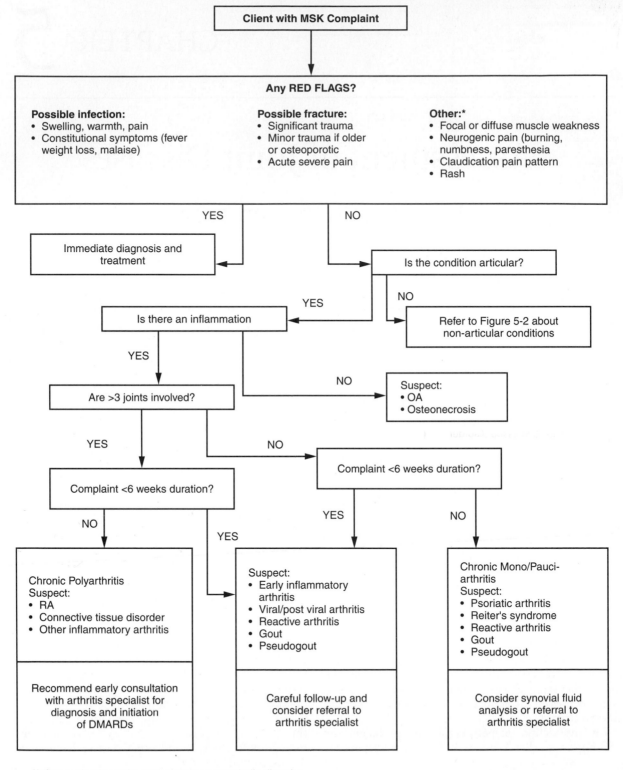

Figure 5-1. Algorithm for the initial assessment of musculoskeletal (MSK) complaints. (Adapted from *Ontario Treatment Guidelines for Osteoarthritis and Rheumatoid Arthritis and Acute Musculoskeletal Injury*. Toronto, Publications Ontario, Toronto, 2000, p 8.)

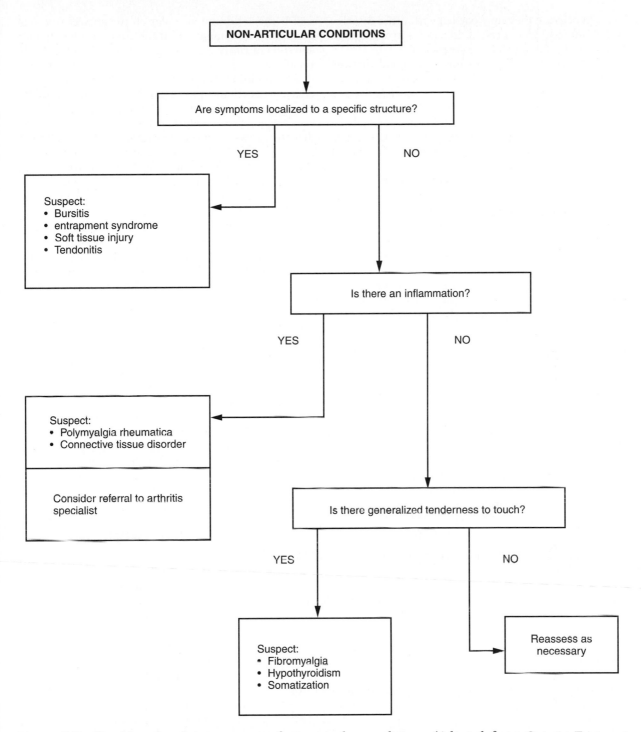

Figure 5-2. Algorithm for the assessment of nonarticular conditions. (Adapted from *Ontario Treatment Guidelines for Osteoarthritis and Rheumatoid Arthritis and Acute Musculoskeletal Injury*. Toronto, Publications Ontario, 2000, p 9.)

but also because they may coexist with other diseases and, if unrecognized, present difficulties in assessment and the risk of inappropriate treatment.

In the section on assessment of spinal disease, the phenomena associated with referred pain are described, as are the skills needed to localize the site of origin of spinal pain or restriction of movement. Different disease entities affect different parts of the spine. Therapy for the mechanical problems requires recognition of the pathogenetic forces acting at vulnerable levels.

We define a screening examination, for those with few complaints, as well as a thorough exploration for clients with more challenging problems. This examination is quickly completed when there are few findings and comprehensive when there are many. It is important to first rule out conditions or "red flags" that require immediate care. Examples are possible joint infections; trauma; and neurological, vascular, or cutaneous symptoms (Figure 5-1).[1] The examiner should then ask: Is the condition articular? If the answer is yes, is there joint inflammation? If the condition is articular and inflammatory, are more than three joints involved? Finally, are the articular symptoms acute or chronic? If the condition is nonarticular the clinician should check whether symptoms are localized to a specific structure; if there is inflammation, is tenderness to touch regional or widely distributed (Figure 5-2)?[1] The diagnostic classification of Schumacher,[2] in the *Primer on the Rheumatic Diseases,* is difficult to memorize; a simplified grouping is offered in Table 5-1, which gives a basic division into inflammatory, degenerative, metabolic, and nonarticular syndromes, and Table 5-2, which gives a subclassification of the inflammatory types. The group of seronegative forms of chronic polyarthritis associated with the antigen HLA-B27 and the common but neglected "benign polyarthritis" group are separated from the seropositive diseases because the genetic and immunological features are so different.

Table 5-1. Musculoskeletal Disorders

Inflammatory joint diseases
Traumatic, mechanical, and **degenerative** disorders
Metabolic disorders with skeletal manifestations
Nonarticular rheumatic syndromes
Miscellaneous disorders

The Rheumatological History

A client's clinical history has led to a provisional diagnosis, and the prognosis and plan of management were implicit in this label. The shortcomings of this approach are very apparent in the chronic musculoskeletal disorders. A diagnosis of rheumatoid arthritis (RA) is consistent with any prognosis from the most benign to the most severe, and the variety of treatment programs that may be appropriate is very wide.

Table 5-2. Subclassification of Inflammatory Joint Diseases

Group	Examples
1. Seropositive chronic polyarthritis (rheumatoid arthritis and variants)	Rheumatoid arthritis
	Sjögren's syndrome
2. Diffuse connective tissue disorders ("collagen") diseases	Systemic lupus erythematosus
3. Seronegative chronic polyarthritis HLA B27-associated diseases	Ankylosing spondylitis
	Reiter's syndrome
Other	Arthritis with psoriasis
4. Juvenile chronic polyarthritis group	Systemic form
	Oligoarticular form
5. Benign polyarthritis group (due to immune mechanisms)	Rheumatic fever
	Serum sickness
6. Due to infectious agents	Gonococcal arthritis
7. Associated with systemic disease	Sarcoidosis
	Hypertrophic osteoarthropathy
8. Crystal-induced synovitis	Gout
	Pseudogout

Table 5-3. Problems and Challenges Facing Clients and Care-Providers

General	Rehabilitation Specific
Uncontrolled polyarthritis	Pain, joint tenderness and effusions
Structural damage and deformity	Joint deformity and limited activities of daily living
Functional loss	Stiffness, decreased range of motion and muscle wasting
Pain amplification syndromes	Sleep disturbances, fatigue, referred pain from neck and back
Inappropriate drug therapy, nonadherence, and side effects	Lack of disease knowledge and its management
Focus on coping or passive therapies rather than on control or cure	Lack of focus on client goals
Extra-articular involvement: nodules, vasculitis, lung fibrosis, pericarditis	Decreased general health and physical fitness
Incorrect or incomplete diagnosis	Incomplete and inappropriate management plan
Exaggerated pain behavior	Inappropriate or inconsistent responses, social role conflicts

When a health professional conducts a quantitative assessment of severity, a more useful objective is the definition of the *problems* challenging the client and care provider. Table 5-3 lists these problems and challenges.

> **While you are assessing a client avoid leading questions.**

While performing the assessment, the observer is constantly making choices, influenced by the interaction of preliminary hypotheses on the nature of the client's problems and the evidence emerging from history and examination. Because each client is unique, the assessment process also will be unique. It is easy to assess the severity of inflammation unless the client has important nonarticular pain. This issue must not be ignored but may be set aside in a few moments if unsupported by the clinical evidence, or it may dominate the assessment process. The *objective of the assessment is to produce a plan of management*. Past treatment efforts are important. Often it emerges that appropriate therapy was discontinued after inadequate trials or for "side effects" not characteristic of that therapy, with decisions made without adequate evidence or advice. Thus, the chosen strategies must be followed consistently over time, with ongoing quantitative monitoring of markers of success, failure, or toxicity, with an information system understood and available to all members of the treatment team and particularly the client. Realistic goal setting and adherence to agreed-upon therapies is important, and the client should be given both full information and a high level of responsibility.

Each treatment plan is a miniature therapeutic trial, presenting difficulties comparable to those arising in controlled studies of new drugs. From these we learn the need to define in advance the duration and objectives of the trial period and to choose numerical measures of treatment effect. These measures permit subsequent decisions to be made on the basis of a quantitative and qualitative evaluation of progress.

Elements of a Rheumatological History

A rheumatological history, when followed by a physical examination of symptoms, will provide the clinician with mounting evidence relating to the nature of the client's complaints, prognosis, impact on lifestyle, and setting of treatment goals. It also helps in establishing a rapport with the client.

History of Present Illness

Ask the client for the year the disease began, which joints were involved, and whether the onset was sudden or gradual. Ask if this was a single episode, a steadily progressive condition with remissions and exacerbations, or a slowly progressive active disease. Review with the client the most recent disease activity, such as the most limiting joint problems and

Table 5-4. Positive Findings in the Review of Symptoms Relevant to Rheumatic Diseases

System/Region	Symptom/Complaint	Diagnosis to Consider
Integument	Nail pitting	Psoriatic arthritis
	Nodules	RA
	Tophi	Gout
	Photosensitivity	SLE, scleroderma
	Rashes	Vasculitis, dermatomyositis, Lyme disease, psoriatic arthritis
Head and neck	Alopecia	SLE, scleroderma
	Dysphagia	Scleroderma, polymyositis
	Dry eyes/mouth	Sjögren's syndrome
	Jaw claudication	Temporal arteritis
	Nasal ulceration	Wegener's granulomatosus, SLE
Chest	Cough	Interstitial pulmonary fibrosis
	Chest pain	Pericarditis, pleuritis, costochondritis
Abdomen	Abdominal pain	Mesenteric vasculitis, peptic ulcer
Genitourinary	Penile ulceration	Behçet's syndrome, Reiter's syndrome
	Penile/vaginal discharge	Reiter's syndrome
	Microscopic hematuria	Lupus nephritis
Neurological	Paresthesias	Carpal tunnel syndrome
	Seizures	Lupus cerebritis
	Headache	Temporal arteritis
Other	Fever	Systemic juvenile arthritis, septic arthritis, vasculitis
	Fatigue	Fibromyalgia
	Weakness	Polymyositis, dermatomyositis

From Nichols LA: History and physical assessment. In Robbins L (ed): *Clinical Care of the Rheumatic Diseases,* ed 2. Atlanta Association of Rheumatology Health Professionals, 2001.
RA = rheumatoid arthritis; SLE = systemic lupus erythematosus.

systemic or extra-articular features. Then inquire about the impact of the disease on activities of daily living and on client and family lifestyles. Ask about treatment history and any changes in treatment: these include hospitalization; drug management, systemic or local; rehabilitative management, such as pain control, exercise, joint protection, and energy conservation tools; surgical measures taken or contemplated; and psychosocial interventions.

Summarize Current Status

In one brief paragraph describe the client by age, sex, disease duration, pattern of joint involvement, systemic features, joint damage, and impact on activities of daily living (ADL). Also include the client's goals.

Systems Review

Because many rheumatic diseases are systemic in nature, a review of all body systems will help the clinician identify important diagnostic symptoms or comorbid conditions. Table 5-4 summarizes findings in a systems review relevant to the rheumatic diseases.[3]

Measures of Inflammatory Activity

A study by the Cooperating Clinics Committee of the American Rheumatism Association (ARA) identified four measures of special value in measuring activity of rheumatoid arthritis[4]; their scheme has been used in a large number of published studies. The scheme consists of the following:

- Duration of morning stiffness, measured in minutes
- Grip strength measured in millimeters of mercury (mm Hg) for right and left hands
- Number of actively inflamed joints
- Blood sedimentation rate measured in millimeters per hour (mm/hr)

In addition, the visual analogue scale (VAS) is an important measure now being used. Clients are asked to score their symptoms as a mark on a 10-cm-long line, anchored at the ends as "no pain" or "pain as bad as it can possibly be." Measuring marks on a line with a millimeter rule can be tedious, and comparable results can be obtained with a numeric intensity scale, by asking clients to put a number to their symptoms, on a 0 to 10 scale, with 10 being the worst possible.

Other measures and indices have become standard.[5] These include disability and quality of life questionnaires, such as the Health Assessment Questionnaire,[6] the second version of the Arthritis Impact Scale,[7] and clients' and observers' global assessments. Strategies for combining multiple individual measures into a single summary measure of severity or treatment outcome also have been reported.[8] More recently the SF-36 Health Status Survey, a general quality of life measure has been validated in a variety of disease groups including the rheumatic diseases.[9] These global measures and indices are generally used to measure outcomes in research studies and are not well suited to measuring change in clinical care. (See Chapter 17 and Appendix II for descriptions and discussions of these global measures.)

> **Simple quantitative measures facilitate communication among clinicians.**

Specific Clinical Techniques

Duration of Morning Stiffness, Pain, and Fatigue

To avoid leading questions, ask "How do you feel when you first get up—is that a good time or a bad time?" "Was this morning typical of the last week?" (If this morning was very unusual, settle for typical or average experience in the past week.) "What time did you get out of bed?" "Five minutes later, what were your symptoms?" For duration of morning stiffness, ask "At what time did the stiffness ease?" Then ask "altogether, for how many minutes did the morning stiffness last after you got out of bed and started moving around?" Ask specifically about pain and fatigue and score as 0 to 10 on a numeric intensity scale. Ask the client to select a number that best describes the intensity of the pain or fatigue. This scale is easy to use, is responsive enough to detect treatment effects, and can be used repeatedly over time to monitor progress.

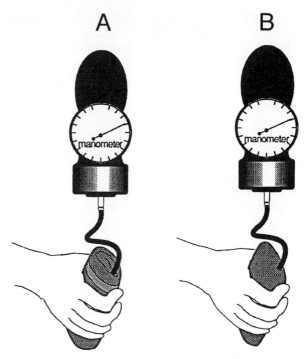

Figure 5-3. *A*, Grip strength using rolled cuff. *B*, Grip strength using a sewn bag. (Copyright H. Smythe, MD, FRCP[C].)

Grip Strength

In RA the symmetric distribution of inflammation in synovial joints of the hand and wrist can lead to a substantial reduction in grip strength due to pain on movement. However, absolute levels of grip strength may be affected by time of day, fitness, deformity, or pain of any origin, so that a single measure of grip strength is not a specific measure of inflammation. Change in grip strength, however, is quite sensitive to treatment effects.

A modified sphygmomanometer is a useful and common device to measure grip strength in RA. Roll the blood pressure cuff loosely (so that an index finger can fit inside) into a cylinder about 6 cm (2.5 inches) in diameter, and secure with two broad rubber bands, 7 × 1 cm. Inflate the system to 100 mm Hg, and then deflate it to 20 mm Hg (Figure 5-3, *A*). Encourage the client to squeeze,—*hard!*—and record the highest level reached and maintained for 3 seconds. For greater sensitivity and reproducibility, the bladder is removed from the original cuff, folded into three equal portions and sewn permanently into a special bag made of ordinary cotton material 14 × 7.5 cm (Figure 5-3, *B*).

The modified blood pressure cuff also is an excellent device for measuring isometric muscle strength in selected muscle groups (see later under "Functional Assessments"). A 20 mm Hg rise in pressure is equal to about 2 kg of force on the bag (about 5 lbs.).[10–12]

Actively Inflamed Joints

The ARA joint count[4] is a brilliant simplification that permits essential information to be gathered in minutes. Active joint inflammation is deemed to be present if *any* of the following three signs are present: *effusion, tenderness,* or *stress pain.* It is often helpful to diagram the distribution of actively inflamed joints as in Figure 5-4 and to count the total number. Rubber

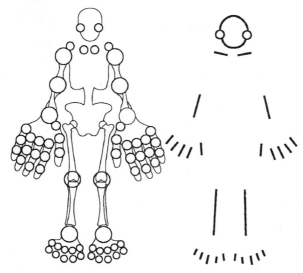

Figure 5-4. Distribution of actively inflamed joints. Provides a visual format for recording data on actively inflamed joints. (Copyright H. Smythe, MD, FRCP [C].)

stamps or printed formats are available for the more elegant drawing, but the stick figure gives comparable information. In reviewing charts over time, the visual display gives more key information than long written accounts. In a validation study, we compared the joint counts taken by four different observers: senior rheumatology fellows, rheumatologically trained physiotherapists, rotating medical residents, and non-medical independent assessors.[13] Agreement levels among the fellows and physiotherapists were significantly higher than those among rotating residents and independent assessors. Among the four types of observers, agreement in the large joints was most common. Standardization of techniques is critical for communication among clinicians. In a study of interobserver variability among six rheumatologists, variability before standardization was 13.8% and after standardization variability was reduced to 3.2%.[14] In other schemes, joints are given scores weighted according to their size or the severity of the inflammation, but the gain in sensitivity in weighted joint counts is offset by greater interobserver variation. Just as important is the ability to communicate information. A statement that there are 15 actively inflamed joints with 6 effusions is easily understood, but few can decipher the meaning of a Lansbury Index value of 56.[15]

> **The presence of excess joint fluid is so central to the recognition of inflammatory disease that effusions are often counted separately.**

Synovial Effusions

The most reliable general sign is the demonstration of *fluctuation.* Because synovial fluid lies in a closed sac,

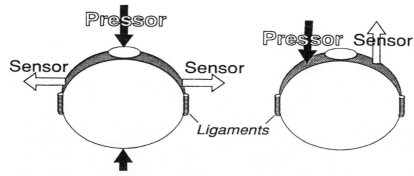

Figure 5-5. Two ways of detecting joint effusions. (Copyright H. Smythe, MD, FRCP[C].)

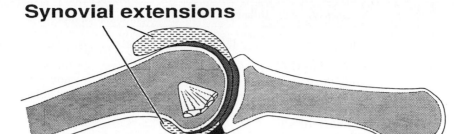

Synovial extensions

Volar Plate

Figure 5-6. Anatomy of metacarpophalangeal or metatarsophalangeal joint. Only the origin of the collateral ligament is indicated; the insertion is into the volar plate and the phalanx. (Copyright H. Smythe, MD, FRCP[C].)

compression of one portion of the sac causes the fluid to shift within the sac and adds to the distention of the sac elsewhere. If an effusion is detected, this is the most reliable sign of inflammation, and tests of joint line tenderness and stress pain are not necessary. Figure 5-5, left, illustrates the *four-finger technique* to detect fluid in an interphalangeal joint. It is relatively easy to learn, but applicable only when the joint can be surrounded. Extending the joint tightens the anterior capsule, so that the fluid moves to the extensor surface and is more readily seen and felt. The placement of the examiner's "sensor" fingers is critical. The collateral ligaments are outside the synovium and prevent the fluid from bulging. The "sensors" must be dorsal to the ligaments and proximal to the base of the middle phalanx (Figure 5-6). For most joints, the examiner must use the *two-finger technique* (Figure 5-5, right), with one finger pressing downward and the other feeling the upward lift. These techniques can be practiced on a fresh, but well-massaged, grape. The push of the pressor finger should be directed slightly away from the sensor finger to prevent a shift of periarticular fat, which gives a false impression of a fluid lift. The score is normal unless there is thoroughly convincing evidence of fluid. Expressions such as "boggy" swelling or "soft tissue" swelling indicate only uncertainty, provided perhaps by a lack of skill and an excess of fat. When fat is deposited about joints, its distribution may mimic an effusion; being fluid at body temperature, fat may fluctuate. If subcutaneous, it can be pinched up to establish that it is superficial to deep fascia. Muscle bellies also will fluctuate across the long axis of the fibers, but not parallel with them.

The *bulge* sign is a sensitive and dramatic indication of a small effusion. In the knee joint, the pouch of synovium medial to the patella is emptied of fluid by a gentle upward stroke and refilled by an upward or downward stroke on the lateral side. A similar sudden bulge can be seen over the radial head when the elbow is gently moved from midflexion to full extension.

> The most reliable sign of synovial effusion is the demonstration of fluctuation.

Specific Joint Line Tenderness

When the clinician studies articular or nonarticular tenderness, it is extremely important to work at "threshold" levels. Unlike the bulge of fluid, tenderness is usually *most marked under the collateral ligaments*. Clients with pain syndromes also may report tenderness of their joints in areas other than the collateral ligaments so the clinician must be sure to control for this. Distinctly more tenderness must be present with firmer pressure on bone or tissue adjacent or at a distance to the joint being tested.

How hard should one press to test for joint line tenderness? Enough pressure must be applied to cause blanching of the examiner's fingernail. The clinician also can determine the client's general level of tenderness by squeezing the triceps and the lower calf muscles and by pressing over the manubrium, metacarpals, and proximal phalanges. The pressure

Table 5-5. Manual Techniques to Assess Actively Inflamed Synovial Joints

Joints	Synovial Effusion	Joint Line Tenderness	Stress Pain
Temporomandibular	Place tip of forefinger anterior to external auditory meatus. As patient opens mouth, effusion fills the normal hollow in that area.	Apply pressure with tips of index and middle fingers along joint line.	Client opens and closes mouth as far as possible.
Sternoclavicular	Palpate with thumbs over both joints for swelling lateral to top of sternum.	Apply pressure with thumb over joint line lateral to top of sternum.	
Acromioclavicular		Locate a small dip at lateral end of clavicle and press with forefinger.	Client adducts arm across chest or shrugs shoulders.
Shoulder	Palpate for fullness over anterior aspect or over bicipital tendon area. Look for fullness on abduction for subacromial bursitis.		With client's arm in 60 degrees abduction, apply overpressure at the limits of passive lateral or medial rotation.
Elbow	Look for fullness or bulge on either side of olecranon process, or below lateral epicondyle. Feel for bulge on extension and rotation of forearm.	Palpate grooves with elbow at 45 degrees flexion.	Apply overpressure at limits of passive flexion and extension.
Wrist	Palpate for effusion distal to the prominence of the ulna or on its radial aspect after compression of ulnar side.	With wrist in neutral apply pressure over dorsal aspect of the joint line.	Apply overpressure at the limit of passive flexion or extension.
Metacarpophalangeal	Thumbs on dorsal aspect of joint line, press with one thumb and detect fluid shift with the other—two-finger technique.	With thumbs in the same position, apply pressure with thumbs on either side.	Hyperextend metacarpophalangeal joints passively, one at time.

Table 5-5. Manual Techniques to Assess Actively Inflamed Synovial Joints—*cont'd*

Joints	Synovial Effusion	Joint Line Tenderness	Stress Pain
Distal and proximal interphalangeal of the hand	Use four-finger fluid shifting, with thumbs and index fingers placed on palmar/dorsal aspect and side to side.	Apply pressure on over medial and lateral aspects of joint line.	Apply overpressure at the limits of passive extension or flexion.
Hip			Flex hip and knee at 90 degrees; stress joint passively at limit of rotation- medial or lateral.
Knee	Pouch of synovium medial to patella is emptied of fluid with upward stroke and refilled with a downward stroke on lateral side; look for bulge.	Apply pressure over medial and lateral aspect of knee at its joint line with knee in 60 degrees flexion.	Stress the knee at the limits of full flexion or extension.
Ankle	Look for diffuse swelling using two thumbs technique on either side of tibialis anterior and extensor hallucis tendons.	Apply pressure anteriorly at joint line with thumbs.	With knee flexed, apply pressure at the limit of passive dorsiflexion.
Subtalar			With ankle in dorsiflexion passively invert and evert the calcaneum over the talus.
Midtarsal			With ankle in dorisflexion passively invert and evert the midfoot at limit of range.
Metatarsophalangeal		Apply pressure over the joint line dorsally and distal to the metatarsal head with joint slightly flexed, for each individual joint.	Apply traction to the joint, then stress joint at the limit of passive flexion, for each individual joint.
Distal and proximal interphalangeal of the foot		Apply pressure over medial and lateral aspects of joint line.	Apply pressure at the limit of passive flexion, for each individual joint.

Table 5-6. ARA Cooperating Clinics Committee Study of Inflammatory Measures

Measures of Inflammation[†]	Percentile Grade Limits								
	10	20	30	40	50	60	70	80	90
Morning stiffness, minutes	5	30	60	75	90	120	160	220	300
Grip strength, mm Hg									
Males	250	190	160	140	125	105	90	75	55
Females	190	150	130	110	100	85	75	60	50
Number of actively inflamed joints	4	6	9	12	15	20	25	30	36
Sedimentation rate	10	20	28	35	40	50	60	70	90

Data from The Cooperating Clinics Committee of the American Rheumatism Association.[4]
*A typical patient with RA would fall in the 50th percentile and would have morning stiffness of 90 minutes, grip strength of 125 if male or 100 if female, 15 actively inflamed joints, and a sedimentation rate of 40. Similarly, a patient with severe RA would fall in the 80th percentile with morning stiffness of 220, grip strength of 75 if male and 60 if female, 30 actively inflamed joints, and a sedimentation rate of 70.

used on joints should be about 20% less than that to reach the pain threshold elsewhere. When in doubt, record the joint as inactive. The risks of overcounting are greater than those of undercounting, because error may lead to overdiagnosis, overtreatment, and unnecessary complications.

Stress Pain

Stress pain is produced when a joint at the limit of its range of movement is nudged a little further passively. This is especially useful in joints in which effusions are difficult to detect such as the shoulder (limit of medial and lateral rotation), wrists, metacarpophalangeal (MCP) joints, and joints in the ankle region. Pain *during* the arc of movement may be due to bare bone rubbing on bare bone (caused by loss of articular cartilage); it is not a reliable sign of inflammation.

The wrists and ankles include many separate synovial spaces, but each is treated as one. The neck and hips are not tested, because it requires skill and time to determine whether pain in these regions is truly inflammatory in origin. Simpler schemes with even fewer joints have been used. Joint count techniques are described in greater detail in Table 5-5.

Relative Severity

In the ARA Cooperating Clinics Committee study,[4] four measures of inflammatory activity were assessed in 499 clients with peripheral RA. For each measure, the findings were divided into 10 grades of relative severity as shown in Table 5-6. A typical male client

had about 90 minutes of morning stiffness, a grip strength of about 125 mm Hg, 15 actively inflamed joints, and an erythrocyte sedimentation rate (ESR) of about 40 mm/hr. Clients with mild disease had values in the first few columns, and those with very active arthritis would fit in the right-hand side of the table.

The observations were repeated for the same clients 1 week later, without treatment change. Whereas variation of a measure into adjacent grades was common (about 30%), change of more than two grades or more occurred uncommonly (about 5% of clients). Thus, if major changes are observed, these probably reflect real changes in the client's condition and not chance variation.

Composite Indices

The relative severity indicated by any one measure rarely agrees exactly with others (otherwise only one would be needed). In older clients, for example, the ESR tends to be high and may not reflect a changing clinical state. Grip strength is one of the most repeatable and sensitive measures, but it may be affected markedly by age and established deformities. Schemes have been developed to combine separate observations into a single numerical index. Lansbury described both an Articular Index,[15] which gave extra weight to large or more severely involved joints, and an disease Activity Index.[7] The Articular Index was combined with measures of grip strength, morning stiffness, ESR, duration to fatigue, and the need for acetylsalicylic acid. Smythe, Goldsmith, and others have described a Pooled Index,[13,16] in which the various measures were standardized to a common scale of standard deviation units. The Pooled Index and other indices of inflammation are commonly used in clinical trials and have been shown to be responsive to treatment effects.

Destruction and Deformity in Inflammatory Joint Disease

Patterns of Damage

Stiffening may be the outstanding feature of damage. Stiffening results from intra-articular adhesions in the synovial extensions (see Figure 5-6) and deep to the collateral ligaments or from adhesion of surrounding tendons and ligaments to a thickened capsule. Ultimately, this stiffening followed by thinning of the articular cartilage may progress to a bland, painless bony fusion. The first sign will be loss of range of motion, which *must* be treated aggressively as quickly as possible. This sign may seem more characteristic of aging, but it is a severe threat in juvenile-onset arthritis. Damage also may result in instability or *loosening*. Destruction of supporting structures may allow displacement of controlling tendons and joint structures. Finally, loss of articular cartilage will leave bare bone, with characteristic *bone-on-bone crepitus*.

> **Stiffening of damaged joints can be a severe threat in juvenile-onset arthritis.**

The *mechanisms of damage* vary and are affected by the anatomy and function unique to each joint. To produce *angular deformities*, there must be a *deforming force* and *damage to a supporting structure*. For ulnar deviation at the MCP joints to occur, radial collateral ligaments must be attenuated or destroyed by the inflammatory process, which is most aggressive between collateral ligaments and bone. The pull of flexor tendons is the deforming force, and the angular deformity progresses more rapidly if the flexor or extensor tendons are themselves displaced by damage to *their* supporting ligaments.

In the MCP joints of the hands, the structures attached to the volar plate determine the patterns of deformity. The volar plate is a fibrocartilaginous extension of the articular surface of the base of the proximal phalanx (see Figure 5-6), to which it is firmly attached. The flexor tendon is held close to the volar plate by the tendon sheath, thickened here to form a pulley or sling ligament. With flexion grip, the palmar pull of the flexor tendon is transmitted through the volar plate to the collateral ligaments. When these stretch, the base of the proximal phalanx is displaced in a palmar direction. The angle of pull of the second tendon means that this deforming force falls mostly on the radial collateral ligament. If the sling ligament stretches, the tendon is pulled to the ulnar side of the joint. Superficial to the collateral ligaments are the transverse fibers of the extensor hood, also anchored to the volar plate. These keep the extensor tendon centered over the center of the dorsal aspect of the joint and, if damaged, also will allow ulnar subluxation of the extensor tendons. The displaced flexor and extensor tendons now are powerful ulnar deviators.[17] In the fifth finger, the ulnar pull of the short flexors in the hypothenar eminence overpowers the weak radial pull of the long flexor.

In the metatarsophalangeal (MTP) joints of the feet, displacement of the flexor tendons from under the metatarsal heads permits the unopposed extensors to pull the proximal phalanx into hyperextension. The unsupported metatarsal heads prolapse, cutting through the protective fatty-fibrous pad and, eventually, the skin. Calluses form to prevent skin penetration.

In addition to inflammation, *shear instability* in joints produces rapid loss of articular cartilage. Severe crushing forces develop in joints that are *locked*, because of capsular adhesions, or because they are loaded at the limit of their normal range of travel.

Quantifying Damage

Joint destruction may be assessed clinically or radiologically. In evaluating rheumatoid damage, osteoarthritic changes in the terminal interphalangeal, fifth proximal interphalangeal, first carpometacarpal, and first MTP joints are ignored. No simple method of describing these often complex changes has yet achieved international acceptance. For clinical use, we recommend a simple count of damaged joints, applying to this problem the same technique we have used for quantifying inflamed joints. On a skeleton diagram (see Figure 5-4), signs of damage such as loss of range, lax collaterals, bone or tendon subluxation, malalignment, metatarsal prolapse, hammer toes, or bone-on-bone crepitus are recorded. Crepitus must be distinguished from the snapping sensations that occur when some normal joints move under load—because the contours of the bony components rarely match—from the localized fine painless crepitus of deteriorating cartilage or the villous crepitus of hypertrophied synovium. Bony crepitus is hard, may cause sudden pain, and may be felt well away from the joint line as vibration down the shaft of the bone.

Damage-Duration Index

The number of "damaged" joints is related to the duration of the disease and its aggressiveness. The count of damaged joints is divided by the disease duration in years, giving an index of the rate of destruction. Obviously, a client with 10 damaged joints after only 2 years of disease (damaged-duration index = 5) is much more threatened by aggressive disease than a client with 10 damaged joints after 40 years of disease (damage-duration index = 0.25). These two examples illustrate the extreme values seen in clinical studies. A median value for the index is about 0.75.

> The number of "damaged" joints is related to the duration of the disease and its aggressiveness.

Use of These Measures in Prognosis and as a Guide to Treatment

Inflammatory joint disease may have a benign, malignant, or intermediate course, with each requiring different approaches to treatment and follow-up. Guides to determine prognosis early in the course of the disease are needed. Age and sex have relatively little predictive value. An abrupt, severe onset, forcing the client to bed within weeks of the onset, paradoxically suggests a rather favorable course. The following factors are of some value and may indicate a more unfavorable outlook:

- Rapid accumulation of damage to date, assessed clinically or radiologically
- The presence of extra-articular features, such as nodules or nailfold infarcts
- A psychologically adverse passive reaction to disease, particularly when symptoms are used to manipulate family or health care workers
- High levels of rheumatoid factor

Extra-articular Features

Each group of arthropathies has its own pattern of extra-articular features. In rheumatoid disease, look for tendon sheath involvement, tendon nodules, subluxation, or rupture and Baker's cyst. Also look for other nodular sites such as the posterior border of the ulna, heels, or base of the skull, Raynaud's phenomenon,

nailfold infarcts (appearing as dark slivers about the base of the nails), peripheral neuropathy, palmar erythema, and leg ulcers; all of these indicate vasculopathy. Dry or inflamed eyes, pleural pain, or lung fibrosis can occur. Check for anemia clinically (compare pallor of the palm with your own, check the nailbed, and look inside the eyelid), or by reviewing the hemoglobin levels in relevant reports.

In patients with ankylosing spondylitis or Reiter's syndrome, inquire about urethritis or colitis and look for conjunctivitis, iritis, skin and mucosal lesions, and enthesitis (tender spurs) at the heel or elsewhere. Figure 5-7 provides a polyarthritis assessment form designed for clinical use.

Functional Assessments

A number of schemes have been developed to measure a client's ability to function. They consist of the following:

- Clinical measures of impairment such as joint range of movement (ROM) passive or active, and tests of muscle strength and endurance
- Functional status measures or the ability to do the usual self-care ADL such as eating, dressing, and grooming
- Health status, a broader measure than functional status, which encompasses total physical, social, and mental status
- Quality of life (QOL), a more comprehensive and abstract measure than either functional status or health status
- Health-related QOL, a combination of functional status, disease symptoms, social roles, and activities, such as work or school, and emotions and mood.[18]

Because the focus of this chapter is clinical strategies, we will discuss the first two measures listed above. Measures of health status and QOL, which are better suited to measure outcomes of health care trials, will be covered in Chapter 17.

Joint Range

Active movement testing provides information about the status of both contractile and noncontractile structure of the joints. If on active movement the client obtains full active range, the clinician can continue with the resisted testing portion of the examination. If the active range is limited, the clinician should proceed to passive ROM testing to determine which structures are causing the restriction.

POLYARTHRITIS ASSESSMENT

Patient's Name_____ Age_____ Assessment Date _____

Inflammatory Activity

Duration of morning stiffness, hours   _____

Grip strength, mm. of Hg.   Right   _____/20

                            Left   _____/20

Number of active joints   _____

Sedimentation Rate   _____

Active Joints

Joint Pain Now (Circle number):

No Pain: 0 — 1 — 2 — 3 — 4 — 5 — 6 — 7 — 8 — 9 — 10 :*Worst possible*

Damaged Joints: Include lax collaterals, subluxation, bone on bone crepitus, malalignment, loss of more than 20 % of normal passive range of motion. Exclude Heberden's nodes.

Extra-Articular Features

Nodules

Eye

Vasculitis

Other (Specify) _____

"FIBROMYALGIC" POINT COUNT

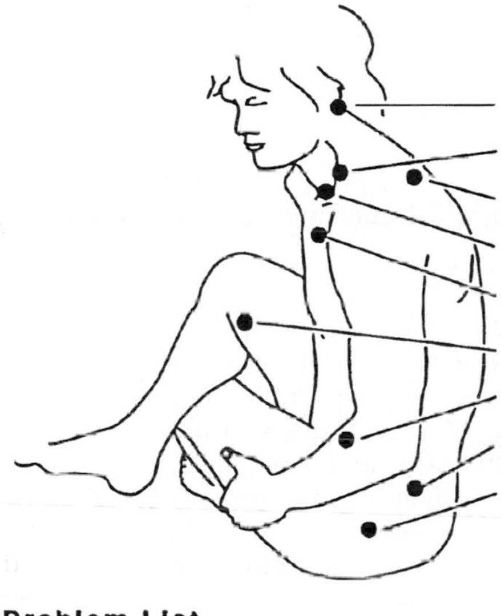

Point Count

	Right	Left
Occiput	_____	_____
Trapezius	_____	_____
Supraspinatus	_____	_____
Low neck	_____	_____
2nd rib	_____	_____
Inner knee	_____	_____
Outer elbow	_____	_____
Gluteus	_____	_____
Trochanter	_____	_____
Total (of 18)	_____	

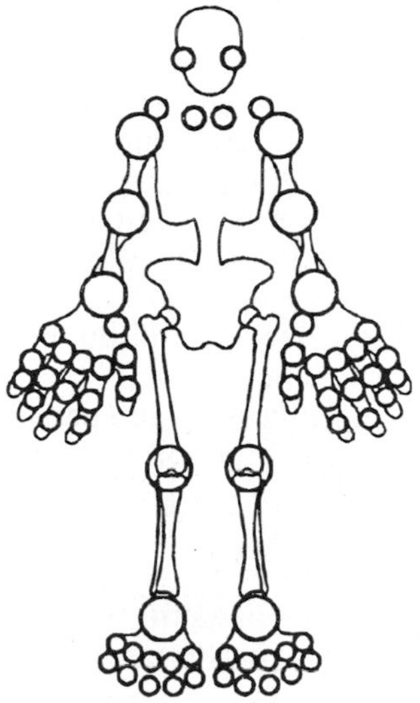

Number active _____

Damaged Joints

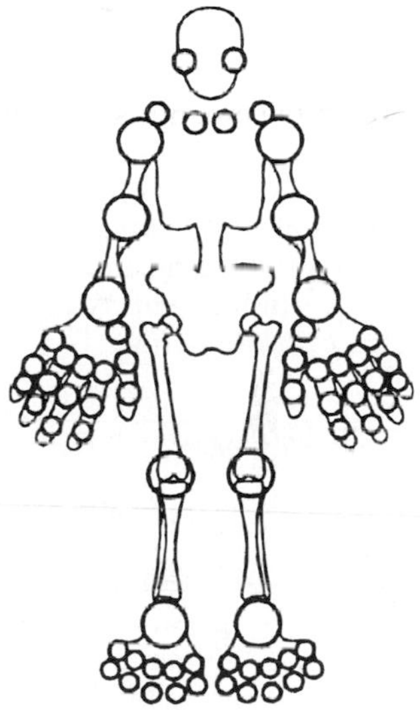

Number damaged _____

Problem List _____

_____

_____

_____

Functional Class

Extend to one decimal place. Best possible score is 1.0, worst is 4.9.   Class:_____

1. COMPLETE ability to carry on all usual duties without handicaps.
2. ADEQUATE FOR NORMAL ACTIVITIES despite handicap of discomfort or limited motion.
3. LIMITED only to little or none of duties of usual occupation or self-care.
4. INCAPACITATED. Bedridden or confined to a wheelchair; little or no self-care.

Observer: _____

Figure 5-7. Polyarthritis assessment form. (Copyright H. Smythe, MD, FRCP[C].)

Passive testing of ROM is used to provide information about the state of the noncontractile elements of a joint (ligaments, capsule, fascia, bursae, etc.). These structures are stretched or stressed as the joint is taken to the end of the available range. The scheme recommended by the American Academy of Orthopedic Surgeons (AAOS) in 1966[19] is commonly used, despite the fact that no serious attempts to validate the technique have been attempted since its inception. There are scatterings of poorly conducted observer variation studies and anecdotal information that reports poor observer agreement due to inconsistencies of anatomical points of reference. In a recent review minor modifications were proposed for the original concepts.[20]

To gently assess full passive ROM using a standard goniometer, the client is placed in a secure, comfortable non–weight-bearing position to remove restrictions due to muscular contractions. Be sensitive to hypermobility as well as stiffness and pain on movement. Record range in degrees, using the anatomical position, with palms forward, as the zero starting point. A fully extended knee is at 0 degrees, not 180 degrees. Avoid use of the ambiguous minus sign. Is a knee at −15 degrees hyperextended or demonstrating a loss of full extension? If it is hyperextended use 15–0–140 as an example, with 0 as the starting point, hyperextension being 15 degrees and flexion being 140 degrees. To measure ROM of all joints that show signs of inflammation or destruction can be time consuming and results are subject to diurnal variation and observer error. Clinicians should select and measure joints likely to have a major impact on ADL or joints targeted for surgical reconstruction.

Muscle Strength

Accurate estimates of muscle strength are important in the rheumatic diseases, both as a diagnostic and as a prognostic tool and as a guide to evaluate the effects of medical, surgical, and rehabilitative interventions. The measures commonly used are the British Medical Research Council (MRC) scale and simple weight-lifting techniques. More recently sophisticated computerized devices such as the isokinetic dynamometer have been introduced. The 0 to 5 MRC scale describes the quality of a contraction and therefore lacks precision: a score of 4 is not twice as strong as a score of 2. Weight-lifting techniques are cumbersome and require an assortment of weights that can be awkward to attach to the distal parts of a limb. Although computerized devices have been shown to be valid, they are expensive, cumbersome, and lack the

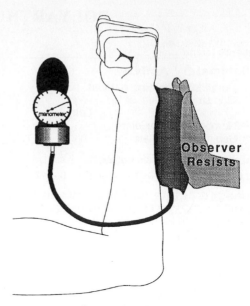

Figure 5-8. Use of modified blood pressure cuff to measure isometric triceps strength. (Copyright H. Smythe, MD, FRCP[C].)

mobility required in clinical situations or services in the home. Any method used should be *quantitative*, so that numbers may be produced; *objective,* so that observer impressions do not affect the measurement values; *responsive* to changes in muscle strength; *reliable,* in that the instrument is free from defects and does not require frequent maintenance; *reproducible* in the hands of different observers; *adaptable* to different muscle groups and clinical situations; *portable* so that it may be used in different settings; and lastly *fast, safe, comfortable,* and *inexpensive.*

A variety of hand-held dynamometers that meet some of the above criteria have been introduced recently, but most of these, with the exception of the *modified sphygmomanometer* (MS), have not been properly validated.[10–12] The modified MS shown in Figure 5-3, originally used to measure grip strength, has been successfully adapted to measure isometric muscle strength as shown in Figure 5-8 (see cuff preparation earlier in this chapter). Several reports attest to its precision, accuracy, and responsiveness.[10–12,21]

Measurement Technique

The bag is inflated to 100 mm Hg to remove wrinkles in the bladder, the pressure is then reduced to 20 mm Hg, and the valve is closed tightly. This produces a measurement interval of 20 to 300 mm Hg. The inflated cuff is placed on the required lever point,

Table 5-7. American College of Rheumatology Revised Criteria for Classification of Functional Status in Rheumatoid Arthritis*

	Class Description
Class I	Completely able to perform usual activities of daily living (self-care, vocational, and avocational)
Class II	Able to perform usual self-care and vocational activities, but limited in avocational activities
Class III	Able to perform usual self-care activities, but limited in vocational and avocational activities
Class IV	Limited ability to perform usual self-care, vocational and avocational activities

From Hochberg MC, Chang RW, Dwosh I et al: The American College of Rheumatology 1991 revised criteria for the classification of global functional status in rheumatoid arthritis. *Arthritis Rheum* 35:498–502, 1992.
*Usual self-care activities include dressing, feeding, bathing, grooming, and toileting. Avocational (recreational and/or leisure) and vocational (work, school, homemaking) activities are patient desired and age- and sex-specific.

and the scale is positioned so that it is visible to the observer, but masked to the client. The limb is brought to the starting position at the required joint angle, and the client is asked to hold that position. The observer applies pressure on the bag gradually with the palm of the hand, reaching the maximum that the client can hold to the count of 5 seconds. The part is held in this maximal position for a further 2 seconds to allow the needle's momentum to settle, at which time the scale is read by the observer. Pressure is applied with the flat of the hand placed along the longitudinal axis of the cuff. *Avoid gripping the cuff* because this will falsely elevate the reading. The muscle strength is the highest force recorded on the scale (in mm Hg) that the client is able to sustain without movement. A fine muscle tremor may precede an abrupt cessation of muscle power due to the Golgi tendon organ inhibitory effect. This tremor is accepted both as an end point of the test and evidence that the client is producing maximal effort and is referred to as a *make contraction*. In contrast to a *break contraction* (in which the maximal hold is broken), a make contraction is preferable in the rheumatic diseases because it is less likely to damage joint or muscle structures compromised by the disease process.

Precautions

The measurement is valid only if it is painless. The client must be cooperative and prepared to attempt a maximal contraction. The test objectives should be carefully explained, and a trial run should precede the test.

Limitations

The range of the instrument is from 20 to 300 mm Hg. Exceptional strength may exceed the scope of the instrument, and the examiner must be strong enough to be able to resist the client's strength. This technique is not suitable for measuring small muscle groups acting on short lever points.

Description of Techniques

Figure 5-9, *A* to *J*, illustrates the methods used to measure muscle groups commonly targeted in the rheumatic diseases. The starting positions are selected to ensure client safety and to produce valid results. Although the techniques shown test muscle groups in one plane, they can be adapted to three-dimensional testing using spiral diagonal patterns of movement advocated in proprioceptive neuromuscular facilitation.

Functional Status and Activities of Daily Living

Several approaches have been used to assess self-care ADL: direct observation, such as the Keitel Index; clinician global estimate of function, such as the ACR functional classes; and client- or clinician-directed questionnaires. Although the Keitel Index has been shown to be sensitive to short-term change, it is time consuming (10 to 15 minutes) and can only be administered by trained observers.[18] The clinician global assessment is subjective and depends on the clinician's interpretation of symptoms. The revised ACR criteria for classification of function in RA[22] shown in Table 5-7 has too few grades to measure small changes in function and works better if a decimal place is used to indicate variation within the classes. Thus, a "good" 2 might be scored as 2.2, and a "bad" 2 as 2.9.

In clinician- or client-directed questionnaires, the essential dimensions of function commonly used are mobility, such as walking, use of stairs, and body

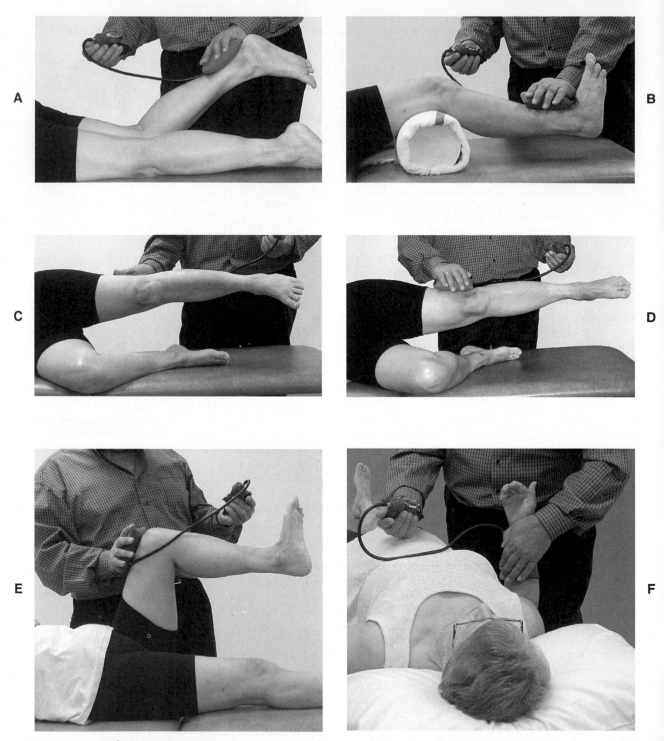

Figure 5-9. Techniques to measure isometric muscle strength in selected muscle groups using the modified sphygmomanometer. **A,** Right knee flexors. **B,** Right knee extensors. **C,** Left hip extensors. **D,** Left hip abductors. **E,** Left hip flexors. **F,** Right elbow flexors. (Photography courtesy of Gail Paterson, BSc.PT; photo editing courtesy of James Crouse, MASc, Dalhousie University Physiotherapy.) *Continued.*

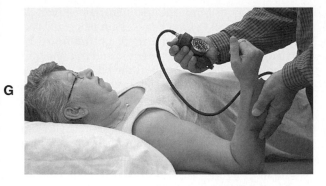

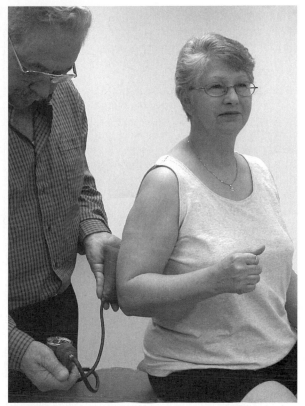

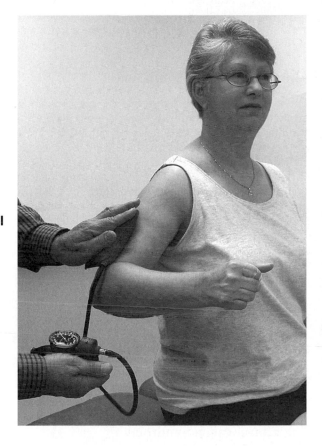

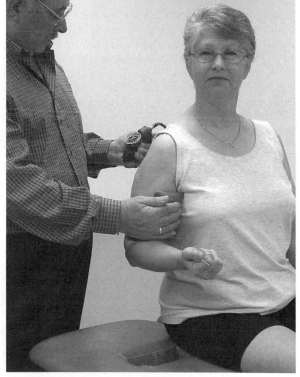

Figure 5-9. *Continued* **G,** Right elbow extensors. **H,** Right shoulder extensors. **I,** Right shoulder abductors. **J,** Right shoulder flexors. (Photography courtesy of Gail Paterson, BSc.PT; photo editing courtesy of James Crouse, MASc, Dalhousie University Physiotherapy.)

Table 5-8. Assessment of Function*

Mobility (walking, climbing stairs, transfers)
Self-care (eating, dressing, washing, grooming, toilet use)
Hand/arm function (door handles, keys, coins, jar tops, pen, scissors, carrying light/heavy objects)
Work/play activities (work at home or outside home, light/heavy housework, hobbies)
Use of transport (driving, public transport)
Other

*Activity scores: Normal, With difficulty, Unable to do. Provide a narrative description regarding changes to perform specific functions.

transfers; self-care, such as eating, dressing, washing, grooming, use of toilet; hand functions, such as managing door handles, keys, coins, jar tops, pens, scissors, and carrying objects; work/play activities, such as work outside the home, light and heavy work in the house, hobbies, and sports.[23]

By using these dimensions of function as a guide, more information can be gathered quickly about the needs of an individual client by thoughtful, less rigidly structured inquiry. Hence in clinical situations, it is critical to survey components of failing function to direct clinical strategies to correct or overcome such difficulties. A simple Assessment of Function sheet, shown in Table 5-8, provides a thorough inventory of the dimensions of function and enables clinicians to score, as well as comment on, areas of difficulties. A narrative description can emphasize recent changes in ability to perform specific functions. Using such a narrative clinicians can define reasons for loss of function (i.e., pain, stiffness, weakness, instability, fatigability) or any of these increasing with duration of disease activity.

Exaggerated Pain Behavior and Disability Assessment

Health professionals are increasingly asked by third parties to make judgments about disability that can be difficult if the complaints seem to be out of proportion to evidence of disease or if there are words or actions that seem inappropriately dramatic. Given the rise in costs associated with disability awards over the past decade, it is evident that these assessments are an important responsibility and that clinicians do not do them well. Signs of "exaggerated" pain behavior have been described[24] but not validated, not informed by knowledge of referred pain patterns, and not sensitive to cultural effects that may affect the observer and the client. An early well-designed study on pain behavior[25] did not assume that pain behavior is necessarily abnormal. In a study of clients with fibromyalgia, markers of pain behavior did not predict treatment outcome.[26] We have found (unpublished data) that quantitative scoring of a list of adjectives describing the client's reactions to examination to be a valuable assistance to masked observers asked to judge whether volunteer clients were giving honest responses or exaggerating their tenderness in a modest way. These adjectives are included in the format for recording findings on the assessment of spinal disease at the end of this chapter (see Figure 5-15).

Pain Amplification Syndromes

There is increasing interest in the specific neural mechanisms that modulate the response to painful stimuli. Endorphins ease pain and substance P is involved in pain mediation, but knowledge of the neurobiochemical mechanisms by which pain is increased remains inadequate. Many pain amplification syndromes have been recognized. Although not inflammatory in nature, all can occur in clients with RA, enormously complicating assessment and treatment. These include the following:

- Referred pain syndromes
- The "fibromyalgia" syndrome
- Reflex dystrophy syndromes
- The painful shins of steroid therapy
- Narcotic withdrawal pain

In a recent review, functional somatic syndromes were identified by medical specialty (Table 5-9), showing that considerable overlap existed between individual syndromes and that the similarities outweigh the differences.[27]

The Fibromyalgia Syndrome

The most common and best studied of these syndromes is now termed *fibromyalgia* (FM), formerly "fibrositis." Arising from major studies over two decades, new, internationally recognized criteria for the diagnosis of FM have emerged.[28] The combination of *widespread pain* and *tenderness at 11 or more of 18 defined bilateral sites* (Figure 5-10) yielded sensitivity of 88% (88% of clients preselected with this diagnosis met these criteria) and specificity of 81% (meaning that 19% of

Table 5-9. Functional Somatic Syndromes by Specialty

Specialty	Functional Somatic Syndrome
Gastroenterology	Irritable bowel syndrome, nonulcer dyspepsia
Gynecology	Premenstrual syndrome, chronic pelvic pain
Rheumatology	Fibromyalgia
Cardiology	Atypical or noncardiac pain
Respiratory medicine	Hyperventilation syndrome
Infectious diseases	Chronic (postviral) fatigue syndrome
Neurology	Tension headache
Dentistry	Temporomandibular joint dysfunction, atypical facial pain
Ear, nose, and throat	Globus hystericus—a lump in the throat
Allergy	Multiple chemical sensitivity.

From Wessely S, Nimnuan C, Sharpe M: Functional somatic syndromes: one or many? *Lancet* 354:936–939, 1999.

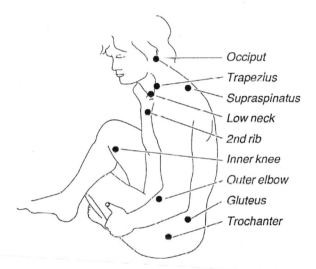

Occiput
Trapezius
Supraspinatus
Low neck
2nd rib
Inner knee
Outer elbow
Gluteus
Trochanter

Figure 5-10. The tender points in the American College of Rheumatology criteria set; possible total of 18 points bilaterally.

clients with other pain syndromes met these criteria). The statistical power of the criteria came from the addition of the disciplined tender point count. Think of it as *fibromyalgia* translating as widespread pain and *fibrositis* as points of tenderness.

The primary purpose of these criteria was to define groups of clients for research studies. They are only a guide to diagnosis and assessment of severity. Symptoms of fatigue, headache, and sensitivity to a variety of stimuli in the external and internal environ-ment were common and are important in the clinical assessment.

The *pathogenesis* of these features also can be summarized simply. The *location* of the pain and the different locations of the tender points are determined by the patterns of referred pain associated with mechanical problems in the spine. *Upper body tender points relate to mechanical problems in the neck and lower body points to problems in the low back.* The *severity* of the pain and the presence of the ac-companying symptoms are further influenced by *amplifying factors,* such as sleep disturbance and physical deconditioning. In brief, FM is about necks, backs, sleep and fitness.

It follows that diagnosis depends on the under-standing that nonarticular pain, "numbness," or "swelling" may often be due to *referred pain mechanisms.* Assessment of such clients requires a systematic examination for characteristic patterns of unexpected tenderness and nontenderness and a knowledgeable search for the sources of referred pain. The commonly overlooked relevant findings are marked tenderness in the low anterior neck and great difficulty in performing a sit-up due to profound abdominal muscle weakness.

In the client with RA, concomitant FM often leads to serious overestimation of the amount of inflam-matory activity. The client with FM and concomitant RA (or other joint disease) may describe point pain, stiffness, fatigue, and even "swelling." When joint effusions cannot be demonstrated, the clinician must recognize that these symptoms *may* reflect the FM rather than uncontrolled inflammation and may require totally different treatment strategies (see Chapter 12).

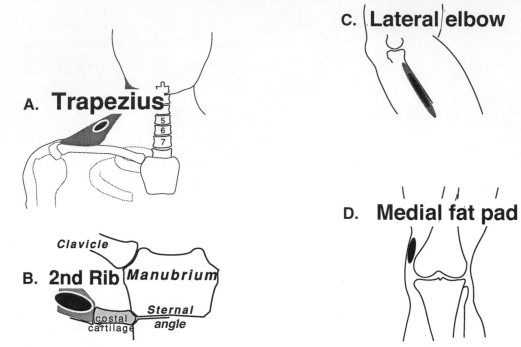

Figure 5-11. Sites for screening examination. **A,** Trapezius, the tender point is in the muscle at the midpoint of the upper border. **B,** Second rib, the tender point is in the origin of the pectoralis major muscle, near the costochondral junction. **C,** Lateral elbow, the tender point is about 3 to 6 cm from the epicondyle, in the extensor muscle of the middle finger, rotating with the radius. **D,** Medial fat pad located 3 to 6 cm above the knee joint line, just posterior to the vastus medialis.

Evaluation of the Client with Chronic Pain

Assessment for the purpose of diagnosis can be simple, because most of the information about tenderness is contained in a subset of eight of the ACR points (Figure 5-11).[29] Often, as part of the treatment strategy the assessment must include an educational component. The client needs to learn the relevance of neck support, sit-up exercises, and aerobic fitness, and the interview becomes more complex and time-consuming. Evaluation of relative severity of pain is even more demanding, especially if there are insurance or medicolegal issues. Evidence of exaggerated pain behavior should be recorded but interpreted with caution. An opinion about prognosis may be requested. In this section we will concentrate on an efficient basic examination, with indications of elements of more extensive approaches.

Examination for Tenderness

The equivalent of 4 kg of pressure is the recommended amount that should be applied at the location of tenderness. Applying the correct amount of pressure is a learned skill. Observer variation can be halved with training, and it is helpful to have a dolorimeter to practice on. The pressure is delivered perpendicularly through your terminal phalanx. The clinician should learn not only the feel of 4 kg of pressure but also observe the associated degree of blanching in and beside the nailbed.

Measuring Tenderness

Tender points can be counted as present or absent, scored for severity, or measured by dolorimetry, in terms of the kilograms of force required to reach pain threshold. With a limited number of points, a tenderness score can function well statistically and is easily translated into counts. Variation among examiners can be a problem with any of these techniques, and formal testing of interobserver variation can identify difficulties and provide feedback that ensures uniformity of technique, The following scoring technique has been used extensively:

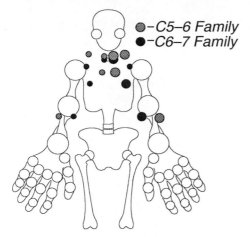

Figure 5-12. Distribution of tender points associated with chronic neck strain. The location and quality of the pain are variable, but the location of the tenderness is different, constant, and predictable, with a different pattern of points related to the C6–C7 level from those defined in the American College of Rheumatology criteria.

0 = none
1 = mild; expressed, but no withdrawal
2 = moderate; expressed plus withdrawal
3 = severe; immediate exaggerated withdrawal
4 = client untouchable; withdraws without palpation

For the ACR 18-point count, circle tender points shown on Figure 5-10 for right and left sides.

Possible Neck Problems

With the client lying supine, tenderness at the upper body sites as defined in the ACR criteria study is determined (see Figure 5-10). These are at the *key site* in the low anterior neck just above the inner end of the clavicle and at the C6–C7 sites, coracoid tip, lateral pectoral, and medial epicondyle (Figure 5-12).

Possible Low Back Problems

Check for abdominal muscle weakness, locked lumbar hyperextension, and the accessory sites of referred tenderness shown in Figure 5-13. Check for limited forward flexion in terms of finger-floor distance, limited straight leg raising, pain on dorsiflexion of the foot, popliteal nerve tenderness, muscle weakness, and reflex loss.

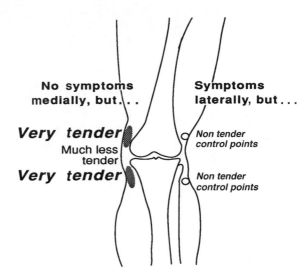

Figure 5-13. Tender and control sites near the left knee with referred pain from the back.

Assessment of Spinal Disease

The approach presented here is a supplement to standard approaches to spinal assessment. In what structures does the client's pain originate? What is the nature of the pathological changes? How much investigation is appropriate for the client?

Referred Pain: Why Is It So Hard to Diagnose?

Diagnosis of the nature and site of origin of deep pain is difficult because the involved structures are not represented in the brain (Figure 5-14) or in our body image. If a finger is hurt, the pain is felt in a fraction of a second, localized to within millimeters, and the quality of the injury is recognized as sharp, burning, or crushing. None of this is true of pain of deep origin. Deep pain is referred, that is, misinterpreted as arising in tissues other than its site of origin, especially to muscles and bony prominences, usually sharing the same segmental nerve supply. Awareness of the injury may be *delayed* for hours or days, and the *quality* of the distress may vary from aching, to burning, swelling, or numbness, according to the region to which it is referred.

Secondary reflex changes often develop, which may be thought of as being protective in intent. Hyperalgesia also may develop and is often more pronounced in deep structures than in skin, with local

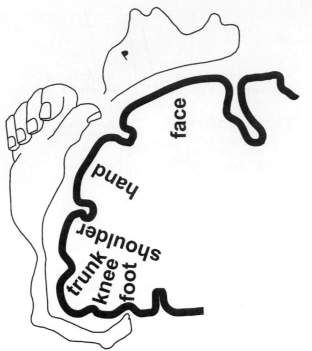

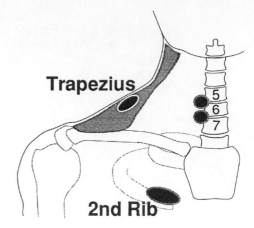

Figure 5-15. Referred points in the neck. (Copyright H. Smythe, MD, FRCP[C].)

Figure 5-14. The somatosensory cortex reflecting Penfield's vision of representation. Note that the hands and feet are represented, but deep structures are not. (Adapted from Strong J, Unruh AM, Wright A et al [eds]: *Pain, a Textbook for Therapists.* Philadelphia, Churchill Livingstone, 2002, p 32. With permission.)

points of referred deep tenderness. Circulation may increase. Muscle spasm occurs to splint the part and prevent movement, but voluntary muscle action also is inhibited. All of these signs can lead to an erroneous diagnosis of injury in the area of reference, and the deep, central primary pathological condition may be overlooked. As a rule, pain is referred distally rather than proximally. Knowledge of the common patterns of pain reference can be quickly gained, and the search for the primary site of pathologic change may be challenging but is usually rewarding.

Regional Tenderness

Exactly the same sites become tender in regional pain syndromes associated with spinal problems as in the general pain syndrome of FM. Lateral elbow pain, aggravated by use, may be called "tennis elbow." Dissatisfaction with localized therapies may lead to

closer evaluation. The tenderness is not found at the lateral epicondyle, but about 5 cm distally, at the origin of the extensor carpi radialis brevis muscle, close to and rotating with the radius (see Figure 5-11, *C*). The marked and sharply localized tenderness still suggests a local pathological condition, but further examination reveals equally marked, unsuspected sites of tenderness at other characteristic sites (Figure 5-15), much more marked on the symptomatic side and unassociated with lower body pain or tenderness. The lateral elbow tenderness and nearby pain are part of a referred pain syndrome. Full examination for referred pain patterns of tenderness is essential for correct diagnosis and effective treatment of "overuse" syndromes.

Overuse Syndromes

The pain may not be restricted to the elbow but may extend distally and be associated with a sense of numbness or tingling in the hand, strange in that it is often mixed with pain. If the texture of cloth can still be recognized, despite the "numb" feeling, nerve compression is unlikely. These symptoms may disturb sleep and also are aggravated by use at work or at play. Two (or more) factors are contributing. Loads on the arms are equally loads on the neck. In addition, the pull of a muscle on its very tender origin by the elbow is the mechanical equivalent of the pressure of the examiner's finger—it hurts. Again full examination for referred pain patterns of tenderness is essential for correct diagnosis and effective treatment of these syndromes.

Symptom Patterns

Mechanical Lesions

Mechanical lesions include chronic strain, disk disease, apophyseal joint osteoarthritis, spondylolysis, and spondylolisthesis. The most common problems are mechanical in origin; begin abruptly; and improve quickly with a brief period of rest, analgesic (*not* anti-inflammatory) therapy, and early mobilization. If recovery is delayed or interrupted by recurrences, identification of continuing pathogenetic forces may be the key to therapy. Nearly all of the mechanical problems affect either the lower cervical spine or the two lower lumbar vertebrae, and these two areas will eventually cause symptoms in virtually every member of the population. Why does this occur? The lower lumbar spine is locked at the extreme range of hyperextension in virtually everyone with low back pain problems and close to the extreme range in all individuals.[30] The lower neck is vulnerable for a variety of reasons, of which the most important and neglected are compressive and shearing stresses arising during sleep.

Inflammatory Back Pain

Ankylosing Spondylitis

Early recognition of ankylosing spondylitis (AS) is important because aggressive anti-inflammatory treatment can prevent damage. Radiological changes in the sacroiliac joints may be delayed, so that diagnosis may depend on recognition of characteristic symptoms and signs. Involvement of the low lumbar spine is not common in the early stages, so midline lumbosacral pain is uncommon. Buttock pain of insidious onset, with night pain and morning pain and stiffness that ease with exercise are characteristic. Midlumbar paravertebral pain, arising at the thoracolumbar junction and aggravated by turning during sleep, is often the next symptom and is uncommon in mechanical problems. Precipitation by gastrointestinal or genitourinary infection, heel pain, lower limb arthritis, ocular inflammation, painless mucosal lesions, or a family history may make the diagnosis easy. Physical findings will be discussed later.

Spinal Osteomyelitis, Discitis, or Tumor

These are much less common and their diagnosis is difficult but essential. Only occasionally is infection linked with clear evidence of systemic sepsis. Often the onset is insidious. With spondylitis, night pain is common, and the thoracolumbar junction is a favored site; this is missed with routine spine films, because the lesions may be too low to be seen on the thoracic films and too high for the lumbar films. Pain and tenderness at sites other than the low cervical and low lumbar spine lead to appropriate diagnostic investigations.

Polymyalgic Syndromes

Widespread pain, not clearly restricted to swollen or damaged joints, may occur in FM, polymyalgia rheumatica, viral or other infection ("influenza"), autoimmune disease, or tumor. The differential diagnosis is as broad as that for fever of unknown origin.

Important Other Diagnoses

These include osteoporosis and other metabolic bone disease, neurological disorders, and pain referred from viscera. It is, fortunately, unusual for any of these conditions to be primarily located or restricted to the lower cervical spine or lumbosacral angle. Pain and stiffness are often worse during or after rest, and evidence of systemic disease may be present. Pain arising in the midlumbar spine associated with morning stiffness could be due to a mechanical problem, but the overwhelming probability of this diagnosis that would be associated with lumbosacral angle pain is not present, so that the diagnostician must be especially alert. If the anatomical site is wrong, if the pattern of pain does not fit with mechanical aggravation, or if symptoms or signs of other disease are present, beware of missing an important other diagnosis.

Red Flags

Most pain syndromes are mechanical in origin and are unassociated with nerve root damage or other serious disease. Complex investigations are not warranted, and treatment for active recovery of function should be stressed. However, uncommon but serious problems will be seen and must not be missed. Night pain, weight loss, fever, sweats, or tenderness in the spine between C7 and L4 are all *red flags*, indicating the need for fuller investigation. Look for the following:

- Evidence of nerve root pressure
- Inflammatory back pain
- Important other diagnoses
- Exaggerated pain behavior

Techniques of Spinal Examination

Map Pain, Hyperesthesia, Deep Tenderness, and Pain on Movement

The position illustrated in Figure 5-16 is used to relax tight antigravity muscles and open lordotic curves to

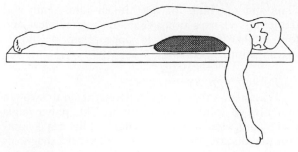

Figure 5-16. Relaxed prone position. A pillow eliminates lumbar lordosis and releases tight ligaments. (Copyright H. Smythe, MD, FRCP[C].)

allow better identification of bony landmarks. Clients should be totally relaxed during this examination. A spinal map may be used to record findings.

Hyperesthesia

Test for deep hyperesthesia by gently raising and rolling a skin fold to create traction on the deep fascia. Where this creates pain, deep pressure and movement must be done warily. Reactive reddening of the skin often develops in an area of referred pain and tenderness, and this dermatographia helps document the contribution of reflex factors to a continuing pain syndrome.

Deep Tenderness

When deep tenderness over interspinous ligaments is elicited without moving the deep vertebral structures, it is referred deep tenderness. After this is recognized, understanding the nature of other sites of referred deep tenderness is easier.

Pain on Movement

The necessary techniques must be safe, using traction or gliding movements rather than crushing forces. Because the orientation of the apophyseal joints is different in each of the cervical, thoracic, and lumbar regions, this determines the direction of movement.

Regional Range of Movement

Measures, such as finger-floor distance, assess overall function of a great number of spinal and extraspinal structures. They are useful in screening and are sensitive to treatment effects.[31] To identify the anatomical structures involved, the approach must be regional. We wish to determine the maximum range that the condition of the joints permits, and this is achieved with the muscles totally relaxed and the

joints not bearing weight. In general, the client should be lying or otherwise securely supported, and movements carefully assisted by the examiner (i.e., passive range should be recorded). It is not necessary to record every possible movement of every joint. Certain great simplifications can focus and increase rather than sacrifice precision. A spinal disorder assessment sheet for recording results of assessment is shown in Figure 5-17.

Lateral flexion of the cervical spine cannot occur for anatomical reasons between the skull and C2; thus, limited lateral flexion is often the most sensitive indicator of lower cervical pathological changes. When rotation is restricted, the site of pain or deep tenderness helps indicate whether the upper or lower cervical spine is involved. The orientation of the apophyseal facets prevents rotation in the lumbar spine, and about one half of the total range occurs between T8 and L1. Fix the pelvis by having the client sit astride the examining table or facing the back of a chair. The shoulder blades get in the way: Have the client place her or his hands on opposite shoulders to move the scapulae laterally, and assist rotation by gentle pressure on the opposite elbow. Do not use the shoulder line as a measure of rotation—movement of the scapulae over the thorax invariably occurs and leads to gross errors. Locate the angles of the ribs at T1, and using a tape measure record range of rotation between T1 and the posterior superior iliac spine. Most of this rotation occurs between T7 and T12, because the attachments of the ribs to the sternum will limit rotation in the upper thoracic spine.

In ankylosing spondylitis, flexion-extension range is first lost at the thoracolumbar junction and last in the lower lumbar spine. The three 10-cm segment method illustrated later is much more sensitive to the effects of spondylitis than the older Schober techniques.[31]

Stress Pain in Deep Structures

In the lower thoracic spine, the most useful technique may be resisted rotation. With the client prone or in the sitting position facing the back of a chair, the examiner's thumb is placed on one side of the interspinous process to register rotation at each level in turn while torque is applied to the upper trunk. Also with the client in the sitting position, pain on long-axis compression may indicate the level of serious bone or disk pathological changes in the lumbar spine. Further, with the client prone and totally relaxed, firm quick thrusts on the spinous processes produce anteroposterior movement on each segment in turn and permit very accurate localization of pain.

Assessment of Spinal Disorders

Patient's Name_____ Age_____ Assessment Date _____

1. Posture, Spinal Curves and Gait :

Little flexion takes place in the upper thoracic spine, which is curved to accommodate the heart and lungs. The erect posture forces secondary curves in the low cervical and lumbar spine. The neck is resting on T1, which is inclined forward to a greater or lesser degree. Loss of occiput-wall distance often reflects changes in thoracolumbar spine, or even hips.

- cervical
  — occiput-to-wall distance (neck extended),_____ cm.
- thoracic, curve flat or accentuated?
- lumbar
- leg length inequalities
- Gait abnormalities.

2. Map hyperesthesia, tenderness, pain on motion.

Spinal Pain Now (Circle number):

None: 0 — 1 — 2 — 3 — 4 — 5 — 6 — 7 — 8 — 9 — 10 :*Worst possible*

3. Mobility

			Results	Normal
Cervical	upper	flexion-extension	_____ °	90°
	lower	flexion extension	_____ °	90°
	(patient	rotation, right	_____ °	80°
	supine)	left	_____ °	80°
	lateral	right	_____ °	> 50°
	flexion	left	_____ °	> 50°
Thoracic	chest expansion	infra-mammary	_____	> 5 cm
	rotation	pelvis to T1	_____ °	> 40°

4. Thoracolumbar flexion-extension

In the Schober test, marks are made over the S1 spine and 10 cm higher, with the subject standing. The distance between the 2 marks is remeasured after full flexion, and normally increases by 5 cm.

The 10 cm segment test, has proved more sensitive in measuring losses due to age or disease. Changes of >2.5 cm occur normally in the upper 2 segments, >3 cm in the lowest.

1. Spinal Curves

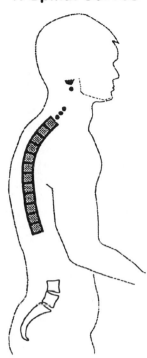

2. Pain Diagram

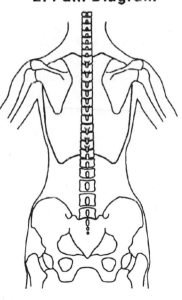

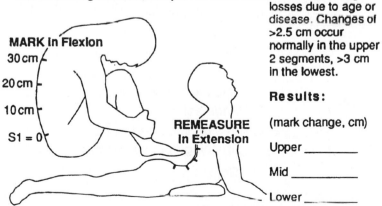

MARK In Flexion
30 cm
20 cm
10 cm
S1 = 0

REMEASURE In Extension

Results:

(mark change, cm)

Upper _____

Mid _____

Lower _____

Figure 5-17. Spinal disorders assessment form. *Illustration continued on following page.* (Copyright H. Smythe , MD, FRCP[C].)

5. Restricted Range

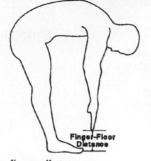

Finger-floor distance, _____cm

7. Three Phase Straight Leg Raising

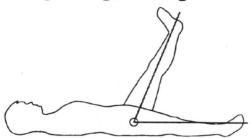

Phase one: Mark location of any pain.
    Right _____° Left _____°
Phase two, drop 15° dorsiflex foot.
    Pain? Right _____° Left _____°
Phase three; drop another 15°, dorsiflex foot
    Pain? Right _____° Left _____°

11. Suck-in Situps

Safety: The exercise must be painless.
    The spine must form a smooth, C-shaped curve, with no movement at the belt line. Begin with a strong pelvic tilt, then tilt the head forward until the chin is on the chest. Smoothly bring the elbows to the knees, and lay back pushing the belt line down.

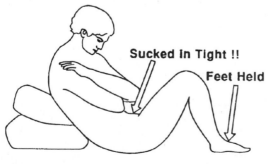

Sucked In Tight !!

Feet Held

6. Locked Hyperextension

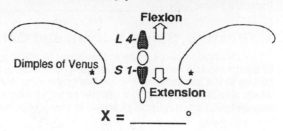

$X = $ _____°

8. Bow-String Sign
Popliteal nerve tenderness
    Tender? Right _____ Left _____

9. Reflexes
Score 0 — 4; normal 2.

Site	Right	Left
Knee (L3-4)		
Hamstring (L5)		
Ankle (S1)		

10. Exaggerated Pain Behaviour

(score each 0-4).   1) grimacing __
2) bracing __ 3) sighing __ 4) rubbing __
5) guarding __ 6) leap __ 7) alert, passive,
anticipation __ 8) inconsistency __
9) groans __10) histrionic __ 11) tremor __
12) Other, score __ and describe.

Situp Scoring Scale:

0. Can't do a sit-up.
1. Needs 2 or more pillows.
2. Flat, arms stretched toward knees.
3. Hands to opposite elbows.
4. Hands to opposite shoulders.
5. Hands behind neck.
6. Arms behind head, fingers
    touching opposite ears.

    Score _____

Observer: _____

Figure 5-17. *Continued*

Tests of Nerve Compression

Limitation of Straight Leg Raising

This may occur when excursion of a nerve root is limited as it tightens over a protruding disk or alternatively because of reflex muscle spasm or apprehension on the part of the client. The limitations produced by the check-rein effect of root pressure are mechanically consistent; whereas muscle spasm or apprehension will vary under different circumstances.

The *three-phase straight leg raising (SLR) test* is more informative than the unmodified test. In phase one, gentle elevation of the relaxed, straight limb is continued until stopped by pain; the angle is recorded. In phase two, the limb is dropped 10 to 15 degrees until pain is relieved, and only then is the foot sharply dorsiflexed. Discomfort in the calf may be due to stretching of the muscle, but pain in the posterior thigh or back counts as a positive test result. In phase three, this observation is controlled by lowering the limb a further 15 degrees, at which point sharp dorsiflexion of the foot will not cause nerve root pain but will still place traction on a calf that is tender because of venous thrombosis or rupture of synovial fluid from the knee.

If results are doubtful, mechanical consistency can be further measured by a *three-phase finger-to-floor test*, first with the feet together, again with the "involved leg" back, and finally with the "involved leg" forward. In the absence of root pressure, slight improvement usually occurs with each repetition. If root pressure is present, advancing the involved leg (equivalent of SLR) worsens performance. Another modification of SLR can be taught to the client and used later when there is concern about continuing back pain. Here the client sits on the edge of a chair with knees straight and gently slides the fingertips down the front of the shin. If he or she can reach within 15 cm of the ankle, continuing nerve root pressure is unlikely.

In the rare instances when only the L3–L4 lumbar roots are involved, SLR will ease rather than aggravate pain, as the femoral nerve trunk passes in front of the hip joint. In the *three-phase femoral stretch test* there is reproduction of pain by passive hyperextension of the hip, relief by slight flexion, and further aggravation by flexion of the knee.

Nerve Trunk Tenderness

Nerve trunk tenderness consistently accompanies nerve root pressure. This is best exemplified by the "bowstring sign," in which the popliteal nerve is found to be sharply more tender than the adjacent hamstring muscles, which are used as a control. In the L3–L4 root syndrome, the femoral nerve will be sharply tender, and in cervical disk disease, the brachial plexus will be tender.

Impairment of Nerve Root Function

Impairment of nerve root function must be sought with care. Loss of power must be tested using adequate resistance. Calf power should be tested by having the client stand on one foot and rise up on the "toe" 10 times. Weakness of dorsiflexion of the ankle can be tested with the client sitting, heels on the ground, foot in dorsiflexion, and maximal resistance applied manually on the dorsum of the foot. Weakness of great toe extension may be a more sensitive test of the L5 root damage. Sensory testing is often inconsistent when the client is apprehensive. The cold edge of a tuning fork may give a more consistent sensory stimulus and thus more consistent results than the most skillfully wielded pin, and the client who is exaggerating may report cold while denying heat, equating cold with numbness. Loss of vibration sense is a sensitive test for neuropathy.

Reflex Loss

The commonly damaged nerve root is L5, so the medial hamstring reflex is added to the usual list. If the client is fully relaxed, reinforcement techniques are rarely necessary. *Record reflexes* on all routine examinations, and then one can tell if a reflex is newly lost.

Ongoing Mechanical Factors

The special vulnerability of the lower lumbar spine is due to a posture of extreme hyperextension. With the client sitting on a chair fully flexed, place your index finger and thumb firmly on the L4 and S1 vertebra, and feel the movement of the spinous processes as the client rises slowly, by extending his or her spine (Figure 5-17, item 6). At first there is little movement; extension is occurring at the hips. Then the two vertebral spines come together until the extreme of hyperextension is reached, after which no further movement in this region occurs. This end point is often reached with the client's upper trunk still 20 degrees flexed, so record $X = 20$ degrees. Locked lumbar hyperextension is usually due either to postural habit or to weak abdominal muscles, both reversible with some effort. Other less obvious and less treatable causes are excessive thoracic curves and loss of hip extension due to intrinsic hip disease or to tight ligamentous and capsular structures anteriorly about the hip. These are common in obesity, diffuse idiopathic skeletal hyperostosis, diabetes, and in large-boned individuals.

Summary

The quantitative measures of inflammation, damage, and function described in this chapter have been extensively reported in the literature in terms of their validity, reproducibility, and responsiveness. They are an important component of the curricula of graduate medical trainees in rheumatology and of rheumatologically trained physical and occupational therapists and are part of the undergraduate curricula of these disciplines in certain parts of the United States and Canada. The techniques lend themselves well to communication between specialists and nonspecialists.

Standardization of these measures of inflammation enhances communication within the treatment team that always includes the client. Management of inflammatory arthritis is facilitated by sound assessment that plays an important role in goal setting and treatment plans.

References

1. *Ontario Treatment Guidelines for Osteoarthritis and Rheumatoid Arthritis and Acute Musculoskeletal Injury,* Toronto, Publications Ontario, 2000.
2. Schumacher HR Jr (ed): *Primer on the Rheumatic Diseases,* ed 10. Atlanta, Arthritis Foundation, 1993.
3. Nichols LA: History and physical assessment. In Robbins L (ed): *Clinical Care of the Rheumatic Diseases,* ed 2. Atlanta, Association of Rheumatology Health Professionals, 2001.
4. The Cooperating Clinics Committee of the American Rheumatism Association: A seven-day variability study of 499 patients with peripheral rheumatoid arthritis. *Arthritis Rheum* 8:302–335, 1965.
5. Felson DT, Anderson JJ, Boers M et al: The American College of Rheumatology preliminary core set of disease activity measures for rheumatoid arthritis trials. *Arthritis Rheum* 36:729–740, 1993.
6. Fries JF: Toward an understanding of patient outcome measurement. *Arthritis Rheum* 26:697–704, 1983.
7. Meenan RF, Mason JH, Anderson JJ et al: AIMS2: the content and properties of a revised and expanded arthritis impact measurement scales health status questionnaire. *Arthritis Rheum* 35:1–10, 1992.
8. Conference on outcome measures in rheumatoid arthritis clinical trials: Maastrich, the Netherlands, April 29–May 3, 1992. *J Rheumatol* 20:525–603, 1993.
9. Hoopman WM, Towheed T, Anastassiadis T et al: Canadian normative data for the SF-36 Health Survey. *Can Med Assoc J* 163:265–271, 2000.
10. Helewa A, Goldsmith CH, Smythe HA: The modified sphygmomanometer—an instrument to measure muscle strength: validation study. *J Chronic Dis* 34:353–361, 1981.
11. Helewa H, Goldsmith CH, Smythe HA: Patient, observer and instrument variation in the measurement of strength of shoulder abductor muscles in patients with rheumatoid arthritis using a modified sphygmomanometer. *J Rheumatol* 13:1044–1049, 1986.
12. Helewa A, Goldsmith C, Smythe H et al: An evaluation of four different measures of abdominal muscle strength: patient, order, and instrument variation. *J Rheumatol* 17:965–969, 1990.
13. Smythe HA, Helewa A, Goldsmith CH: Independent assessor and pooled index as techniques for measuring treatment effects in rheumatoid arthritis. *J Rheumatol* 30:175–180, 1977.
14. Klinkhoff AV, Bellamy N, Bombardier C et al: An experiment in reducing interobserver variability of the examination of joint tenderness. *J Rheumatol* 15:492–494, 1988.
15. Lansbury J: Methods for evaluating rheumatoid arthritis. In Hollander JL (ed): *Arthritis and Allied Conditions.* Philadelphia, Lea & Febiger, 1966.
16. Goldsmith CH, Smythe HA, Helewa A: Interpretation and power of a pooled index. *J Rheumatol* 20:575–578, 1993.
17. Smith EM, Juvinall RC, Bender LF et al: Flexor forces and rheumatoid metacarpophalangeal deformity. *JAMA* 198:130–134, 1966.
18. Hawley DJ: Functional ability, health status and quality of life. In Robbins L (ed): *Clinical Care of the Rheumatic Diseases,* ed 2. Atlanta Association of Rheumatology Health Professionals, 2001.
19. American Academy of Orthopedic Surgeons: *Joint Motion: Method of Measuring and Recording.* Edinburgh, Churchill Livingstone, 1966.
20. Gerhardt JJ, Rondinelli RD: Goniometric techniques for range of motion assessment. *Phys Med Rehabil Clin North Am* 12:507–537, 2001.
21. Kaegi C, Thibault MC, Giroux F et al: The inter-rater reliability of force measurements using the modified sphygmomanometer in elderly subjects. *Phys Ther* 78:1095–1103, 1998.
22. Hochberg MC, Chang RW, Dwosh I et al: The American College of Rheumatology 1991 revised criteria for the classification of global functional status in rheumatoid arthritis. *Arthritis Rheum* 35:498–502, 1992.
23. Helewa A, Goldsmith CH, Smythe HA: Independent measurement of functional capacity in rheumatoid arthritis. *J Rheumatol* 9:794–797, 1982.
24. Waddell G: Understanding the patient with back pain. In Jayson MIV (ed): *The Lumbar Spine and Back Pain,* ed 4. Edinburgh, Churchill Livingstone, pp 469–485, 1992.
25. Richards JS, Nepomuceno C, Riles M et al: Assessing pain behaviour: the UAB pain behaviour scale. *Pain* 14:393–398, 1982.
26. Clark S, Burckhardt C, Campbell S et al: Pain behaviour and treatment outcomes in fibromyalgia patients. *Arthritis Rheum* 35:S350, 1992.
27. Wessely S, Nimnuan C, Sharpe M: Functional somatic syndromes: one or many? *Lancet* 354:936–939, 1999.

28. Wolfe F, Smythe HA, Yunus MB et al: The American College of Rheumatology 1990 criteria for the classification of fibromyalgia: report of the Multicentre Criteria Committee. *Arthritis Rheum* 33:160–172, 1990.

29. Smythe HA, Buskila D, Gladman DD: Performance of scored palpation, a point count, and dolorimetry in assessing unsuspected non-articular tenderness. *J Rheumatol* 20:352–357, 1993.

30. Helewa A, Goldsmith CH, Lee P et al: Does strengthening the abdominal muscles prevent low back pain: a randomized controlled trial. *J Rheumatol* 26:1808–1815, 1999.

31. Miller MH, Lee P, Smythe HA et al: Measurement of spinal mobility in the sagittal plane: new skin contraction technique compared with established methods. *J Rheumatol* 11:507–511, 1984.

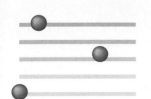

CHAPTER 6

Pharmacology

Priti Flanagan, BSP, PharmD
Joan M. Walker, PhD, PT

<table>
<tr><td>

Drugs for the Treatment of Osteoarthritis and Rheumatoid Arthritis
Acetaminophen
Salicylic Acid Derivatives
Nonsteroidal Anti-Inflammatory Drugs
Corticosteroids
  Systemic Therapy
  Intra-articular Therapy
Disease-Modifying Antirheumatic Drugs
Antimalarial Agents

</td><td>

Gold Compounds
Penicillamine
Sulfasalazine
Cytotoxic Agents
  Methotrexate
  Azathioprine
  Cyclophosphamide and Chlorambucil
  Cyclosporine
Leflunomide
Biologic Agents
Etanercept
Infliximab

</td><td>

Drugs for the Treatment of Crystal-induced Arthritis (Gout)
Colchicine
Allopurinol
Uricosuric Agents
Adherence and Cost Issues
Iontophoresis
Complementary and Alternative Medicine
Pharmacogenomics
Areas of Research
Summary
References

</td></tr>
</table>

Treatment goals and objectives for clients with arthritis may include one or more of the following: (1) reduction of joint pain, (2) reduction of inflammation, (3) preservation of joint function, (4) prevention of disease progression, and (5) maintenance of lifestyle. Goals and objectives will be prioritized depending on the actual disease state and condition of the client. Pharmacological therapy plays an important role in the achievement of these goals and objectives.

The physical therapist and occupational therapist should be familiar with a client's drug regimen for a number of reasons. Drug therapy may influence treatment timing and response, and therefore the therapist can play a role in monitoring the efficacy of drug therapy. The therapist also can monitor for any side effects of medications and a client's adherence to a prescribed drug therapy regimen. By providing information to clients about their medication and reinforcing the need to adhere to their medication regimens, a therapist can help to enhance adherence. Furthermore, a therapist can ensure that drug containers can be easily manipulated by the client who has arthritis that involves the hands.

A therapist's role in drug therapy is as follows:

- Monitor intake
- Monitor adverse reactions
- Monitor ability to open containers

PHYSICAL REHABILITATION IN ARTHRITIS, Joan M. Walker, PhD, PT, and Antoine Helewa, MSc(Clin Epid), PT, Elsevier Inc. © 2004.

- Contribute to client's drug education
- Consider client's drugs in timing of treatment and effect of modalities

Most arthritis conditions have multifactorial etiology; thus, drug therapy is often complex, involving several interventions simultaneously. Drug therapy in some instances is efficacious; at other times it can be harmful. Careful monitoring of response is essential.

In this chapter we will focus on the various drugs used in the pharmacological management of arthritis. This will include a review of the pharmacology and pharmacokinetics of the drugs, their adverse effects and drug interactions, and the availability and administration of the products. For further detail, readers are referred to Chapter 4 and individual product monographs.[1,2]

Drugs for the Treatment of Osteoarthritis and Rheumatoid Arthritis

There are many different pharmacological agents used in the treatment of arthritis. Some provide symptomatic relief, whereas the goal of others is to slow or arrest the disease process. Acetaminophen, aspirin and its derivatives, and nonsteroidal anti-inflammatory drugs (NSAIDs) provide relief from the pain associated with arthritis. Aspirin, NSAIDs, and steroids provide symptomatic relief from the inflammation. Pharmacological agents to slow disease progression in rheumatoid arthritis (RA) are referred to as disease-modifying antirheumatic drugs (DMARDs) and include antimalarial agents, gold compounds, penicillamine, sulfasalazine, and cytotoxic agents such as methotrexate and azathioprine. Three new DMARDs are leflunomide, infliximab, and etanercept (the latter two are sometimes termed biologic agents in the literature). Steroids also play a role in slowing the progression of RA. Some of these drugs also are used in the treatment of other forms of arthritis, such as systemic lupus erythematosus (SLE). Combinations of these drugs can be used to simultaneously provide symptom relief and slow or arrest the disease process. Drugs such as colchicine, allopurinol, and uricosuric agents are used in the treatment of gout and hyperuricemia. In this chapter we will focus on the common drugs used in the treatment of arthritis. Pharmacology, pharmacokinetics, adverse drug reactions, drug interactions, and availability and administration of the agents will be discussed. The actual approach to treating a particular disorder and role of these drugs in that treatment are discussed in

Chapter 4. Special considerations for therapists are included at the end of each drug or drug category.

Acetaminophen

Pharmacology and Pharmacokinetics

Acetaminophen is an agent that effectively reduces pain (analgesic effect) and reduces fever (antipyretic effect). It is believed to produce its analgesic effect by a mechanism similar to that of acetylsalicylic acid (ASA or aspirin); however, the exact site and mechanism of action are still not clearly understood.[3] Unlike aspirin, acetaminophen possesses no clinically significant anti-inflammatory activity.[3] It differs also from aspirin in that it does not affect uric acid levels and does not inhibit platelet activity.[3,4]

Acetaminophen is used for its analgesic activities in the treatment of arthritis and may be used in conjunction with anti-inflammatory therapy. A dose of acetaminophen of 650 mg given four times daily provides analgesia similar to that of an equal dose of aspirin.[5]

The dosage form determines the pharmacokinetics of acetaminophen. Acetaminophen is rapidly absorbed from the gastrointestinal (GI) tract after oral administration, with peak plasma concentrations occurring within 10 to 60 minutes for the immediate-release tablets and 60 to 120 minutes for the extended-release tablets.[4] The absorption of the extended-release formulation may be delayed by food.[4] It has a half-life in the range of 1 to 3 hours. This may be prolonged in neonates, in clients with liver disease, and after ingestion of toxic doses.[4]

Adverse Effects and Drug Interactions

Acetaminophen is generally well tolerated. Mild, reversible elevations in liver enzyme levels may occur, but levels return to normal when the drug is discontinued.[6] At higher doses, clients may become excited, disoriented, and/or dizzy. Excessive doses of acetaminophen (7.5 to 10 g) can cause liver toxicity and may be fatal.[4] Early symptoms of toxicity may include nausea, vomiting, and abdominal pain.[6] Acetylcysteine is a specific antidote used to treat acetaminophen toxicity.

Chronic abuse of alcohol may increase the toxicity of acetaminophen.[4] Concurrent administration of barbiturates, carbamazepine, rifampin, isoniazid, phenytoin, or sulfinpyrazone may increase the risk of liver toxicity.[3,4] There is some evidence that acetaminophen may potentiate the effect of warfarin, which may warrant increased monitoring of blood coagulation (e.g., international normalized ratio testing).[4,7,8]

Availability and Administration

Acetaminophen is available in a wide variety of dosage forms (tablet, liquid, suppository) and in a number of combination products with other medications. The usual oral or rectal dose of acetaminophen for adults is 325 to 650 mg every 4 to 6 hours.[4] The maximum dose is 4 g/day.[4] The extended-release formulation is available in 650-mg tablets and is taken every 8 hours.[4] The maximum recommended extended-release dose is 3.9 g/day.[4]

> ## Acetaminophen, Considerations for Therapists
>
> - Acetaminophen will only reduce pain—not inflammation.
> - Acetaminophen should provide an analgesic effect within 30 to 60 minutes after oral administration.
> - Acetaminophen rarely causes adverse effects.
> - Clients exhibiting symptoms of toxicity should be referred immediately for medical attention.
> - Acetaminophen is found in combination with other medicinal ingredients in both nonprescription and prescription drugs, so clients may be taking more acetaminophen than they realize. This may increase the risk of adverse effects.
> - Clients with arthritis find it easier to do their exercises after the drug has had an effect, but must be cautioned not to overexert.

Salicylic Acid Derivatives

Pharmacology and Pharmacokinetics

ASA is the prototype of the salicylates and is used to reduce pain (analgesic effect), inflammation (anti-inflammatory effect), fever (antipyretic effect), and platelet aggregation (antithrombotic effect).[4]

ASA exerts its anti-inflammatory activity primarily by inhibiting prostaglandin synthesis (Figure 6-1). Phospholipids are released from cells in response to tissue injury and are converted to arachidonic acid, which is further metabolized via the lipoxygenase and cyclooxygenase pathways. The end products (leukotrienes, prostaglandins, thromboxane) help to mediate the inflammatory response to tissue injury.

ASA exerts its anti-inflammatory activity by irreversibly inhibiting the activity of the cyclooxygenase enzyme.[6] This enzyme also is found in platelets. Because platelets cannot resynthesize cyclooxygenase, the effect of ASA lasts the entire life span (about 7 days) of the platelet and thus interferes with platelet aggregation. This will result clinically in an increased risk of bleeding and easy bruising. The analgesic effect of ASA is in part mediated by its anti-inflammatory activity. However, it is believed to also suppress pain at the subcortical level.[6]

> **Many medications in addition to ASA may result in an increased risk of bleeding and easy bruising. Consider this when handling clients manually and applying apparatus or splints.**

The salicylates are rapidly absorbed from the *stomach and small intestine* after oral administration, with peak plasma levels occurring within 15 to 120 minutes, depending on the specific dosage formulation. ASA is partly converted to salicylate during absorption, and both ASA and salicylate produce anti-inflammatory effects.[4]

Adverse Effects and Drug Interactions

Despite its wide availability, the use of ASA is limited in many clients because of its high incidence of adverse effects (Table 6-1). At doses used to alleviate inflammation, the major adverse effect of ASA is gastric intolerance, which may manifest as dyspepsia, nausea, indigestion, or heartburn. Gastric irritation may be decreased by taking aspirin with a large glass of water or milk or by taking it with food.[4] ASA also has been buffered and enteric coated to help decrease adverse GI effects. The enteric-coated preparations are most commonly prescribed for the treatment of arthritis, because they cause less GI irritation than the uncoated ASA products.[9] ASA also may cause mucosal erosion and ulceration and fecal blood loss.[6] This is due to direct irritation of the GI mucosa and decreased production of prostaglandins, which protect the gastric mucosa. Therapies to reduce development of ulcers due to aspirin are discussed later under NSAIDs.

At high doses ASA also can have negative effects on the central nervous system (CNS) by causing tinnitus, altered hearing, and vertigo, which may cause balance problems. These are reversible when the dose is reduced. At doses less than 2 g/day, serum uric acid levels may be increased, whereas levels will decrease at doses greater than 4 g/day.[6] ASA may rarely cause liver toxicity. Because prostaglandins play a role in

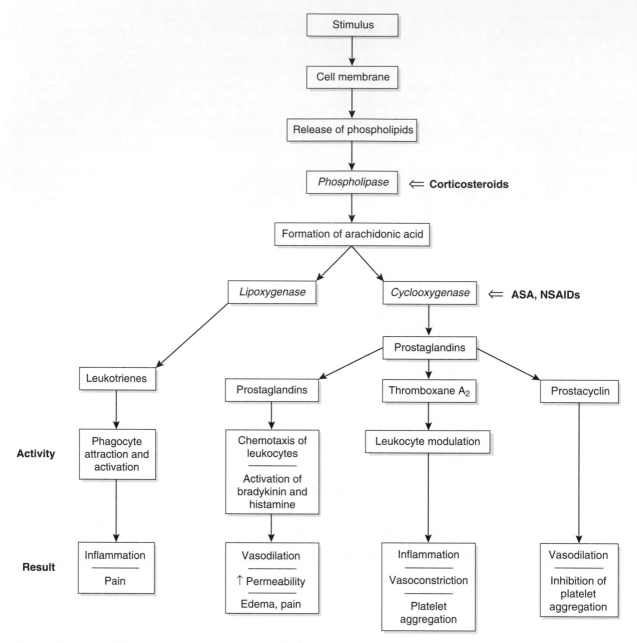

Figure 6-1. Simplified schematic diagram of the inflammatory process. Site of action of corticosteroids, acetylsalicylic acid, and nonsteroidal anti-inflammatory drugs. When drugs are effective, subsequent effects in the inflammatory process are minimized. (Data from Payan DG, Shearn MA: Nonsteroidal anti-inflammatory drugs; nonopioid analgesics; drugs used in gout. In Katzung BG [ed]: *Basic and Clinical Pharmacology,* ed 4. Norwalk, CT, Appleton & Lange, 1989, pp 431-450; and Schuna AA, Coulter L, Lee SS: Rheumatoid arthritis and the seronegative spondyloarthropathies. In DiPiro JT, Talbert RL, Hayes PE et al [eds]: *Pharmacotherapy, a Pathophysiologic Approach.* Norwalk, CT, Appleton & Lange, 1993, pp 1313–1329.)

Table 6-1. Adverse Effects of Acetylsalicylic Acid (ASA)*

Cardiovascular effects	Hematological effects
Pulmonary edema	Leukopenia
Central nervous system effects	Thrombocytopenia
Tinnitus	Pancytopenia
Altered hearing	Purpura
Vertigo	Hepatic effects
Dizziness	Hepatotoxicity
Dermatological effects	Hypersensitivity effects
Skin eruptions and lesions	Urticaria
Gastrointestinal effects	Angioedema
Dyspepsia	Bronchospasm
Heartburn	
Nausea	
Vomiting	
Diarrhea	
Indigestion	
Ulceration	

Data from Repchinsky C (ed): CPS 37th edition. Ottawa, Canadian Pharmacists Association, 2002.
*This list is not all-inclusive; it includes effects that are most likely to occur, or, if do occur, may be serious.

maintaining normal kidney function, in some instances use of aspirin may lead to impaired renal function ranging from elevation of serum creatinine levels to acute renal failure.[4] ASA may cause hypersensitivity reactions (urticaria, angioedema, bronchospasm) in clients with asthma and nasal polyps. As mentioned previously, ASA irreversibly impairs platelet aggregation and prolongs bleeding time. Because new platelets must be released before bleeding time will return to normal and this can take up to 7 days, it is generally recommended that ASA be discontinued about 7 days before any surgery.[9]

Tinnitus, dizziness, and vertigo may result from high doses of aspirin and cause balance problems. These side effects may require dosage adjustments that result in suboptimal benefit for pain and inflammation.

Potential interactions of ASA with other drugs are presented in Table 6-2. Clients who are taking any of these drugs concurrently with ASA should be monitored for the potential effects of these interactions.

Availability and Administration
ASA is available in several dosage forms (tablets, effervescent tablets, suppositories) manufactured by various companies and in both immediate- and long-acting preparations. Most products are available over the counter without a physician's prescription. A usual oral dose for ASA is 325 to 650 mg every 4 hours; however, higher doses of 3.2 to 5.4 g/day (in divided doses) may be needed for arthritis. The exact dose is tailored to the specific client and will be adjusted based on the client's response and adverse effects. Dosing also may be guided by measurement of salicylate levels.[4] Measurement of drug levels can be useful in evaluating drug absorption and client adherence. In children with juvenile RA (JRA) the usual initial dose is 60 to 130 mg/kg in those weighing 25 kg and 2.4 to 3.6 g/day in those weighing more than 25 kg.[4] The various salicylic acid derivatives available are presented in Table 6-3.

Several nonacetylated salicylates (choline magnesium trisalicylate, salsalate, diflunisal) are available as options for anti-inflammatory and analgesic therapy. These agents may be safer in those with asthma, GI upset, and bleeding tendencies.[5,6]

Nonsteroidal Anti-Inflammatory Drugs

Pharmacology and Pharmacokinetics
NSAIDs were developed in response to the need for aspirin-like drugs without the toxicities of aspirin. There are currently several NSAIDs available in the

Table 6-2. Drug Interactions with Acetylsalicylic Acid (ASA)*

Drugs	Effects
Affecting ASA	
Ascorbic acid, ammonium chloride	↓ salicylate excretion
Antacids	↓ salicylate activity
Corticosteroids	↑ salicylate clearance
Affected by ASA	
Angiotensin-converting enzyme inhibitors	↓ antihypertensive effect
Anticoagulants	Prolonged bleeding time
β-Blockers	↓ antihypertensive effect
Methotrexate	↑ methotrexate blood levels
Nonsteroidal anti-inflammatory drugs (NSAIDs)	↓ NSAID blood levels and ↑ risk of gastrointestinal toxicities

Data from Cada DJ Facts and Comparisons. St. Louis, Facts and Comparisons Inc, 2002.
*This list is not all-inclusive; it includes interactions that are likely to occur, or, if do occur, may be serious.

Table 6-3. Nonsteroidal Anti-Inflammatory Drugs*

Class	Brand Name[†]	Dose[‡] and Dosing Schedule	Analgesic Effect (hours)		Anti-inflammatory Effect	
			Onset	*Duration*	*Onset (days)*	*Peak (weeks)*
Acetic acid derivatives						
Diclofenac	Voltaren (USA and CAN)	75–100 mg in 3 divided doses	—	—	—	2
Indomethacin	Indocid (USA and CAN)	75–100 mg in 3 divided doses	0.5	4–6	Within 7	1–2
Tolmetin Na	Tolectin (USA and CAN)	600–1,800 mg in 3–4 divided doses	—	—	Within 7	1–2
Ketorolac	Toradol (USA and CAN)	100 mg q⁴–6h (oral) 10–30 mg q⁴–6h (IM)	IM: 10 min	IM: up to 6	—	—
Etodolac	Lodine (USA)	800–1200 mg in divided doses	0.5	4–6	—	—
Nabumetone	Relafen (USA)	1000 mg as a single dose	—	—	—	—
Fenamates						
Mefenamic acid	Ponstel (USA), Ponstan (CAN)	250 mg q6h	—	—	—	—
Meclofenamate Na	Meclomen (USA)	200–400 mg/day in 3 or 4 doses	1	4–6	Few days	2–3

Table 6-3. Nonsteroidal Anti-Inflammatory Drugs*—cont'd

Class	Brand Name[†]	Dose[‡] and Dosing Schedule	Analgesic Effect (hours)		Anti-inflammatory Effect	
			Onset	*Duration*	*Onset (days)*	*Peak (weeks)*
Indole derivatives						
Sulindac	Clinoril (USA and CAN)	20 mg once daily	1	48–72	7–12	2–3
Oxicams						
Piroxicam	Feldene (USA and CAN)	20 mg once daily	1	48–72	7–12	2–3
Tenoxicam	Mobiflex (CAN)	10–20 mg once daily	—	—	—	—
Meloxicam	Mobic (USA), Mobicox (CAN)	7.5–15 mg once daily	—	—	—	—
Propionic acid derivatives						
Fenoprofen	Nalfon (USA and CAN)	1.8–2.4 g in 3–4 divided doses	—	—	2	2–3
Flurbiprofen	Ansaid (USA and CAN)	200–300 mg in 3 divided doses	—	—	—	—
Ibuprofen	Motrin (USA and CAN)	800–1200 mg in 3–4 divided doses	0.5	4–6	Within 7	1–2
Ketoprofen	Orudis (USA and CAN)	150–200 mg in 3–4 divided doses	—	—		—
Naproxen	Naprosyn (USA and CAN)	750–1000 mg in 2 divided doses	1	Up to 7	Within 14	2–4
Naproxen Na	Anaprox (USA and CAN)	275 mg q6–8h	1	Up to 7	Within 14	2–4
Tiaprofenic acid	Surgam (CAN)	600 mg in 2–3 divided doses	—	—	—	—
Pyrazolon derivatives						
Phenylbutazone	Butazolidin (CAN)		—	—	—	—
Salicylic acid derivatives						
ASA	Various	2.6–5.4 g in 3–4 divided doses	—	—	—	—
Choline, magnesium trisalicylate	Trilisate (USA and CAN)	1–1.5 g twice daily	—	—	—	—

Continued

Table 6-3. Nonsteroidal Anti-Inflammatory Drugs*—cont'd

Class	Brand Name[†]	Dose[‡] and Dosing Schedule	Analgesic Effect (hours)		Anti-inflammatory Effect	
			Onset	Duration	Onset (days)	Peak (weeks)
Difluinsal	Dolobid (USA and CAN)	500–1000 mg in 2 divided doses	1	8–12	—	—
Salsalate	Disalcid (USA)	3000 mg in divided doses	—	—	—	—
Selective COX-2 inhibitors						
Celecoxib	Celebrex (USA and CAN)	OA: 100 mg twice daily or 200 mg once daily; RA: 100–200 mg twice daily				
Rofecoxib	Vioxx (USA and CAN)	12.5–25 mg once daily				
Valdecoxib	Bextra (USA)	10 mg once daily				
Other						
Floctafenine	Idarac (CAN)	200–400 mg q6–8h	—	—	—	—

*Data from Repchinsky C (ed): *CPS*, ed 37. Ottawa, Canadian Pharmacists Association, 2002,[1] Connor EP (product manager): *Physicians' Desk Reference.* Montvale, NJ, Medical Economics Data Production Company, 2002,[2] Cada DJ (ed): *Facts and Comparisons.* St Louis, 2002, Facts and Comparisons.[3] McEvoy GK (ed): *AHFS Drug Information.* Bethesda, MD, American Society of Hospital Pharmacists, 2002.[4]
[†]Common brand name in United States (USA) and Canada (CAN).
[‡]Usual anti-inflammatory dose except for ketorolac, mefenamic acid, etodolac, and idarac: Doses adjusted based on response and occurrence of adverse effects.
[§]Information not available.
COX-2, cyclooxygenase-2; IM = intramuscular; OA = osteoarthritis; RA = rheumatoid arthritis.

United States and Canada (see Table 6-3) that are divided into several chemical classes. The anti-inflammatory effect of NSAIDs is mediated through their ability to inhibit the activity of the cyclooxygenase (COX) enzyme (see Figure 6-1). The COX enzyme is responsible for the conversion of arachidonic acid into prostaglandins. Two forms of this enzyme, cyclooxygenase-1 (COX-1) and cyclooxygenase-2 (COX-2), exist, and they have different physiological functions. COX-1 is a constitutive form of the enzyme that is present in many cells of the body, including platelets, mucosal cells of the GI tract, and the endothelium. Conversely, COX-2 is an inducible form because its production can be increased greatly in response to inflammation. Through its actions, pain, swelling, and stiffness can occur. The traditional NSAIDs inhibited both forms of the COX enzyme to varying degrees.

With the availability of the COX-2 specific inhibitors, also referred to as the coxibs, it was felt that the analgesic and anti-inflammatory benefits of the NSAIDs would be retained with less toxicity.

Adverse Effects and Drug Interactions

Adverse effects associated with NSAID use are similar to those seen with the salicylates. The coxibs have been reported to cause less severe GI events and have less effect on platelet function[10–12]; however, data from long-term investigations are needed to establish their relative risk of toxicity compared with the traditional NSAID drugs. Risk factors for GI perforation, ulceration, and bleeding among users of NSAIDs and salicylates are previous peptic ulcer disease, advanced age, concomitant use of warfarin, corticosteroids, or other NSAIDs, chronic alcoholism, and comorbid

Salicylic Acid Derivatives, Considerations for Therapists

- ASA and its derivatives will reduce pain and inflammation.
- Avoid aggressive mobilization at peak analgesic activity. Consider duration of analgesic activity because pain decrease may allow excessive motion and cause further trauma to joint structures.
- Onset and peak anti-inflammatory activity must be considered in planning physical activity because this can negate drug effects by promoting further release of enzymes that destroy cartilage.
- CNS effects (i.e., tinnitus, dizziness) may affect a client's ability to respond to and participate in physical therapy (PT) and/or occupational therapy (OT). Be observant for new balance problems.
- Clients taking high doses of ASA may bruise easily; use care in applying apparatus, in some massage techniques (e.g., deep transverse frictions), and mobilization techniques.
- Clients may experience GI irritation and/or ulceration, which may add to their discomfort.
- ASA is found in combination with other medicinal ingredients in both prescription and nonprescription drugs, so clients may be taking more aspirin than they realize. This may increase the risk of adverse effects. Monitor both prescription and over-the-counter drug intake.

illness.[13] Those at risk for adverse GI events such as ulceration may receive concomitant misoprostol, histamine-2 receptor antagonists (e.g., ranitidine, famotidine), or a proton pump inhibitor (e.g., omeprazole, lansoprazole, pantoprazole) to minimize this risk. Because NSAIDs do inhibit platelet function, they should be discontinued approximately 24 hours before any surgery to allow bleeding times to return to normal.[14]

The COX-2 enzyme is responsible for maintenance of kidney function and therefore its inhibition can result in adverse renal effects. Furthermore, edema and hypertension are effects that could be expected with both the traditional and coxib NSAIDs. Because

Table 6-4. Drug Interactions with Nonsteroidal Anti-Inflammatory Drugs (NSAIDs)*

Drugs	Effects
Affecting NSAIDs	
Cimetidine	↑ or ↓ NSAID blood levels
Probenecid	↑ blood levels of NSAIDs
Salicylates	↓ blood levels of NSAIDs and ↑ risk of GI toxicities
Affected by NSAIDs	
Anticoagulants	Prolonged bleeding time
Angiotensin-converting enzyme inhibitors	↓ antihypertensive effect
β-Blockers	↓ antihypertensive effect
Cyclosporine	↑ risk of nephrotoxicity
Phenytoin	↑ phenytoin levels
Lithium	↑ lithium levels
Loop diuretics	↓ effect of diuretic
Methotrexate	↑ risk of toxicity
Thiazide diuretics	↓ effect of diuretic

Data from Cada DJ (ed): Facts and Comparisons. St. Louis, Facts and Comparisons Inc, 2002.[3]
*This list is not all-inclusive; it includes interactions that are likely to occur, or, if do occur, may be serious.

of the possibility of renal toxicity, the NSAIDs should be used cautiously in clients at high risk (e.g., those with congestive heart failure), and renal function should be carefully monitored.[14]

Since several drugs may interact with NSAIDs (Table 6-4), clients taking concomitant drugs should be monitored carefully. Not all of the available NSAIDs will interact with concurrently administered drugs to the same degree.

Availability and Administration

Table 6-3 lists the NSAIDs currently available along with the most common brand name, usual dose and dosing interval, and onset of analgesic and anti-inflammatory activity. If one NSAID is not effective, another may be tried. It is not unusual for clients to try several NSAIDs before an effective one is found. As noted in Table 6-3, some NSAIDs are given once daily whereas others must be given three to four times a day. Frequency of dosing may influence adherence with drug therapy, because adherence tends to decrease as the number of doses increases. Most of the NSAIDs require a prescription.

NSAIDs, Considerations for Therapists

- NSAIDs will reduce pain and inflammation but are not equipotent in their activity.
- Familiarity with the onset and duration of analgesic activity is important.
- Pain intensity should decrease with the decrease in inflammation.
- Because onset of anti-inflammatory activity is gradual, treatment should be progressed slowly over several weeks.
- CNS adverse effects (i.e., dizziness) may affect a client's ability to respond to and participate in OT and/or PT.
- Clients may experience GI irritation and ulceration which will add to their discomfort.
- Some NSAIDs, such as ibuprofen and naproxen sodium, are available without a prescription, so clients may be taking several NSAIDs or more ibuprofen or naproxen than they realize. This may increase the risk of adverse effects.

Corticosteroids

Corticosteroids are used in the treatment of arthritis because of their anti-inflammatory and immunosuppressive effects. They come in various dosage forms and strengths and may be administered as short- or long-term drug therapy. In this section, systemic and intra-articular administration will be discussed separately. Corticosteroids also may be delivered as intravenous (IV) boluses in some forms of arthritis as intra-articular injections and are often used topically in SLE.

Systemic Therapy

Pharmacology and Pharmacokinetics The adrenal cortex produces and releases various hormones into the circulation. They are divided into three main groups: (1) glucocorticoids (primarily responsible for regulation of fat, carbohydrate, and protein metabolism), (2) mineralocorticoids (primarily responsible for maintaining water and electrolyte balance), and (3) sex hormones (i.e., androgens, testosterone, estradiol).[15] Natural and synthetic versions of these hormones are used in the treatment of a wide variety of disorders, particularly inflammatory and immunological diseases.

Corticosteroids exert their anti-inflammatory effect by inhibiting the activity of phospholipase in the arachidonic acid cascade (see Figure 6-1), which decreases production of prostaglandins and leukotrienes.[16] Corticosteroids cause an increase in the number of neutrophils, resulting in an overall decrease in the number of cells available at the inflammation site.[16] Corticosteroids also cause a decrease in the number of lymphocytes, monocytes, eosinophils, and basophils, resulting in a decreased ability to respond to antigens.[16] The immunosuppressive activity of corticosteroids is due to a combination of the effects described above.[16]

Studies have shown that corticosteroids reduce both pain and stiffness in clients with RA.[17] Although not typically considered disease modifying, there is some evidence that the use of corticosteroids is associated with reduced joint damage in clients with RA, which continues to occur after the corticosteroid therapy is stopped.[18,19]

Adverse Effects and Drug Interactions Because the adrenal hormones affect so many functions within the body, administration of exogenous corticosteroids has the potential to cause numerous adverse effects, some of which can be very serious (Table 6-5). With short courses of high doses, clients may experience elevations in serum glucose levels and in white blood

Table 6-5. Adverse Effects of Corticosteroids*

Cardiovascular effects	Gastrointestinal effects
Arrhythmias	Nausea
Hypertension	Vomiting
Atherosclerosis	$\uparrow$ appetite
Central nervous system effects	Weight gain
Convulsions	Peptic ulcer
Vertigo	Pancreatitis
Headache	Musculoskeletal effects
Neuritis	Muscle weakness
Steroid psychosis	Muscle wasting
Dermatological effects	Osteoporosis
Impaired wound healing	Aseptic necrosis
Thin fragile skin	Delayed skeletal development
Petechiae	Ophthalmic effects
Ecchymoses	Cataracts
Purpura	$\uparrow$ intraocular pressure
Striae	Glaucoma
Acneform eruptions	Exophthalmos
Urticaria	Other effects
Edema	$\uparrow$ susceptibility to infection
Focal atrophy	Hypothalamic-pituitary-adrenal axis
Endocrine effects	suppression
Amenorrhea	Agranulocytosis
Cushingoid syndrome	Coagulation disturbances
Hyperglycemia	Nephrolithiasis
Secondary adrenocortical and pituitary	$\uparrow$ white blood cell counts
unresponsiveness	
Fluid and electrolyte effects	
Sodium retention	
Edema	
Hypokalemia	
Hypertension	
Alkalosis	
Hypocalcemia	

Data from Cada DJ (ed): Facts and Comparisons. St. Louis, Facts and Comparisons Inc, 2002,[3] and McEvoy (ed): AHFS Drug Information. Bethesda American Society of Hospital Pharmacists, 2002.
*This list is not all-inclusive; it includes effects that are most likely to occur, or, if do occur, may be serious.

cell counts. Corticosteroids cause potassium loss and sodium retention (which may manifest clinically as elevated blood pressure and edema). Psychosis, if it occurs, usually does so within 15 to 30 days of starting therapy; the risk appears to increase with higher doses.[3] Corticosteroids also may cause GI irritation and ulceration.

These same adverse effects also may occur with longer courses of drug therapy, in addition to other potential complications. Continued therapy with corticosteroids results in suppression of the natural hypothalamic-pituitary-adrenal axis, even after as little as 1 week of medication. As a result, the corticosteroid should not be stopped abruptly to prevent adrenal insufficiency or the reappearance of disease or symptoms. Those who have successfully discontinued their corticosteroid therapy may require supplemental corticosteroid during stressful events such as surgery. Long-term corticosteroid treatment may result in Cushing's syndrome, with puffiness of the face,

Table 6-6. Drug Interactions with Nonsteroidal Anti-Inflammatory Drugs (NSAIDs)*

Drugs	Effects
Affecting Corticosteroids	
Barbiturates	↓ pharmacologic effect of corticosteroid
Cholestyramine, antacids	↓ absorption of corticosteroid
Oral contraceptives	↑ corticosteroid effects
Phenytoin	↓ corticosteroid effects
Ketoconazole	↑ corticosteroid effects
Macrolide antibodies	↑ corticosteroid effects
Rifampin	↓ corticosteroid effects
Affected by Corticosteroids	
Anticoagulants	Dose of anticoagulant may need to be altered
Cyclosporine	↑ levels of both drugs
Digoxin	↑ risk of digoxin toxicity
Isoniazid	↓ isoniazid levels
Diuretics	↑ risk of hypokalemia
Salicylates	↓ salicylate levels
Theophylline	Alteration in activity of either drug may occur

Data from Cada DJ (ed): Facts and Comparisons. St. Louis, Facts and Comparisons Inc, 2002.
*This list is not all-inclusive; it includes interactions that are likely to occur, or, if do occur, may be serious.

redistribution of fat from the extremities to the trunk and face, insomnia, acne, increased hair growth, and increased appetite.

With prolonged administration, muscle weakness, thinning of the skin, easy bruising, and osteoporosis may occur. Healing of wounds is often impaired. Corticosteroid use also may result in visual complications, such as development of cataracts and glaucoma.

Avascular necrosis (necrosis due to loss of blood supply) has been reported, particularly in clients taking corticosteroids for the treatment of SLE. These clients may be more at risk because of an associated rheumatoid arteriolar vasculitis occurring in the affected bone. Avascular necrosis usually occurs in the head of the femur. Aseptic necrosis (necrosis without infection) of the hip, knee, or shoulder also may occur in clients receiving high doses.

Parenteral administration of corticosteroids may result in scarring, induration, inflammation, paresthesia, and irritation at the site of injection. Hyperpigmentation or hypopigmentation as well as atrophy, sterile abscesses, burning, and tingling also have been reported.[3]

Corticosteroids have the potential to interact with several other medications (Table 6-6). Barbiturates, phenytoin, and rifampin will enhance the clearance of corticosteroids and decrease their pharmacological effect. Response to vaccinations and toxoids may be decreased, because corticosteroids inhibit the body's antibody response.

Availability and Administration There are several corticosteroids on the market for use in arthritis (Table 6-7). Orally administered corticosteroids are usually intended as temporary therapy until the disease is controlled or a therapeutic response from another drug is obtained. They may be used long term, at the lowest dose possible, if clients fail to show a response to other treatment. It is usually recommended that the corticosteroid be administered once daily in the morning to mimic the natural release of adrenal hormones and to minimize hypothalamic-pituitary-adrenal axis suppression.[9] With higher doses, the total daily dose may be divided and administered twice daily to provide better symptomatic relief.[9]

Intra-Articular Therapy

With intra-articular therapy, the corticosteroid is injected directly into the affected joint. This will reduce pain and inflammation, with benefit lasting for a few weeks.[20] Intra-articular therapy may be preferable for RA that affects only a few joints because the risk of systemic adverse effects is minimized compared with oral therapy.[9]

Table 6-7. Common Corticosteroids Used in Arthritis*

Corticosteroid	Equivalent Dose (mg)	Relative Anti-Inflammatory Potency	Relative Mineralocorticoid Potency	Examples of Products Available
Short-acting				
Cortisone	25	0.8	2	Cortone tablets (CAN and USA)
Hydrocortisone	20	1	2	Solu-Cortef injection (CAN and USA), Cotrel tablets (CAN)
Intermediate-acting				
Prednisone	5	4	1	Deltasone tablets (USA)
Prednisolone	5	4	1	Various: injection, tablets
Triamcinolone	4	5	0	Kenalog (CAN and USA), Aristospan (CAN and USA) injection
Methylprednisolone	4	5	0	Depo-Medrol (CAN and USA) injection, Medrol (CAN and USA) tablets
Long-lasting				
Dexamethasone	0.75	25-30	0	Decadron tablets (CAN and USA)
Betamethasone	0.6-0.75	25	0	Celestone injection (CAN and USA); tablets (USA)

Data from Repchinsky C (ed): CPS, 29th edition. Ottawa, Canadian Pharmaceutical Association, 2002.[1] McEvoy GK (ed): AHFS Drug Information. Bethesda, American Society of Hospital Pharmacists, 2002.[4]
*This is not a comprehensive list of all brand names and dosage forms for these corticosteroids available in the United States (USA) and Canada (CAN).

Intra-articular corticosteroid therapy is contra-indicated in clients with local infection, generalized infection with bacteremia, and recent serious injury at the injection site. Potentially, the most serious complication of intra-articular administration is the introduction of infection to the joint, which fortunately, occurs very rarely.[21] Other possible effects of intra-articular therapy include crystal-induced synovitis, cutaneous atrophy, osteonecrosis, steroid arthropathy, and tendon rupture. The risk of systemic effects is low, but they may occur and the risk increases with the frequency of injections.[4] Local adverse reactions, such as postinjection flare, may occur; the pain can be alleviated by local application of ice and oral analgesics. The reaction will usually subside within a few hours.[21]

There are several corticosteroids that may be injected into the affected joint (see Table 6-7). The rate of absorption and duration of action are related to the solubility of the compound injected; the least water-soluble compounds (i.e., triamcinolone) have the longest duration of action. The actual agents used and the dose depend on the physician's experience, size of the joint, degree of inflammation, and amount of fluid present in the joint.

Corticosteroids, Considerations for Therapists

- Corticosteroids will provide symptomatic relief.
- Corticosteroids may cause GI irritation.
- A once-daily morning dose of a corticosteroid is preferred, but clients may be taking divided doses spread out evenly over the day to provide symptomatic relief.
- Clients should not stop taking long-term corticosteroids abruptly, because symptoms of the disease may reappear or worsen or symptoms of adrenal suppression may occur.
- Corticosteroids may impair vision and cause osteoporosis, weight gain, edema, muscle weakness, dizziness, low blood glucose levels, and easy bruising. These and other adverse effects may affect the client's ability to respond to or participate in OT and/or PT.
- Caution should be exercised in treatment of clients receiving long-term corticosteroid therapy (RA, JRA) because of the high potential for fractures with minimal stress.
- After corticosteroid therapy intra-articular injection of weight-bearing joints, bed rest, or non-weight bearing on crutches will be required for a period of about 5 days.
- Monitor skin condition when splints, braces, and apparatus are used to attach resistance equipment, because of skin fragility and easy bruising.

Disease-Modifying Antirheumatic Drugs

Antimalarial Agents

Pharmacology and Pharmacokinetics

Hydroxychloroquine and its parent drug chloroquine are two antimalarial drugs that have been used in the treatment of RA. They are considered to be DMARDs. Although their exact mechanism of action is unknown, it is believed that they have both anti-inflammatory and immunosuppressive activities.[6]

Adverse Effects and Drug Interactions

When these drugs are used as antimalarials, the adverse effects are usually mild and reversible. However, more serious and sometimes irreversible adverse effects can occur with higher doses used for longer durations, such as those used in the treatment of RA.[4] After oral administration, adverse GI effects such as epigastric discomfort, nausea, vomiting, diarrhea, and cramps may occur. These may be minimized when the drugs are taken with food or a glass of milk. Clients may experience pruritus, skin rash, pigmentary changes of the skin, bleaching of the hair, or hair loss.[4] The CNS may be affected with the client complaining of symptoms such as headache, fatigue, and nervousness. Confusion, personality changes, and depression also may occur. Rarely, peripheral neuritis, neuromyopathy, and adverse hematological effects may occur.[4]

> Clients taking antimalarial drugs who experience new eye problems should be immediately referred to their physician.

A major concern with the antimalarial drugs is their ability to cause visual toxicities, such as keratopathy and retinopathy. Keratopathy, including transient edema or deposits in the cornea, have been reported in 30% to 70% of clients. It can occur within just a few weeks of the beginning of therapy and is reversible when the drug is discontinued. It may be asymptomatic in up to 50% of clients; however, other clients may experience visual halos, focusing difficulties, blurred vision, or photophobia.[4]

The risk of retinopathy increases with increasing doses.[9] Symptoms of retinopathy include blurred vision, night blindness, light flashes and streaks, and photophobia. Occasionally, retinal changes are reversible if detected early, but they are usually permanent and may result in blindness. The retinal damage may occur even after the drug is stopped. Routine examinations are necessary to monitor for these visual toxicities. Long-term therapy with high doses of hydroxychloroquine has been associated with fewer adverse effects than similar treatment with chloroquine.[4]

The antimalarial agents should not be used concurrently with phenylbutazone, gold compounds, or penicillamine, because of the increased risk of severe skin reactions. They should be used cautiously with drugs that cause hepatotoxicity, because hydroxychloroquine concentrates in the liver and may cause toxicity. Levels of digoxin may be increased if it is used concomitantly with hydroxychloroquine.[3]

Availability and Administration

Hydroxychloroquine is available in both the United States and Canada as Plaquenil, 200-mg tablets. Treatment for RA is usually initiated at a dose of 400 mg/day, and when a good response is obtained the dose may be reduced by about 50% to 200 mg/day.[1] It may take 1 to 6 months before an effect is seen, and therefore an adequate trial of the drug should be given.[22] It is not currently approved for use in JRA, because its safety in children for this indication has not been proven.[1] Hydroxychloroquine also is used in the treatment of SLE. Baseline and periodic eye examinations and blood counts should be obtained to monitor for toxicities while clients are being treated with hydroxychloroquine.

Antimalarials, Considerations for Therapists

- Hydroxychloroquine is a DMARD, and it may not provide relief for 1 to 6 months.
- Hydroxychloroquine is generally well tolerated; any GI irritation may be reduced when the drug is taken with food or milk.
- Doses used in the treatment of RA may cause serious visual toxicities that may be asymptomatic or cause changes, such as blurred vision, visual halos, difficulty in focusing, photophobia, and fog before the eyes. Permanent damage and blindness may occur. Clients experiencing these effects should be referred to their physician.

Gold Compounds

Pharmacology and Pharmacokinetics

Gold therapy, or chrysotherapy, has been available for the treatment of RA since the 1920s.[6] Gold therapy is believed to have an immunosuppressive effect by inhibiting the maturation and function of mononuclear phagocytes and T cells.[23] In addition, gold has minimal anti-inflammatory effects. Gold is classified as a DMARD and will slow the progression of RA and provide some symptom relief.[6,23]

The two injectable formulations, gold sodium thiomalate (water-soluble) and aurothioglucose (oil-soluble), are both intended for intramuscular administration. Gold sodium thiomalate is rapidly absorbed after injection, whereas aurothioglucose is absorbed slowly and irregularly. With oral gold therapy only

Table 6-8. Adverse Effects of Gold Compounds*

Gastrointestinal effects
  Diarrhea
  Abdominal cramping and pain
  Nausea
Hematological effects
  Leukopenia
  Thrombocytopenia
  Aplastic anemia
  Eosinophilia
  Agranulocytosis
  Pancytopenia
Mucocutaneous effects
  Rash
  Pruritus
  Erythema
  Ulceration of oropharynx
  Metallic taste
  Exfoliative dermatitis
Renal effects
  Proteinuria
  Hematuria
  Glomerulonephritis
  Nephrotic syndrome
Other effects
  ↑ liver enzyme levels
  Hepatitis
  Headache
  Dizziness
  Peripheral neuropathy
  Nitritoid reaction
  Interstitial pneumonitis
  Anaphylactic reaction
  Conjunctivitis

Data from McEvoy GK (ed): AHFS Drug Information. Bethesda, American Society of Hospital Pharmacists, Inc, 2002.[4]
*This list is not all-inclusive; it includes effects that are most likely to occur, or, if do occur, may be serious.

approximately 25% of the dose is absorbed.[1] Both oral and intramuscular formulations can take 3 to 6 months to be beneficial for RA.[22]

Adverse Effects and Drug Interactions

Although similar adverse effects (Table 6-8) occur with all gold therapy, the incidence does differ, depending on the formulation. The common adverse effects, up to 60% to 80%, of intramuscular gold therapy are mucocutaneous in nature, ranging from erythema to exfoliative dermatitis.[24] Some clients complain of lumps at the site of injection, as well as increased joint symptoms for a day or two after receiving an injection.[9,20] Stomatitis may occur and will sometimes be preceded by a metallic taste. With oral gold therapy the most common adverse effect, up to 40%, is diarrhea, whereas 16% will experience GI irritation in the form of nausea, vomiting, or abdominal cramping.[25] Skin complications will occur in about 25% of clients receiving auranofin.[25] Exposure to sunlight or artificial ultraviolet light may exacerbate any skin rashes.[4]

All gold compounds can cause renal and liver toxicities. Renal effects, if recognized early, are usually mild and reversible. However, if gold therapy is continued, the renal effects can become serious and chronic.[4] Bone marrow suppression is the most serious complication of chrysotherapy and may present as leukopenia, thrombocytopenia, or pancytopenia in 1% to 10% of clients.[6] Aplastic anemia is another serious, but rare, side effect.[6] Up to 40% of clients may develop eosinophilia, which often accompanies or precedes other toxic reactions.[26] Vasomotor (or nitritoid) reactions consisting of flushing, weakness, dizziness, sweating, and hypotension may occur with gold sodium thiomalate.[4] If these occurs, aurothioglucose, which is absorbed more slowly, may be used.[4]

Gold compounds may be used safely in conjunction with salicylates, NSAIDs, or corticosteroids. Often one of these anti-inflammatory agents is used concomitantly to alleviate symptoms until the therapeutic effects of the gold compounds occur. Penicillamine, antimalarials, and the cytotoxic drugs cyclophosphamide, azathioprine, and methotrexate should not be used with the gold compounds. The safety of auranofin when used with high doses of corticosteroids or other gold compounds has not been determined.[3]

Availability and Administration

Gold is available in both intramuscular injection and oral formulations. Gold sodium thiomalate (Myochrysine in Canada, Aurolate in the United States) and aurothioglucose (Solganal in the United States and Canada) are both approved for adult and juvenile RA. Auranofin (Ridaura in the United States and Canada) is only approved for use in adults with RA. Auranofin may be preferred by some because it can be administered orally and its adverse effect profile is more favorable. However, others prefer the injectable preparations, because they may be more effective than the oral product but with them clients are required to visit the physician's office regularly for follow-up and injections.[9] The efficacy of this drug therapy appears to be affected by duration of disease, because those who have had RA for less than 5 years respond better to gold therapy than those who have had the disease

longer.[27] Gold has been administered intra-articularly; however, it does not appear to have any therapeutic advantage over corticosteroids.[21]

Chrysotherapy can be continued as long as the client responds favorably to the drug and does not experience intolerable or toxic adverse effects. Baseline urinalysis and blood counts should be obtained before drug therapy is initiated and regularly thereafter.[22] Clients should report to their physician if they notice any pruritus, skin rashes, stomatitis, fever, sore throat, or unusual bruising. If any toxicity is noticed, gold therapy should be discontinued, and after the toxicity has resolved, the client should be reevaluated for reinstitution of gold therapy.

Gold Compounds, Considerations for Therapists

- **Gold therapy is a DMARD and may not provide relief for up to 3 to 4 months.**
- **If clients complain of rashes, stomatitis, pruritus, fever, sore throat, or easy bruising they should be referred to their physician, because these symptoms may be indicative of more serious toxicities.**
- **Because skin rashes may be aggravated, ultraviolet light therapy should not be given to clients taking gold compounds.**

Penicillamine

Pharmacology and Pharmacokinetics

Penicillamine, although a degradation product of penicillin, has no antibacterial activity. It is believed to work in the treatment of RA through both immunosuppressive and anti-inflammatory activities.[6] Penicillamine is well absorbed after oral administration, with peak concentrations occurring within 1 hour.[4] The benefit of penicillamine in RA may take 3 to 6 months to be realized.[22]

Adverse Effects and Drug Interactions

The incidence of adverse effects is high with penicillamine (Table 6-9) with the most common being skin rashes, occurring in up to 50% of clients.[28] Rashes occurring early in drug therapy may require discontinuation of penicillamine. After the rash resolves, the drug can usually be restarted at a lower dose without any further problems.[4] Rashes with pruritus, occurring 6 months or more after the onset of therapy, do not resolve as easily. The rash may

Table 6-9. Adverse Effects of Penicillamine*

Allergic/immunological effects	Bone marrow suppression
Pruritus	Agranulocytosis
Drug eruptions	Aplastic anemia
Urticaria	Hepatic effects
Exfoliative dermatitis	Hepatic dysfunction
Thyroiditis	Jaundice
Gastrointestinal effects	Toxic hepatitis
Anorexia	Mucocutaneous effects
Nausea	Skin rash
Vomiting	↑ skin friability
Epigastric pain	Excessive skin wrinkling
Diarrhea	Oral ulcerations
Hematological effects	Renal effects
Leukopenia	Proteinuria
Thrombocytopenia	Hematuria
	Glomerulopathy

Data from McEvoy GK (ed): AHFS Drug Information. Bethesda, American Society of Hospital Pharmacists, Inc, 2002.[4]
*This list is not all-inclusive; it includes effects that are most likely to occur, or, if do occur, may be serious.

persist for weeks after the drug is discontinued and may recur if penicillamine is restarted.[4]

Thrombocytopenia and leukopenia are hematological adverse effects that can occur as a result of penicillamine therapy; they usually occur during the first year of treatment, often after 6 months.[28] The most common renal effect is proteinuria, seen in up to 20% of clients.[6] Penicillamine has been associated with inducing the autoimmune syndromes of myasthenia gravis and SLE.[9]

Administration of penicillamine may cause GI irritation in the form of nausea, vomiting, diarrhea, and epigastric pain. Some clients will complain of blunted taste perception, especially for salt and sweets. This is usually self-limiting, resolving after 2 to 3 months of therapy.[1]

Because of similar hematological and renal effects, penicillamine should not be used with gold therapy, antimalarial agents, phenylbutazone, or cytotoxic agents. The absorption of penicillamine will be decreased by the coadministration of iron salts, antacids, and food. Penicillamine may cause a decrease in serum digoxin levels, thereby potentially decreasing its pharmacological effects.[3]

Availability and Administration

Penicillamine, available as Cuprimine 125- and 250-mg capsules in both the United States and Canada, is approved for the treatment of RA in adults. It is not currently approved for use in children with JRA,

because its safety and efficacy have not yet been established.[4] Therapy is started with 125 to 250 mg/day, which may be increased by 125 to 250 mg/day at 1- to 3-month intervals. If there is no benefit of the drug at a dose of 1 to 1.5 g/day for 3 to 4 months, the drug should be stopped because further use will probably not produce any benefit.[1] Penicillamine should be taken on an empty stomach so that its absorption is not affected by food or other medications. Baseline blood counts and urinalysis should be performed and repeated every 2 weeks until the dose is stable and then every 1 to 3 months thereafter.[22]

Penicillamine, Considerations for Therapists

- **Penicillamine is a DMARD and may not provide relief for 3 to 6 months.**
- **Clients complaining of fever, sore throat, or easy bruising should be referred to their physician, because these symptoms may be indicative of more serious toxicities.**
- **Monitor for skin rashes.**

Sulfasalazine

Pharmacology and Pharmacokinetics

Sulfasalazine (SZ), a conjugate of a sulfapyridine

Table 6-10. Adverse Effects of Sulfasalazine*

Dose-Related Effects	Idiosyncratic Effects
Hematological effects	Dermatological effects
Heinz body anemia	Skin rash
Glucose-6-phosphate dehydrogenase (G-6-PD)	Exfoliative dermatitis
deficiency hemolytic anemia	Gastrointestinal effects
Leukopenia	Colitis exacerbation
Megaloblastic anemia	Hepatotoxicity
Other effects	Pancreatitis
Nausea	Hematological effects
Vomiting	Agranulocytosis
Anorexia	Hemolytic anemia
Headache	Pulmonary effects
Fever	Bronchospasm
Arthralgia	Eosinophilia
Cyanosis	Pulmonary infiltrate
Reversible male infertility	Other effects
Tachycardia	Systemic lupus erythematosus
Neonatal kernicterus	Raynaud's phenomenon

Data from Duncan BS. In Koda-Kimble MA, Young LY, Kradjan WA et al (eds): Applied Therapeutics, The Clinical Use of Drugs, 7th ed. pp 26-1–26-20. Philadelphia, Lippincott Williams & Wilkins, 2001.
*This list is not all-inclusive; it includes effects that are most likely to occur, or, if do occur, may be serious.

and 5-aminosalicylic acid, was originally synthesized in the 1930s.[9] A high incidence of adverse effects with minimum efficacy led to its disuse.[29] There has recently been renewed interest in and use of the drug in the treatment of RA, using lower doses that cause fewer adverse effects. The exact mechanism of action of SZ in RA remains unclear, but the drug may have anti-inflammatory and immunomodulatory activities.[6] SZ is poorly absorbed in the GI tract after oral administration. In the colon, SZ is broken down into its two components and the sulfonamide is absorbed. Most of the salicylate portion of the drug stays in the colon.[4]

Adverse Effects and Drug Interactions

Adverse effects occur in up to 21% of clients receiving SZ and can be divided into dose-related and idiosyncratic (Table 6-10).[30] Dose-related adverse effects tend to occur at doses greater than or equal to 4 g/day and early in the course of therapy. Clients often experience nausea, vomiting, anorexia, headache, arthralgias, cyanosis, and tachycardia. These adverse effects can be minimized by an initial low dose and a slow increase in dosage. The idiosyncratic reactions, although rare, are much more serious and toxic. These adverse reactions include effects such as agranulocytosis, skin rashes, hepatic toxicities, and lung diseases.[30]

Absorption of SZ can be reduced by concomitant administration of ferrous sulfate or cholestyramine. SZ may interfere with folic acid absorption and may decrease digoxin concentrations by up to 25%.[30] Warfarin and oral hypoglycemic agents may compete with sulfapyridine for its protein binding sites. Methotrexate may be displaced, thus increasing the risk of toxic effects.

Availability and Administration

The enteric-coated formulations of SZ (Salazopyrin EN-Tab in Canada, Azulfidine EnTabs in the United States) are used for the treatment of RA and JRA. Therapy is initiated at 500 mg/day and increased by 500 mg/day at weekly intervals to a maximum of 2 g/day. The onset of effect will not occur for several weeks to months; an adequate trial is necessary.[9] Baseline blood counts should be obtained and repeated periodically during therapy.

> ## Sulfasalazine, Considerations for Therapists
>
> • **Sulfasalazine is a DMARD that may not provide relief for 1 to 3 months.**

Table 6-11. Adverse Effects of Methotrexate*

Dermatological effects	Hematological effects
Rashes	Leukopenia
Dermatitis	Thrombocytopenia
Urticaria	Anemia
Acne	Hemorrhage
Alopecia	Hepatic effects
Gastrointestinal effects	↑ liver enzyme levels
Gingivitis	Hepatic fibrosis
Glossitis	Hepatic cirrhosis
Stomatitis	Pulmonary effects
Enteritis	Pneumonitis
Ulcerations	Pulmonary fibrosis
Anorexia	
Nausea	
Vomiting	
Diarrhea	
Pancreatitis	

Data from McEvoy GK(ed): AHFS Drug Information. Bethesda, American Society of Hospital Pharmacists, 2002.[4]
*This list is not all-inclusive; it includes effects that are most likely to occur, or, if do occur, may be serious.

- Clients may experience dose-related adverse effects (i.e., nausea, vomiting, headache, arthralgias) early in the course of drug therapy.
- Clients complaining of rashes, sore throat, or easy bruising should be referred to their physician, because these symptoms may be indicative of more serious toxicities.

Cytotoxic Agents

Methotrexate

Pharmacology and Pharmacokinetics Methotrexate (MTX) is an antimetabolite that has been used in the treatment of RA since the 1950s.[20] As an antimetabolite it acts as a folic acid antagonist, thus decreasing the production of a coenzyme vital to the cell life cycle; without this coenzyme the result is cell death. In the treatment of RA its exact mechanism of action is unclear, but it is believed to act primarily as an immunosuppressive agent. It also may have some anti-inflammatory activity.[28] MTX is well absorbed after oral administration, with peak concentrations occurring within 1 to 4 hours.[4]

Adverse Effects and Drug Interactions The frequent adverse effects with MTX therapy include nausea, vomiting, diarrhea, and dizziness (Table 6-11). These effects usually occur on the days that MTX is administered. Because MTX affects rapidly dividing cells, it also can cause mouth and GI ulceration, dermatitis, alopecia, leukopenia, and thrombocytopenia.[20] MTX may cause acute and chronic liver toxicity. Dry nonproductive cough, dyspnea, fever, and chest pain may be indicative of pulmonary toxicity, and the drug should be discontinued. Some of the common adverse effects of MTX therapy, such as nausea, mouth ulceration, and anorexia, also are indicative of folic acid deficiency. This has led to the supplementation of folic acid 1 mg daily or 5 mg once weekly. This supplementation has been shown to reduce these adverse effects without altering the efficacy of MTX.[31]

Clients receiving MTX should avoid all alcohol, because this will increase the risk of development of chronic hepatotoxicity. Drugs that may displace MTX from its protein-binding site and therefore increase the risk of toxicity should be used cautiously. Examples include salicylates, SZ, sulfonamides, sulfonylureas, phenytoin, phenylbutazone, tetracyclines, and chloramphenicol. The risk of toxicity also may increase with concomitant use of NSAIDs.

Availability and Administration MTX therapy, approved for adults with RA, can be administered orally, subcutaneously, or intramuscularly. Parenteral dosing is used for doses greater than 15 mg because oral bioavailability is reduced with larger doses.[20] MTX can be started orally with 7.5 mg once weekly given as a single dose or in three divided doses spaced every 12 hours. This "pulse" type of therapy has been carried over from the MTX regimen used in the treatment of psoriasis and appears to be less toxic.[32] The dose may be increased by 2.5 mg/wk every 6 weeks, if no response is seen in 6 to 8 weeks. Generally doses do not exceed a weekly dose of 20 mg.[1] A response to therapy may be seen as early as 3 weeks.[33] Baseline and periodic blood counts, urinalysis, renal and liver function tests, and chest x-ray films should be obtained to monitor for adverse effects.[1]

Methotrexate, Considerations for Therapists

- Methotrexate is a DMARD and may not provide relief for up to 1 to 2 months.
- On the day (or days) the client is taking MTX, she or he may experience nausea, vomiting, diarrhea, and dizziness. It might be best to avoid scheduling OT or PT on these days.
- Clients complaining of nonproductive cough, dyspnea, fever, chest pain, or easy bruising should be referred to their physician, because these symptoms may be indicative of more serious toxicities.

Azathioprine

Pharmacology and Pharmacokinetics Azathioprine is an immunosuppressive agent approved for the treatment of RA in adults. Although its exact mechanism of action in RA is unclear, it does provide symptomatic relief, probably through its immunosuppressive activities.[28] After oral administration it is rapidly absorbed from the GI tract.[20] Azathioprine is eliminated renally.

Adverse Effects and Drug Interactions The usual adverse effects with azathioprine are GI and hematological. GI irritation in the form of nausea, vomiting, and diarrhea may be reduced by taking azathioprine with food and dividing the doses.[20] Hematological effects, such as leukopenia and thrombocytopenia, may

occur with higher doses.[33] Use of azathioprine may increase the risk of malignancies, but this risk appears to be relatively low with the doses used in the treatment of RA.[20] Azathioprine also may increase the risk of infection. Liver toxicity and hepatitis may occur.

The dose of azathioprine may need to be reduced in clients also receiving allopurinol. Clients receiving azathioprine and other bone marrow suppressive agents should be monitored carefully for signs of toxicity.

Availability and Administration Azathioprine (Imuran in the United States and Canada) is approved for the treatment of RA in adults. Therapy should be started with a low dose of 1 mg/kg/day and increased by 0.5 mg/kg/day in clients who do not respond in 6 to 8 weeks.[20] A 12-week trial is needed to determine effectiveness of this drug therapy.[20] Doses should be reduced in those with impaired renal function (e.g., creatinine clearance <50 ml/min).[20] Clients should have baseline and periodic blood counts throughout the course of drug therapy to monitor for adverse effects.

Azathioprine, Considerations for Therapists

- Azathioprine is a DMARD and may not provide relief for up to 12 weeks.
- Clients may experience GI irritation that may be reduced when the dose is taken with food and dividing the doses.
- Clients complaining of infections, sore throat, or easy bruising should be referred to their physician, because these symptoms may be indicative of more serious toxicities.

Cyclophosphamide and Chlorambucil

Cyclophosphamide (Cytoxan in the United States and Canada) and chlorambucil (Leukeran in both the United States and Canada) are both immunosuppressive agents that have been used in the treatment of RA. These agents may be used as a last resort for clients with RA who have active disease unresponsive to other treatment modalities.[34] As with other cancer chemotherapeutic agents, adverse effects may be toxic and very serious. The common adverse effects are bone marrow suppression and GI irritation in the form of nausea and vomiting. These agents also may cause malignancies, particularly leukemias. Therefore, if these drugs are used in the treatment of RA, clients should be informed of all potential toxicities and monitored very carefully for adverse effects.

Cyclosporine

Cyclosporine, an immunosuppressive agent, has been used for several years in organ and bone marrow transplantation. It also has been evaluated in the treatment of RA. Cyclosporine has been shown to reduce symptoms of arthritis. In studies, doses less than 10 mg/kg/day have been shown to successfully provide symptomatic relief.[34] Its role in slowing the disease progression or inducing a remission is not yet known.

The major disadvantage of routine use of cyclosporine is its high incidence of serious adverse effects, which range from hypertension to nephrotoxicity. Clients receiving this medication need to be monitored carefully and at regular intervals. Although cyclosporine may prove to be a very useful addition to therapy for RA, currently benefits of drug therapy must be weighed carefully against the known risks and toxicities associated with this agent.

Leflunomide

Pharmacology and Pharmacokinetics

Leflunomide is a new DMARD approved for use in the treatment of RA. It is an immunosuppressive drug that inhibits primidone synthesis, resulting in reduced proliferation of autoimmune T cells and production of autoantibodies by B cells.[3,6] It also has some anti-inflammatory effect.[3] Leflunomide is taken orally and nearly completely absorbed.[6] Most of the activity of leflunomide is due to its active metabolite.[3]

Adverse Effects and Drug Interactions

The common adverse effects of leflunomide are diarrhea, liver function test abnormalities, nausea, and vomiting.[1] Reports of hepatotoxicity and death associated with the use of leflunomide have highlighted the need for regular monitoring of liver function tests.[35] In addition, other effects that require monitoring are alopecia, rash, headache, and infection related to immunosuppression.[22]

The amount of active metabolite of leflunomide is reduced by the coadministration of cholestyramine, but is increased by the coadministration of rifampin.[3] The administration of leflunomide with other drugs, such as methotrexate, that can cause liver damage may increase the amount of damage.[3]

Availability and Administration

Leflunomide (Arava in the United States and Canada) is available as a tablet for oral administration. Therapy is initiated with a loading dose of 100 mg/day for 3 days and then continued at 20 mg/day. If this dose is not tolerated, a 10 mg/day dose can be used.[1,22] The benefit of leflunomide treatment is apparent within 4 to 12 weeks after it is started.[22]

Leflunomide, Considerations for Therapists

- The benefit of leflunomide therapy for RA may take 4 to 12 weeks to become apparent.
- Because leflunomide can impair the body's ability to fight infection, it may be inadvisable for clients to attend OT and/or PT during the flu season.
- Advise clients to contact their physician if you or they notice unusual tiredness, if they experience nausea or vomiting, or if they are jaundiced because these symptoms may indicate liver damage.

Biologic Agents

Etanercept

Pharmacology and Pharmacokinetics Etanercept is a biologic agent that is a product of recombinant DNA technology. It binds to tumor necrosis factor–alpha (TNF-α), thereby inhibiting its action.[1] As a result, etanercept acts to reduce the inflammatory process that leads to further joint destruction in RA. Etanercept has been studied for the treatment of RA and has demonstrated benefit in clients whose RA has not responded adequately to other DMARDs.[36]

Adverse Effects and Drug Interactions Because of its parenteral route of administration, etanercept can cause injection site reactions. The most serious adverse effect of this drug is the potential for recipients to develop infections due to its inhibition of TNF-α, which is part of the body's defense system against infection. Use of etanercept has been associated with the development of malignancies and also neurological effects such as demyelinating disorders and changes in mental status.[22]

Availability and Administration Etanercept is available as Enbrel in the United States and Canada. It is approved for the treatment of RA (United States and Canada) and JRA (United States). For RA, the recommended etanercept dose is 25 mg given subcutaneously twice a week (72 to 76 hours between injections).

> ### Etanercept, Considerations
> ### for Therapists
>
> - Benefit may be noticed in a few days, but may take up to 12 weeks.
> - This drug can impair the body's ability to fight infections. Therefore, clients should be encouraged to notify their physician if they develop signs or symptoms of an infection and to avoid public places in the flu season.
> - Be alert to unusual joint or muscle stiffness or muscle rigidity, which may indicate the development of a demyelinating disorders which etanercept therapy has been associated with and advise clients to contact their physician.

Infliximab

Pharmacology and Pharmacokinetics Infliximab is a biologic agent that is an antibody to TNF-α. It is produced through the fusion of mouse and human immune proteins.[20] Infliximab binds to TNF-α, preventing its interaction with its receptor. This prevents an inflammatory reaction and subsequent joint damage in RA.[36]

Adverse Effects and Drug Interactions Clients receiving infliximab may experience a reaction related to its administration with symptoms including fever, chills, pruritus, and rash within the first 2 hours.[20] The most common adverse effect with infliximab therapy is the increased risk of upper respiratory infections.[20] Similar to etanercept, those who receive this drug are at risk of other infections, as well as the development of malignancies and neurological effects such as demyelinating disorders and changes in mental status.[22] Furthermore, its use has been associated with increased mortality and hospitalization due to worsened heart failure in those with moderate to severe congestive heart failure.

> **Therapists should be aware of the risk of infections with the newer DMARDs.**

Availability and Administration Infliximab is available as Remicade in the United States and Canada and is approved for the treatment of RA.[37] It is administered in combination with methotrexate to prevent the formation of antibodies to the mouse portion of the drug.[20] The recommended dose for RA is 3 mg/kg given as an intravenous infusion, followed by the same dose 2 and 6 weeks later and then every 8 weeks thereafter.[1]

> ### Infliximab, Considerations
> ### for Therapists
>
> - Infliximab is a newer DMARD with a wide onset of action ranging between a few days to up to 4 months.
> - An increased risk of respiratory infections should be considered when scheduling OT and/or PT.
> - Caution clients to seek medical attention if they develop an allergic reaction or hives, experience flushing, difficulty breathing, or chest pain, or develop an infection; these may be drug related.

Drugs for the Treatment of Crystal-Induced Arthritis (Gout)

NSAIDs are a good choice for clients with acute gouty arthritis because an effect is obtained within a few hours. Other drugs used at different stages in the treatment of gout are colchicine, allopurinol, and uricosuric agents.

Colchicine

Pharmacology and Pharmacokinetics

Colchicine may be used for prophylaxis and for treatment of acute gout, although less today than previously. Although its exact mechanism of action is unknown, it does provide symptomatic relief by reducing the body's inflammatory response to the deposition of urate crystals in the affected joint. Colchicine also decreases lactic acid production, thereby interfering with urate deposition. Colchicine is absorbed from the GI tract after oral administration and is partially metabolized in the liver. Peak plasma concentrations of colchicine occur within 1 to 2 hours. Colchicine has a short plasma half-life of only 20 minutes after IV administration.[4]

Adverse Effects and Drug Interactions

The common adverse effects from colchicine are nausea, diarrhea, abdominal pain, and vomiting. Bone marrow suppression (agranulocytosis, thrombocytopenia, leukopenia, aplastic anemia), loss of body and scalp hair, rashes, peripheral neuritis or neuropathy, myopathy, renal damage, and increased liver function test results may occur with long-term use of colchicine. Swelling, redness, and pain may occur at the injection site when colchicine is administered intravenously.[4,38]

With chronic administration or high doses, colchicine may impair the absorption of vitamin B_{12}. Colchicine should be used cautiously with any drug that may cause GI toxicities or diseases of the blood because of the possible potentiation of adverse effects. Concurrent use of alcohol also may increase the risk of GI toxicities. In addition, alcohol is known to increase serum uric acid levels.

Availability and Administration

Colchicine is available only in tablet form in Canada, and in both tablet and IV formulations in the United States. To treat acute attacks of gout, colchicine is most effective when it is started as soon as an attack is suspected. Pain and swelling should begin to subside within 12 hours and are usually gone within 48 to 72 hours. With IV administration, relief should be apparent within 6 to 12 hours.[39]

Colchicine, Considerations for Therapists

- Clients presenting with an inflamed joint characteristic of gout (a constant squeezing pressure type of pain of increasing intensity usually in one joint) should be referred immediately to the physician because therapy (with colchicine) is most effective when given as soon as possible.
- Severe diarrhea, nausea, and vomiting may be early signs of toxicity; clients should be referred to their physician.
- Elderly clients may be more susceptible to toxicity and should be watched carefully for adverse effects (i.e., GI symptoms, unusual bruising, prolonged bleeding).

Allopurinol

Pharmacology and Pharmacokinetics

Allopurinol is used in the treatment of gout. It works by inhibiting an enzyme involved in the synthesis of uric acid. It effectively decreases serum and urine concentrations of uric acid.[35] Allopurinol is well absorbed after oral administration, with peak plasma levels occurring within 2 to 6 hours. Serum uric acid concentrations usually begin to fall within 24 to 48 hours, with the maximum effect seen in 1 to 3 weeks. Improvement in clinical symptoms, such as a decrease in the size of tophi, may take up to 6 months.[39]

Elderly clients may be more susceptible to toxic effects of medications. They should be monitored carefully and referred to their physician when unexplained symptoms are present.

Adverse Effects and Drug Interactions

Allopurinol is generally well tolerated, with fewer than 1% of clients experiencing an adverse effect.[4] However, adverse effects may occur (Table 6-12). Allopurinol may exacerbate symptoms of acute gout during the first few months of therapy because uric acid is released from the tissues into the blood. Clients may receive colchicine or an NSAID concurrently with allopurinol for the first few months of allopurinol therapy to alleviate these symptoms.[4]

The risk of bone marrow suppression is increased if clients are taking allopurinol and a cytotoxic agent, such as azathioprine or cyclophosphamide. Alcohol and diuretics may increase serum uric acid levels, thus decreasing the effectiveness of allopurinol. Clients taking captopril and other similar agents may be predisposed to severe hypersensitivity reactions. An increased incidence of dermatological reactions occurs in clients taking ampicillin or amoxicillin with allopurinol.[4,39]

Availability and Administration

Allopurinol is available in tablets for oral administration in 100-mg and 200-mg strengths in the United States and 100-mg, 200-mg, and 300-mg strengths in Canada. The starting dose is often 100 mg/day for 2 weeks, and then the dose is increased to whatever is needed to lower serum uric acid levels to below 6.5 mg/100 ml. The higher the dose of allopurinol, the greater is the effect on the serum uric acid levels. Maintenance doses vary from 200 to 600 mg/day.[39]

Table 6-12. Adverse Effects of Allopurinol*

Central nervous system effects
    Peripheral neuropathy
    Headache
    Somnolence
Dermatological effects
    Rash
    Severe dermatitis
Gastrointestinal effects
    Nausea
    Vomiting
    Diarrhea
    Abdominal pain
    Gastritis
    Dyspepsia
Hematological effects
    Bone marrow suppression
	Hepatic effects
	    ↑ liver enzyme levels
	    Hepatitis
	    Hepatocellular damage
	Hypersensitivity effects
	    Fever, chills
	    Leukopenia or leukocytosis
	    Eosinophilia
	    Arthralgia
	    Rash
	    Pruritus
	    Nausea
	    Vomiting
	    Exfoliative dermatitis

Data from McEvoy GK (ed): AHFS Drug Information. Bethesda, American Society of Hospital Pharmacists, Inc, 2002.[4]
*This list is not all-inclusive; it includes effects that are most likely to occur, or, if do occur, may be serious.

Allopurinol, Considerations for Therapists

- **GI irritation can be reduced when allopurinol is taken with food.**
- **Maximum effectiveness may not be seen for up to 6 months.**
- **Clients noticing a rash or complaining of infections, sore throat, or unusual bruising should be referred to their physician, because these may be indicative of more serious toxicities.**

Uricosuric Agents

Probenecid, sulfinpyrazone, and large doses (>4 g/day) of ASA are all uricosuric agents. They all work in the kidney to enhance the urinary excretion of uric acid. Therapy is usually initiated slowly, because excretion of a large amount of uric acid increases the risk of urate stone formation in the kidney. Initiation of uricosuric therapy also has been associated with acute gout attacks. Therefore, colchicine is often used concurrently to alleviate symptoms of acute gouty attacks.

The common adverse effects with probenecid therapy are nausea, vomiting, and anorexia. Less commonly, rash and hypersensitivity reactions can occur. Sulfinpyrazone is an analog of phenylbutazone but has no anti-inflammatory activities.

Adherence and Cost Issues

Adherence with therapeutic drug regimens is often a problem in clients with chronic diseases and is also a concern of many health professionals in the treatment of arthritis. Medications used in treatment are often quite expensive. The drug itself may be costly, and cost may increase with number of doses needed per day and with drugs that require routine monitoring of laboratory parameters. If the client does not have insurance to cover these costs, doses may be skipped in an attempt to make the prescription last longer, or the prescription may never be filled. Generic versions of aspirin and many of the NSAIDs are now available, which helps to lower the costs. However, many of the DMARDs have no generic equivalents, and they are generally quite expensive. Exact costs of medications can be obtained by calling a local pharmacy in the area.

As mentioned earlier, many of these drugs have bothersome and often intolerable adverse effects. These are just some of the factors that may outweigh any benefits clients derive from the medications and may lead to nonadherence. Studies in clients with RA have found an adherence rate with medications ranging from 51% to 78%.[40] This may be due to the factors mentioned earlier or to other client-specific factors, such as lack of understanding of the disease and unrealistic expectations of the drug therapy.

Solutions to adherence problems are not easy owing to the many factors that may be involved.[41] It is important that the health care provider listen to the client to determine the possibility of nonadherence and the reasons for it. These should be discussed with the client and possible solutions identified. Any instructions should be clear and easy to understand. If complexity of drug therapy is a problem, alternatives should be sought. It may be possible to simplify regimens, or adherence aids such as medication calendars may be used. If financial difficulties are contributing to nonadherence, generic equivalents may be available. It may be possible to switch a client's medication to drugs that do not require routine, costly laboratory monitoring.

Iontophoresis

As discussed, most drugs used in the treatment of arthritis are administered orally. Gold is given intramuscularly, and corticosteroids often are injected directly into the inflamed tissue. Another mode of administration, although not widely used, is iontophoresis—electromotive drug administration (EMDA) (also transdermal drug administration).[42–44] This involves the topical administration of active drug ions that pass through the skin with the aid of a continuous direct current. Dexamethasone, ketorolac, etofenamate, and tenoxicam are some of the drugs that have been applied in this manner in clients with both inflammatory and degenerative arthritis and have been shown to offer longer-lasting pain relief than a placebo. There has been a greater interest in EMDA in Europe. Of 39 articles located in a PubMed search since 1975, 69% were of European origin, and only one was a double-masked study.[44] Although the technique is sterile, painless, and noninvasive,[42] specificity of action and cost effectiveness of EMDA compared with oral administration requires demonstration. Topical NSAID preparations may be used as couplants during ultrasonic treatment, which, theoretically, may enhance skin penetration of the NSAID and improve drug efficacy while avoiding the GI irritative effect.[45] Interested readers should consult references[42,43,46] for detail on dosages, techniques, indications, and contraindications.

Complementary and Alternative Medicine

Complementary and alternative medicine is a broad classification that includes natural or herbal products. It is important to be aware of the use of these products to treat diseases and symptoms, including the pain and inflammation associated with arthritic conditions. Consumers may be eager to try natural products either because they find no relief from traditionally available medications or because they find the side effects intolerable. Another reason some turn to the use of natural products is because they believe natural products are safer and are free of adverse effects. This, however, is not necessarily true. Because fewer regulations govern these products in terms of both claims about benefit and safety compared with traditionally available medications, there may be greater risk of adverse effects. It is important for the health care professional to ask clients about the use of these products. Clients also must be instructed that use of these products, similar to use of traditionally available medications, must be monitored by the client and health care personnel for both benefit and harm.

> Natural products are marketed by many manufacturers and typically are governed by fewer regulations than traditional drugs. One brand cannot easily be noted to be superior to another.

Natural products that may be used by those with arthritis include herbal treatments, nutritional supplements, and complementary medicines. These products include glucosamine and chondroitin, S-adenosylmethionine, collagen, and tumeric.[47] Although many claims are made about products that have benefit for the treatment of arthritis and its symptoms, few are supported by good scientific evidence. In general, there is a lack of good scientific research on these products and their use in arthritic conditions.

Glucosamine and chondroitin are natural products that have been tested in clinical trials. Pooled results from these trials have been evaluated, and overall these products appear to be beneficial for the treatment of osteoarthritis.[48,49] Glucosamine is a substance that is produced in humans and is important for the production of some of the key components of cartilage.[47] The use of glucosamine in osteoarthritis is thought to help with the regeneration of cartilage.[50] The reported side effects of glucosamine are generally mild and could include stomach upset and itching.[50] Its use may affect glucose regulation.[47] There are no known drug interactions.[47,51] Chondroitin is another natural product that is important for cartilage function.[47,51] Although there are no known severe adverse effects of chondroitin, it may cause stomach upset.[52] Chondroitin and glucosamine may work synergistically; however, this remains to be confirmed through clinical trials. With both of these products, it is important to note that even though they have been studied, the benefit may be specific to the formulations of these natural products used in the clinical trials and not to all brands.

Several sources of information are available to help consumers and health care professionals evaluate the use of these products. One resource is a web site from the Arthritis Foundation (http://www.arthritis.org), which has information about herbs and supplements that are claimed to help in treatment of arthritic symptoms and potential interactions of these products with other drugs. Other useful web sites that provide evaluations of some of the products for which benefit for arthritic conditions is claimed are those produced by the Mayo Clinic (http://www.mayoclinic.com) and the Cochrane Collaboration Consumer Network (www.cochraneconsumer.com).

Pharmacogenomics

Pharmacogenomics is a newer area of drug use and refers to the study of genetic variations that affect individuals' response to drug therapy. Currently, the most well-known application of the use of genetic variation in drug response is in the area of drug metabolism and the variations in the cytochrome P450 enzymes. The use of pharmacogenomics in the development of drugs could lead to optimization of drug therapy to maximize benefit, while limiting toxicity.

The use of genetic information is new in the field of rheumatology. However, there may be applications of genomics in the diagnosis and prognosis of diseases.[53] These may lead to the use of pharmacogenomic explorations for treatment of rheumatological disorders such as RA.

Areas of Research

The following are some areas for future research:

- Are therapy outcomes improved in clients with rheumatoid arthritis when PT (or OT) is combined with anti-inflammatory drug therapy?

- Do adverse reactions to medications impact the client's ability to participate in and respond to OT and/or PT?
- Is adherence to a medication schedule increased when occupational or physical therapists actively monitor drug intake as part of rehabilitation?
- Are adverse effects of medications detected earlier and decreased in severity when occupational or physical therapists actively monitor drug side effects as part of rehabilitation?
- In monoarticular arthritis is there a difference in the response rate and cost effectiveness between intra-articular injection, iontophoresis, or phonophoresis?

Summary

Clients may have to try several drugs before they find the one most effective for them, and they may be taking a combination of drugs. The PT and OT should be knowledgeable about the following aspects of a client's drug therapy:

- What drug(s) are being taken?
- What is the frequency of the dose's speed of action (minutes, days, weeks)?
- What are the physiological side effects of the drugs?

The therapist has a responsibility to understand potential interactions between the effects of a client's medications and their response to OT and/or PT, both in a general sense and to specific modalities. Appropriate modifications should be made to the delivery of PT; for example, aggressive mobilization or strengthening should not be performed at the peak period of pain relief or in the presence of active inflammation. It also is the therapist's responsibility to advise the client to see or contact her or his physician if adverse effects of drug therapy are suspected.

References

1. Repchinsky C (ed): *CPS,* ed 37. Ottawa, Canadian Pharmacists Association, 2002.
2. Connor EP (product manager): *Physicians' Desk Reference.* Montvale, NJ, Medical Economics Data Production Company, 2002.
3. Cada DJ (ed): *Facts and Comparisons.* St Louis, Facts and Comparisons, 2002.
4. McEvoy GK (ed): *AHFS Drug Information.* Bethesda, MD, American Society of Hospital Pharmacists, 2002.

5. Boh LE, Elliott ME: Osteoarthritis. In DiPiro JT, Talbert RL, Yee GC et al (eds): *Pharmacotherapy: A Pathophysiologic Approach,* ed 5. New York, McGraw-Hill, 2002, pp 1639–1656.

6. Furst DE, Munster T: Nonsteroidal antiinflammatory drugs, disease-modifying antirheumatic drugs, nonopioid analgesics, and drugs used in gout. In Katzung BG (ed): *Basic and Clinical Pharmacology,* ed 8. New York, McGraw-Hill, 2001, pp 596–623.

7. Hylek EM, Heiman H, Skates SJ et al: Acetaminophen and other risk factors for excessive warfarin anticoagulation. *JAMA* 279:657–662, 1998.

8. Shek KL, Chan LN, Nutescu E: Warfarin-acetaminophen drug interaction revisited. *Pharmacotherapy* 19:1153–1158, 1999.

9. Chen SW, Gong WC: Rheumatic disorders. In Koda-Kimble MA, Young LY, Kradjan WA et al (eds): *Applied Therapeutics, the Clinical Use of Drugs,* ed 7. Philadelphia, Lippincott Williams & Wilkins, 2001, pp 41-1–41-41.

10. Silverstein FE, Faich G, Goldstein JL et al: Gastrointestinal toxicity with celecoxib vs nonsteroidal antiinflammatory drugs for osteoarthritis and rheumatoid arthritis. The CLASS study: a randomized controlled trial. *JAMA* 284:1247–1255, 2000.

11. Bombardier C, Laine L, Reicin A et al: Comparison of upper gastrointestinal toxicity of rofecoxib and naproxen in client with rheumatoid arthritis. *N Engl J Med* 343:1520–1528, 2000.

12. Catella-Lawson F, Reilly MP, Kapoor S et al: Cyclooxygenase inhibitors and the antiplatelet effects of aspirin. *N Engl J Med* 345:1809–1817, 2001.

13. Tannenbaum H, Peloso PMJ, Russell AS et al: An evidence-based approach to prescribing NSAIDs in the treatment of osteoarthritis and rheumatoid arthritis. the second Canadian consensus conference. *Can J Clin Pharmacol* 7(suppl A):4A–16A, 2000.

14. Amadio P, Cummings DM, Amadio P: Nonsteroidal antiinflammatory drugs. Tailoring therapy to achieve results and avoid toxicity. *Postgrad Med* 93:73–97, 1993.

15. Gums JG, Terpening CM: Adrenal gland disorders. In DiPiro JT, Talbert RL, Yee GC et al (eds): *Pharmacotherapy, a Pathophysiologic Approach.* New York, McGraw-Hill, 2002, pp 1379–1393.

16. Chrousos GP, Marjioris AN: Adrenocorticosteroids and adrenocortical antagonists. In Katzung BG (ed): *Basic and Clinical Pharmacology,* ed 8. New York, McGraw-Hill, 2001, pp 660–678.

17. Arnold M, Schrieber L, Brooks P: Immunosuppressive drugs and corticosteroids in the treatment of rheumatoid arthritis. *Drugs* 36:340–363, 1988.

18. Kirwan JR, the Arthritis and Rheumatism Council Low-Dose Glucocorticoid Study Group: The effect of glucocorticoids on joint destruction in rheumatoid arthritis. *N Engl J Med* 333:142–146, 1995.

19. Hickling R, Jacoby RK, Kirwan JR, the Arthritis and Rheumatism Council Low Dose Glucocorticoid Study Group: Joint destruction after glucocorticoids are withdrawn in early rheumatoid arthritis. *Br J Rheumatol* 37:930–936, 1998.

20. Schuna AA: Rheumatoid arthritis. In DiPiro JT, Talbert RL, Yee GC et al (eds): *Pharmacotherapy, a Pathophysiologic Approach.* New York, McGraw-Hill, 2002, pp 1623–1637.

21. Schumacher HR Jr (ed): *Primer on Rheumatic Diseases,* ed 10. Atlanta, Arthritis Foundation, 1993.

22. American College of Rheumatology Subcommitte of Rheumatoid Arthritis Guidelines. *Arthritis Rheum* 46:328–346, 2002.

23. Roberts LJ, Morrow JD: Analgesic-antipyretic and antiinflammatory agents and drugs employed in the treatment of gout. In Hardman JG, Limbird LE (eds): *Goodman & Gilman's The Pharmacological Basis of Therapeutics,* ed 10. New York, McGraw-Hill, 2001, pp 687–731.

24. Penneys NS, Ackerman AB, Gottlieb NL: Gold dermatitis: a clinical and histopathological study. *Arch Dermatol* 109:372–376, 1974.

25. Heuer MA, Pietrusko RG, Morris RW et al: An analysis of worldwide safety experience with auranofin. *J Rheumatol* 12:695–699, 1985.

26. Davis P, Hughes GRV: Significance of eosinophilia during gold therapy. *Arthritis Rheum* 17:964–968, 1974.

27. Luukkainen P, Kajander A, Isomaki H: Effect of gold on progression of erosions in rheumatoid arthritis. *Scand J Rheumatol* 6:189–192, 1977.

28. Pugh MC, Pugh CB: Current concepts in clinical therapeutics: disease-modifying drugs for rheumatoid arthritis. *Clin Pharmacol* 6:475–491, 1987.

29. Anonymous: Sulfasalazine in rheumatoid arthritis therapy. *Clin Pharmacol* 6:921, 1987.

30. Duncan BS: Inflammatory bowel disease. In Koda-Kimble MA, Young LY, Kradjan WA et al (eds): *Applied Therapeutics, the Clinical Use of Drugs,* ed 7. Philadelphia, Lippincott Williams & Wilkins, 2001, pp 26-1–26-20.

31. Chambers M: Rheumatoid arthritis. *Pharm Pract* 9(7)CE1:3–7, 1993.

32. Letendre PW, DeJong DJ, Miller DR: The use of methotrexate in rheumatoid arthritis. *Drug Intell Clin Pharm* 19:349–358, 1985.

33. Hartnett M: DMARDs in rheumatoid arthritis. *On Contin Pract* 16(2):11–14, 1989.

34. Arnold M, Schrieber L, Brooks P: Immunosuppressive drugs and corticosteroids in the treatment of rheumatoid arthritis. *Drugs* 36:340–363, 1988.

35. Schuna AA: Hepatoxicity of leflunomide causing concern. *Am Pharm Assoc Drug Info Line* 3:1, 2002.

36. Pisetsky DS, St Clair EW: Progress in the treatment of rheumatoid arthritis. *JAMA* 286:2787–2790, 2001.

37. Important drug warning on remicade. Available at http://www.hc-sc.gc.ca/hpfb-dgpsa/tpd-dpt/remicade_e.html. Accessed Sept 18, 2002.

38. Brater DC: *USPDI, Drug Information for the Health Care Professional,* vol 1. Greenwood Village, CO, Micromedex, 2002.

39. Young LY, Campagna KD: Gout and hyperuricemia. In

Koda-Kimble MA, Young LY, Kradjan WA et al. (eds): *Applied Therapeutics, the Clinical Use of Drugs*, ed 7. Philadelphia, Lippincott Williams & Wilkins, 2001, pp 40-1–40-21.

40. Deyo RA: Compliance with therapeutic regimens in arthritis: issues, current status, and a future agenda. *Semin Arthritis Rheum* 12:233–244, 1982.

41. Boza RA, Milanes F, Slater V et al: Client noncompliance and overcompliance. *Postgrad Med* 81:163–170, 1987.

42. Cummings J: Iontophoresis. In Nelson RM, Currier DP (eds): *Clinical Electrotherapy*. Norwalk, Appleton & Lange, 1991, pp 317–329.

43. Belanger A-Y: *Evidence-Based Guide to Therapeutic Physical Agents*. Philadelphia, Lippincott Williams & Wilkins, 2002, pp 1–25.

44. Saggini R, Zoppi M, Vecchiet F et al: Comparison of electromotive drug administration with ketorolac or with placebo in clients with pain from rheumatic diseases: a double-masked study. *Clin Ther* 18:1169–1174, 1996.

45. Benson HAE, McElnay JC: Topical non-steroidal anti-inflammatory products as ul, rasound couplants: their potential in phonophoresis. *Physiotherapy* 80:74–76, 1994.

46. Banga AK, Panus PC: Clinical applications of iontophoretic devices in rehabilitation medicine. *Crit Rev Phys Med Rehab* 10:147–179, 1998.

47. LaValle JB, Krinsky DL, Hawkins EF et al: *Natural Therapeutics Pocket Guide*. Hudson, OH Lexi-Comp, 2000.

48. McAlindon TE, LaValley MP, Gulin JP et al: Glucosamine and chondroitin for treatment of osteoarthritis: a systematic quality assessment and meta-analysis. *JAMA* 283:1469–1475, 2000.

49. Towheed TE, Anastassiades TP, Shea B et al: Glucosamine therapy for treating osteoarthritis (Cochrane Review), *The Cochrane Library*, Issue 3, Oxford Update Software, 2002. Available at http://www.cochranelibrary.com. Accessed Oct 12, 2002.

50. DerMarderosian A, Beutler JA: *The Review of Natural Products*. St Louis, Facts & Comparisons, 2002.

51. Boon H: Glucosamine. In Chandler F (ed): *Herbs: Everyday Reference for Health Professionals*. Ottawa, Canadian Pharmacists Association and Canadian Medical Association, 2000.

52. Rotblatt M, Ziment I: *Evidence-Based Herbal Medicine*. Philadelphia, Hanley & Belfus, 2001.

53. Cope AP, Schulze-Koops H: Meeting report: 22nd European Workshop for Rheumatology Research, Leiden, The Netherlands, 28 February–3 March, 2002. *Arthritis Res* 4:276–279, 2002.

CHAPTER 7

Surgical Interventions

Mary Ann Keenan, MD
Douglas Palma, MD

Although arthritis in the majority of clients will be successfully managed with nonsurgical approaches, surgical intervention plays an important role in the management of both inflammatory and degenerative forms of arthritis. A team approach and consultative management is critical in client treatment, particularly for the client with inflammatory arthritis. Unlike osteoarthritis (degenerative arthritis), in which surgery may be needed for only one or two joints, the client with inflammatory arthritis may require surgery for several joints. Also, in inflammatory arthritis, the disease process will continue after surgery.

PHYSICAL REHABILITATION IN ARTHRITIS, Joan M. Walker, PhD, PT, and Antoine Helewa, MSc(Clin Epid), PT, Elsevier Inc. © 2004.

Rheumatoid arthritis (RA) affects all synovial joints, bone, muscle, fascia, ligaments, and tendons. Because it is a systemic disease it also can affect internal organs.[1] Immune mechanisms are involved as evidenced by the presence of large numbers of lymphocytes in the synovial tissue and by the presence of rheumatoid factor (immunoglobulin M antibodies) in the serum and synovial fluid of 80% of clients. These antigen-antibody reactions activate the complement system and attract neutrophils to the joint fluid. The immune complexes then are phagocytized and lysosomal enzymes are released into the synovial fluid. These enzymes and the inflammatory synovial pannus are, in part, responsible for the destruction of articular cartilage and periarticular structures. Tendons also are directly invaded by the inflammatory synovium and may attenuate and rupture. Ligaments and joint capsules become weakened by the chronic inflammatory process and may become stretched by repeated joint effusions. (See also Chapters 3 and 4.)

The erosion of articular cartilage is greatly enhanced by the superimposition of mechanical derangements on a joint weakened by chronic inflammation and enzymatic deterioration. Osteoporosis results from the hyperemia of inflammation. Disuse of limbs secondary to pain, weakened muscle action, and mechanical derangements enhance the osteoporosis.[2,3]

Optimum management requires an interdisciplinary team approach involving many specialists. The orthopaedic surgeon should be involved early in the course of the client's disease and not merely be called upon when medical management has failed to be effective. Knowledge of biomechanics, gait dynamics, and energy requirements can be useful in preserving function for the client. Because the disease is an ongoing and progressive process, the goal of management is to prevent deformities and maintain function for the client over a lifetime.

Factors in the Decision Process

Many factors must be considered in the decision of whether to intervene surgically in the management of the client with arthritis. Each client is unique, an individual, with a differing set of perceptions, expectations, socioeconomic needs, and reactions to disability. The risk/benefit balance must be carefully considered, and the client must be fully involved in the decision process. Questions that the orthopaedic surgeon must ask are (1) Will surgery alleviate the symptoms related to weakness, instability, and pain? (2) Will surgery make the client more independent, more self-sufficient? (3) Will surgery stabilize the client's condition and prevent further loss of function? (4) Will surgery enable the client to continue or return to employment? (5) Will surgery facilitate care giving? In selected situations early surgical intervention may prevent excessive deterioration of joint structure and function. Synovectomy has been shown to be effective in preventing tendon rupture in the hand.[4,5] Arthroscopic synovectomy and débridement of cartilage lesions of the knee and shoulder show promise for slowing joint destruction.[6–11] Fusion of an unstable cervical spine can prevent the disastrous effect of a spinal cord injury.[12–18]

The majority of surgical interventions are reconstructive. Because relief of pain is the most consistent result of reconstructive surgery, pain is the primary indication for surgery. Restoration of motion and function with correction of deformity are additional indications for surgical intervention.[19] Preoperative assessment is a meticulous process. The surgeon must attempt to elicit sufficient information from the client, family, and therapists, in addition to clinical examination and radiographic evaluations, to ascertain which deformities are causing the greatest functional losses. The client can only tolerate a finite number of surgical procedures, and these must be carefully staged to obtain the maximal result.

> **Pain is the primary indication for surgery because relief of pain is the most consistent result of reconstructive surgery.**

Joint scoring systems are available and used in the assessment of the client's suitability for surgery. The Harris scoring system is commonly used for total hip replacements.[20] It was developed by a team of orthopaedic surgeons and physical therapists to incorporate objective values of functional tasks into the scoring system. The indication for surgery is not based on a single, cumulative total preoperative score, and the scoring systems used should include consideration of the factors in the following sections.

Pain
Is the client's pain associated with movement or weight bearing? Does the pain require control with narcotic drugs? Pain that is not easily controlled is a strong indicator for surgery.

Function and Activities of Daily Living
Clients should be assessed or questioned about their ability to perform required activities of daily living (ADL) and to participate in recreational activities. Quantitative tests appropriate to the involved joint(s) should be used whenever possible. These include measures such as distance walked; gait velocity; number of stairs ascended/descended; and ability to get in and out of a car, to manipulate objects, and to dress. Function in ADL has a significant impact on the client's quality of life. Quantitative tests allow for assessment of the surgical intervention that may follow.

Ability to Work
Is the client employed? Has the client had to reduce her or his level of employment or cease employment altogether?

Joint Condition
Assessment of a joint encompasses range of motion (ROM), stability, and the presence and degree of

deformity or malalignment. The status of contiguous joints also must be assessed, because their condition may have a significant impact on success of surgery. For example, when knee surgery is contemplated, the surgeon needs to assess whether the foot can be placed plantigrade. Can the contralateral limb support the operative leg during postoperative rehabilitation, and can ambulatory aids be managed by the upper limbs?

Age

The client's physiological age is more important than chronological age. Age is a critical factor in the potential life of the planned procedure and in the client's expectations of surgery.

Weight

Particularly in patients with osteoarthritis (OA) in whom a limited number of joints are affected, obesity has a negative impact on the success of surgical interventions of lower limb joints. Morbid obesity is a relative contraindication to hip or knee arthroplasty.

Ability of the Client to Cooperate

Ultimately, a positive outcome from surgical interventions depends on the client's ability to actively cooperate with postoperative rehabilitation. In some clients, however, when surgical intervention may facilitate care, surgery may be undertaken despite the perception that the client will not be cooperative.

Because relief of pain is the most consistent result of reconstructive surgery, pain is the primary indication for surgery.

Client Perceptions and Expectations

It is important to establish clearly what the client perceives surgery may accomplish and what her or his expectations of outcome may be. Some clients may see surgery as curative, allowing full resumption of former life and recreational activities. Others may perceive surgery as cosmetic to correct deformity; however, this may be a minor factor in the decision process if adequate function exists despite the presence of deformity. Other clients' main expectation may be improvement in function. It should be established clearly whether these expectations are realistic. Expectations must be viewed in the light of comorbid conditions.

General Health

The presence of coexisting medical conditions will affect the client's ability to participate in postoperative rehabilitation. Cardiovascular and respiratory con-

Table 7-1. Factors that Compromise Surgical Intervention

1. Morbid obesity
2. Active infection
3. Overwhelming poor general health
4. Inadequate motor control (paresis or paralysis)
5. Inadequate bone stock
6. Emotional instability

ditions may present concerns regarding the choice of anesthetic technique. An unstable or rigid cervical spine may necessitate flexible fiberoptic intubation.

Factors that compromise a positive outcome from surgical intervention are given in Table 7-1. The presence of an active infection, obesity, or emotional instability may necessitate a delay in scheduling surgery until an improvement or resolution has been achieved. Other factors, such as inadequate bone stock, may completely negate surgical intervention.

Types of Surgical Procedures

Table 7-2 lists the various surgical procedures that may be performed in clients with arthritis and their goals. Pain relief and improvement in or restoration of function are desired outcomes of all procedures. Procedures may be combined, such as débridement with ligament release or elbow joint synovectomy with radial head excision. The more commonly performed procedures are osteotomy, débridement, arthrodesis (fusion), and arthroplasty (joint replacement surgery).

In clients with inflammatory arthritis who have uncontrolled synovitis and good articular cartilage, a synovectomy is a palliative approach.[4-11] Removal of synovium retards cartilage destruction due to release of cartilage degradative enzymes by the synovium. Synovium, however, tends to regenerate. An osteotomy may delay the need for a total joint replacement and is often used in young, active individuals with degenerative arthritis, in whom extensive destruction of articular cartilage is present.[21-24]

Arthrodesis is a primary procedure when spinal instability associated with intractable pain and/or neural compression is present. In both the cervical and lumbar regions, arthrodesis is combined with neural decompression of either the spinal cord or the nerve roots. Arthrodesis may be the only reasonable

Table 7-2. Surgical Procedures and their Main Purpose

Procedure	Purpose
Débridement	Removal of damaged cartilage fragments, loose bodies, and inflamed synovium; smooth irregular surfaces
Osteotomy	Improve joint or limb alignment to redistribute forces
Arthrodesis	Provide stability, prevent further malalignment and/or compression of neural elements
Arthroplasty	Improve or restore function; decrease disability; eliminate severe pain
Synovectomy	Remove inflamed synovium to protect articular cartilage or tendons from enzymatic damage
Bursectomy	Removal of inflamed bursa (i.e., olecranon)
Tendon transfer	Correct malalignment, restore function, arrest deterioration of tendons
Nerve decompression	Relieve nerve compression (i.e., ulnar nerve transposition at the elbow)
Nodule resection	Cosmesis, pain relief

alternative to arthroplasty or the end result if arthroplasty fails. Local intercarpal fusions provide stability while maintaining some wrist ROM and function. Contiguous joints should be mobile and functional when arthrodesis is considered. When arthrodesis is planned for the hip or knee joint, it is imperative for function that the other large joint has adequate, pain-free motion and motor control. Arthrodesis also is a primary procedure when there is inadequate bone stock for an arthroplasty.

Arthroplasties have been performed on most joints; however, they are mainly used for hip, knee, and shoulder joints. This procedure requires adequate bone stock and motor control and is particularly indicated in the presence of severe pain and disability. A partial joint hemiarthroplasty (i.e., only one surface, such as only the femoral surface at the hip or unicompartmental at the knee) or a total joint arthroplasty may be performed.[25–33] A variety of metal alloys, high-density polymers, and ceramic materials are used to resurface joints. Problems exist in loosening of implants and the creation of wear particles that produce an inflammatory response at the bone impact interface with eventual bone erosion.[34–37]

Surgical Considerations in Inflammatory Arthritis

Surgery in inflammatory arthritis usually is not an isolated event as it may be in OA. RA is a systemic disease and will continue to progress after surgery. In RA, multiple joint involvement is an important factor. The benefit of surgery to one joint may be negated by

Table 7-3. Priority of Surgical Procedures

Lower limb:
    Foot, hip, knee, ankle
Upper limb:
    Wrist, hand, elbow, shoulder
Nondominant before dominant side

the extent of involvement of a contiguous joint. For example, hand surgery is affected by the condition of the elbow and shoulder, and when these joints are severely involved the client may not be able to use any improved hand function. In such cases the priority of operations becomes important.

Priority of Operations

In the client with multiple joint involvement, cervical instability with myelopathy takes priority. Generally operations are performed on the lower limb joints before upper limb joints (Table 7-3). If upper limb function is so poor, however, that the client could not tolerate use of ambulatory aids, then upper limb surgery will take priority over lower limb procedures. Correction of malalignment and contractures may be essential to the outcome of other procedures. For example, malalignment of the ankle/foot complex can affect knee replacement outcome.[38]

Limb dominance must be considered in multiple surgical procedures, not only for scheduling but also for the type of procedure. A wrist arthrodesis may be more appropriate for the "helping hand" (nondominant) and joint replacements to the dominant hand to provide motion. A stable, pain-free wrist is needed for successful hand surgery, and functional motion in the elbow and shoulder is needed for hand and wrist procedures.

Surgical Procedures and Medications

Collaboration and consultation between the orthopaedic surgeon and the rheumatologist are essential throughout planned surgical procedures. A client should achieve maximum benefit from medication before surgery, and the disease should be controlled for a good surgical outcome. Consideration must be given to the client's medications.[1] There is a need to ensure that other joints remain quiescent so the postoperative rehabilitation can be achieved. Use of nonselective nonsteroidal anti-inflammatory drugs (NSAIDs) will need to be stopped 5 days preoperatively to decrease postoperative bleeding. The selective (cyclooxygenase-2 [COX-2]) anti-inflammatory drugs have no effect on platelet function and do not need to be discontinued.[39,40] In the postoperative period, deep vein thrombosis is a complication that can be fatal, and its prophylaxis cannot be overlooked. Thus, use of NSAIDs needs to be balanced with prophylaxis for deep vein thrombosis to avoid bleeding complications and minimize the risks of thrombosis. With lower limb procedures, medication dosage may need to be changed so that the client can properly use ambulatory aids in a relatively pain-free manner.

Surgical Procedures for Specific Anatomic Locations

Spine

Surgery in the spine has the goals of providing stabilization, relief, or prevention of pain and neurological complications. Surgery is indicated in the presence of one or more of the following: intractable pain, excessive instability, or neurological deficit. Involvement of the cervical spine in RA is classically divided into three categories.[12–18,41] The common form of involvement is atlantoaxial instability resulting from erosion of the transverse and alar ligaments. These ligaments normally maintain the odontoid process of the axis within the anterior one third of the ring of the atlas where the two bones articulate with one another. Disruption of the ligaments results in excessive motion between C1 and C2. Forward flexion of the head causes anterior subluxation of the atlas on the axis and possible impingement of the spinal cord or occlusion of the vertebral arteries.

The second common form of arthritic spine disease is subaxial instability. This can be manifested by subluxation occurring between two or more cervical vertebrae below the level of C2. When the degree of subluxation is severe or it appears suddenly, pressure can be exerted on the spinal cord. This pressure may be sufficient to cause permanent and complete quadriparesis. Commonly, the subluxation occurs slowly, and the spine adapts to a severe degree of deformity before clinical symptoms appear.

The least common pattern of cervical spine deformity is superior migration of the odontoid process of C2 resulting from severe bone erosion. As the dens migrates proximally, radiographic detail is lost secondary to the overlapping of bony structures. Computed tomography (CT) is most useful in elucidating the exact nature of the deformities.

Orthotic supports are useful in controlling the client's symptomatology. Posterior cervical fusion is indicated when the spinal cord is at risk of damage. The common level of fusion is C1–C2, supplemented by wire fixation. When the subluxation is irreducible or severe osteoporosis is present, fusion to the occiput may be necessary. Occasionally, it is useful to supplement the bone graft with polymethyl methacrylate (PMMA) fixation.

Cervical spine disease in clients with erosive polyarticular arthritis often presents difficulties in endotracheal intubation at the time of surgery. The stability of the cervical spine should be assessed before any surgical procedure on a client with RA. Lateral flexion-extension radiographs taken within 1 year of surgery are sufficient to detect any significant instability. Use of the flexible fiberoptic bronchoscope for such problems is helpful. The indications for fiberoptic intubation in the client with arthritis are the following:

1. An unstable cervical spine on flexion and extension
2. Limited mobility of the cervical spine
3. Impaired motion of the temporomandibular joints with or without associated micrognathia. When present in clients with severe erosive disease of the cervical spine and proximal migration of the odontoid process, a rotational deviation of the larynx occurs that mandates use of a flexible fiberoptic scope.[16]

In OA with spinal stenosis, decompression is often accomplished using a posterior approach with decompressive laminectomy and foraminotomy. If multiple levels are decompressed or if facet joints are resected, fusion is required, because spinal instability has been created. In addition, fusion is indicated when treating degenerative spondylolisthesis that has not responded to the conservative therapy of rest, NSAIDs, and physical rehabilitation.

Postoperative protocols emphasize mobilization as soon as possible, such as ambulation, but avoidance of any strenuous activity. Clients are followed until fusion is evident by radiography. During this time, they are required to advance their mobility and to avoid any contact activities or aggressive exercise. This may take from 6 months to 1 year.

Upper Extremity

Shoulder

The shoulder is a common site of arthritic involvement.[42-44] Normally, the glenohumeral joint has more motion than any other joint. This motion is rotation, and the glenoid is very shallow to allow greater freedom of motion. In RA, shoulder involvement is generally insidious in onset, with episodic increases in pain. The pain is not constant early in the course of the disease and therefore shoulder disease is often not recognized until a significant amount of destruction is present. It is important to examine the shoulder on a regular basis to detect early loss of motion and function.

The rotator cuff muscles are central to the normal functioning of the shoulder. They provide stability to the humeral head and also provide rotation. In RA, attenuation and rupture of the rotator cuff is common. Trauma or degenerative arthritis also causes rotator cuff tears. When the rotator cuff has ruptured, the humeral head migrates proximally and is subjected to abnormal muscle forces. This results in the rapid deterioration of the glenohumeral joint.

Magnetic resonance imaging (MRI) provides a useful tool for examining the shoulder. The integrity of the rotator cuff, biceps tendon, and glenoid labrum can be assessed. In the client with RA, synovectomy can be performed arthroscopically using motorized shavers or the holmium:yttrium-aluminum-garnet (Ho:YAG) laser with minimal morbidity.[16] Impingement of a chronically inflamed rotator cuff against the undersurface of the acromion also can be treated by arthroscopic acromioplasty.

When the rotator cuff ruptures, repair should be performed. If the rupture is detected early, excessive damage to the glenohumeral joint can be avoided. If extensive joint damage is already present, then repair or reconstruction is done at the time of prosthetic arthroplasty. The extensively damaged glenohumeral joint can be successfully reconstructed by prosthetic arthroplasty.[43,45-48] Preoperative radiographic evaluation should include anteroposterior, lateral, and axillary radiographs to assess the alignment of the glenoid. The glenoid is often eroded asymmetrically and the prosthetic glenoid component must be accurately aligned for optimum functional result and to minimize the abnormal forces that might lead to prosthetic loosening. If the glenoid is abnormal or there is an irreparable rotator cuff tear, then only a hemiarthroplasty is performed (i.e., replacing only the proximal humerus). Pain is effectively alleviated by total shoulder replacement. The functional result depends on the integrity of the soft tissues and muscle function. A careful postoperative therapy program is essential to maximize function. It should emphasize ROM initially and progress to strengthening as the soft tissues heal.

The anterior portion of the deltoid muscle provides forward elevation of the humerus. This is the position of function and the common arc of motion for activities using the upper extremity. It is therefore important to preserve these muscle fibers and their attachments when any surgery of the shoulder is performed. Without a functioning anterior deltoid muscle, shoulder arthroplasty is contraindicated.

The tendon of the long head of the biceps muscle stabilizes the humeral head against riding upward. It also reduces subacromial impingement. The intra-articular portion of the tendon should be preserved whenever possible.

Post-traumatic osteoarthritis is another major cause of glenohumeral joint dysfunction. Degeneration of the joint may occur after multiple dislocations, multidirectional instability, and fracture of the proximal humerus. Pain with motion often is the main symptom for which clients seek medical attention.

Elbow

The elbow joint consists of three separate articulations: the radiocapitellar, ulnotrochlear, and radioulnar. These articulations allow the hand to rotate 180 degrees around the longitudinal axis of the forearm. Hand function depends on the hand being placed correctly in space as required for use. The elbow is the most important joint for positioning the hand. Unlike the shoulder or wrist, if the elbow is fused the functional loss is great. The goal of treatment is to maintain a painless arc of motion.

Subcutaneous rheumatoid nodules are common along the extensor surface of the ulna. These often cause problems with pressure when the arm is rested on any surface. They may interfere with the use of forearm troughs on walking aids. If bothersome, they should be surgically excised, but the client must be advised that they can recur.

Radiocapitellar arthritis often is the predominant feature of elbow involvement after radial head fractures and can cause marked pain and decreased ROM. The pain is most pronounced with pronation and supination of the forearm. Radial head excision and synovectomy are effective in relieving the pain and often result in an improved arc of motion.

Ulnohumeral arthritis does not always require surgical intervention. When the joint destruction is severe, but ligamentous stability remains, prosthetic arthroplasty can be done.[49–51] Several designs of elbow prostheses are available. They can be classified into semiconstrained and unconstrained designs. An unconstrained design is preferable, because the mechanical forces leading to loosening are not directly transferred to the bone. The shoulder should be evaluated carefully before prosthetic elbow arthroplasty. In a client with limited shoulder motion greater forces will be exerted on the elbow in an effort to compensate for the decrease in shoulder function.

Wrist and Hand

Reconstructive hand surgery can be considered for the client with inflammatory or degenerative arthritis. Evaluating a client with hand deformities and developing a rational plan for treatment can be a complex task. Many joints, tendons, and ligaments are involved in a linked system of structure and function.

Synovitis Dorsal tenosynovitis is common in RA. It is significant because it often results in rupture of the extensor tendons.

Extensor tendon ruptures occur as the result of attenuation of the tendon from chronic inflammation, ischemia secondary to interference with the normal circulation to the tendon, attenuation of the tendon from rubbing against abnormal bony surfaces that are prominent secondary to ligamentous laxity, and direct invasion of the tendon by synovium. Tenosynovectomy should be performed in clients who have persistent synovitis for a 4- to 6-month interval that has not been responsive to medical treatment. Recurrence of the synovitis is rare after synovectomy and the procedure has been shown to prevent extensor tendon rupture.[4,5,52]

The tendons that commonly rupture in order of frequency are the extensors of the fifth finger, the extensor of the ring finger, and the extensor pollicis longus (EPL). The results of surgical repair by tendon transfer are inversely proportional to the number of tendons involved. Prompt diagnosis and treatment are essential for a successful outcome. For a single tendon rupture in the fifth and ring fingers, a side-to-side repair using the adjacent extensor tendon is advised.

The extensor indicis tendon also may be transferred for repair of the EPL tendon or for rupture of two finger extensors. For more complex ruptures, the wrist extensors or flexor digitorum superficialis tendons (FDS) may be transferred dorsally to restore function.

Synovitis in the flexor tendon sheaths is manifested by crepitation palpable in the palm with finger flexion and extension. Triggering of the fingers may result from the inflamed synovial tissue catching on the flexor pulleys with motion. Carpal tunnel syndrome also may occur secondary to the swelling within the carpal canal, which causes pressure on the median nerve. Early treatment consists of local steroid injection to reduce the inflammation, splinting, and medical management of the underlying synovitis. Persistent synovitis may require carpal tunnel release and synovectomy. Rupture of the flexor tendons is rare.

Wrist The wrist joint is a common site of synovitis. The wrist begins to deviate in a radial direction and subluxate volarly. The radioulnar joint is commonly inflamed and painful. Radial deviation of the carpus can be rebalanced by transfer of the extensor carpi radialis longus tendon to the extensor carpi ulnaris.

RA is a systemic disease and will continue to progress after surgery.

When the wrist becomes unstable, several choices of surgical treatment are available. If the deformity is mild, bone stock can be preserved and motion maintained by a limited carpal fusion. The lunate and scaphoid are fused to the distal radius to prevent further displacement of the carpus. The distal ulna can be fused to the distal radius to provide a platform to support the wrist. A segment of the ulna is removed just proximal to the fusion to allow for pronation and supination of the forearm. If the intercarpal joints are severely involved by the arthritis, the base of the capitate can be removed and a spacer can be inserted to preserve motion at the intercarpal row.

Another option is to perform a prosthetic arthroplasty of the wrist. More bone stock is removed with this procedure, but revision is still possible if the prosthesis fractures. Several designs of total joint prosthesis have been developed for the wrist.[53–55]

Fusion of the wrist joint provides a stable and pain-free joint and remains a reasonable surgical choice for selected individuals. Fusion may interfere with personal hygiene tasks and so it is advisable to avoid fusing both wrist joints. Several conditions

146

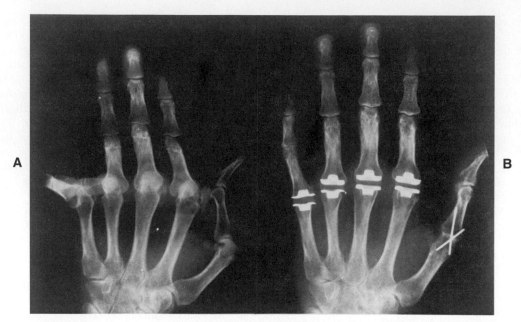

Figure 7-1. **A,** Preoperative radiograph of a client with rheumatoid arthritis that shows a boutonnière deformity of the thumb. The metacarpophalangeal (MCP) joints of the fingers are dislocated volarly and the fingers are ulnarly deviated. **B,** Postoperative radiograph showing reconstruction of the hand using Silastic interposition arthroplasties of the MCP joints and fusion of the MCP joint of the thumb. (Courtesy Wright Medical Technology, Inc, Arlington, TN 38002.)

requiring limited fusions include chronic instability patterns of the wrist, fixed flexion contractures, and developmental deformations.[3,56,57]

Wrist and finger deformities commonly occur together in a collapsing zigzag pattern. The wrist deviates in a radial direction and the fingers then drift ulnarward at the metacarpophalangeal (MCP) joint level. When both deformities are present, it is important to realign the wrist before the finger deformities are corrected or the ulnar deviation of the fingers will recur.

Metacarpophalangeal Joints Ulnar deviation and volar subluxation of the fingers at the MCP joint level is common (Figure 7-1, *A*). In RA with ulnar deviation, the extensor tendons subluxate into the valleys between the metacarpal heads. This can be confused with extensor tendon rupture. When the joint surfaces are preserved, a synovectomy, soft-tissue release of the volar capsule, and realignment of the extensor tendons will improve function.[5] If the joint surfaces are destroyed, a Silastic interposition arthroplasty is indicated (Figures 7-1, *B* and 7-2). If the joints are unstable secondary to ligament loss, it may

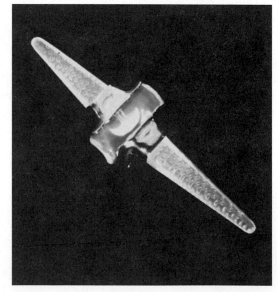

Figure 7-2. A Silastic prosthesis used for interposition arthroplasties of the MCP joints. (Courtesy Wright Medical Technology, Inc, Arlington, TN 38002.)

be necessary to reconstruct the radial collateral ligament using a portion of the volar plate to provide a stable pinch. Tightness of the intrinsic tendons occurs in conjunction with the subluxation of the MCP joints. When this occurs, a release of the intrinsic tendons is performed along with the arthroplasty. Dynamic splinting of the fingers to maintain alignment while allowing motion is used continuously for 6 weeks after surgery and then for an additional 6 weeks at night.

Proximal Interphalangeal Joints Continued synovitis causes gradual attenuation of the capsular and ligamentous structures, with resulting tendon imbalance. The fingers can develop either a flexion or an extension type of deformity.

A flexion deformity of the proximal interphalangeal (IP) joint results from rupture or attenuation of the central slip of the extensor mechanism with gradual volar displacement of the lateral bands. As the lateral bands subluxate volarly, a hyperextension deformity of the distal IP joint results. This flexion malalignment also is called a boutonnière deformity (see Figure 3-8, B). A boutonnière deformity interferes with grasping large objects but does not usually impede pinch function used for picking up small items.

Interposition arthroplasty using a Silastic spacer has given unpredictable results in the proximal IP joints. Fusion of the IP joints gives dependable results when the boutonnière deformity is fixed (see Figure 7-1, B). In the index and long fingers, stability for pinch is required for good function rather than a large arc of motion. Motion is more important in the ring and small fingers to provide a functional grasp. When arthroplasty is considered, the ring and fifth fingers are usually selected.

Hyperextension ("swan-neck") deformities can be either primary or secondary (see Figure 3-8, A). Primary deformities are due to stretching of the volar plate from synovitis or rupture of the FDS tendon. A flexion deformity of the MCP joints with tightness of the intrinsic muscles proximally combined with a mallet deformity distally results in a secondary swan-neck deformity. Swan-neck deformities interfere with picking up of small objects but do not cause much difficulty with grasping larger objects. If the deformity is treated early and is secondary to intrinsic tightness, a release of the intrinsic tendons will correct the imbalance. When the deformity is seen late and is rigid, the choices of surgical treatment are fusion or arthroplasty.

Derangements of the distal IP joints are either mallet deformities secondary to rupture of the extensor tendon or lateral deformities from loss of capsular and ligamentous support. When the deformities interfere with function, fusion of the joint is indicated.

Thumb Flexion of the thumb MCP joint with extension of the IP joint is the equivalent of a boutonnière deformity (see Figure 7-1, B). The reverse deformity also can be seen with extension of the MCP joint and flexion of the IP joint. An adduction deformity of the metacarpal joint places increased stress on the MCP joint, producing lateral instability and hyperextension. Adduction of the thumb occurs when the carpometacarpal joint has subluxed radially.

Arthritic derangements of the first carpometacarpal joint are a common disorder with a higher incidence in women. The clinical symptoms include pain and weak grasp. This condition can be treated with fusion, but arthroplasty is desirable to maintain motion. Interpositional arthroplasty can be performed by excising the trapezium and inserting soft tissue in its place.

> Careful postoperative therapy programs are essential to maximize function gained from surgical procedures.[38]

Lower Extremity

Hip

Total joint replacement has vastly improved the quality of life for the client with arthritis. Special problems exist in the client with RA when total hip arthroplasty is being considered. Osteoporosis is very pronounced, and fracture can occur easily during the surgery. Protrusio acetabuli also is common and may require bone grafting. Delayed wound healing can occur, especially if the client has been taking systemic steroids. The risk of infection also is increased in this population. In the client with juvenile rheumatoid arthritis, excess femoral anteversion may be present, distorting the anatomy. Also, the small size of the bone may require a special prosthesis. Despite these problems, total joint arthroplasty remains the treatment of choice for the arthritic hip.[59-65] Total joint arthroplasty provides a stable joint with excellent functional potential. Fixation of the prosthetic components may be obtained using PMMA or by bony ingrowth into a porous surface. The following case study illustrates a typical sequence of treatment.

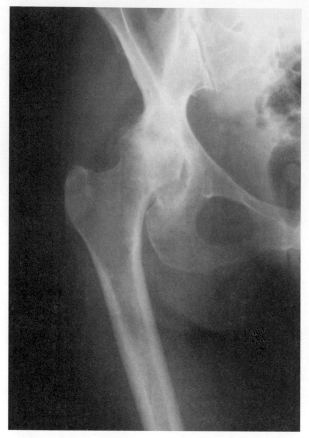

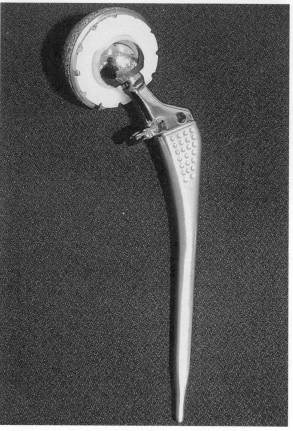

Figure 7-3. Preoperative radiograph of the hip showing extensive osteoarthrosis with femoral head collapse, subchondral sclerosis, and osteophyte formation. (Courtesy Wright Medical Technology, Inc, Arlington, TN 38002.)

Figure 7-4. A modular total hip prosthesis that has a porous surface on the acetabular components allowing for fixation by bony ingrowth. The femoral component has a surface precoated for maximal fixation to polymethyl methacrylate cement.

Case Study

LB is a 76-year-old woman with the initial complaint of right groin pain. She had a history of poliomyelitis without bulbar involvement diagnosed in 1924. She had been functioning reasonably well and presented in 1992 to our clinic. She initially underwent a conservative management program of NSAIDs and activity modification. This nonoperative therapy was successful until 1998. At this time, she stated that her pain had progressed and severely limited her normal daily activities. She had constant groin pain that worsened with ambulation and had prevented her from going up or down stairs. She was not obtaining relief from NSAID therapy and ambulated at home with crutches. She chose at this point to undergo a right total hip replace-

ment. Her preoperative radiographs demonstrate severe OA with flattening of both the femoral head and acetabulum (Figure 7-3). Her surgery was uncomplicated. She underwent a hybrid total hip arthroplasty in which the acetabular component has a porous surface to allow fixation by bony ingrowth (Figure 7-4). The femoral component was cemented because her significant osteoporosis would not give adequate bony fixation. Her postoperative rehabilitation began on day 2 with gait training and ROM exercises. She was discharged to in-client rehabilitation at that time and 2 weeks later to home after achieving independent ambulation. At 2 years after the operation, her hip replacement was painless, and she was able to perform her ADLs (Figure 7-5).

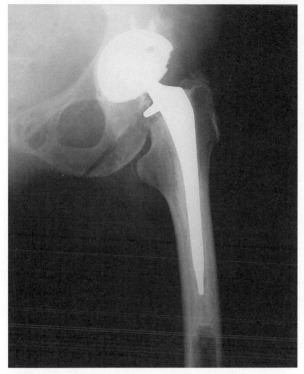

Figure 7-5. Postoperative radiograph taken 2 years after hybrid total hip arthroplasty. There is excellent apposition of the bone surfaces against the acetabular component and good contact between the cement, bone, and femoral prosthesis. (A hybrid total hip has an acetabular component with a porous backing to allow bony ingrowth for fixation while the femoral stem is cemented into position.)

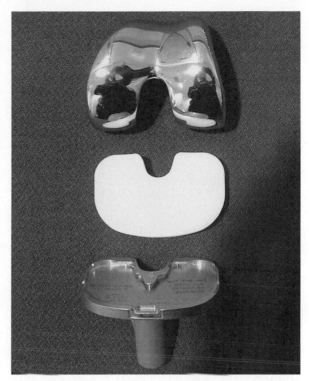

Figure 7-6. A modular total knee prosthesis that can be inserted using polymethyl methacrylate cement fixation or as a porous ingrowth device.

Knee

Valgus deformity is commonly seen in the client with RA. This is the result of a valgus deformity of the hindfoot that then places excessive stress on the knee proximally. Mild medial knee pain can be relieved with the use of an ankle-foot orthosis that corrects hindfoot valgus. Knee flexion deformity also is common. In the presence of a joint effusion, the intra-articular pressure and therefore the pain are minimized by placing the knee in 30 degrees of flexion. This encourages the formation of flexion contractures.

When evaluating a client with OA of the knee, the physician must determine which joint spaces are involved. There are three potential compartments: the medial, the lateral, and the patellofemoral. Often a client has involvement only of the medial or lateral joint space. If the client is younger than 55 years of age, has no systemic disease, is active and has no varus or valgus thrust while walking, has at least 90 degrees of knee flexion, and has less than a 15-degree flexion contracture, then a high tibial osteotomy is indicated.[21,22,24,28] This procedure will change the mechanical axis of the leg such that during weight bearing, the mechanical axis will pass through the unaffected compartment and often will delay the need for total knee arthroplasty for up to 10 years.

Arthroscopic evaluation of the knee has demonstrated the importance of the meniscus in the degeneration of the knee. In the client with RA, the synovium directly invades the body of the meniscus, which causes tears. The mechanical derangement resulting from the torn meniscus then causes rapid deterioration of the articular surfaces, which have been rendered abnormal by the action of enzymes. Synovectomy of the joint line and partial meniscectomy are easily accomplished under arthroscopic control

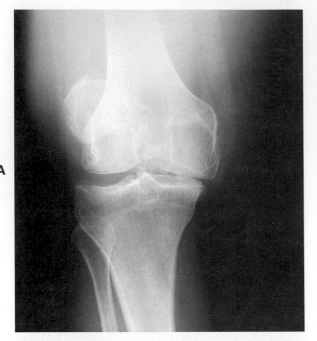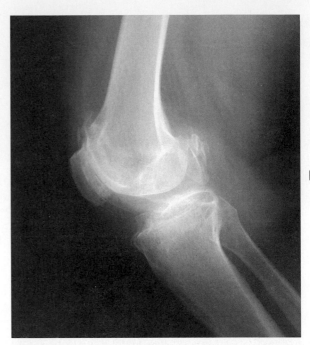

Figure 7-7. A, Preoperative anterior-posterior radiograph of a knee showing extensive osteoarthrosis with loss of the medial joint space and varus malalignment. **B,** Lateral radiograph shows extensive patellofemoral arthritis and loose bodies in the posterior joint space.

and may have a role in preventing articular damage in the rheumatoid knee.[6,8,10,11,66] In the mildly osteoarthritic knee, arthroscopic débridement is very successful in alleviating painful symptoms. With the advent of the Ho:YAG laser, rough, fraying articular cartilage can be smoothed, and loose bodies can be removed. Finally, the degradative enzymes of the inflammatory process can be washed from the joint.

Total knee arthroplasty has proved to be an effective procedure to restore knee alignment and motion and to relieve pain (Figures 7-6, 7-7, and 7-8).[25,66–73] When a valgus deformity is present, serial soft tissue releases should be done to realign the limb before cutting the bone for insertion of the prosthetic components. The lateral retinaculum, popliteus tendon, proximal iliotibial band, posterolateral capsule, and lateral collateral ligament can be released in this sequence to provide soft tissue balance. A flexion deformity is corrected at the time of arthroplasty by release of the posterior capsule from the femur or by removing additional bone from the distal femur in severe cases. The following case study illustrates a typical scenario.

Case Study

AG is a 57-year-old woman with advanced bilateral degenerative arthritis of both knees. She had been doing a home exercise program and taking a variety of NSAIDs without relief. In August 1999, she had an arthroscopic débridement of the left knee, which gave minimal relief of her symptoms. At this point, she reported increasing difficulty with ambulation and performing her ADLs due to the pain. The limited motion of her knees was aggravating the degenerative arthritis in her spine. After meeting with the surgeon, nurse, and therapists, she elected to proceed with a total knee arthroplasty (Figure 7-6). Her preoperative radiographs demonstrated severe OA and valgus malalignment of her knees (Figure 7-7).

Her postoperative rehabilitation began on day 2 with gait training and ROM exercises. She was discharged to in-client rehabilitation at that time and 2 weeks later to home after achieving independent ambulation. At 2 years after the operation, her right knee replacement was painless and she was able to perform her ADLs with significant improvement in her ROM (Figure 7-8). In addition, she had some improvement but not complete resolution of her chronic back pain.

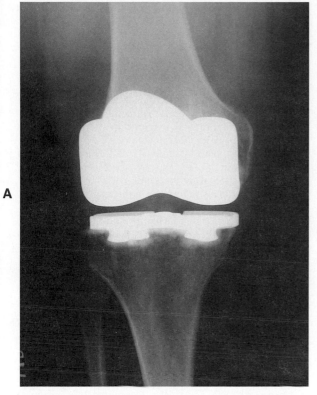
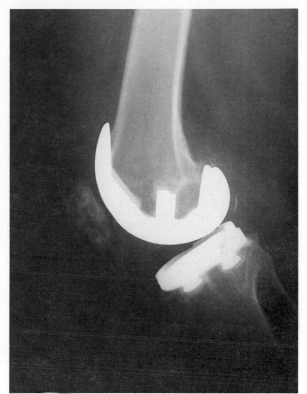

Figure 7-8. A, Anteroposterior radiograph of knee showing a total knee arthroplasty. The normal valgus alignment has been restored by the surgery. B, Lateral radiograph of a total knee arthroplasty.

Foot

Forefoot involvement is common in RA. Claw toe deformities with plantar subluxation of the metatarsal heads result in painful callosities on the plantar surface of the forefoot. This is usually accompanied by a hallux valgus deformity. Skin ulcerations may form over bony prominences. Forefoot pain prevents the client from transferring body weight over the foot during terminal stance and results in a shortened step-length. Extra-depth shoes with wide toe boxes and moulded pressure-relieving inserts may be sufficient to relieve pain and improve gait (see Chapter 14). When the deformities are marked, resection of the metatarsal heads in conjunction with fusion of the metatarsophalangeal joint of the great toe is indicated.

Hindfoot involvement also is common and results in a planovalgus or pronation deformity.[38,74,75] A longitudinal arch support or similar shoe insert is not sufficient to hold the hindfoot in alignment. When the deformity is supple, an ankle-foot orthosis with a well-moulded arch support will control the position of the heel and subtalar joint during gait. This also will reduce the valgus thrust on the knee joint. If the deformity is fixed, a triple arthrodesis will align the hindfoot.

Summary

Arthritis is a disease that can be extremely debilitating. When conservative medical therapy has failed, however, surgical intervention can significantly alleviate the symptoms of arthritis and either stabilize or improve function. When indicated, surgical intervention is an effective and powerful tool used for the treatment of arthritis.

References

1. Katz W: Modern management of rheumatoid arthritis. *Am J Med* 79(suppl 4C):24–31, 1985.
2. Belt EA, Kaarela K, Lehto MU: Destruction and arthroplasties of the metatarsophalangeal joints in

seropositive rheumatoid arthritis. A 20-year follow-up study. *Scand J Rheumatol* 27(3):194–196, 1998.

3. Belt EA, Kaarela K, Lehto MU: Destruction and reconstruction of hand joints in rheumatoid arthritis. A 20-year follow up study. *J Rheumatol* 25(3):459–461, 1998.

4. Ryu J, Saito S, Honda T et al: Risk factors and prophylactic tenosynovectomy for extensor tendon ruptures in the rheumatoid hand. *J Hand Surg Br* 23(5):658–661, 1998.

5. Sekiya I, Kobayashi M, Taneda Y et al: Arthroscopy of the proximal interphalangeal and metacarpophalangeal joints in rheumatoid hands. *Arthroscopy* 18(3):292–297, 2002.

6. Bynum CK, Tasto J: Arthroscopic treatment of synovial disorders in the shoulder, elbow and ankle. *Am J Knee Surg* 15(1):57–59, 2002.

7. Gendi NS, Axon AJ, Carr KD et al: Synovectomy of the elbow and radial head excision in rheumatoid arthritis. Predictive factors and long term outcome. *J Bone Joint Surg Br* 79(6):918–923, 1997.

8. Gibbons CE, Gosal HS, Bartlett J: Long term results of arthroscopic synovectomy for seropositive rheumatoid arthritis: 6–16 year review. *Int Orthop* 26(2):98–100, 2002.

9. Horiuchi K, Momohara S, Tomatsu T et al: Arthroscopic synovectomy of the elbow in rheumatoid arthritis. *J Bone Joint Surg Am* 84-A(3):342–347, 2002.

10. Klug S, Wittmann G, Weseloh G: Arthroscopic synovectomy of the knee joint in early cases of rheumatoid arthritis: Follow up results of a multicenter study. *Arthroscopy* 16(3):262–267, 2000.

11. Takagi T, Koshino T, Okamoto R: Arthroscopic synovectomy for rheumatoid arthritis using a holmium:YAG laser. *J Rheumatol* 28(7):1518–1522, 2001.

12. Casey AT, Crockard HA, Bland et al: Surgery on the rheumatoid cervical spine for the non-ambulant myelopathic patient: too much, too late? *Lancet* 347(9007):1004–1007, 1996.

13. Collins DN, Barnes CL, FitzRandolph RL: Cervical spine instability in rheumatoid patients having total hip or knee arthroplasty. *Clin Orthop* 272:127–135, 1991.

14. Dunbar RP, Alexiades MM: Decision making in rheumatoid arthritis. Determining surgical priorities. *Rheum Dis Clin North Am* 24(1):35–54, 1998.

15. Kandziora F, Mittlmeier T, Kerschbaumer F: Stage-related surgery for cervical spine instability in rheumatoid arthritis. *Eur Spine J* 8(5):371–381, 1999.

16. Keenan MA, Stiles SC, Kaufman RL: Acquired laryngeal deviation associated with cervical spine disease in erosive polyarticular arthritis. *Anesthesiology* 58:441–449, 1983.

17. Pham XV, Bancel P, Menkes CJ et al: Upper cervical spine surgery in rheumatoid arthritis: retrospective study of 30 patients followed for two years or more after Cotrel-Dubousset instrumentation. *Joint Bone Spine* 67(5):434–440, 2000.

18. Van Asselt KM, Lems WF, Bongartz EB et al: Outcome of cervical spine surgery in patients with rheumatoid arthritis. *Ann Rheum Dis* 60(5):448–452, 2001.

19. Charter RA, Nehemkis AM, Keenan MA et al: The nature of arthritis pain. *Br J Rheumatol* 24(1):53–60, 1985.

20. Harris WH: Traumatic arthritis of the hip after dislocation and acetabular fractures: treatment by mold arthroplasty. An end-result study using a new method of result evaluation. *J Bone Joint Surg Am* 51(4):737–755, 1969.

21. Tigani D, DelBaldo A, Trentani P et al: Closed-wedge tibial osteotomy: conventional technique versus a new system of compression dynamic fixation. *Orthopedics* 25(11):1265–1268, 2002.

22. Kanamiya T, Naito M, Hara M et al: The influences of biomechanical factors on cartilage regeneration after high tibial osteotomy for knees with medial compartment osteoarthritis: clinical and arthroscopic observations. *Arthroscopy* 18(7):725–729, 2002.

23. Cooke TD, Harrison L, Khan B et al: Analysis of limb alignment in the pathogenesis of osteoarthritis: a comparison of Saudi Arabian and Canadian cases. *Rheumatol Int* 22(4):160–164, 2002.

24. Adili A, Bhandari M, Giffin R et al: Valgus high tibial osteotomy. Comparison between an Ilizarov and a Coventry wedge technique for the treatment of medical compartment osteoarthritis of the knee. *Knee Surg Sports Traumatol Arthrosc* 10(3):169–176, 2002.

25. Argenson JN, Chevrol-Benkeddache Y, Aubaniac JM: Modern unicompartmental knee arthroplasty with cement: a three to ten year follow up study. *J Bone Joint Surg Am* 84-A(12):2235–2239, 2002.

26. Deshmukh RV, Scott RD: Unicompartmental knee arthroplasty for younger patients: an alternative view. *Clin Orthop* 404:108–112, 2002.

27. Deshmukh RV, Scott RD: Unicompartmental knee arthroplasty: long-term results. *Clin Orthop* 392:272–278, 2001.

28. Stukenborg-Colsman C, Wirth CJ, Lazovic D et al: High tibial osteotomy versus unicompartmental joint replacement in unicompartmental knee joint osteoarthritis: 7–10 year follow up prospective randomized study. *Knee* 8(3):187–194, 2001.

29. Yun AG, Martin S, Zurakowski D et al: Bipolar hemiarthroplasty in juvenile rheumatoid arthritis: long-term survivorship and outcomes. *J Arthroplasty* 17(8):978–986, 2002.

30. Pandit R: Bipolar femoral head arthroplasty in osteoarthritis. A prospective study with a minimum 5 year follow up period. *J Arthroplasty* 11(5):560–564, 1996.

31. Bhan S, Malhotra R: Bipolar hip arthroplasty in ankylosing spondylitis. *Arch Orthop Trauma Surg* 115(2):94–99, 1996.

32. Prieskorn D, Burton P, Page BG et al: Bipolar hemiarthroplasty for primary osteoarthritis of the hip. *Orthopedics* 17(12):1105–1111, 1994.

33. Torisu T, Utsunomiya K, Masumi S et al: Bipolar hip arthroplasty in rheumatoid arthritis. *Clin Orthop* 244:188–197, 1989.

34. Zhu YH, Chiu KY, Tang WM: Review article: polyethylene wear and osteolysis in total hip arthroplasty. *J Orthop Surg (Hong Kong)* 9(1):91–99, 2001.

35. Miura H, Higaki H, Nakanishi Y et al: Prediction of total knee arthroplasty polyethylene wear using the wear index. *J Arthroplasty* 17(6):760–766, 2002.

36. Terefenko KM, Sychterz CJ, Orishimo K et al: Polyethylene liner exchange for excessive wear and osteolysis. *J Arthroplasty* 17(6):798–804, 2002.

37. Dumbleton JH, Manley MT, Edidin AA: A literature review of the association between wear rate and osteolysis in total hip arthroplasty. *J Arthroplasty* 17(5):649–661, 2002.

38. Keenan MA, Peabody JK, Gronley J et al: Valgus deformities of the feet and characteristics of gait in patients who have rheumatoid arthritis. *J Bone Joint Surg Am* 73(2):237–247, 1991.

39. Dionne RA, Khan AA, Gordon SM: Analgesia and COX-2 inhibition. *Clin Exp Rheumatol* 19(6 suppl 25):S63–S70, 2001.

40. Gordon P, West J, Jones H et al: A 10 year prospective follow up of patients with rheumatoid arthritis 1986–96. *J Rheumatol* 28(11):2409–2415, 2001.

41. Chandler DR, Nemeje C, Adkins HA et al: Emergency cervical spine immobilization. *Ann Emerg Med* 21(10):1185–1188, 1992.

42. Zeman CA, Areand MA, Cantrell JS et al: The rotator cuff deficient arthritic shoulder: diagnosis and surgical management. *J Am Acad Orthop Surg* 6(6):337–348, 1998.

43. Waldman BJ, Figgie MP: Indications, technique, and results of total shoulder arthroplasty in rheumatoid arthritis. *Orthop Clin North Am* 29(3):435–444, 1998.

44. Van Den Ende CH, Rozing PM, Dijkmans BA et al: Assessment of shoulder function in rheumatoid arthritis. *J Rheumatol* 23(12):2043–2048, 1996.

45. Trail IA, Nuttall D: The results of shoulder arthroplasty in patients with rheumatoid arthritis. *J Bone Joint Surg Br* 84(8):1121–1125, 2002.

46. Torchia ME, Cofield RH, Settergren CR: Total shoulder arthroplasty with the Neer prosthesis: long-term results. *J Shoulder Elbow Surg* 6(6):495–505, 1997.

47. Lehtinan JT, Belt EA, Kauppi MJ et al: Bone destruction, upward migration, and medialisation of rheumatoid shoulder: a 15 year follow up study. *Ann Rheum Dis* 60(4):322–326, 2001.

48. Boardman ND, Cofield RH, Bengtson KA et al: Rehabilitation after total shoulder arthroplasty. *J Arthroplasty* 16(4):483–486, 2001.

49. Gill DR, Morrey BF: The Coonrad-Morrey total elbow arthroplasty in patients who have rheumatoid arthritis. A ten to fifteen year follow-up study. *J Bone Joint Surg Am* 80(9):1327–1335, 1998.

50. Schemitsch EH, Ewald FC, Thornhill TS: Results of total elbow arthroplasty after excision of the radial head and synovectomy in patients who had rheumatoid arthritis. *J Bone Joint Surg Am* 78(10):1541–1547, 1996.

51. Tanaka N, Kudo H, Iwano K et al: Kudo total elbow arthroplasty in patients with rheumatoid arthritis: a long term follow-up study. *J Bone Joint Surg Am* 83-A(10):1506–1513, 2001.

52. Stein AB, Terrono AL: The rheumatoid thumb. *Hand Clin* 12(3):541–550, 1996.

53. Carlson JR, Simmons BP: Total wrist arthroplasty. *J Am Acad Orthop Surg* 6(5):305–315, 1998.

54. Divelbliss BJ, Sollerman C, Adams BD: Early results of the universal total wrist arthroplasty in rheumatoid arthritis. *J Hand Surg Am* 272:195–204, 2002.

55. Gellman H, Hontas R, Brumfield RH et al: Total wrist arthroplasty in rheumatoid arthritis: a long-term clinical review. *Clin Orthop* 342:71–76, 1997.

56. Houshian S, Schroder HA: Wrist arthrodesis with the AO titanium wrist fusion plate: a consecutive series of 42 cases. *J Hand Surg Br* 26(4):355–359, 2001.

57. Hartigan BJ, Nagle DJ, Foley MJ: Wrist arthrodesis with excision of the proximal carpal bones using the AO/SFIF wrist fusion plate and local bone graft. *J Hand Surg Br* 26(3):247–251, 2001.

58. Johnstone BR: Proximal interphalangeal joint surface replacement arthroplasty. *Hand Surg* 6(1):1–11, 2001.

59. Creighton MG, Callaghan JJ, Olejniczak JP et al: Total hip arthroplasty with cement in patients who have rheumatoid arthritis. A minimum ten year follow-up study. *J Bone Joint Surg Am* 80(10):1439–1446, 1998.

60. Jana AK, Engh CA, Lewandowski PJ et al: Total hip arthroplasty using porous-coated femoral components in patients with rheumatoid arthritis. *J Bone Joint Surg Br* 83(5):686–690, 2001.

61. Keisu KS, Orozeo F, McCallum FJ et al: Cementless femoral fixation in the rheumatoid patient undergoing total hip arthroplasty: minimum 5-year results. *J Arthroplasty* 16(4):415–421, 2001.

62. Ranawat CS: Surgical management of the rheumatoid hip. *Rheum Dis Clin North Am* 24(1):129–141, 1998.

63. Severt R, Wood R, Cracchiolo A et al: Long term follow-up of cemented total hip arthroplasty in rheumatoid arthritis. *Clin Orthop* 265:137–145, 1991.

64. Tang WM, Chiu KY: Primary total hip arthroplasty in patients with rheumatoid arthritis. *Int Orthop* 25(1):13–16, 2001.

65. Thomason HC, Lachiewicz PF: The influence of technique on fixation of primary total hip arthroplasty in patients with rheumatoid arthritis. *J Arthroplasty* 16(5):628–634, 2001.

66. Sculo TP: The knee joint in rheumatoid arthritis. *Rheum Dis Clin North Am* 24(1):143–156, 1998.

67. Bellemans J, Victor J, Westhovens R et al: Total knee arthroplasty in the young rheumatoid patient. *Acta Orthop Belg* 63(3):189–193, 1997.

68. Chmell MJ, Scott RD: Total knee arthroplasty in patients with rheumatoid arthritis. An overview. *Clin Orthop* 366:54–60, 1999.

69. Gill GS, Joshi AB: Long term results of retention of the posterior cruciate ligament in total knee replacement in rheumatoid arthritis. *J Bone Joint Surg Br* 83(4):510–512, 2001.

70. Konig A, Kirschner S, Walther M et al: Hybrid total knee arthroplasty. *Arch Orthop Trauma Surg* 118(1–2):66–69, 1998.

71. Laskin RS, O'Flynn HM: The Insall Award. Total knee replacement with posterior cruciate ligament retention in rheumatoid arthritis. Problems and complications. *Clin Orthop* 345:24–28, 1997.

72. Rodriguez JA, Bhendi H, Ranawat CS: Total condylar knee replacement: a 20 year follow up study. *Clin Orthop* 388:10–17, 2001.

73. Schai PA, Scott RD, Thornhill TS: Total knee arthroplasty with posterior cruciate retention in patients with rheumatoid arthritis. *Clin Orthop* 367:96–106, 1999.

74. Tillmann K: Surgery of the rheumatoid forefoot with special reference to the plantar approach. *Clin Orthop* 340:39–47, 1997.

75. Toolan BC, Hansen ST: Surgery of the rheumatoid foot and ankle. *Curr Opin Rheumatol* 10(2):116–119, 1998.

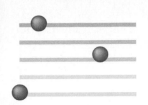

CHAPTER 8

Management of the Child and Adolescent with Juvenile Rheumatoid Arthritis

F. Virginia Wright, MSc(Clin Epid), PT
Elaine Smith, MSW, RSW

PHYSICAL REHABILITATION IN ARTHRITIS, Joan M. Walker, PhD, PT, and Antoine Helewa, MSc(Clin Epid), PT, Elsevier Inc. © 2004.

Table 8-1. Manifestations of JRA

Joint pain and stiffness
Muscle spasm and atrophy
Joint contractures
Systemic manifestations (i.e., rash, pericarditis, lymphadenopathy)
Skeletal growth disturbances
Osteoporosis (primary or as a result of drug therapy)
General failure to grow (primary or as a result of drug therapy)
Eye involvement (chronic iridocyclitis in pauciarticular JRA)
Nutritional deficiencies
Fatigue
Fibrositis
Aerobic deconditioning

Data from Melvin and Atwood, 1989[8] Klepper and Scull, 1999[7] and Mier et al, 2000.[5]

Juvenile rheumatoid arthritis (JRA) belongs to a large group of connective tissue disorders that occur in children and adolescents. Although many of these disorders also occur in adults, their clinical prognosis and presentation tend to be vastly different in children. Incidence for JRA varies internationally from 1.3 to 22.6 per 100,000 children younger than 16 years of age.[1]

Recently, a new classification of pediatric arthritis has been developed by the International League of Associations for Rheumatology to create more homogeneous subgroups of disease and facilitate communication between rheumatologists internationally.[2,3] The new umbrella term is *juvenile idiopathic arthritis* (JIA), representing six subtypes of JIA: pauciarticular arthritis; polyarticular (rheumatoid factor negative) arthritis; polyarticular (rheumatoid factor positive) arthritis; oligoarthritis; enthesitis-related arthritis; and psoriatic arthritis.[3] The focus of this chapter is on the disease manifestations and functional limitations associated with the three subgroups of JIA most often seen by physical therapists, i.e., pauciarticular (fewer than five joints involved in the first 6 months of arthritis), polyarticular (at least five joints involved in the first 6 months of disease), and systemic arthritis (chronic arthritis with systemic features).[4] These three subgroups previously were known as *juvenile rheumatoid arthritis* (JRA) according to American College of Rheumatology criteria.[1,3] In the remainder of the chapter JRA is used rather than the broader umbrella term JIA.

Diagnosis

Criteria for diagnosis and classification of JRA are presented in Chapter 4 along with medical manage-

ment of the disease. Although the majority of children with JRA are rheumatoid factor–negative (seronegative), 10% will have later-onset seropositive polyarticular disease, which has the same aggressive course as adult rheumatoid arthritis (RA).

Relevance of Disease Course and Prognosis

It is important that the physical therapist and occupational therapist recognize the differences between the subtypes of JRA with respect to manifestations and prognosis. Seronegative JRA is essentially unique to childhood and is characterized by soft tissue swelling, early connective tissue contracture in response to joint stiffness and pain, rapid loss of muscle strength, juxta-articular osteoporosis, local growth disturbances, and later joint destruction (Table 8-1).[5–8] There is a tendency for ankylosis, particularly at the cervical spine apophyseal, carpal, and tarsal joints.[9] There is evidence that the young cartilage offers resistance to erosions into bone with the possibility for healing because of its thickness and growth potential.[10] This disease picture differs from the proliferative synovitis, ligamentous laxity, and rapid destructive patterns of adult RA or seropositive JRA.

The prognosis for children with pauciarticular onset before 5 years of age to regain full joint mobility and functional ability is generally considered to be excellent unless the disease progresses to a polyarticular course.[11] Iridocyclitis may occur as a serious ocular complication of pauciarticular JRA that can lead to blindness if untreated and requires careful monitoring

Table 8-2. Overall Management of JRA

Objectives	Management Components
Decrease inflammation	Drug management
Control/reduce pain	Pain management strategies
Increase and maintain range of motion (prevent/reduce deformity)	Exercise/modalities/hydrotherapy
Increase and maintain strength	Rest/joint protection/splinting positioning
Maintain and optimize function	Orthopedic surgery interventions (tendon releases, osteotomies, joint replacement)
Encourage independence in daily activities	Guidance/adaptations regarding functional activities, school, and recreation
Encourage positive psychosocial and emotional development	Psychological and psychosocial support/counseling
Increase child's and family's understanding of JRA and its management	Education about JRA

Data from Scull, 2000[16] Mier et al, 2000[5] Emery et al, 1995[15] and Melvin and Atwood, 1989.[8]

by the rheumatology team.[8,12] The prognosis is more guarded for seronegative polyarticular JRA. Poor functional outcomes are related to hip involvement or to a prolonged disease course, and up to 35% of these individuals may still have active disease as adults.[13,14] Children with systemic-onset disease also have a poorer prognosis,[13,14] particularly in conjunction with extensive visceral involvement and long-term corticosteroid use.

However, with the advent of new drug management options and provision of optimal overall treatment, the prognostic pictures of the past may change for the better.[13] Overall, in more than 50% of children JRA will be in complete remission by late adolescence although their ultimate functional status is extremely variable.[3,13] Losses in joint mobility, bony damage, osteoporosis, and growth abnormalities that remain at the time of remission will persist as primary and significant factors limiting mobility. The others will have disease that continues into adulthood or relapses from time to time. For both of these groups, joint replacements may be indicated when bone growth nears completion in late adolescence.[13,15]

Goals and Components of Overall Management

Management objectives and components are presented in Table 8-2.[5,15,16] An overall picture of management is provided in the Algorithm for JRA (JIA) Management (Figure 8-1). The management team consists of in-dividuals representing the child's community, school, and local hospital, as well as the tertiary care center's rheumatology program (Figure 8-2), whose understanding and experience with children with JRA probably vary considerably. In small communities, the child may be the only one with JRA. Service providers have to develop strong communication strategies between themselves and with the child and family to ensure coordinated and effective care (see Case Study later in this chapter). The physical and occupational therapists need to be aware of the roles of physicians, nurses, and social workers in particular. All should draw on their expertise when they consider issues such as pain and stress management, knowledge about JRA, medications, adherence to intervention routines, nutrition, sleep issues, healthy lifestyle choices, peer relationships and developmental issues, splinting and energy conservation, sexuality, family coping, and financial and community resources.

Drug Management and Implications

Pharmacological agents are used in JRA to decrease and control overall inflammation and systemic manifestations, and to relieve pain (see Chapters 4 and 6). They act in tandem with physical management efforts to reduce or prevent joint contractures, damage, and disability. Treatment algorithms, such as that of the British Pediatric Rheumatology Group, demonstrate the earlier use of disease-modifying (i.e., second-line) agents than in previous years.[4] Drug

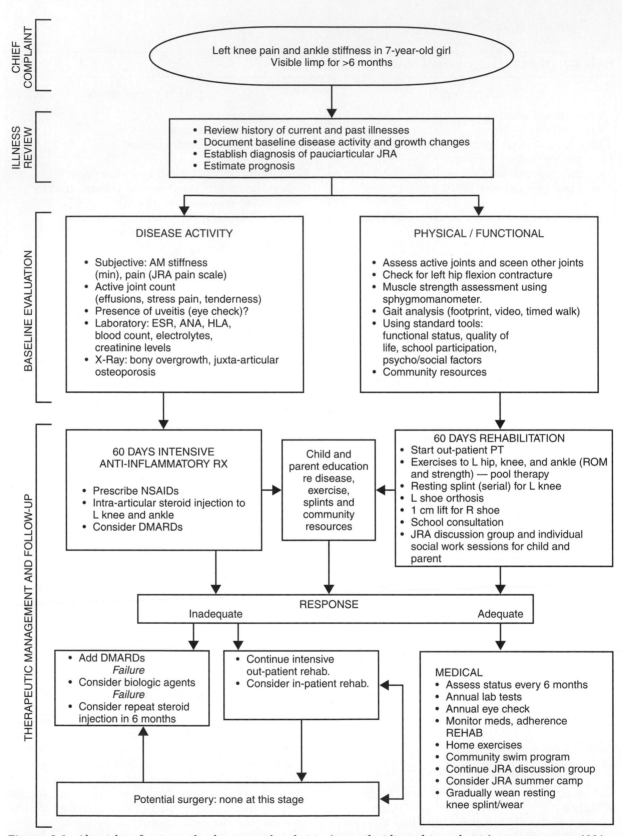

Figure 8-1. Algorithm for juvenile rheumatoid arthritis (juvenile idiopathic arthritis) management. ANA = antinuclear antibodies; DMARDs = disease-modifying antirheumatic drugs; ESA = erythrocyte sedimentation rate; JRA = juvenile rheumatoid arthritis; L = left; NSAIDs = nonsteroidal anti-inflammatory drugs; R = right; ROM = range of motion.

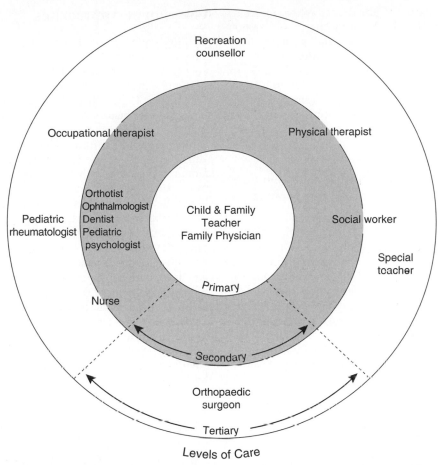

Figure 8-2. The arthritis team. Three levels of care are shown. Primary care providers are the family members/personal caregivers, family physician, and teacher. Team members for secondary and tertiary care may be located in a hospital, clinic, home, or school. Tertiary care team members may be located only in large urban centers where specialist care is provided.

management in JRA changed drastically in the early 1990s with the introduction of methotrexate as a second-line agent.[17,18] More recently, etanercept (e.g., Embril) has been introduced in pediatric rheumatology[3,19,20] and its effects have been described as revolutionary.[17] It is classified as a biologic agent, specifically a tumor necrosis factor inhibitor, and has been used successfully in children with uncontrolled polyarticular disease[17,20] and also in combination with methotrexate.[21] For children with severe systemic disease, cyclosporine, a cytotoxic drug, may be another option.[17,22] In addition to drugs to manage the arthritis, children also may be taking special medications and following dietary regimens for osteoporosis and generalized growth delay.[6]

The critical issue for physical and occupational therapists in relation to drug management is awareness

of the child's medication profile. This requires close reciprocal communication with the child's rheumatologist and nurse for information and feedback. Issues relating to cost and access have arisen with these new drugs, many of which are extremely expensive and may require nursing or social work staff to help with provision, funding, and monitoring.

Therapists must have a clear understanding of the goals of drug management and the expected timelines and patterns of change. For example, a child who starts taking methotrexate requires a thorough rehabilitation assessment at baseline, followed by identical sequential assessments at 3- to 4-month intervals for the first year to determine effectiveness. A child scheduled for intra-articular steroid injections will require pre-injection assessment with emphasis on the physical and functional status of the joints to be injected. This should be followed by postinjection assessments, initially at 2, 6, and 12 weeks and then at more extended intervals as dictated by other aspects of the child's treatment. There also should be a 3- to 6-week period of intensive therapy after injections to try to resolve joint contractures and improve strength and function (see Case Study later in this chapter).

Assessment and treatment protocols should be strongly influenced by the drug management program.

The team also needs to be aware of use of alternative treatments such as naturopathic and homeopathic treatments, chiropractic treatments, and acupuncture and share precautionary information regarding any possible side effects or interactions with traditional medications and therapies. Preliminary work has identified the relatively high rate of their use in JRA.[23] It is critical that the child and parent feel comfortable in sharing information on use of alternative therapies so that all components of the management scheme work in tandem.

Outcome Measures for JRA

Many of the impairment-based outcome measures used in JRA have been imported directly from adult rheumatology and are presented in Chapter 5 (e.g., active joint count, range of motion (ROM), muscle strength testing, gait or footprint analysis,[24] and timed walk). The main difference in their use in pediatrics is the need for modification of instructions provided to the child and for interpretation of results using pediatric normative values where available.

Assessment of JRA differs from that of adult RA in its use of age- and content-specific child- and parent-report functional status questionnaires. The measures that differ in JRA are the self-report measures. Given the emergence of a strong emphasis on client-centered practice, self-report measures have arisen as a way to enlist the client's viewpoint on functional abilities, pain, psychosocial status, self-efficacy, and quality of life. They have been developed according to physical and psychosocial developmental perspectives to ensure a focus relevant to a child's priorities and capabilities in the home, school, and community settings.

Assessment Approaches

The child's physical and occupational therapists may find that working together during the evaluation process reduces the assessment burden on the child and family, providing a more cohesive and integrated assessment of the child. After establishment of the child's medical history and subjective details (obtained from child and parent), the physical and occupational therapists should proceed together with the active joint count. Use of the joint man (homunculus) is a standard way of recording information on effusions, stress pain, damage and deformity for each joint (Figure 8-3). Joint counts always should be completed before other aspects of the physical assessment are undertaken to ensure that findings are put into an appropriate perspective.

Comprehensive assessment of ROM, strength, gait, fine and gross motor skills, and functional abilities may require several assessment sessions over a few weeks, particularly in a child with multiple joint involvement. Assessment sessions also can be integrated with initial therapy to allow concurrent work on primary problem areas. The assessment time provides an excellent opportunity for education of the child and parent about the findings and any changes since the last assessment. Diagrams of muscles and joints and use of a skeleton are helpful to explain the assessment information to the child and family.

Assessment periods also can be profitably used for disease education of the child and the parents.

Identification of an Active Joint

Criteria to identify an active joint in a child with confirmed JRA are similar to those used in an adult, as discussed in Chapter 5. Joints should be examined bilaterally for comparative symmetry, contour, muscle wasting, deformity, and ligamentous stability. Occasionally there may be a "dry synovitis" in which ROM is restricted and stress pain is evident even though there is no effusion.

Watching for nonverbal clues in young clients can be more informative than questions.

In some circumstances a child may be afraid to tell the team about pain or functional problems because

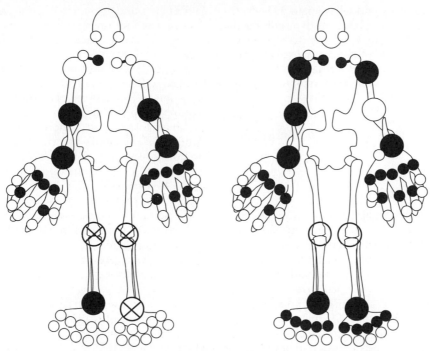

Figure 8-3. Example of an active joint count in a child with polyarticular disease. A joint is actively inflamed if effused, tender on pressure, or painful when stressed. The left figure shows 22 active joints, of these three are effused (×); the right figure shows 33 active joints (•) not counting effusions separately.

of anticipation of consequences of admitting to pain. This might result in recommendations for inpatient hospitalization or increased outpatient therapy appointments, the possibility of intra-articular injections, or restriction of activities and sports.

Impact of Hypermobility

It is important to recognize that up to 10% of all children are hypermobile.[25] This tendency to hypermobility will mask an early joint contracture and adds to the difficulty in early diagnosis. Bilateral comparisons of joint ROM and an overall check for signs of hypermobility are important aspects of joint assessment in pediatrics. For example, a hypermobile child with pauciarticular JRA may have 15 degrees of hyperextension of the right elbow while the left elbow extends only to neutral. Although there is no stress pain or effusion in the left elbow, the difference in ROM and radiological evidence of overgrowth at the left radial head strongly suggests a previous active inflammation at the elbow joint.

Evaluation of Pain

A new understanding of the prevalence of pain in JRA has emerged with the advent of pediatric-specific pain assessments that permit children's rating of pain in ways that are suitable to their cognitive stage.[26–29] Evaluation consists of careful observation during assessment and treatment, and for school-aged children also can be obtained through a self-report pain measure. This might consist of the use of body diagram outlines that the child colors in to identify the location and intensity of pain[27] or visual analogue scales to indicate the magnitude of pain at selected joints during various activities and at rest or to rate global pain. Alternatively, there are multifaceted measures of the different components of pain. For example, the Varni-Thompson Pediatric Pain Questionnaire (PPQ)[28] or the Abu-Saad Pediatric Pain Assessment Tool have been validated in children (4 to 16 years of age) with chronic pain. These pain scales require 30 and 45 minutes for a school-aged child to complete after an initial explanation from the therapist.

It is essential to be aware of the child's pain before, during, and after therapy treatment and also to identify the factors that aggravate and relieve pain. However, a balance needs to be struck between determining the child's pain and helping him or her manage it and work through it. Overuse of pain measures (e.g., use of visual analogue pain scales during each visit) may result in too much focus on pain symptoms rather than on methods of handling the pain.

> **Children are reliable reporters of their pain.**

Evaluation of Function

Changes in functional capabilities often are far more important to a child than the gains in ROM and strength that may underlie these improvements.[30] There was a flurry of activity through the 1990s in the development of client-report functional/health status questionnaires for JRA and pediatrics.[31–33] These measures generally have shown good reliability and validity,[34–39] although for most of them responsiveness to change continues to be evaluated.[32,40–43] The decision as to which of the client-report measures to use is complex because they may serve different purposes.[30,44] Clinicians need to be closely acquainted with the content and properties of each measure so that they can select the one most appropriate to the situation. Most can be obtained at minimal or no cost through their developer.

Of the child and parent-report functional measures, the Child Health Assessment Questionnaire (CHAQ)[36] has been used most often in drug trials. Its brevity and reliability have been identified as its primary assets. It has been translated into more than 30 languages, making it an international standard.[45] The primary limitations of the CHAQ are its ceiling effect and concerns about responsiveness to clinically meaningful change.[40,46–48] From a physical or occupational therapist standpoint, it provides limited information for problem identification and goal setting. Other measures such as the Juvenile Arthritis Functional Status Index (JASI),[38] the Juvenile Arthritis Quality of Life Questionnaire (JAQQ),[34] and the Child Health Assessment Profile[37] are much more comprehensive but may be too lengthy to be feasible in all clinical situations.

An alternative is to use an observational measure such as the Juvenile Arthritis Functional Assessment Scale (JAFAS)[35] or the Turner Observed Functional Test (TOFT).[41] The limitations of observational measures are the time required to administer them and their failure to be truly representative of the broad range of daily activities. They may, however, be useful to help occupational and physical therapists gain a better understanding of performance and quality issues related to function.[41]

There may be lack of agreement between the responses of parents and children on client-report measures. This should not necessarily raise concerns because different contexts, environments, and expectations affect scoring. The optimal situation is to acquire responses from both child and parent and use these to arrive at a more comprehensive understanding of the child's functional abilities in different circumstances.

Some of the JRA functional measures for school-aged children (e.g., the JASI[38]) do not have age-appropriate content for a young child. Instead, other pediatric functional measures that were designed for evaluation of young children with physical disabilities may be more suitable, i.e., measures such as is the Pediatric Evaluation of Disability Inventory (PEDI), a developmentally based functional questionnaire.[49]

Evaluation of Priority Functions

Evaluation of a child's individual functional priorities should be added to a functional evaluation.[30] Three measures that address priority activities are the MACTAR patient preference questionnaire (See Appendix II), for which the wording has been adapted for use by children,[38] the Canadian Occupational Performance Measure (COPM),[50] and Goal Attainment Scaling (GAS).[51] The functional priority lists are valuable for client-centered treatment goal setting and may prove to be especially responsive to important changes in status.

Psychosocial Issues That Influence Management

Initial Reactions to Diagnosis

The inherent difficulty in diagnosing JRA often causes delays in initiation of appropriate management. A child may have spent the weeks during which diagnosis is being determined on an acute-care ward with children with life-threatening diseases (e.g., leukemia), and families may have fears associated with this experience. Although the diagnosis of JRA will relieve concerns about mortality, its unpredictable course and prognosis may put parents and children on an emotional roller coaster. This makes it difficult for them to assimilate the extensive information provided by the health care team, and families may initially have difficulty following recommendations. New information must be provided in small sections and reiterated to facilitate easier understanding and acceptance.[52] Therapists and nurses all have strong ongoing roles in this regard given their close, long-term involvement with the child.

Stages of Grief

Children and their families will go through various stages of grief after the diagnosis of JRA: shock and disbelief, isolation, anger, resentment and bargaining, self-blame, depression, and then, potentially, acceptance.[53] Grief may be cyclical in nature,[54] reemerging with each new complication, new life experience, and transition through the developmental stages. Response to illness will vary within families themselves, further intensifying family stress.

The Child's Response to the Disease

Through the extended course of the disease, the child's mood and ability to adhere to therapy may fluctuate in response to many factors. Overall, the child may feel a lack of control over life, because many decisions and intrusive treatment procedures become a daily and unavoidable experience. Defiance and hopelessness can be a child's ways of fighting back against lack of control over the disease. These may manifest as a refusal to take medications, participation in activities that are physically risky, failure to attend therapy sessions or demonstration of apathy during therapy, or lack of adherence with home programs. The variable nature of the arthritis can be confusing and disturbing, and recurrent periods of pain and restriction can be difficult to cope with and understand. For example, dramatic and rapid physical improvement often occurs after multiple intra-articular steroid injections. These gains may be followed by a sudden return of the symptoms, pain, and limitations. At the time of injection, the child and family must be warned of this possibility so that appropriate goal setting, follow-up, and support can be put in place.

The severity of the arthritis does not necessarily link with the child's ability to adapt. Some children with severe JRA cope well, whereas others with "mild" pauciarticular involvement demonstrate greater adjustment problems.[55] The latter children may have considerable fear of deterioration of physical capabilities and difficulties in fitting in with a peer group. These children may perceive themselves as belonging neither to the group of children who are severely physically disabled nor to the group of their non-physically challenged peers.

Emerging fears, emotions, and behaviors are outlined in Table 8-3.[56,57] Lack of mobility, time, or energy for peer activities can increase isolation and

Table 8-3. Emotions and Behaviors That May Occur in a Child with JRA

Anxiety about:
- Long-term dependence on family
- Outcome of the disease
- Academic success and future career planning
- Severe illness or death
- Handling of chronic pain
- Intrusive and painful medical procedures
- Side-effects/long-term impact of medications

Potential resultant behaviors and emotions:
- Anger
- Depression
- Withdrawal and isolation
- Low energy
- Sadness
- Passivity
- Inferiority
- Low self-esteem
- Denial

Data from Unruh and McGrath, 2000[57] and Black et al, 2000.[56]

sadness and reduce self-confidence. One contributor to stress is the child's perception of being a burden by causing major lifestyle changes for her or his family. For example, the need for an accessible school and regular access to medical care may require that a family move to a different city even when it means that one parent has to stay behind to continue at a job.

Another issue that needs to be considered is the impact of having arthritis during adolescence, which in itself is a time of special challenges.[58] This brings about a double crisis in that fears about loss of physical abilities, difficulties in separating from parents, the experience of being different from peers, and uncertainty about short- and long-term health compound the existing developmental challenges.[58,59] Reactions to the disease may be very difficult to discern in an adolescent. A tough or cynical exterior or an overly accepting attitude may mask concern about the disease and the future, regardless of the severity of the disease. Awareness of these reactions helps the health care team members to be sensitive to potential problems. Adolescents with JRA have described ways of dealing with the issues including hanging in, trying not to make the illness their first priority, trying to make the best of the situation and maintaining a positive attitude, and finding someone to talk to, e.g., a peer support group.[58]

Table 8-4. Potential Impact of JRA on the Family

One parent giving up his or her job to meet increased care requirements
Changes in caregiver roles and responsibilities
Rearrangement or elimination of social activities and interests causing family isolation
Increased transportation requirements for appointments and travel to school
New set of expenses for drugs, splints, and transportation that compound the effects of lost salary
Treatment and appointment time requirements
Home therapy time demands
Loss of time for family activities
Lack of sleep (both parent and child) in response to illness demands
Emotional stress of dealing with a child's behaviors and adherence
Need to develop strategies to manage pain
Challenges of splinting regimens and adherence
Physical demands on parent to assist with child's mobility
Handling of issues related to the child's emerging independence

Data from Atwood, 1989[63] and Allaire et al, 1992.[62]

Suggestions for Helping a Child to Deal with Feelings

Children need to develop a way of dealing with feelings of fear and anxiety. If unexpressed, these may emerge as negative behaviors, emotional insecurity, or poor adjustment to the disease and its management. Even children who appear to successfully cope with the disease may have a high level of underlying psychological or physiological strain.[60] Consequently, social support is critical in JRA, regardless of the level of stress reported. This may take the form of esteem/emotional support, informational support, or companionship.[61] The team, in particular the social worker, can provide a forum for a child's or adolescent's expression of these fears and stresses. Play activities utilizing doll houses, puppets, or stories; individual counseling; music; and art can all facilitate the expression of feelings. Group sessions for exercise or discussion may reduce the sense of isolation and provide a sense of belonging, shared goals, and a safe environment to express feelings and facilitate effective problem solving.[52] Role playing may be of particular value for adolescents. Participants in our program have initiated role-playing topics (e.g., physician, patient, and parent at the clinic; patients receiving injections and blood work; or the demanding or protective parent/therapist/teacher).

Impact on the Family

Having a child with JRA brings about changes in family lifestyle and dynamics that must be recognized when the rehabilitation program is planned (Table 8-4 and Case Study).[62,63] Lifestyles may be altered in social, financial, time, energy, emotional, and behavioral areas, thereby increasing family stress. Impacts on families can be extremely variable,[64] with some families reporting a tremendous range of issues[54,65] whereas others appear high in cohesion.[60] JRA may be most disruptive in the first year after diagnosis[66] when previously-used coping mechanisms are no longer adequate. Table 8-5 provides a list of family-related factors that illustrate the potential for involvement of team members.[54,67]

Open and frequent communication with the child and family is essential so that potential difficulties can be anticipated and handled quickly. The child or family members may require psychosocial counseling with a social worker to facilitate adjustment to the disease and its impact, to encourage expression of feelings, to assist in development of coping strategies, and also to help the family identify and focus on positive aspects of their life.

Parenting Issues

Overall it appears that a healthy parent-child relationship is a critical factor in promoting positive outcomes.[67] One key concept in parenting and caring for a child with JRA is that discipline must be maintained as close to the family's usual routine as possible. In some families there may be overprotection of a child with JRA, whereas others may place unrealistic demands on the child to achieve physical gains (e.g., several hours of therapy every day). Episodic

Table 8-5. Family-Related Factors that Affect Coping with JRA

Nature of the relationships within the family (parent with child with JRA, marital, siblings)
Physical and emotional strengths and weaknesses of the child and other family members
Family members' level of sharing of care responsibilities
Physical dependence of the child and associated care burden on parents/caregiver
Availability of extended family supports
Parenting skills
Problem-solving skills of child and family members
Communication skills within and beyond the family unit
The family's belief system (spiritual, cultural, relating to illness)
Life experiences concerning illness and medical care
Financial impact of the care requirements
Availability and level of specialization of local health care resources

Data from Frank et al, 1998[67] and Britton, 1999.[54]

behavioral changes, in which the child becomes demanding or manipulative, may seem to the child to be the only way to exert control over the environment. If parents ignore the child's inappropriate behaviors, making special concessions, the child learns that people behave differently toward him or her and may take advantage of this. Behavioral limits still must be set regardless of chronic disease with some choices to allow the child a sense of personal control. The issue of dependence versus independence, which is difficult anyway as a child develops, may become an arena for parent-child conflict. Nonadherence issues also have potential for eliciting parent-child conflict.

Parents often have considerable misunderstanding about the prognosis of the disease and aims of therapy.[54] Education programs that focus on exercise, pain, and medical and social support management issues have led to significant gains in parents' perceptions of competency in handling their child's arthritis.[68] Support can come through formal groups that are organized and facilitated by members of the health care team, e.g., social work and nursing, and also may take the form of community-based self-help parent groups.[69]

Developmental Considerations

In addition to changes related to the child's arthritis over time, there will be changes related to developmental maturation and in the family's responses to both. Summaries of developmental stages and issues related to JRA have been outlined in detail elsewhere.[56] The process of continuous developmental change (physical, cognitive, psychosocial) always must be

considered when rehabilitative approaches are planned, implemented, and evaluated. For example, an approach that worked well when the child was 5 years old may meet resistance once the child is in grade 1 and begins to assert independence. Issues that may need to be addressed include the child's resistance to wearing wrist splints to school, unhappiness about leaving school early to attend therapy, and fatigue from spending an entire day at school. If these issues are not recognized and handled promptly, the therapy program is susceptible to failure.

The impact of JRA on psychosocial development and well-being has been the object of considerable research. For example, there may be a tendency for family, friends, teachers, and others to treat adolescents with JRA whose growth has been stunted as one would a child of a younger age. Although it is clear that psychosocial issues vary greatly among children, it is important for all physical therapists to be aware of the potential impact of a chronic disease on a child's developing socialization, independence (locus of control), and self-concept.

Sexuality

Sexuality, which is one component of the transition process to adulthood, is an area that has received little attention in literature on JRA or in the pediatric chronic disease literature overall.[70] Teens with disabilities need to go through the transition process to adulthood just as their peers do.[71] For normal development, they need to be aware of issues of puberty, boy/girl friends, and sexuality and to be positively supported by parents and others in social activities and in developing a health self-concept.[72] Teens with JRA will have the same questions as their peers, as well as additional uncertainties related to arthritis, e.g., will I get a boyfriend or girlfriend, will I be able to have sex, will I be able to have a child and will this child have arthritis? They need to have access to education on issues related to sexuality and have the opportunity to talk about their questions and worries.

Given all of the other competing issues related to disease management, prognosis, and financial coping, parents and perhaps the teens themselves may not see sexuality as an area that needs to be addressed.[73,74] There may be limited opportunities to achieve independence from parents, explore new skills, excel at physical tasks, socialize with peers, make decisions, or take responsibility for oneself.[56,71,74]

Because exposure to sex education at school can be quite variable,[70] health care professionals should be an important source of information on sexuality. They need to be aware of the issues and have knowledge of correct information and ways to assist the teen in understanding sexuality and issues related to JRA.[74] Nurses in particular have a strong role in advising teens about issues related to pregnancy and medications and social safety issues, e.g., alcohol use,[75] street-proofing, bullies, and school safety.

Team Considerations

Differences in beliefs and value systems of arthritis team members also affect the care of the child with JRA. Team members must be aware of their feelings about the disease process, potential outcomes, and the attitudes they project. Staff may see children with complex disease for whom successes are slow in coming, gains are barely visible, and the disease process is unpredictable with flare-ups and regression. Staff and families may sometimes feel helpless and discouraged about a particular child's condition. Occasionally, the family's frustration about the unpredictability of arthritis is expressed as anger toward various team members, often the ones they see the most frequently. Team members need to retain objectivity. Issues behind the anger should be recognized and managed. The team also should recognize the difficulties associated with temporarily aggravating pain during exercise sessions and sharing difficult information and the effect of these on the relationship with the family.

Team members need to set realistic expectations not only for the child but also for themselves. Prevention of deterioration of a child's physical capabilities is often a major accomplishment when disease is aggressive and persistent. It is essential to recognize the work of the child, parents, and team and give credit!

The child's adjustment may be strongly influenced by the reactions of others close to them. Team members who have close association with a child over several years should not underestimate the positive impact they can have on the child's development and perceptions through their actions and suggestions. Open communication between team members and the family is essential to share different viewpoints, to gain a full understanding of progress, and to identify accomplishments.

> **Respect should be given to the disease process and its ability to frustrate the best treatment plan. The team, the child, and the family need to remember they cannot work miracles.**

Principles of Physical Treatment and Rehabilitation

The therapeutic management of a child or adolescent must be relevant to their developmental and emotional maturity. Differences between JRA and adult RA also dictate a different physical management strategy in terms of the nature and goals of treatment. Physical and occupational therapeutic exercise and splinting approaches in JRA emphasize stretching of soft tissue contractures, strengthening of surrounding musculature to regain or maintain joint mobility, encouragement of optimal positioning of joints that are susceptible to fusion, and facilitation of function.

The physical and occupational assessment and treatment approaches must be proactive. Although the course of JRA is difficult to predict, a child's disease pattern often establishes itself over time (e.g., recurrent joint inflammation at hips and knees whereas other joints and systemic disease remain inactive). An understanding of the pattern and type of disease helps therapists focus clearly on the primary goals of treatment. Contractures and weakness can be anticipated based on the typical patterns of restriction and overgrowth in JRA (Table 8-6) and preventative treatment programs can be instituted.[5,7,15,16,63,76–78] Joint endfeels and a radiograph review are key factors in guiding intervention decisions. The therapist should be alert to the child's response to anti-inflammatory and disease-modifying drugs to ensure that overly intensive therapy is not administered in the presence of overt inflammation.

It is essential also to recognize and treat secondary contractures (i.e., those that arise in a joint adjacent to one with arthritis). For example, a hip flexion con-

Table 8-6. Pain Reduction Approaches

Relaxation training with techniques such as progressive muscle relaxation, tension relaxation, or relaxed breathing techniques

Stress management (daily hassles) training

Art, music, and play

Hypnosis

Problem-solving approaches

Cognitive coping strategies include distraction, visual or guided imagery, and negative thought stopping, cognitive refocusing, and restructuring

Behavioral strategies such as use of positive reinforcement

Data from Unruh and McGrath, 2000[57] von Weiss et al, 2002[61] Rapoff and Lindsley, 2000[81] and Thastum et al, 2001.[83]

tracture may develop due to a knee flexion contracture in a child with knee arthritis only. The knee synovitis and flexion contracture should respond fully to early treatment, but unless attention also is directed to the hip, a hip flexion contracture and compensatory lumbar lordosis may become the primary problem.

Pain Management

Pain in JRA has a potential for functional, social, and psychological morbidity and can have a dramatic effect on the quality of life of the child through the critical developing years.[79] It has been estimated that up to 30% of children with JRA have moderate to severe pain[80] and that most children have daily episodes of mild pain.[81] The impact of the child's pain on the child's family can be also considerable.[79,82] All members of the rheumatology team must be cognizant of pain issues related to JRA and should work in tandem to help the child and family cope.[57] Because physical and occupational therapy practitioners provide the primary rehabilitation services for children with rheumatological diseases and their family members, they are well suited to ensure appropriate evaluation and management of pain, thus reducing the potential for disability and handicap.[57]

The multidimensional aspects of pain in JRA have been described as a puzzle in which nociception, feelings, thoughts (cognitions), and behavior all interrelate.[81] Consequently a multidimensional approach needs to be taken to pain management, including a strong focus on the more recently advocated cognitive approaches[81] by a social worker or psychologist who has been trained to do this work. It is critical that the approaches used be age appropriate.

Reactions to Pain

The influence of pain and stiffness on the child's ability to participate in home, school, and recreational activities can be profound. Fatigue, reluctance to walk, irritability, interrupted sleep at night, and muscle tenderness all may originate from uncontrolled or chronic pain and synovitis and translate into reduced quality of life. "Catastrophizing" is a common and harmful response to pain and is an excellent target for cognitive restructuring approaches.[81,83] A dramatic positive change in affect is often noted after the child's pain is controlled. It is not unusual for team members and families to be extremely surprised when the child experiences a positive behavioral change in response to reduction of pain.

The child and family may find it difficult to push through the day's activities and therapy demands when pain is present. An important consideration is the parents' and child's fears of what the pain means. They may question whether further damage occurs by encouraging the child to perform the painful exercises or activities. Therapists also may have difficulty working a child through pain that occurs during treatment and make exceptions and offer special privileges out of sympathy for the child.

Problem Solving Related to Pain

Identification of pain should facilitate interpretation of the source of pain and allow clinical judgment to determine whether the particular treatment should be continued as is or modified. It also should help to reduce the child's and parents' concerns about the implications of pain and allow them to work through it. Often the pain experienced during therapy is muscular in nature and resolves immediately after the stretching or strengthening exercise. Many children need help to differentiate between pain and stiffness and between muscle and joint pain. Some pain occurs when new physical activities are started and is usually temporary (e.g., severe foot pain in a child who has been minimally ambulatory before multiple joint corticosteroid injections and who is starting to walk greater distances).

Management of Pain

Selection and provision of pain interventions need to be a team endeavor to determine who on the immediate or extended team has the skills to provide the selected approach. The use of pharmacological and physical therapeutic pain-relieving modalities has been covered extensively in Chapters 6 and 9, and these principles generally can be applied with children. In our clinical experience, most children tolerate and may prefer ice to heat as long as it has been introduced positively and gradually with a clear explanation about its purpose. For use of any electrotherapy modality the child must be old enough to be able to appreciate and describe sensations associated with the modality (i.e., at least 6 years of age).

Other Pain Management Techniques

As with adults with RA, pain management strategies should extend beyond application of modalities (i.e., a direct reaction to pain) into use of cognitive-behavioral (cognitive) approaches by a social worker or psychologist who has been trained to do this work. The cognitive approach states that behavior and affect are mediated by cognitive function and is focused on modifying distorted perceptions.[84] Recently, there has been recognition of a number of techniques that are described in greater detail by experts in the area.[57,81] The overall goal is to provide the child with a means to personally control or handle their pain and permit more complete and happy participation in daily life.

Pain intervention work needs to take place within a positive and supportive environment.[57] Possible individual or group interventions[61,57,81] that can be provided by those with training in the techniques are outlined in Table 8-6. Cognitive strategies that focus on helping the child to gain an understanding of their disease and then apply methods to alter or reduce their pain form an important part of the JRA group psychoeducational and camp programs that are offered by various rheumatology programs.[52,85] It is important that children be given age-appropriate explanations about the pain they are experiencing, what they might anticipate in response to various interventions or activities, and how the techniques

can help in managing the pain.[52,57] Parents also need to be included in discussions about pain and its management so that they are better able to react appropriately and provide support because pain-coping strategies of parents and children seem to be linked.[66,83] It is clear that any interventions that take place within a group context need to be tailored carefully to the characteristics of participants in the group so that the material does not cause anxiety.[52] Numerous resources exist in the health literature on various techniques for pain management in general populations, and several sources that apply well to JRA are listed in Appendix I.

It has been suggested that strategies that teach pain mastery and self-efficacy be used with children early in the course of the disease before maladaptive patterns develop.[80] A clear relationship exists between use of coping strategies early on in the course of the disease and better long-term outcomes.[80] Questionnaires on strategies for coping with pain may be useful at the time of initial assessment to assist in identifying those who may be at risk for pain management issues and to evaluate the impact of cognitive approaches.[80] These include the Coping Strategies Questionnaire adapted for children,[80] and the Pain Coping Questionnaire,[86] which is currently undergoing further validation work in JRA. Both extend beyond assessment of pain status and focus on a direct assessment of a child's ability to manage pain. As an extension to these, several other questionnaires to examine the perceived abilities of the child or parent to manage the child's arthritis are available, and each of these contains a pain management component.[87–89]

Exercise in JRA

Basic Concepts

Grading of Exercise Based on Disease Activity

Detailed guidelines are presented in the JRA literature for the type of exercise appropriate to the stage of disease activity[7,15] (i.e., acute, subacute, chronic). Unfortunately research has not been sufficient in rigor, quantity, or scope to permit the development of evidence-based clinical practice guidelines. Although it generally is agreed that exercise must not be so vigorous that inflammatory activity is aggravated or joint instability is encouraged, the causal relationship between levels of physical activity and inflammation is unclear. Unless a child has severe systemic illness or is experiencing an acute episode of generalized joint spasm and pain, bed rest and immobilization of joints should be avoided. It is essential to recognize that different levels of disease activity may exist within various joints at any one time. In the presence of acute synovitis, the recommended therapy consists of gentle active-assisted and passive exercises for the targeted joints with an emphasis on the concurrent use of modalities such as ice, hot packs, or wax for relief of pain and swelling. If inflammation is subacute or chronic, the treatment program is progressed to include active and strengthening exercises, functionally based gross motor activities, and conditioning exercises.[7] Daily exercise programs that take each joint through a full active ROM traditionally have been advocated, because routine activity does not always require that a joint move to its limit.[7] For lack of other empirical evidence, conclusions from the RA studies still form the basis of exercise protocol decisions in JRA (see Chapter 9). Ultimately, decisions regarding the appropriate intensity of exercise and physical activity are based on the therapist's judgment and clinical experience and on careful monitoring of the child's response to therapy.[7]

Suspension Systems   One approach to ROM and strength improvements that has garnered little attention in the JRA physical therapy literature is the use of sling suspension systems.[90] The standard gym sling set-up can be modified to allow use at home, i.e., installation of a ceiling hook over the child's bed to allow hook up of a rope and sling set. These set-ups are particularly useful for gravity-eliminated ROM work for hip flexion/extension, hip abduction, and knee flexion/extension, and springs can be added to provide graded resistance at the end of range. This set-up lends itself well to a child's independent exercise and in our experience, children find it to be extremely useful to painlessly mobilize stiff joints. It is especially useful in situations in which pool therapy is not available.

Management of Specific Joints

Details on restriction and adaptation of the various joints are presented in Table 8-7 in association with the typical patterns of contracture and bony change. Surgical interventions, covered in Chapter 7, usually are a later-stage management strategy. The primary exception to this is use of soft tissue releases at the hip joint. Because about 33% of children with JRA will eventually develop serious hip involvement, surgical lengthening of contracted hip flexors and adductors may be an important preventative strategy in younger children.[91]

Soft Tissue Management for Young Children

The greater soft tissue flexibility and hypermobility in children younger than 8 years of age and the earlier stage of disease of younger children point to the need

Table 8-7. Clinical Manifestations and Patterns of Contracture and Restriction*

Clinical Manifestations	Restriction/Adaptation
Cervical Spine	
In polyarticular and systemic JRA	Loss of extension, rotation, and side flexion
Narrowing then fusion of apophyseal joints, specifically C2 and C3	May develop torticollis
Dysplasia of vertebral bodies	Eye movements compensate for lack of neck ROM
Odontoid process instability (less common than in adult RA)	
Temporomandibular Joint	
Undergrowth (micrognathia) and altered occlusion of teeth	Restriction of mouth opening, pain, and difficulty when chewing
Mandibular asymmetry if unilateral	Greater functional restriction when cervical spine involved and extension is restricted
Less common in PA JRA	
Shoulder Region	
Overgrowth of humeral head with irregular shape and shallow glenoid fossa	Insidious loss of GL-H ABD, and flexion, tightening of pectorals and protractors
Subluxation may occur	More dysfunction when elbow and wrist involved

Continued

Table 8-7. Clinical Manifestations and Patterns of Contracture and Restriction*—Cont'd

Clinical Manifestations	Restriction/Adaptation
Elbow	
Occurs in all subtypes	Extension lost early
Overgrowth of radial head restricts ROM	Shoulder ROM initially compensates for supination ↓
Ulnar nerve entrapment possible	Wrist involvement accentuates pronation, supination losses
Wrist	
All subtypes, starts early	Rapid loss extension
Accelerated carpal maturation	Marked weakness extensors
Undergrowth of ulnar styloid, with severe changes may migrate dorsally	Tend to rest in flexion and ulnar deviation with notable spasm of wrist flexors
Radio- and intercarpal fusion	Distal R-U disease causes loss of pronation and supination
Carpal tunnel syndrome	
Hand	
Premature epiphyseal fusion and growth abnormalities	PIP (especially fourth) more common than DIP contractures
Flexor tenosynovitis may be dramatic	Loss of MCP flexion (especially second), loss of MCP hyperextension
Involvement later in PO and S-JRA than in PA-JRA	Marked ↓ grip strength
MCP and CMP subluxation	Boutonnière < swan neck deformities
Thoracolumbar Spine	
Unusual site in JRA	Kyphosis in association with neck and shoulder involvement
Steroid drug therapy may cause osteoporosis, wedging vertebral bodies, small compression fractures	Lumbar lordosis due to hip flexion contractures
	Scoliosis secondary to lower limb asymmetries
Hip	
Femoral head overgrowth	Flexion contracture-may be masked by lumbar lordosis
Osteoporosis	Marked spasm of ADDs and flexors
Trochanteric growth changes	Loss of ABD and rotations, eventually flexion
Shallow acetabulum and reduced femoral neck angle, especially if weight bearing limited	May have marked pain on weight bearing
Lateral subluxation of femoral head aggravated by tight ADDs	Secondary deformities of contracted hip, knees, lumbar spine
Potential for protrusion acetabuli, avascular necrosis	
Primary cause of ROM ↓ and dysfunction	
Occurs in PO and S-JRA after a few years	
Knee	
Most common joint involved in all subtypes, involved early	Rapid development of flexion contracture

Table 8-7. Clinical Manifestations and Patterns of Contracture and Restriction*—Cont'd

Clinical Manifestations	Restriction/Adaptation
Distal femoral overgrowth (medial) may cause leg length discrepancy in unilateral disease	Rapid atrophy of quadriceps
Knee valgus aggravated by tight hamstrings, iliotibial band	Loss of patella mobility due to adhesions
Posterior tibial subluxation due to prolonged joint involvement or excessive correction of knee flexion contracture	Risk of femoral fracture associated with falling due to flexion loss and osteoporosis
Ankle/Foot	
Altered growth produces bony changes in tarsals, potential fusion	Loss of flexion (often only 90 degrees)
Hindfoot valgus/varus due to ankle involvement or to knee valgus	Secondary development of hip flexion contracture
MTP subluxation	Early loss of inversion, eversion
Hallux valgus	Later loss of dorsiflexion and plantar flexion, specifically in minimally ambulatory children
IPs: growth changes due to premature epiphyseal closure	Altered gait, loss of MTP hyperextension affects toe-off
	Overlapping of IPs (specially with hallux valgus)

Data from Atwood, 1989[63] Emery et al, 1995[15] Libby et al, 1991[77] Reed and Wilmot, 1991[9] Scull, 2000.[16] Mier et al, 2000[5] and Laxer and Clarke, 2000.[16]

*The listing is not inclusive; features characteristics of JRA are given.

ABD = abduction/abductors; ADD = adduction/adductors; CMP = carpometacarpal-phalangeal; DIP = distal interphalangeal; GL-H = glenohumeral; IP = interphalangeal; MCP = metacarpophalangeal; MTP = metatarsophalangeal; PA = pauciarticular; PO = polyarticular; S = systemic; ↓ = decreased; ↑ = increased.

for intensive therapy early in the disease course. It may be tempting to allow the focus of therapy for young children to be on play-directed or developmentally based activity rather than on joint ROM and strengthening. The lack of joint-specific mobilization and stretching, however, may result in establishment of very resistant contractures that subsequently require soft tissue releases or reconstructive surgery. In our clinical experience, preschool children can participate in JRA group pool and gym therapy sessions (Figure 8-4) and tolerate soft tissue stretches and splinting. Age-appropriate adherence-enhancing strategies (i.e., stickers and games) should be built into their program.

Special Considerations for Children with Pauciarticular JRA

There may be a tendency to regard the joint involvement of a child with pauciarticular JRA as less serious than multiple joint involvement in a child with polyarticular disease. Deformity of even one or two joints in a child with pauciarticular JRA can be a serious long-term sequela of the disease. Early intensive rehabilitation efforts are needed for these children with mild involvement. For example, a knee flexion contracture of 15 degrees with a knee valgus deformity of 10 degrees and compensatory hindfoot varus of 5 degrees in a young child cause concern about abnormal pressures across open epiphyses. This altered growth situation is compounded by hyperemia (increased blood flow) that may occur at the distal femur and proximal tibia in conjunction with knee synovitis.[9] Research in adults suggests that increased intra-articular pressure associated with muscle imbalance and shortening may encourage osteoarthritic changes.[92]

> Age-appropriate adherence-enhancing strategies must be built into all aspects of children's programs.

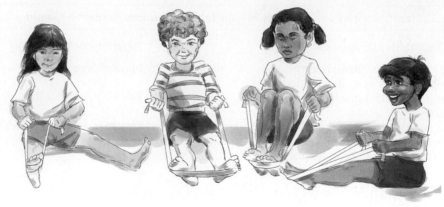

Figure 8-4. Group exercise session.

The Developmental Sequence and Function

The delayed acquisition of complex fine and gross motor skills (i.e., cutting with scissors, pouring from a pitcher, hopping on one leg, one-handed ball catching) sometimes observed in young children with JRA may be due to physical inability to perform the task because of restriction and pain. This delay should not introduce concern; improvement in the child's physical status usually leads to rapid learning of these skills. Ideas on the impact of JRA on skill development are outlined in a recent chapter on occupational therapy in JRA.[56]

Acquired skills occasionally are lost, and effort is required to ensure that they are regained. For example, a child may have achieved dressing independence at age 6 and then temporarily be incapable of performing this task because of a disease flare. In some situations, regaining independence may require effort and problem-solving skills on the part of the health care team and the family.[56]

Hydrotherapy

All JRA rehabilitation publications reviewed mentioned hydrotherapy as a means to relieve pain and encourage joint ROM through active exercises and specific joint stretches. Incorporation of active exercise during hydrotherapy should increase blood flow and muscle core temperature, facilitating maximal contractions due to reduced muscle viscosity and increased biochemical reactions.[93] Despite its widespread acceptance, there have been few published efficacy studies on the topic and no consensus on best practice exists.[94]

Effectiveness of Hydrotherapy in JRA

To evaluate the specific effects of pool therapy (stretching, ROM, strengthening exercises), Bacon et al[95] conducted a one-group pre- and post-test study of 11 children with JRA. Statistically significant improvements occurred only for several hip ROM measures and for heart rate recovery. Insufficient sample size and the reduced validity of a one-group design drastically limited conclusions. Recent studies have tended to combine pool therapy with other exercise modalities so that a study of a pure effect has not been possible.

> **The pool is a safe environment for work on aerobic conditioning.**

Value of Hydrotherapy in JRA

The buoyancy and weight-relieving properties of water are of great importance for children with JRA, allowing painful and stiff joints to move with little force. The pool may be the only place in which a child with severe lower extremity involvement is able to tolerate walking. Hydrotherapy also is of great value in early postoperative stages or after an acute disease flare. Because lower extremity joints are minimally loaded in shoulder-deep water in the pool, it is a safe and fun environment in which to work on aerobic conditioning.

Overview of Hydrotherapy Techniques

Skillful use can be made of water's turbulence, surface tension, and viscosity to safely and comfortably provide varying degrees of resistance.[96] Bad Ragaz lower extremity mobilization and strengthening techniques are highly suitable for children with JRA, with the use of inner tubes or rings for support.[97] This technique combines principles of proprioceptive neuromuscular facilitation with hydrotherapy so that movement and muscular work are facilitated in a controlled manner. Manual techniques and water buoyancy and turbulence produce the desired movement patterns. In general, the incorporation of water wings and other flotation devices to either assist or resist movement adds variety and interest[96] and provides free and secure movement for children with very restricted mobility. This freedom of movement deserves special notice. Observers watching pool groups of children with JRA often remark that it is hard to believe that these children who demonstrate such ease of movement in the water are the same ones who had such difficulty changing for the pool and walking into the water.

Group Pool Sessions

The pool is an ideal medium for group exercise therapy sessions.[95] Group membership may consist of children of diverse ages (3 to 16 years of age) and varying disease activity. A group session integrates ROM, stretching, strengthening, aerobic, and swimming activities. Individual variation in performance according to age and physical ability is taken into account. Those who have attended the group for a long time or are older act as role models and "peer educators" for newer or younger members.

Group sessions also are a way to foster leadership skills. The participants may take turns "running" the group, which provides a chance for them to feel competent physically, cognitively, and socially. Groups also are an opportunity for fun, lively peer interactions, and water sports/games. This may be the one time for children of all ages with JRA in a community to be together. A large number of children can participate in several group pool sessions per week, thereby using PT time more efficiently.

Group pool sessions are an easy way to get a younger child to work hard. Although quality movement should not be expected from young children, they can be expected to follow a sequence of movements as long as they are supported in the water. As the child matures, familiarity with the hydrotherapy protocol will allow a focus on achievement of the optimal range and repetition speed for each exercise.

Stretching of Soft Tissue Structures

In children, lengthening of muscle must occur in tandem with skeletal growth if ROM and flexibility

Table 8-8. Joints Susceptible to Flexion Contractures in JRA

Elbow
Wrist
Metacarpophalangeal
Proximal interphalangeal
Distal interphalangeal
Hip
Knee

are to be maintained. Shortening of muscle and tendon and the resulting joint contractures are early consequences of JRA. The holding and use of joints in positions of physiological flexion mimic the effects of immobilization of the joint and result in decreased length of muscle fibers. The resulting contractures, although initially flexible, may persist through the disease's course and become a major cause of disability.

Table 8-8 lists the joints of greatest concern for flexion contractures in JRA. Resolution of contractures is possible if they are attended to early on in conjunction with local control of synovitis. There is little evidence, however, about which stretching methods are most efficacious. Studies provide evidence that muscle and tendon respond to brief stretching with improved immediate post-treatment flexibility and that heat facilitates stretching.[98–100] The use of proprioceptive neuromuscular facilitation techniques, e.g., contract-relax and hold-relax, has been found by this chapter's physical therapist author to be a pain-free and effective way to help the child work into extremes of the available range without overstressing the joint. In addition, the use of isometric holds in a gravity-eliminated position at the end of the passive ROM is an easy way to help the child focus on activating and strengthening the targeted muscle(s) in the newly acquired range. In JRA there may be more leeway for gain in extensibility in restricted muscle because of opportunities for growth and healing. Conversely, there is also risk of adverse effects including damage to immature epiphyseal areas in the proximity of tendinous attachments.

Suggested Approaches to Brief Stretching

The two main types of stretching to consider in JRA are brief stretch (e.g., 60-second hold during pool PT) and prolonged low-load stretch for several hours (e.g., night splints for hands, elbows, or knees; night hip traction, wrist working splints for day wear). Brief stretching gently mobilizes the joint, temporarily extends muscle fibers, and prepares the tissues for their lengthened position in the splint. This active stretching, ideally in a warm pool, is necessary to assist in gradual breakdown of scar tissue, adhesions, and fibrotic contractures that occur with inflammatory tissue disease.[101]

Stretching pain should be minimized whenever possible so that protective spasm does not sabotage results. For example, passive stretches and gentle grade 1 mobilizations of finger joints are best undertaken in a warm pool after the child has exercised for about 20 minutes. Ideally a static stretch should be maintained for as long as tolerated (i.e., at least 2 minutes) to permit the plastic deformation of connective tissue rather than just a temporary lengthening of elastic myofibrils.[102,103] The child must learn to relax during the stretch. One way to facilitate relaxation is to encourage deep breathing. Active and active-assisted exercises should occur after stretching to promote use of joints and muscles within the new range.

Stretching sessions often are tolerated better if children feel that they are doing warm-up exercises similar to those that their sports heroes do every day. Naming a stretch after a child's hero may be an easy way to increase the child's adherence. Similarly, pre- and poststretch measurements using a tape measure gives a child tangible feedback on immediate gains and easily marks progress over the weeks.

Splinting: An Approach to Prolonged Low-Load Stretching

Basic Concepts

Rationale for Use of Splints

Because connective tissue needs elongation to facilitate permanent lengthening,[104] use of a prolonged low-load stretch via night resting splints is an appropriate option. An additional concern in JRA is the extent of morning stiffness experienced. If a child is allowed to sleep comfortably flexed without splints, the first hours of the day are spent getting the limb "straight" again.

> A child's adherence to stretching can be enhanced by naming a stretch after one of their heroes, such as "the Spiderman knee stretch."

Types of Splints

The splints fabricated for children with JRA are similar to those used in adult RA in terms of their design, materials, and purpose (see Chapter 14). Resting splints for elbows, wrists and hands, knees, and occasionally ankles are provided to ensure optimal positioning through the night and a prolonged low-load stretch. Soft or rigid neck collars, specially designed cervical pillows, and Buck's skin traction for the hips are other devices used to promote an optimal "extended" sleeping posture and encourage relaxation of muscle spasm.

Splints prescribed to support, protect, and optimally position joints during daily activities include wrist working splints, neck collars, and foot orthoses (Figure 8-5). Occasionally dynamic splints are indicated to resolve contractures (i.e., dynamic finger splints). Care should be taken to guard against joint subluxation and epiphyseal damage that may occur due to overzealous corrective force on developing joints.

Manufacture of Splints

Given the frequency of alteration required for many splints, it may be most expedient and cost-effective for occupational and physical therapists to work together in their fabrication and adjustment. Prefabricated splints are not ideal, because they do not conform to joint angles and may not provide the correct support. A splinting session is preceded by a pool therapy treatment in which the soft tissue structures are heated and stretched so that slight reduction of the contracture is achieved before splinting. In other situations when a permanent splint is being fabricated after contracture resolution or when molding to the contracture is difficult, collaboration with an orthotist may be advised. Other issues concerning

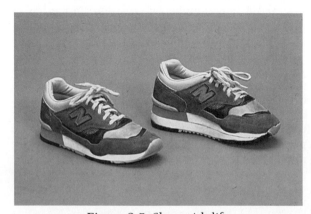

Figure 8-5. Shoe with lift.

splinting materials are given in Chapter 14. Although standard guidelines for positioning of the joint(s) are a helpful starting point, the child's individual contracture pattern, soft tissue extensibility, and radiographic findings should direct the splinting process.

Characteristics of a Good Splint

The splint should contain the joint well, providing up to two-thirds circumferential support along the long bones to prevent the child from inadvertently pulling out of the splint. For example, shallow wrist working splints allow a child to pull over the lateral splint border into ulnar deviation. Overcorrection of contractures should be avoided—a straight knee splint used for a bent knee will not provide adequate support posteriorly to allow the spasm in the soft tissue structures to relax. Furthermore, forcing a knee into a splint that uses a three-point pressure system may simply encourage posterior tibial subluxation.

Serial Splints

The use of serial splinting allows a gradual correction of a flexion contracture. The use of three or four serial splints over a period of 4 to 6 months may allow resolution of a stubborn flexion contracture. The first splint would be molded to conform exactly to the contours of the existing contracture. Subsequent remoldings should permit reduction of the splint angle to reflect improvements of the underlying joint angle as soft tissue structures lengthen. Improvement in flexion contractures may occur more quickly when splinting immediately follows intra-articular joint injections that have reduced joint inflammation and associated muscle spasm. Frequent monitoring and adaptation, possibly every 1 to 2 weeks, is needed for these children.

Serial Casting

There may be times when serial casting using plaster or Hexcelite is preferable to serial splinting with thermoplastic materials. The main drawback to serial splinting is that the splints can be removed by the child. Based on our experience, the most that can be expected is 8- to 10-hours of splint wear-time per day. Serial casting, on the other hand, ensures that the child will wear the cast and maintain the soft tissue lengthening until the cast is removed by the clinician. Joints that are amenable to serial casting procedures are the wrist, knee, and ankle.

One approach to serial casting that does not place undue burden on the child and family is to put the cast on the child's joint on a Friday morning and leave the cast on over the weekend. On the following Monday afternoon the cast is bivalved. This provides 72 hours of gentle soft tissue stretch, support, and accompanying relaxation of the periarticular structures. The child then wears the bivalved cast for at least 20 hours daily over 1 to 2 weeks, at which point a second cast is applied and the entire procedure is repeated. Pool therapy (with the cast removed) is essential during this period to allow the child to actively work the muscles in the new range. The interval between castings allows the soft tissue structures to accommodate to their new length.

As long as there are no adverse effects (i.e., aggravation of joint inflammation), three to four serial casts may be appropriate within the cycle. A thermoplastic splint then is fabricated to maintain the joint in the corrected position. The splint-wearing schedule depends on the joint, the type of splint (resting versus daytime), and the child's tolerance.

Methods to Enhance Splint-Wearing Adherence

Adherence issues are paramount when use of resting and working splints is considered. A splint that is not worn cannot be effective no matter how well it is designed! Table 8-9 presents a summary of potential reasons for nonadherence.[105–107]

Sometimes a full set of splints (wrist working, hand, and knee resting splints) is prescribed for a child during a single clinic visit along with a rigorous wearing schedule. There may be considerable difficulty in the child suddenly being expected to tolerate several splints through the night. From our clinical experience, it is better to gradually introduce the various splints, gaining adherence with one for several weeks before the next is introduced. The decision as to which splint to start with should be based on priority therapy goals. For example, if knee contracture resolution is a primary goal, knee splint wear would be started first, followed by addition of other splints as tolerated.

> It is better to introduce splints gradually, to gain adherence with one before the next splint is introduced.

Many children enjoy helping to make their splints (e.g., cutting out and applying straps, choosing the color of splinting material and straps). Companion

Table 8-9. Reasons for Nonadherence with Splints

Discomfort due to inadequate fit
Restriction of function when in splint
Increased stiffness associated with use
Uneasiness/self-consciousness about peers' reactions to splint
Insufficient understanding (child or parent) about reasons for wearing splint
Unrealistic splint-wearing schedule
Lack of positive reinforcement/recognition for splint wear
Lack of improvement in joint position or function despite previous adherence

Data from Bolding and Sanders, 2000[105] Rapoff, 2000[106] and Wynn and Eckel, 1986.[107]

splints may be made at the same time for the child's favorite stuffed animal (Figure 8-6). The child then takes on the responsibility of ensuring that his or her stuffed friend *also* wears the splint every night!

Positive feedback recognizing adherence is imperative because gains in ROM may be intangible to the child. Acknowledgment of splint wear can take the form of stickers for the splints or a reward point system. Splint wear is expected for the entire night (i.e., until the child gets out of bed in the morning). Otherwise, parent-child confrontations can arise around when the splints can be removed (i.e., 2 AM versus 5 AM versus 7 AM). For young children, parents may be advised to put splints on after the child is asleep.

Some children have difficulties coping with the immobility associated with splint wear at night. Movement of a child with polyarticular JRA who has difficulty turning in bed without splints may be dramatically restricted when the splints are on. Simple movements, such as getting out of bed to go to the bathroom, may be completely limited. Therapists need to help parents work out a system so that assistance to reposition or get up is readily available (i.e., a two-way voice monitor in the child's room or a bell to ring for assistance).

During times in which contracture reduction is being undertaken, splints should be worn every night. When the joint status is stable and the disease is relatively inactive, a program of alternate-night splint wear may be considered. Guidelines should be clear and adherence monitored closely to ensure that splint usage is not abandoned altogether.

A child may be concerned about the profound morning stiffness associated with wearing of night splints. Children's anxiety about this stiffness and reluctance to wear the splint or hip traction device may be reduced if they are warned of the sensation in advance. They should be given measures to help the discomfort resolve (i.e., morning tub bath, gentle

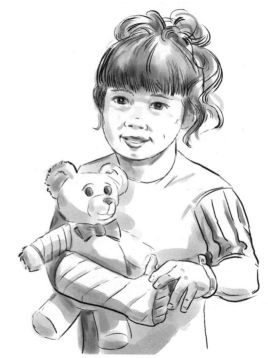

Figure 8-6. Adherence with splint wearing can be enhanced by making a splint for the child's favorite toy.

ROM exercises after splint removal, or a sling suspension set-up over the bed that is used before getting up). A common reason for nonwear relates to the fit of the splint. Children grow quickly, and a splint may be too short or tight within several months of fabrication. The parent and child need to be warned of this on receiving the splint and instructed to come back for adjustments if the borders become snug.

Splint Wear at School

The child may feel that a daytime splint draws attention to their physical disability. For children with mild disease, it may be the only visible sign of arthritis. The team needs to ensure that appropriate support is in place to lessen the anxiety. The person who provides the splint to the child should ask the child and parent(s) what type of support they need to make splint wear more acceptable and suggest different options (e.g., the therapist talking to the teacher or class about splint wear). The child may find that wearing a daytime splint restricts movement to the extent that functional activities such as writing are difficult. In some children splint adjustment may be required, whereas in others, time and practice will reduce the functional difficulties.

Muscle Strengthening

Muscle atrophy in JRA is common and seems to be most closely related to the severity of the disease.[108,109] Other causes of weakness are similar to those seen in adult RA: disuse atrophy, reflex inhibition due to effusion and pain, nonspecific myositis, ultrastructural muscle fiber damage due to the disease process, and drug-induced myopathy have been observed as common muscle changes in adult RA.[109] All JRA publications reviewed recommended isometric exercise as the safe way to increase strength,[7,15,16,110] using evidence from effectiveness and safety in adult RA as justification. There may be greater strength improvement in JRA than in adult RA, given a child's potential for growth and healing and the less destructive nature of the disease. Although there is considerable evidence about the existence of weakness in JRA,[48] few studies have examined muscle strengthening in JRA. There is evidence though that a multifaceted 3-month strength training program can be successful in achieving significant gains in strength in children with JRA along with type II fiber recovery.[111] Recently, there has been more interest in activity and fitness-based programs and their impact on endurance and disease activity. One of the benefits of these programs is the enhancement of muscle strength.[47]

Muscle-Strengthening Protocols

A child with JRA whose muscle weakness has been present for several months may be unable to elicit maximal effort from targeted muscles. Patterns of compensation for certain muscle groups, such as the hip abductors and extensors, often are well established. Some children may be fearful of attempting an anti-gravity hold because they anticipate pain or joint damage. For weak musculature (e.g., grade 3), an active-assisted antigravity lift and gentle support during the isometric hold will reduce the child's fears of the limb painfully dropping and encourage active contraction of the targeted muscle group.

At the beginning of training, methods of providing muscle feedback should facilitate the relearning of maximal muscle activation. Biofeedback via a simple hand-held unit in conjunction with isometric exercise may be useful at this stage. It serves as a comfortable alternative to neuromuscular stimulation, which probably gives sensory rather than motor input given the low intensities that children tolerate.

When progressive resistance exercises are used, evaluation of the child's repetition maximum (RM)[90] is done often at the beginning of training (i.e., every week), and then is determined as appropriate as training progresses. An example of an initial isometric progressive resistance exercise (PRE) program for children with quadriceps weakness might consist of two sets of six isometric contractions, each using a weight that equals a 75% RM for the first set, followed by a 50% RM for the second set.

The RM program lends itself well to home programs both in terms of time required and the ease with which the child can document and see gains. The RM strengthening program can be adapted for use with sling and spring set-ups in which the resistance of the spring is used in calculating the RM. This approach encourages active ROM at large joints, such as the hip, offering light spring resistance at the end of range to facilitate contraction of the target muscle group.

Aerobic Capabilities and Training

Deconditioning has been acknowledged to be a common issue in JRA. In a comparative study of the aerobic capacity of children with JRA and nondisabled control subjects, aerobic capacity of children with JRA was lower ($p < .001$) than that of the age- and sex-matched control group. Up to 20% of children with JRA do not do any physical activity outside of school.[112] A number of recent studies in JRA have indicated the safety and potential benefits of aerobic exercise in JRA[47,113–115]; these results parallel the experience in adult RA. There are, however, issues about the ability of those with active hip involvement to tolerate these programs even when they are modified.[114]

Cross-training, which incorporates a combination of strengthening and endurance exercises has been studied in 10 children with JRA who participated in a training program over a 3-month period.[111] Type II fibers in the quadriceps muscle did demonstrate a tendency to have a more normal electromyographic response pattern after training, although endurance and strength were unchanged. Lack of improvement probably was related to the fact that the sample size was inadequate to detect a significant difference. A child's interest and motivation is heightened if he or she is given access to a computerized bicycling or treadmill system that provides a video course to ride with feedback on speed and distance. There also may be some exciting and creative possibilities for use of adapted dance exercise or martial arts programs. The questions that now arise are about the extended impact of exercises on functional status and quality of life.[47]

> **Remember, a child is not an adult.**

Implications of Osteoporosis

Varying degrees of osteoporosis are commonly seen in JRA. Although osteoporosis is multifactorial in nature,[112] it occurs particularly in children with prolonged corticosteroid use or periods of restricted mobility.[9,116] There is an increased likelihood of pathological fractures in the presence of limited ROM (e.g., a femoral fracture when the child falls and the knee flexion range is less than 90 degrees). There have been a considerable number of studies on enhancement of

bone mineral status in JRA over the last decade. General management principles now include minimization of corticosteroid use, control of disease activity, use of biphosphates, and promotion of weight-bearing activities to increase bone density, encourage growth at epiphyses, and improve flexibility and muscle strength.[112,116] When weight bearing on land is difficult because of lower extremity weakness or pain, a walking program in the therapy pool may be the only means to maintain ambulatory abilities. This should be emphasized until the disease symptoms subside sufficiently to permit use of a walker or crutches on land.

Children who have had arthritis from their early years may have inadequate development of reactive and protective balance responses and have a high risk of a fracture if they fall. Working on standing balance (e.g., use of balance boards or computerized balance systems) may be another way to reduce the risk of falling. Another option is to consider use of Tai Chi Chuan, which has been shown to improve dynamic balance in individuals with physical disabilities.[117]

Despite all efforts to maintain or increase a child's ambulatory abilities, the child still may need an alternate means of mobility for long distances in the community or at school. Available options include tricycles/bicycles (Figure 8-7), battery-powered scooters, or wheelchairs (manual or electric). One important advantage of scooters or bicycles/tricycles

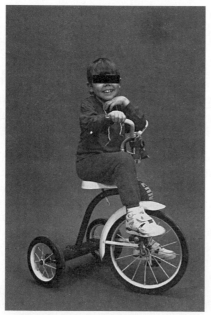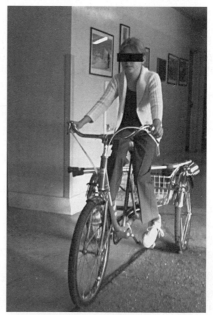

Figure 8-7. Tricycles and bicycles offer an alternate means for mobility over long distances when ambulation is restricted.

is that children are likely to leave them at the classroom door and walk to their desks. With a wheelchair, there is a reduced tendency for the child to get out of it during the day, and consequently the opportunities for short-distance weight bearing are greatly reduced.

Options for Therapy within the Community

There is a need for long-term vigilant follow-up for children with JRA. The therapy program must be flexible and correspond with changes in disease activity. Caution should be observed when including a child with JRA in a group pool or gym session that consists of older adults with arthritis. Unless the differences in disease are clearly explained and understood, new fears about prognosis may arise in the child's mind. It is better to schedule children together to provide a supportive and similar peer group.

Although it is optimal to set up a therapy program within the child's community, there may be a lack of appropriate facilities/services in many outlying and rural areas. Even within urban areas it may be difficult to find clinicians who feel comfortable working with children with JRA. Furthermore, the policy of many acute care hospitals may limit the length of outpatient treatment (i.e., 6 to 8 weeks). This does not address the capricious nature of JRA nor the importance of maximizing ROM and function during the child's growing years. As discussed earlier, change does not always occur in a positive direction. Sometimes tremendous effort must be expended for the child to maintain ROM and ambulatory status. This apparent lack of progress often is used as a reason for not considering a child as meriting continued outpatient intervention.

It is crucial that the pediatric rheumatology team from a tertiary care center forges strong links with the identified treatment team in the child's community and works out the best method of support, both for the local team's needs and for the child and family. Letters of support from the child's rheumatologist that include the rationale for the need for long-term follow-up often are very effective in encouraging extended outpatient care. Teleconferences, computer linkages, or videotapes of therapy assessment and treatment sessions, are effective ways of sharing information.

Home Programs

Careful evaluation of the child's *specific* exercise requirements, coupled with a current understanding of the literature on the effectiveness of these techniques and sensitivity to the family's home situation, will help in development of a plan for exercise that has a chance to succeed. Although the idea of a daily exercise home program of 20 to 30 minutes may seem optimal to the physical therapist, factors such as fatigue after a lengthy school day, the demands of homework, opportunities to spend time after school with friends, and family time constraints may make this impossible. This does not mean that the health care team's principles and better judgment need to be compromised. Flexibility and problem-solving skills need to be used to create and undertake a feasible therapy plan.

Goal Setting and Adherence Enhancement

One of the greatest challenges in designing the rehabilitation program for a child with JRA is the multitude of goals to work on during the child's already limited school and extracurricular time. This is particularly the case for children with polyarticular JRA, in whom 20 or more joints may be identified as problems at any one time. There is always a sense that gains must be made as early and quickly as possible. This, however, must be tempered by a consideration of what the child and family can actually cope with at any point and within their lifestyle.

There is evidence that older children and adolescents are interested and able to participate in decision making in relation to their care and that adherence may be enhanced when this process is allowed.[118] The problems and goals identified by the child, team, and parent(s) may not always correspond in terms of content, priority, or expression. It is important to take the time to listen to, understand, and respond to the various viewpoints.[119] Nonadherence may result if a child and parent(s) do not understand how the goals are to be attained or are not cognizant of the ongoing results of care.[59]

Barriers to Adherence

The extended months or years over which the child and family are expected to adhere to treatment regimens can lead to boredom and indifference and wear down child and family adherence. Lack of improvement often translates into a reduction in adherence. Frustration is encountered if progress that was anticipated does not materialize even after the child and family adhered to treatments and made recommended lifestyle changes. The family may ask many questions pertaining to the perceived failure. Was there not more that could have been done by staff or family? Were the decisions that were made about medications

Table 8-10. Factors That May Influence Adherence

Parental Factors
Level of awareness of the importance of different aspects of the child's care
Attitudes toward the individual or facility providing the care
Belief in the efficacy of treatment
Financial and support resources
Family function

Therapist Factors
Level of sensitivity to child's/family's lifestyle and belief system
Ability to provide positive reinforcement
Flexibility to changes in child's status
Willingness to explain/provide education during assessment and treatment sessions

Child/Adolescent Factors
Time restrictions due to school, work, and social life
Discouragement/boredom with long-term treatment programs
Emerging independence and autonomy
Satisfaction with care/service providers

Data from Wynn and Eckel 1986,[107] Mayo 1978,[121] and Rapoff 2000.[106]

the right ones? The physical and occupational therapists need to help the child and family understand that in some circumstances maintaining the physical and functional status quo is an accomplishment in itself. It is critical to consider client and family factors, disease factors, and regimen factors when attempting to solve issues related to adherence.[106]

Importance of Positive Reinforcement

Recently there has been more emphasis on strategies that focus on self-management and positive reinforcement.[106,120] Therapists must recognize the importance of feedback during therapy. An honest, positive comment always can be found even when change is not happening as anticipated. The physical and occupational therapists may be among the few people who actually remark on the effort put forth by the child and family for exercise and splint wear adherence. Use of goal-specific contracts with a meaningful incentive at the end do not have to be equated with bribery; rather, the physical gains gradually achieved from improved adherence in splint wear or exercise may mean very little to the child, necessitating a tangible reward from time to time.

Methods to Enhance Exercise Adherence

Factors that influence adherence and simple ways to enhance exercise adherence are outlined in Tables 8-10 and 8-11.[105–107,121] Realistic, achievable goal setting is important to both family and team outcomes. Parents who are actively involved in encouraging their child's regular use of medications and exercise enhance their child's adherence to the regimens. There is evidence that exercise adherence is less than that for medication and tends to be lower in adolescents than in children.[64] A decrease in reported adherence for adolescents corresponds with the shift of personal responsibility from parent to adolescent. Although transfer of responsibilities to the adolescent is an important part of the transition process, it should occur gradually along with individualized adherence strategies, support, education, and follow-up.

Education and Education About JRA

A child's individual understanding of disease and treatment must be evaluated; comprehension levels on the basis of the child's age, disease duration, and previous educational interventions should not be assumed.[121] There is evidence that children and teens with arthritis have lower than expected knowledge about their diseases and numerous misconceptions.[122] These misconceptions may have serious implications for a child's willing participation in therapeutic regimens.

The child's ability to handle uncomfortable questions from peers and others may depend on understanding of the disease, its manifestations, and its management.

Table 8-11. Adherence-Enhancing Strategies for Exercise Programs

Clearly written, age-appropriate home exercise programs
Education and reeducation about rationale for intervention and skill to carry out
Daily journals to track exercise adherence
Child participates in design and writing of own exercise program and exercise calendar
Child allowed to make choices within exercise program on order of exercises, selection of exercises, number of repetitions, etc.
Personalized exercise videotapes
Regular phone calls or e-mails from physical or occupational therapist to children in remote areas to support/encourage/reduce isolation
Opportunities to participate in JRA/pediatric orthopedic exercise groups
Inclusion of sibling or friend in exercise session at therapy facility or home
Short-term admissions to rehabilitation facility for "tune-up" from time to time
Participation in JRA summer camps
Incentives such as stickers, and cumulative rewards after several weeks of sticker acquisition

Data from Rapoff, 2000[106] and Bolding and Sanders, 2000.[105]

The team nurse will probably be the individual most extensively involved in this long-term education process. The clinic may not be the best setting for education about disease and its management because the stress and anxiety of the clinic visit and any treatment decisions made there can interfere with processing of information. Repetition of information presented at the clinic and review of treatment choices should occur at therapy follow-up sessions. Families may be more inclined to ask questions and retain valuable information in this more relaxed environment.

Discussion of treatment priorities and accomplishments can be built easily into each therapy assessment and treatment session. This provides informal education and review of the child's understanding and adherence with their exercise and splinting regimens. The formation of psychoeducational discussion groups with other children with JRA may be an even better way to provide new information about JRA and coping strategies. These groups also can be used to explain previously provided verbal and written information, providing support and reassurance as well as social contact with others with similar issues and questions.[52] Use of a multidisciplinary team (physical therapist, occupational therapist, nurse, social worker) to run these children's or parents' groups helps to ensure a comprehensive educational approach. It also is critical to recognize that children and teens with arthritis have considerable understanding and expertise about their condition through their experience living with it. They must be included in the planning of the content and focus of psychoeducational programs if the material is going to be relevant to those who receive it.[52]

Educational Materials

The language used by adults to describe JRA may be too abstract for children. It is essential to choose age-appropriate words and materials carefully to explain concepts to a child. Recently, arthritis organizations (Canadian and American) have recognized the need for an individualized, consumer-friendly teaching approach. Several fun workbooks are available to facilitate a child's interest in learning more about his or her arthritis (see Appendix I). These booklets also may be helpful for the siblings of the child with arthritis who may be easily overlooked in terms of their importance in the family unit. Siblings may have unspoken fears about what is happening to their brother or sister. Materials focused for parents with a self-help focus are given in Appendix I. Parents may want to share these materials with other family members, such as grandparents, whose perception may be that arthritis is an elderly person's disease that inevitably leads to permanent and severe disability.

> It is essential to select age-appropriate words and materials carefully to explain concepts to a child.

Participation in School Activities

There is considerable interest in identifying the challenges that children with JRA face in the school setting. This focus is appropriate given that school is the occupation of childhood and is an essential contributor to academic and psychosocial development. Difficulties encountered by a child with JRA include writing problems, mobility restrictions and limitations in participation in physical education, functional restrictions, and problems with self-esteem and peer relationships.[123]

In middle childhood, the peer group exerts a strong influence on a child; feedback and support from friends are essential for a child to gain independence from parents.[61] In JRA a conflicting situation exists because the illness itself creates dependence. Therapists can help to devise strategies that will encourage maximum and realistic independence at home and school according to the child's capabilities. Interactions with a peer group also have a strong impact on self-image and expectations and provide an opportunity for children to receive feedback on accomplishments. Children have a need to be the same as others and will be apprehensive about obvious differences from peers. Changes in abilities and appearances (e.g., short stature, cushingoid features due to prednisone use) may invite comments from peers. The child may need assistance from the arthritis team in learning to handle questions and difficult situations.[52,61]

Suggestions for Adaptations within the School Environment

Children with JRA require understanding and support in the school system if they are to succeed academically and keep pace with their peer group developmentally and socially. A child with JRA may be the only one with the disease in his or her school.[124] Misconceptions about the disease and its prognosis are plentiful. Therapists often have a strong role within the school to provide support and education (written materials, in-service session) to school personnel and the child's class. The team also has a role in working with the child and parents to help them prepare to share information and deal with issues at school. Specific physical problems of a child with JRA can be identified using a school checklist, such as the 39-item list described by Atwood.[124] This list may be a useful tool within the Individualized Education Plan that should be implemented if problems encountered are considered more than minor in nature. Items in the list include rating of ability to get to and from school, the impact of stiffness on various activities, mobility within the school, tolerance of the school day, writing and activity of daily living skills, and the extent of understanding and empathy of classmates and teachers. The child and physical therapist can share the completed list with the teacher to assist in the problem-solving process. Two more extensive measures might prove useful in identifying issues related to the student's integration and maximum participation in the school setting, specifically the School Function Assessment[125] and the School Setting Interview.[126]

Adaptations may be required for children with mobility limitations to ensure safe and full access to the school's key facilities (i.e., cafeteria, washrooms, library, gymnasium).[126] Ideas to ease the physical stress of the child's day are listed in Table 8-12.[63,126,127] Children with mild disease may simply need a slight

---

Table 8-12. Suggestions for Reduction of Physical Stress during Child's School Day

Modifications to the child's school schedule (i.e., altered course load, timetable, classroom location)
Provision of a place to lie down for a rest during lunch or recess
Opportunity to do own exercises during gym class
Environmental modifications
Permission to use the school elevator
Permission to leave each class a few minutes early to avoid hallway rush
Assignment of a classroom buddy to help with carrying books
Physical assistance by a teacher's assistant
Provision of note for classes missed
Availability of a computer for note taking in the classroom or duplicate notes
Frequent opportunities to stand/walk in classroom to counteract lower extremity stiffness
Disability awareness education for teacher/class
Provision of school transportation

Data from Spencer et al 1995,[123] Atwood 1989,[63] Szer and Wright 2000,[127] and Hemmingson and Borell 2000.[126]

modification of gym class to allow full participation in the day. Children with more severe disease may require an assistant to help them in the washroom or to assist in getting them from the school bus to class, as well as physical modifications to the school environment.[126]

The availability of personal computers has been one of the greatest sources of help to children with arthritis of the upper extremities. Use of laptop computers can relieve note-taking and essay-writing burdens, and greater availability of computers in schools may mean that the child does not even have to carry the laptop along from class to class. The only concern about extensive computer use, either for school or for recreational games, is encouragement of flexion contractures at the neck, fingers, and thumbs. It is important that therapists work with the child and teacher to develop optimal seating and positioning arrangements so that excessive neck flexion and shoulder protraction are not overly encouraged or prolonged and that joint support is adequate. The therapist also should teach the child relaxation/stretch positions that can be incorporated every 20 minutes or so into the child's keyboard use. Note that similar education should be given to the child concerning use of hand-held or desktop computer video games.

Barriers to Academic Achievement

One potential obstacle to academic achievement is the amount of time that a child with JRA misses from school due to illness or medical and therapy appointments. Decreased school attendance often creates a number of realistic fears about academic accomplishment and future career planning.[128] Wherever possible, therapy appointment times should be kept to after school hours or occur at the beginning or end of the school day. A family may have a difficult time deciding when it is appropriate to keep their child home from school (e.g., does prolonged morning stiffness necessitate a day at home?), and guidance from the health care team often is warranted. A letter from the child's rheumatologist to school personnel may clarify questions relating to participation in physical education, recess activities, and attendance at school.

Absence from school, poor health, difficulties in concentration due to pain, and low energy levels during class time cause gaps in the child's academic performance. Children having difficulty at school may benefit from psychological assessment to identify their strengths and weaknesses. The information gained then can be used to provide support to the child and guidelines for the school in establishing academic programs. One concern is that the child who is academically capable may be slotted into a lower stream at school because he or she is behind due to poor attendance. It is important that a child who might ultimately be physically restricted has the opportunity to achieve full academic potential so that career paths are not further limited.

For high school students, a lower course load may be necessary to avoid high levels of stress and anxiety that actually incapacitate the student. The team can help school personnel during a student's early high school years to assist in career planning in conjunction with realistic goal setting related to the arthritis and its prognosis.

Recreational and Extracurricular Activities

Time should be made available for the child to participate in recreational and extracurricular activities along with the peer group. Activities that are minimally affected by the physical limitations imposed by JRA such as music, art, crafts and hobbies, drama, and computer activities will give the child greater opportunities to excel. The disadvantage of these more sedentary activities that always should be kept in mind, however, is the potential negative impact on flexion contractures and on fitness and endurance levels. Health professionals can assist the family, child, and teachers identify a balance of activities that will maximize participation, enjoyment, and physical activity within the child's tolerance and schedule.

Individuals with JRA are generally encouraged to participate in all activities within their capability and tolerance. This assumes, however, that they are able to limit their own activities. It is important to encourage safe participation in sports: Lists are available outlining the most suitable and highest risk sports for children and teens with JRA.[16] Physical activities that do not provide jarring impacts on joints are ideal, e.g., swimming, bicycling, walking, Tai Chi or gentle yoga, synchronized swimming, or horseback riding. Other physical activities can be modified to allow a child with arthritis to participate, e.g., a neighborhood game of goal shooting with a hockey stick or basketball, baseball with a partner to run the bases, or a low impact (i.e., nonjumping) boxercise routine at the local community center. Depending on which joints are involved, some children with pauciarticular JRA are able to continue with skiing, skating, modified ballet lessons, or gymnastics. Physical and occupational therapists have a key role in activity analysis related to the sport that the child wants to continue to participate in or try. In this analysis the child's active and damaged joints and the possibilities for stress and injury on these joints related to rapid, forceful, unexpected, or repetitive movements associated with the activity need to be considered. For example, a child with predominantly hand and wrist involvement would not be expected to have difficulties playing soccer whereas one with knee and ankle involvement could experience joint injury and joint flare as a result of playing soccer.

A child who has had prolonged early-onset JRA with marked restriction may never be tempted to try activities beyond his or her tolerance. Activity modification will be particularly difficult for an older child with recent-onset JRA, or one who was previously extremely athletic (see Figure 8-1). The child may be willing to take the risk of temporary pain but ultimately may be immobilized by pain for several days. Children with multiple joint involvement who have been receiving oral steroids or have had periods of reduced weight bearing are at the greatest risk for bony injury such as femoral fractures as a result of physical contact or falling. Thus, the suitability of their participation in contact sports or higher-risk activities such as skiing and skating needs to be considered very carefully.

The physical and occupational therapists have a role in helping the child to better gauge his or her activity tolerance and to learn how to grade participation in demanding school and extracurricular activities. A meeting between the therapists and the school's physical education teacher often helps to dispel myths about the child's potential activity level. It also allows the setting of clear guidelines for physical activity so that the child feels supported in decisions to participate in or refrain from specific gym and recess activities. Self-management strategies should be provided to help the child manage mild stiffness and pain that occurs after some activities.

Future Research Directions

One of the issues related to the paucity of rehabilitation research in JRA is that childhood rheumatic diseases are relatively rare, and the numbers of clients in any one center are generally too small to permit conclusive results. Multicenter trials and use of a common core set of outcome measures within the long-term follow-up of children are needed. Sound research is now possible with the validated functional outcome measures that have direct relevance to the goals of rehabilitation. There also is a need for more intervention-based rather than purely correlational research as a way of looking more closely at cause and effect relationships.[106] Research questions worthy of focus relate to basic impairment, e.g., the effectiveness of interventions to increase extensibility of soft tissue

structures (perhaps in conjunction with use of intra-articular steroid injections) or impact of muscle strengthening on muscle strength and function, as well as the impact of community-based fitness programs including modified martial arts programs and Tai Chi on fitness, functional life, and quality of life.

From a team perspective, questions for further study include evaluation of psychoeducational interventions (e.g., cognitive strategies in reducing pain or the impact of education programs on self-efficacy). Research could include qualitative methodologies to explore children's perceptions of their experiences with participation in long-term physical/occupational therapy programs or their experiences in growing up with JRA.

Summary

Despite the stresses and difficulties, children with JRA and their parents generally demonstrate a positive spirit. Strong personal attributes such as determination, courage, and resilience can develop through the course of treatment. Certain characteristics may be heightened (i.e., empathy, caring, sense of humor), and adolescents with JRA often express career goals that are within the helping professions (i.e., nurse, social worker, teacher).

It is important to remember that the needs of children with JRA are extremely different from those of adults with RA. The majority of children will reach adulthood without arthritis, but the impact of the disease during childhood and any persisting contractures, joint damage, functional loss, and participation limitations will have a dramatic impact on quality of adult life. The management team must be sensitive to the particular requirements of the child and the family and respond to changes associated with both the disease and developmental process. Overall a health promotion approach should be considered to allow the children and teens more personal control over their health.[71] A strong partnership between the child, family, and the extended rheumatology team is critical if therapy goals are to be realized.[129]

Case Study

Michelle is a 13-year-old girl with JRA who lives in a rural community of 3000 people that has few health care resources. The nearest pediatric hospital is 700 miles away.

History.
- Michelle has had polyarticular arthritis since 3 years of age with a serious flare 6 months ago involving 40 joints.

She is receiving methotrexate and a nonsteroidal anti-inflammatory drug.

- Her physical condition has markedly deteriorated with reduced independence in functional abilities and sudden loss of walking abilities for distances beyond 5 feet. She is starting to use a wheelchair outside of the home. Most buildings in her community are not wheelchair accessible. Her home is also not accessible, and the family cannot afford renovations.

- Previously Michelle went to school by a 30-minute bus ride. Now she cannot climb the stairs of the bus, so her parents drive her to school. A ramp was recently built at her school to enable Michelle to get in and out of the school using her wheelchair. In the school, classroom areas are accessible, but the library and gymnasium-cafeteria can be only reached by stairs. She is isolated from her peer group in school during breaks, gym, and assemblies. She has missed 50 days of grade 8 since the flare of her arthritis and receives home tutoring for 3 hours per week.

Psychosocial Status.

- Michelle is depressed and angry about her arthritis coming back after 3 years of minimal disease.
- Her mother is overwhelmed with the added physical and emotional demands. She feels torn in several directions: she has to be with Michelle but also wants to be with her husband and Michelle's sister Renee. Both parents had difficult childhoods with significant losses and have many fears about the future. Her father worries about Michelle's future but does not like to show emotion and does not understand why Michelle is ill again. Her sister Renee is 8 years of age. She worries about Michelle but also feels jealous and sad. She is often left behind with relatives for several weeks when Michelle goes to the pediatric hospital.
- There are few community resources for therapy. The family has great difficulty in planning financially for needs. Social Services (SS) is assisting with costs of medical needs, transportation to the pediatric hospital, and extra drug costs. The family is uncomfortable asking for help. They do not initiate requests for money for food or lodging and requests to SS often are made too late to get approval for funding.

Plan, 4 Weeks after Admission to Pediatric Hospital's Rheumatology Program.

- A new medication regimen (Embril) was established. Michelle received intra-articular steroid injections under conscious sedation to her shoulders, wrists, hips, knees, and ankles to relieve synovitis and pain. A consultation with an orthopedic surgeon revealed extensive damage to Michelle's hip joints, which will probably require total hip replacements in next 5 years.
- Michelle and her mother are overwhelmed by the hospital admission. Her mother cries a lot, and Michelle takes her

anger out on her mother. Michelle's mother received counseling from a social worker to help her deal with the grief process and her feelings and gain self-confidence. She made connection with a local church as another source of emotional and spiritual support.

Progress.

- Michelle was admitted to the pediatric hospital's rehabilitation center for 3 months of intensive therapy. A social worker worked with home SS to arrange accommodation and funding for her mother to stay near the center. Her father was able to take vacation days to allow a visit at the end of the second month, and a family meeting was held to plan for discharge. One goal of the meeting was to answer her father's questions and gain his support. He admitted to having a difficult time accepting Michelle's disease and recognizing gains.

- Michelle's arthritis responded quickly to steroid injections. She attended daily group and individual pool and gym therapy, working most intensively on hip and knee mobility and strength and walking with a wheeled walker and trough crutch attachments. Her primary complaint of ankle pain when walking gradually subsided as walking endurance improved. By discharge 12 weeks later, she had only 10 active joints and a marked decrease in hip pain, her 45 degree hip flexion contractures resolved to 15 degrees, and she was walking 500 feet with trough crutches. She still tended to rely on her mother's help for dressing, but with a new sock aid and reaching device and work with the occupational therapist, she was able to dress independently when encouraged. Wrist day splints were provided, but adherence was only minimal because she is self-conscious about their appearance. She wears her resting hand splints throughout the night, so wrist and hand joints are positioned well for at least 8 hours per day. Her occupational and physical therapists called her local school and during the discussion prepared a list of mobility and accessibility ideas.

- Michelle attended the center's school and got caught up on four of her grade 8 courses. In recreation's art and drama program, she demonstrated increasing levels of confidence, self-image, and leadership abilities. The recreation staff helped her locate a teen drama club in her community.

- She attended formal and informal education sessions by nursing, occupational therapy, physical therapy, and social work staff. She was seen by the social worker for individual counseling regarding separation, adjustment to disability, dependence on others for self-care and mobility, fears, depression, family dynamics, and peer interaction. The social worker addressed upcoming issues and problem-solving and helped guide Michelle in suitable ways of assuming more personal responsibility. Michelle participated in arthritis discussion groups for the first time with several other teens with JRA who faced similar challenges.

With the help of community social services and a local community service club, funding was obtained to purchase a second-hand electric scooter for school and community mobility use.

Discharge Planning 3 Weeks Before Discharge.

- A 1-hour teleconference was held with a local school teacher and the principal and the rehabilitation center's teacher, nurse, occupational therapist, physical therapist, and social worker. Accessibility and mobility needs were reviewed, and the home school indicated that they had been able to make some of the inexpensive changes (e.g., a grab rail in washroom). The problem with stairs in the school and the bus were not yet resolved although funding was applied for to install an elevator. Because Michelle now can manage stairs with crutches, this is not an immediate problem. Michelle will walk to all class-rooms and use her scooter for longer hallway distances. She was given permission to do exercises in the school nurse's office rather than going to gym class.

- A community care nurse will visit Michelle's home twice weekly to supervise physical therapy exercises because the nearest physical therapist is 90 miles away. A physical therapy video for use at home was made at the rehabili-tation center, and a diary designed on computer was to be mailed back monthly to the physical therapist. Michelle's parents will set up a sling and pulley system over her bed to allow hip exercises daily.

- Ongoing counseling and support was arranged with a local SS agency. The rehabilitation center's social worker will call Michelle every 3 weeks to provide support and monitor progress with exercises, splint wear, medications, and walking. A local physician will monitor blood levels and current medications and send results via facsimile to the pediatric rheumatologist. Michelle will return to the pediatric rheumatology clinic in the city in 4 months and be admitted to the rehabilitation center for a 2-week "tune-up."

Skeleton Case Study

Age: 11
Gender: Male
Diagnosis: Systemic-onset JRA
Occupation: Grade 5
Onset: 18 months of age
State: Subacute
Severity: Severe
Adherence: Moderate
Pharmacological management: Reducing dose of oral prednisone, methotrexate, recent multiple joint intra-articular steroid injections
Ethnic group: Spanish

References

1. Gare BA: Juvenile arthritis—who gets it, where and when? A review of current data on incidence and prevalence. *Clin Exp Rheumatol* 17:367–374, 1999.
2. Foeldvari I, Bidde M: Validation of the proposed ILAR classification for juvenile idiopathic arthritis. *J Rheumatol* 27:1069–1072, 2000.
3. Kulas DT, Schanberg L: Juvenile idiopathic arthritis. *Curr Opin Rheumatol* 13:392–398, 2001.
4. Hull RG: Guidelines for management of childhood arthritis. *Rheumatology* (*Oxford*) 40:1309–1312, 2001.
5. Mier RJ, Wright FV, Bolding DJ: Juvenile rheumatoid arthritis. In Melvin J, Wright FV (eds): *Pediatric Rheumatic Diseases*. Bethesda, MD, American Occu-pational Therapy Association, 2000, pp 1–43.
6. Rooney M, Davies UM, Reeve J et al: Bone mineral content and bone mineral metabolism: changes after growth hormone treatment in juvenile chronic arthritis. *J Rheumatol* 27:1973–1981, 2000.
7. Klepper SE, Scull SA: Juvenile rheumatoid arthritis. In Tecklin JS (ed): *Pediatric Physical Therapy*, ed 3. Philadelphia, Lippincott Williams & Wilkins, 1999.
8. Melvin JL, Atwood M: Juvenile rheumatoid arthritis. In Melvin JL (ed): *Rheumatic Disease in Adult and Child: Occupational Therapy and Rehabilitation*, ed 3. Philadelphia, FA Davis, 1989, pp 135–187.
9. Reed MH, Wilmot D: The radiology of juvenile rheumatoid arthritis: a review of the English language literature. *J Rheumatol* 18:2–22, 1991.
10. Brewer EJ, Giannini EH: Juvenile rheumatoid arthritis. *Clin Rheum Dis* 9:629–640, 1983.
11. Petty RE: Prognosis in children with rheumatic diseases: justification for consideration of new therapies. *Rheumatology* (*Oxford*) 38:739–742, 1999.
12. Prieur AM, Chedeville G: Prognostic factors in juvenile idiopathic arthritis. *Curr Rheumatol Rep* 3:371–378, 2001.
13. Oen K, Malleson PN, Cabral DA et al: Disease course and outcome of juvenile rheumatoid arthritis in a multicenter cohort. *J Rheumatol* 29:1989–1999, 2002.
14. Zak M, Pedersen FK: Juvenile chronic arthritis into adulthood: a long-term follow-up study. *Rheumatology* (*Oxford*) 39:198–204, 2000.
15. Emery HM, Bowyer S, Sisung CE: Rehabilitation of the child with a rheumatic disease. *Pediatr Clin North Am* 42:1263–1283, 1995.
16. Scull SA: Physical therapy for the child and adolescent with juvenile rheumatoid arthritis. In Melvin J, Wright FV (eds): *Pediatric Rheumatic Diseases*. Bethesda, MD, American Occupational Therapy Association, 2000, pp 199–222.
17. Bloom BJ: New drug therapies for the pediatric rheumatic diseases. *Curr Opin Rheumatol* 13:410–414, 2001.
18. Takken T, Van Der NJ, Helders PJ: Methotrexate for treating juvenile idiopathic arthritis. *Cochrane Database System Review* CD003129, 2001.

19. Kietz DA, Pepmueller PH, Moore TL: Therapeutic use of etanercept in polyarticular course juvenile idiopathic arthritis over a two year period. *Ann Rheum Dis* 61:171–173, 2002.

20. Lovell DJ, Giannini EH, Reiff A et al: Etanercept in children with polyarticular juvenile rheumatoid arthritis. Pediatric Rheumatology Collaborative Study Group. *N Engl J Med* 342:763–769, 2000.

21. Schmeling H, Mathony K, John V et al: A combination of etanercept and methotrexate for the treatment of refractory juvenile idiopathic arthritis: a pilot study. *Ann Rheum Dis* 60:410–412, 2001.

22. Gerloni C, Cimaz R, Gattinara M et al: Efficacy and safety profile of cyclosporin A in the treatment of juvenile chronic (idiopathic) arthritis. Results of a 10-year prospective study. *Rheumatology* 40:907–913, 2001.

23. Hagen FM, Schneider R, Stephens D et al: The use of complementary and alternative medicine (CAM) by pediatric rheumatology patients. *Arthritis Rheum* 44:S276, 2001.

24. Wright V, Liu G, Milne F: Evaluation of the reliability of measurement of time-distance parameters of gait: a comparison in children with juvenile rheumatoid arthritis and children with cerebral palsy. *Physiother Can* 51:191–200, 1999.

25. Gedalia A, Person DA, Brewer EJ et al: Hypermobility of the joints in juvenile episodic arthritis/arthralgia. *J Pediatr* 107:873–876, 1985.

26. Abu-Saad HH, Uiterwijk M: Pain in children with juvenile rheumatoid arthritis: a descriptive study. *Pediatr Res* 38:194–197, 1995.

27. Savedra MC, Tesler MD, Holzemer WL et al: Pain location: validity and reliability of body outline markings by hospitalized children and adolescents. *Res Nurs Health* 12:307–314, 1989.

28. Varni JW, Thompson KL, Hanson V: The Varni/Thompson pediatric pain questionnaire. I. Chronic musculoskeletal pain in juvenile rheumatoid arthritis. *Pain* 28:27–38, 1987.

29. Wilkie DJ, Holzemer WL, Tesler MD et al: Measuring pain quality: validity and reliability of children's and adolescents' pain language. *Pain* 41:151–159, 1990.

30. Wright FV: Measurement of outcome in juvenile rheumatoid arthritis. In Melvin J, Wright FV (eds): *Pediatric Rheumatic Diseases.* Bethesda, MD, American Occupational Therapy Association, 2000, pp 231–248.

31. Duffy CM, Tucker L, Burgos-Vargas R: Update on functional assessment tools. *J Rheumatol* 27(suppl 58):11–14, 2000.

32. Tucker L: Whose life is it anyway? Understanding quality of life in children with rheumatic diseases. *J Rheumatol* 27:8–11, 2000.

33. Murray KJ, Passo MH: Functional measures in children with rheumatic diseases. *Pediatr Clin North Am* 42:1127–1154, 1995.

34. Duffy CM, Arsenault L, Watanabe et al: The Juvenile Arthritis Quality of Life Questionnaire—development of a new responsive index for juvenile rheumatoid arthritis and juvenile spondyloarthritides. *J Rheumatol* 24:738–746, 1997.

35. Howe S, Levinson J, Shear E et al: Development of a disability measurement tool for juvenile rheumatoid arthritis. The juvenile arthritis functional assessment report for children and their parents. *Arthritis Rheum* 34:873–880, 1991.

36. Landgraf J, Abetz L, Ware JE: *The CHQ User's Manual,* ed 1. Boston, Health Institute, New England Medical Center, 1996.

37. Singh G, Athreya B, Fries J et al: Measurement of health status in children with juvenile rheumatoid arthritis. *Arthritis Rheum* 37:1761–1769, 1994.

38. Tucker LB, Denardo BA, Abetz LN et al: The Childhood Arthritis Profile: validity and reliability of the condition specific scales. *Arthritis Rheum* 38:S138, 1995.

39. Wright FV, Law M, Longo Kimber J et al: The Juvenile Arthritis Functional Status Index (JASI): a validation study. *J Rheumatol* 23:1066–1079, 1996.

40. Young NL, Yoshida K, Williams JI et al: The role of children in reporting their physical disability. *Arch Phys Med Rehabil* 76:913–918, 2002.

41. Feldman BM, Brown T, Lang B et al: Sensitivity to change of functional measures for juvenile arthritis. *Arthritis Rheum* 44:S168, 2001.

42. Tennant A, Kearns S, Turner F et al: Measuring the function of children with juvenile arthritis. *Rheumatology (Oxford)* 40:1274–1278, 2001.

43. Duffy CM, Tucker L, Burgos-Vargas R: Update on functional assessment tools. *J Rheumatol* 27(suppl 58):11–14, 2000.

44. Tucker LB: Outcome measures in childhood rheumatic diseases. *Curr Rheumatol Rep* 2:349–354, 2000.

45. Ruperto N, Ravelli A, Psitorio A et al: Cross-cultural adaptation and psychometric evaluation of the Child-hood Health Assessment Questionnaire (CHAQ) and the Child Health Questionnaire (CHQ) in 32 countries. Review of the general methodology. *Clin Exp Rheumatol* 19:S1–S9, 2001.

46. Dempster H, Porepa M, Young N et al: The clinical meaning of functional outcome scores in children with juvenile arthritis. *Arthritis Rheum* 44:1768–1774, 2001.

47. Takken T, Van Der NJ, Helders PJ: Do juvenile idiopathic arthritis patients benefit from an exercise program? A pilot study. *Arthritis Rheum* 45:81–85, 2001.

48. Wessel J, Kaup C, Fan J et al: Isometric strength measurements on children with arthritis: reliability and relation to function. *Arthritis Care Res* 12:238–246, 1999.

49. Haley SM, Coster WJ, Ludlow LH: Paediatric functional outcome measures. *Phys Med Rehabil Clin North Am* 2:689–723, 1991.

50. Law M, Baptiste S, McColl M et al: The Canadian Occupational Performance Measure: an outcome measure for occupational therapy. *Can J Occup Ther* 57:82–87, 1990.

51. Ottenbacher KJ, Cusick A: Goal attainment scaling as a method of clinical evaluation. *Am J Occup Ther* 44:519–525, 1990.

52. Barlow JH, Shaw KL, Harrison K: Consulting the 'experts': children's and parents' perceptions of psycho-educational interventions in the context of juvenile chronic arthritis. *Health Educ Res* 14:597–610, 1999.

53. Sabbeth B: Understanding the impact of chronic childhood illness on families. *Pediatr Clin North Am* 31:47–69, 1984.

54. Britton C: A pilot study exploring families' experience of caring for children with chronic arthritis: views from the inside. *Br J Occup Ther* 62:534–542, 1999.

55. Quirk ME, Young MH: The impact of JRA on children, adolescents, and their families: current research and implications for future studies. *Arthritis Care Res* 3:36–43, 1990.

56. Black J, Murray-Weir M, Sanders MA: Developmental perspectives in evaluation and treatment. In Melvin J, Wright FV (eds): *Pediatric Rheumatic Diseases*. Bethesda, MD, American Occupational Therapy Association, 2000, pp 103–126.

57. Unruh AM, McGrath PJ: Pain in children: psychosocial issues. In Melvin J, Wright FV (eds): *Pediatric Rheumatic Diseases*. Bethesda, MD, American Occupational Therapy Association, 2000, pp 141–168.

58. Woodgate RL: Adolescent's perspectives of chronic illness: "It's hard." *J Pediatr Nurs* 13:210–223, 1998.

59. Kyngas H: Compliance of adolescents with chronic disease. *J Clin Nurs* 9:549–556, 2000.

60. Huygen AC, Kuis W, Sinnema G: Psychological, behavioural, and social adjustment in children and adolescents with juvenile chronic arthritis. *Ann Rheum Dis* 59:276–282, 2000.

61. von Weiss RT, Rapoff MA, Varni JW et al: Daily hassles and social support as predictors of adjustment in children with pediatric rheumatic disease. *J Pediatr Psychol* 27:155–165, 2002.

62. Allaire SH, DeNardo BS, Szer IS et al: The economic impact of juvenile rheumatoid arthritis. *J Rheumatol* 19:952–955, 1992.

63. Atwood M: Treatment considerations. In Melvin J (ed): *Rheumatic Disease in Adult and Child: Occupational Therapy and Rehabilitation,* ed 3. Philadelphia, FA Davis, 1989.

64. Degotardi PJ, Revenson TA, Ilowite NT: Family-level coping in juvenile rheumatoid arthritis: assessing the utility of a quantitative family interview. *Arthritis Care Res* 12:314–324, 1999.

65. Manuel JC: Risk and resistance factors in the adaptation in mothers of children with juvenile rheumatoid arthritis. *J Pediatr Psychol* 26:237–246, 2001.

66. Timko C, Stovel KW, Moos RH: Functioning among mothers and fathers of children with juvenile rheumatic disease: a longitudinal study. *J Pediatr Psychol* 17:705–724, 1992.

67. Frank RG, Hagglund KJ, Schopp LH et al: Disease and family contributors to adaptation in juvenile rheumatoid arthritis and juvenile diabetes. *Arthritis Care Res* 11:166–176, 1998.

68. Andre M, Hagelberg S, Stenstrom CH: Education in the management of juvenile chronic arthritis. *Scand J Rheumatol* 20:323–327, 2001.

69. King G, Stewart D, King S et al: Organizational characteristics and issues affecting the longevity of self-help groups for parents of children with special needs. *Qual Health Res* 10:225–241, 2000.

70. Cheng MM, Udry JR: Sexual behaviour of physically disabled adolescents in the United States. *J Adol Health* 31:48–58, 2002.

71. Stewart DA, Law MC, Rosenbaum P et al: A qualitative study of the transition to adulthood for youth with physical disabilities. *Phys Occup Ther Pediatr* 21:3–21, 2002.

72. Howland CA, Rintala DH: Dating behaviours of women with physical disabilities. *Sexuality Disabil* 19:41–70, 2001.

73. Ulrich G, Mattussek S, Dressler F et al: How do adolescents with juvenile chronic arthritis consider their diseases related knowledge, their unmet service needs, and the attractiveness of various services? *Eur J Med Res* 29:8–18, 2002.

74. Walter LJ, Nosek MA, Langdon K: Understanding of sexuality and reproductive health among women with and without physical disabilities. *Sexuality Disabil* 19:167–176, 2001.

75. Nash AA, Britto MT, Lovell DJ et al: Substance abuse among adolescents with juvenile rheumatoid arthritis. *Arthritis Care Res* 11:391–396, 1998.

76. Laxer RM, Clarke HM: Rheumatic disorders of the hand and wrist in childhood and adolescence. *Hand Clin* 16:659–671, 2000.

77. Libby AK, Sherry DD, Dudgeon BJ: Shoulder limitation in juvenile rheumatoid arthritis. *Arch Phys Med Rehabil* 72:382–384, 1991.

78. White PH: Growth abnormalities in children with juvenile rheumatoid arthritis. *Clin Orthop* 259:46–50, 1990.

79. Song KM, Morton AA, Koch KD et al: Chronic musculoskeletal pain in childhood. *J Pediatr Orthop* 18:576–581, 1998.

80. Schanberg LE, Lefebvre JC, Keefe FJ et al: Pain coping and the pain experience in children with juvenile chronic arthritis. *Pain* 73:181–189, 1997.

81. Rapoff MA, Lindsley CB: The pain puzzle: a visual and conceptual metaphor for understanding and treating pain in pediatric rheumatic disease. *J Rheumatol* 27(suppl 58):29–33, 2000.

82. Truckenbrodt H: Pain in juvenile chronic arthritis: consequences for the musculoskeletal system. *Clin Exp Rheumatol* 11:S59–S63, 1993.

83. Thastum M, Zachariae R, Herlin T: Pain experience and pain coping strategies in children with juvenile idiopathic arthritis. *J Rheumatol* 28:1091–1098, 2001.

84. Brown T, Delisle R, Gagno N et al: Juvenile fibromyalgia syndrome: proposed management using

a cognitive-behavioural approach. *Phys Occup Ther Pediatr* 21:19–36, 2001.

85. Perron M, Driesman D, Smith E et al: Juvenile arthritis summer camp improves knowledge, satisfaction and health status. *Arthritis Rheum* 44:S276, 2001.

86. Reid GJ, Gilbert CA, McGrath P: The Pain Coping Questionnaire: preliminary validation. *Pain* 76:83–96, 1998.

87. Andre M, Hedengren E, Hagelberg S et al: Perceived ability to manage juvenile chronic arthritis among adolescents and parents: development of a questionnaire to assess medical issues, exercise, pain, and social support. *Arthritis Care Res* 12:229–237, 1999.

88. Barlow JH, Shaw KL, Wright CC: Development and preliminary validation of a self-efficacy measure for use among parents of children with juvenile idiopathic arthritis. *Arthritis Care Res* 13:227–235, 2000.

89. Barlow JH, Shaw KL, Wright CC: Development and preliminary validation of a children's arthritis self-efficacy scale. *Arthritis Rheum* 45:159–166, 2001.

90. Kisner C, Colby LA: *Therapeutic Exercise-Foundations and Techniques*, ed 4. Philadelphia, FA Davis, 2002.

91. Nestor BJ, Figgie MP, Melvin J et al: Surgical treatment of juvenile rheumatoid arthritis. In Melvin J, Wright FV (eds): *Pediatric Rheumatic Diseases*. Bethesda, MD, American Occupational Therapy Association, 2000, pp 249–265.

92. Barrie HJ: Unexpected sites of wear in the femoral head. *J Rheumatol* 13:1099–1104, 1986.

93. Walmsley RP, Swann I: Biomechanics and physiology of muscle strengthening. *Physiother Can* 28:197–200, 1976.

94. Dumas G, Francesconi S: Aquatic therapy in pediatrics: annotated bibliography. *Phys Occup Ther Pediatr* 20:63–79, 2002.

95. Bacon MC, Nicholson C, Binder H et al: Juvenile rheumatoid arthritis: aquatic exercise and lower extremity function. *Arthritis Care Res* 4:102–105, 1991.

96. Jamison L, Ogden D: *Aquatic Therapy using PNF Patterns*. Tucson, AZ, Therapy Skill Builders, 1994.

97. De Deyne PG: Application of passive stretch and its implications for muscle fibers. *Phys Ther* 81:819–827, 2001.

98. Boyle A-M: The Bad-Ragaz ring method. *Physiotherapy* 67:265–268, 1981.

99. Etnyre BR, Abraham LK: Gains in range of ankle dorsiflexion using three popular stretching techniques. *Am J Phys Med* 65:189–196, 1986.

100. Henricson AS, Fredericksson K, Persson I et al: The effect of heat and stretching on the range of hip motion. *J Orthop Sports Phys Ther* 6:110–115, 1984.

101. Magyar E, Talerman A, Mohacsy J et al: Muscle changes in rheumatoid arthritis. *Virchows Arch [A]* 373:267–278, 1972.

102. Feland JB, Myrer JW, Schulthies SS et al: The effect of duration of stretching of the hamstring muscle group for increasing range of motion in people aged 65 years or older. *Phys Ther* 81:1100–1117, 2001.

103. Godges JJ, MacRae PG, Engelke KA: Effects of exercise on hip range of motion, trunk muscle performance, and gait economy. *Phys Ther* 73:468–477, 1993.

104. Williams PE: Use of intermittent stretch in the prevention of serial sarcomere loss in immobilised muscle. *Ann Rheum Dis* 49:316–317, 1990.

105. Bolding DJ, Sanders MA: Occupational therapy for children and adolescents with juvenile rheumatoid arthritis. In Melvin J, Wright FV (eds): *Pediatric Rheumatic Diseases*. Bethesda, MD, American Occupational Therapy Association, 2000, pp 169–198.

106. Rapoff MA: Evaluating and enhancing adherence to regimens for pediatric rheumatic diseases. In Melvin J, Wright FV (eds): *Pediatric Rheumatic Diseases*. Bethesda, MD, American Occupational Therapy Association, 2000, pp 127–140.

107. Wynn KS, Eckel EM: Juvenile rheumatoid arthritis and home physical therapy program compliance. *Phys Occup Ther Pediatr* 6:55–63, 1986.

108. Hedengren E, Knutson LM, Haglund-Akerlind Y et al: Lower extremity isometric joint torque in children with juvenile chronic arthritis. *Scand J Rheumatol* 30:69–76, 2001.

109. Lindehammar H, Sandstedt P: Measurement of quadriceps strength and bulk in juvenile chronic arthritis. A prospective, longitudinal 2 year survey. *J Rheumatol* 25:2240–2248, 1998.

110. Giannini JM, Protas EJ: Comparison of peak isometric knee extensor torque in children with and without juvenile rheumatoid arthritis. *Arthritis Care Res* 6:82–88, 1993.

111. Oberg T, Karsznia A, Gare BA et al: Physical training of children with juvenile chronic arthritis. Effects of force, endurance and EMG response to localized muscle fatigue. *Scand J Rheumatol* 23:92–95, 1994.

112. McDonagh JE: Osteoporosis in juvenile idiopathic arthritis. *Curr Opin Rheumatol* 13:399–404, 2001.

113. Klepper SE: Effects of an eight-week physical conditioning program on disease signs and symptoms in children with chronic arthritis. *Arthritis Care Res* 12:52–60, 1999.

114. Wright V, Raman S, Bar-OR O et al: An evaluation of the feasibility of fitness training for children with juvenile rheumatoid arthritis. *Arthritis Rheum* 43:S169, 2000.

115. Feldman BM, Wright FV, Bar-OR O et al: Rigorous fitness training and testing for children with polyarticular arthritis. *Arthritis Rheum* 43:S120, 2000.

116. Rabinovich CE: Bone mineral status in juvenile rheumatoid arthritis. *J Rheumatol* 27(suppl 58):34–37, 2000.

117. Chan WW, Bartlett DJ: Effectiveness of Tai Chi as a therapeutic exercise in improving balance and postural control. *Phys Occup Ther Geriatr* 17:1–22, 2000.

118. Taylor L, Adelman HS, Kaser-Boyd N: Perspectives of children regarding their psychoeducational decisions. *Prof Psychol Res Prac* 14:882–894, 1983.

119. Petr CG: Adultcentrism in practice with children. *Fam Soc* 73:408–416, 1992.

120. Lemanek KL, Kamps J, Chung NB: Empirically supported treatments in pediatric psychology: regimen adherence. *J Pediatr Psychol* 26:253–275, 2001.

121. Mayo NE: Patient compliance: practical implications for physical therapists—a review of the literature. *Phys Ther* 58:1083–1090, 1978.

122. Berry SL, Hayfors JR, Ross CK et al: Conceptions of illness by children with juvenile rheumatoid arthritis: a cognitive developmental approach. *J Pediatr Psychol* 18:83–97, 1993.

123. Spencer CH, Fife RZ, Rabinovich CE: The school experience of children with arthritis. *Pediatr Clin North Am* 42:1285–1298, 1995.

124. Atwood M: Developmental assessment and integration. In: Melvin J (ed): *Rheumatic Disease in Adult and Child: Occupational Therapy and Rehabilitation,* ed 3. Philadelphia, FA Davis, 1989, pp 188–214.

125. Mancini MC, Coster WJ, Trombly CA et al: Predicting elementary school participation in children with disabilities. *Arch Phys Med Rehabil* 81:339–347, 2000.

126. Hemmingson H, Borell L: Accommodation needs and student-environment fit in upper secondary schools for students with severe physical disabilities. *Can J Occup Ther* 67:162–172, 2000.

127. Szer IS, Wright FV: School integration. In Melvin J, Wright FV (eds): *Pediatric Rheumatic Diseases.* Bethesda, MD, American Occupational Therapy Association, 2000, pp 223–230.

128. Whitehouse R, Shope JT, Sullivan DB et al: Children with juvenile arthritis at school-functional problems, participation in physical education. *Clin Pediatr* 28:509–514, 1989.

129. Hanna K, Rodger S: Towards family-centred practice in paediatric occupational therapy: a review of the literature on parent-therapist collaboration. *Austr Occup Ther J* 49:14–24, 2002.

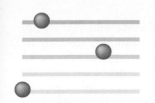

CHAPTER 9

Management of Persons with Rheumatoid Arthritis and Other Inflammatory Conditions

Antoine Helewa, MSc(Clin Epid), PT

Rheumatoid arthritis (RA) and other related syndromes are characterized by inflammation of the synovium and connective tissues of diarthrodial joints and, to a lesser extent, the related tissues—tendons and their sheaths and bursal and periarticular subcutaneous tissues. The systemic and extra-articular manifestations suggest use of the term *rheumatoid disease*; however, these manifestations are less frequent and severe than lesions in the joints.[1]

The joint inflammation of RA is, with minor variation, similar in its effects to that found in other

inflammatory arthritis syndromes, such as juvenile idiopathic arthritis (JIA), ankylosing spondylitis (AS), Reiter's syndrome, and psoriatic arthritis. Whereas systemic disease manifestations are the chief problem in systemic lupus erythematosus (SLE), the features of joint inflammation, although seen less often, are similar to those of RA.

The management of persons with JIA and AS is covered extensively in Chapters 8 and 10. This chapter will focus primarily on the management of persons with RA, and because the joint inflammation in RA shares common features with that of Reiter's syndrome, psoriatic arthritis, and SLE, by extension, the management of these conditions also will be covered. Distinctions in the management of conditions other than RA, where they exist, will be noted.

PHYSICAL REHABILITATION IN ARTHRITIS, Joan M. Walker, PhD, PT, and Antoine Helewa, MSc(Clin Epid), PT, Elsevier Inc. © 2004.

The chapter will begin with a description of the elements in the management of inflammatory joint disease, followed by management objectives. Aspects of management then will be discussed under the following broad strategies: analgesic modalities, rest and activity, therapeutic exercise, restoration of function, pre and postsurgical management, goal setting and contracting.

The chapter will conclude with a list of research questions important to physical management, one case study, and a skeleton case study template as an educational tool.

Elements of Physical Management

Physical therapy (PT) and occupational therapy (OT) are essential physical treatment strategies for clients with RA and other inflammatory arthritic syndromes. Any client with inflammatory joint disease must receive therapy at one time or another regardless of disease stage and severity, but preferably in the early stages of the disease. Because early medical diagnosis is frequently difficult to reach, clients often are referred to therapy after joint manifestations and problems with physical function have become established. There also is a misconception that therapy can do little for these clients in the early stages of the disease or when the inflammation is raging; thus, important early treatment strategies designed specifically to reduce impairment and disability are ignored.

It is preferable that clients with inflammatory joint disease receive therapy in the early stages of the disease. Exposure of clients with RA to PT and OT as health disciplines is important rather than isolated exposure to any of their individual modalities. The best results are achieved when therapy is delivered as a package, custom tailored to the client's needs and encompassing elements of disease education, counseling, assessment, treatment, and independence in activities of daily living (ADL). Three basic elements form the core of PT and OT practice for clients with RA:

- To help nature restore normal physical function, such as the application of therapeutic exercise to restore muscle strength
- To ensure that the body's own healing processes do not become a source of the difficulty (e.g., scarring, contracture, pannus, degenerative changes)
- To apply strategies that will prevent further deterioration of function in a chronic, unrelenting lifelong disease

Therapy techniques are seldom applied singly but rather in combination. For example, therapeutic exercise could be preceded by the application of cold packs to antagonistic muscle groups to enhance the response of the agonists. Disease education and its impact on dysfunction would precede training in joint protection and energy conservation where appropriate. If joint inflammation is uncontrolled, therapy should be applied in association with some medical therapies, such as anti-inflammatory medications, disease modifying medications, analgesic medications, or surgery.

Management Objectives

To achieve success, management of clients with RA must be accompanied by an accurate diagnosis; quantitative assessment of disease activity, impairment, and function; effective anti-inflammatory therapy; and in the presence of joint deformities and destruction, judicious use of rheumatoid surgery. The features and diagnosis of RA are covered extensively in Chapters 3 and 4. Assessment strategies are discussed in detail in Chapter 5, surgical interventions are addressed in Chapter 6. Figure 9-1 illustrates the essential components of RA management, highlighting the relative roles of medical and rehabilitative strategies and demonstrating how they are intertwined.

Generally, the objectives of PT and OT in the management of clients with RA are to do the following:

- Control pain
- Increase and maintain joint mobility and muscle strength
- Maintain cardiopulmonary fitness
- Protect joints, conserve energy, and preserve function
- Educate clients and their caregivers about disease processes and its self-management

To accomplish these objectives, physical and occupational therapists use a variety of treatment techniques. Central to all these techniques is the judicious application of therapeutic exercise and other rehabilitation strategies to restore optimal function, tailored to the client's needs. Most other techniques are primarily adjuncts to these and may include the application of heat, cold, and electrical muscle stimulation.[2] Table 9-1 provides a summary of the techniques commonly used in the treatment of clients with RA, listed by objective and physiological effects sought. Table 9-2 outlines general principles to follow when a therapist plans a treatment program.

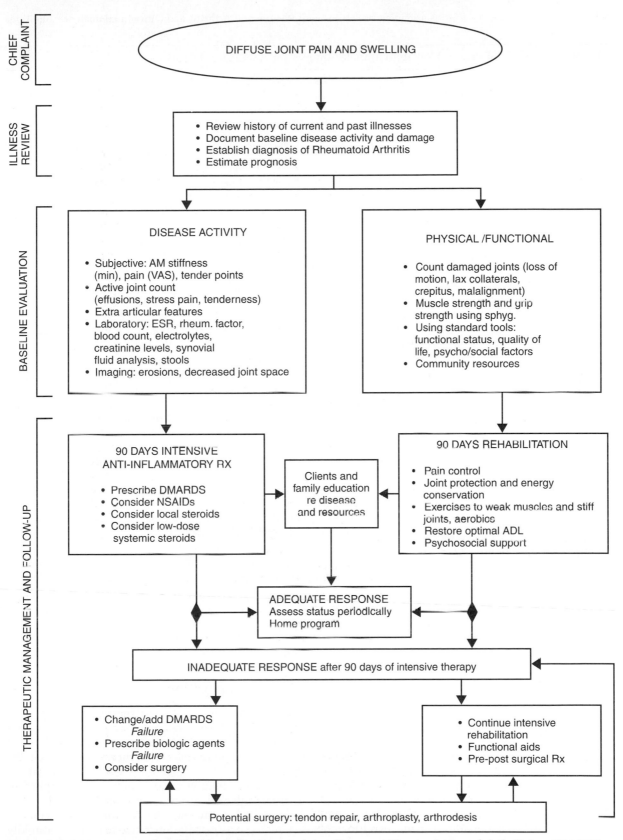

Figure 9-1. Management algorithm for inflammatory joint disease. ADL = activities of daily living; DMARDs = disease-modifying antirheumatic drugs; ESR = erythrocyte sedimentation rate; NSAIDs = nonsteroidal anti-inflammatory drugs; VAS = visual analogue scale.

Table 9-1. Summary of Physical Rehabilitation Techniques for Rheumatoid Arthritis

Modality	Effects	Objective	Comments
Analgesics			
Cold	Inhibits nerve conduction	Controls pain and muscle spasm	Best for active joints*
			Applied to muscles in spasm (flexors)
Heat	Increases nerve conduction	Controls pain and muscle spasm	Best for chronic joints
			Applied to muscles in spasm (flexors)
TENS	Inhibits nerve conduction	Controls pain	Limited to one or two sites
Facilitatory			
Electrical muscle stimulation or ice massage	Facilitatory	Preserves or restores muscle strength	Precedes strengthening exercises
Therapeutic exercise			
Mobilizing	Elasticity of joint and soft tissue structures	Preserves or restores joint range	Active joint: exercise to pain tolerance
Strengthening (isometric/isotonic)	Facilitatory	Preserves or restores muscle strength	Active joint: submaximal isometric
Conditioning (aerobic)	Muscle endurance, cardiopulmonary fitness	Preserves or restores physical fitness	Low-impact or water aerobics
Joint protection and energy conservation	Diminish joint stress	Protect joints and enhance ADL	Encourage adherence

Adapted from Helewa A, Smythe HA: Physical therapy in rheumatoid arthritis. In Wolfe F, Pincus T (eds): *Rheumatoid Arthritis. Pathogenesis, Assessment, Outcome and Treatment.* New York, Marcel Dekker, 1994, pp 415–433.
*Exercise should not be applied to joints anesthetized by cold.
ADL = activities of daily living; TENS = transcutaneous electrical nerve stimulation.

Analgesic Physical Therapy

Analgesic PT modalities alone are not effective in the management of the acutely inflamed joints of uncontrolled RA. When applied with determined anti-inflammatory therapy clients will obtain relief of pain due to raging disease. In general, pain-relieving PT modalities offer short-term relief of pain lasting 1 or 2 hours, serving to warm-up muscles or to relieve muscle tightness and spasm in preparation for therapeutic exercise or certain activities of daily living. Given alone, they serve a very limited purpose and raise unduly a client's hopes of obtaining the sought after, long-lasting relief of chronic pain. Two forms of analgesic PT are commonly used: thermal applications and electrical stimulation.

Thermal Applications

The two commonly applied thermal techniques in clients with RA (and by consensus the most sensible) are the application of simple hot or cold packs. Several known therapeutic effects of thermotherapy for RA patients are effects on pain, muscle spasm, circulation, and inflammation. Heat, in general, when applied to actively inflamed joints ("active joint") in RA, has been known to increase nerve conduction. Thus, it can increase pain sensation in active joints. For mildly

Table 9-2. General Principles in Physical Rehabilitation of Rheumatoid Arthritis

1. Treatment plans must be based on an accurate diagnosis and assessment of disease activity and dysfunction.
2. The selection of treatment techniques and dosage specifications must be supported by scientific evidence. If this evidence is unavailable, then the treatment and dosage should make biological sense. Careful assessment and periodic review of treatment results are essential.
3. Treatment techniques should be brief and simple to apply (preferably by the client) and should be adapted for home use.
4. Treatment techniques should be pain free and safe. If joint swelling or pain lasts 2 hours or more after treatment, the therapy should be reviewed or its intensity reduced.
5. Therapeutic exercise has many objectives and is central to PT management; all other techniques are largely treatment adjuncts to treatment.
6. In addition to principles 3 and 4, strategies to improve client adherence should be based on client instruction about the disease and its treatment.
7. Splints, orthotics and assistive devices, and modifications to home/work environment are client specific and enhance overall rehabilitation and disease management.
8. Alleviation of financial stress and provision of home help, play an important role in the client's ability to adhere to therapy and self-manage their disease.

Adapted from Helewa A, Smythe HA: Physical therapy in rheumatoid arthritis. In Wolfe F, Pincus T (eds): *Rheumatoid Arthritis. Pathogenesis, Assessment, Outcome and Treatment.* New York, Marcel Dekker, 1994, pp 415–433.

inflamed joints, moist heat has the advantage of relieving stiffness or the "gel phenomenon."

Cold, on the other hand, has opposite physiological effects, and therefore can be beneficial for intensely inflamed joints. Cold relieves pain by counterirritant effects and endorphin release.[3] Other known effects of cold include reduction of edema formation and joint swelling. The anti-inflammatory effects of cold are mediated through vasoconstriction, which reduces hyperemia, as well as direct effects on abnormal metabolic processes by reduction of the activity of collagenase in the inflammatory reaction.[4,5] Cold also reduces muscle spasm by decreasing the conductivity of the muscle spindles; the stimulus threshold for firing is raised, thus decreasing the afferent firing rate.[3,6]

In contrast, the application of ice cubes, using a few short strokes over a muscle belly, can stimulate muscle response by facilitating α motoneuron discharge.[7] This facilitatory response is very effective when it is applied to muscles inhibited by joint pain or swelling.

In clients with inflamed joints, hot or cold applications are not interchangeable because they have opposite physiological effects. In a randomized, controlled trial (RCT) of clients with RA (30 active knee joints in all), 15 were allocated at random to a control group and 15 to an ice treatment group. All clients rested in bed for 1 week to stabilize their condition before the trial, and both groups received therapeutic exercise during the experimental period. After 5 days of therapy, there was no difference between the groups in joint circumference or thermographic measurement of skin temperature. The small sample size and the possibility of a type II error may have contributed to these results.[8] In another randomized trial of 18 clients with RA and with shoulder pain no difference was seen between results from use of hot or cold packs. But, again the sample size was inadequate.[9]

At first glance these studies suggest that hot or cold applications are interchangeable and that client choice should determine the application of one technique or another. However, a closer analysis showed that the three studies were fraught with methodological problems, such as the lack of a control group in one and small sample sizes in the other two.

A recent systematic review of 7 RCTs (out of a total of 306 potential studies) that met the review's criteria showed that 5 of 7 studies demonstrated that hot or ice applications had no significant effects on objective measures of disease activity, including joint swelling, pain, medication intake, range of motion (ROM), grip strength or hand function compared with effects in control subjects who received no treatment or those receiving alternate treatment.[10] The reviewers concluded that thermotherapy produced neither positive nor detrimental effects on important outcomes or on joint destruction in RA. Based on current information, thermotherapy can be used as a palliative treatment or as an adjunct to therapeutic exercise in clients with RA. These conclusions are limited by the poor methodological quality of these trials and the large number of borderline values. Further, the question of the interchangeability of hot or cold modalities in RA has not been addressed properly in RCTs.

Paraffin Wax

Another form of heat applied to the hands of clients with RA is melted paraffin wax baths (PWBs) heated to 48° C. A systematic review of PWB therapy analyzed the results of four controlled trials with 303 randomly assigned participants. One of these trials was excluded because it gave equivocal results; the remaining three trials reported that 3 to 4 weeks of PWB applications were accompanied by significant improvements in hand function in clients with RA when followed by exercise.[11]

A second systematic review of thermotherapy identified two RCTs.[10] One trial that compared the combination of PWBs and exercise with exercise alone showed statistically significant results for PWBs and exercise on ROM, pain on nonresisted motion, and grip and pinch function; however, there was no effect on grip strength.[12] In the second RCT, which compared the effects of PWBs, faradic baths, and ultrasound (US) to the hands, no statistically significant differences were seen among the modalities for their effects on hand strength, ROM, joint circumference, or functional status.[13] The reviewers concluded that PWBs and exercise can be recommended for beneficial short-term effects on hands in RA; however the conclusions of both reviews are limited by methodological considerations due to major flaws identified in the review process.[11]

Because the most useful effect of a PWB is relief of morning stiffness due to the gel phenomenon, it should be applied by clients in their own homes. However, applications of wax at home are cumbersome and fraught with danger, and unless the wax is heated in a double boiler, it can cause a fire. A simple, safer alternative is to apply mineral oil to the hands, wear rubber dish-washing gloves, and soak hands in hot water from the tap for 5 to 10 minutes (also see Chapter 16).

Short-Wave Diathermy and Microwave

These two modalities were used often in the past for their purported deep heating effects. In an RCT of 131 clients with RA and osteoarthritis (OA), no differences were seen in ROM, walking, and stair climbing time among clients who received exercise and one other modality either shortwave diathermy (SWD), sham SWD, or infrared and electrical muscle stimulation. The improvement seen in all clients was probably the result of the treatments received, plus the encouragement obtained.[14] Another study showed that by raising intra-articular temperature by 2.4° C, SWD can potentially cause harm.[15] There are no reported studies of the effects of microwave therapy on clients with RA.

SWD and microwave devices are very expensive (>$10,000 per unit), and are not economically viable when we consider the alternatives. Further, SWD is likely to aggravate joint pain[15] and slow healing skin burns may result if SWD is not applied carefully. There is consensus that by far hot packs are safer, cheaper, and as effective as SWD or microwave therapy delivered via devices with flashing lights designed to impress clients and therapists. Furthermore, the unwieldy bulk of these devices and their costs mean their use by clients at home is impractical.

Ultrasound

US is rarely used as an adjunct to therapeutic exercise in the management of RA. Through stable cavitation (the vibrational effect on gas bubbles by an US beam), pulsed or continuous US results in diffusional changes along cell membranes and, thus, alters cell function.[16] Stable cavitation also reduces nerve conduction velocity in pain afferent fibers, thereby decreasing transmission of pain sensations. Continuous US also can increase tissue temperature, an effect similar to that seen with other forms of thermotherapy.

A recent systematic review of the efficacy of US in the management of RA identified eight potential articles.[16] Of these, only 2 RCTs involving 80 patients with RA met the review criteria. In the first study,[17] the authors compared three groups: exercises and PWBs, exercises with US, and exercises with US and faradic hand baths. There were no statistically significant differences among the three groups for pain score, grip strength, proximal interphalangeal joint circumference, articular index, ROM, or level of activity. In the second study,[18] US was compared with the hand in water with placebo US. A statistically significant increase in grip strength was found in the US group compared with the placebo US group and to a lesser extent borderline values were seen in the US group for wrist dorsiflexion, duration of morning stiffness, number of swollen joints, and number of painful joints.

The reviewers concluded that the use of US in combination with other modalities is not supported and cannot be recommended, but US alone can be used for its therapeutic effects as an adjunct to therapeutic exercise.[16]

Applying Thermal Packs

On balance, the simple application of hot or cold packs is the most appropriate form of thermal modality in the treatment of RA. Hot or cold packs are usually applied for 15 to 20 minutes with the material wrapped in a damp towel to permit even conduction of thermal energy. Ice should never be applied directly to the skin (ice massage is an exception), nor should the weight of a limb or torso rest on the pack, because this may burn the cold, anesthetized skin.[2] In a clinical setting, crushed ice can be obtained from special ice-making machines. In the home it can be obtained in the form of ice cubes, crushed ice, or a pack of frozen peas, depending on availability. The crushed ice is usually placed longitudinally in the middle one third of a regular damp bath towel forming a rectangle of about 18 × 8 inches, depending on the part to be cooled. The towel is then folded longitudinally, at which point the crushed ice will adhere to the damp towel, preventing its escape. The ends of the towel free from ice are held tightly in a knot with rubber bands to prevent escape from either end. The pack is then applied to the skin overlying the area to be cooled, leaving one layer of toweling between the crushed ice and the skin surface. Other forms of cooling body surfaces that are commercially available are local sprays and cryowraps.[19]

> Ice, with the exception of ice massage, should never be applied directly to the skin.

Cold Therapy Protocols

There are two commonly used cold treatment protocols in RA, illustrated by the following examples. The first involves the treatment of a knee with moderate synovitis, tightness of the knee flexors, and quadriceps muscle atrophy. Treatment begins with a cold pack application to the skin overlying all knee flexors (hamstrings, popliteus, gastrocnemius) for 15 to 20 minutes. This will decrease muscle spasm by reducing muscle spindle activity. This is followed with ice massage, given in short strokes for 1 minute, to the skin overlying the quadriceps muscles to stimulate muscle response by facilitating α motoneuron discharge in muscles inhibited by pain and swelling. This sets the stage for the application of specific therapeutic exercise techniques to enhance this effect, such as hold relax, slow reversals, or slow isometric reversals.

The second protocol involves the management of a severely inflamed knee joint, held in about 30 degrees of flexion (the loose-packed position preferred for the knee with excess synovial fluid). Cold is applied on the skin surfaces surrounding the knee joint, reaching proximally to the upper end of the suprapatellar pouch and distally below the tibial tubercle. Cold over a joint surface increases the pain threshold by directly reducing the activity of pain-conducting fibers and receptors and by supplying competitive sensations, as suggested by the gate-control theory.

Cold also reduces inflammation by decreasing the activity of collagenase in the inflammatory reaction. Because this may result in cold anesthesia, immediate rigorous isotonic exercise to already inflamed and distended ligamentous structures may result in a competing inflammatory response and lead to further pain and ligamentous laxity. Ideally, gentle slow isometric reversals should be applied, followed by one or two free active movements in the pain-free range.

Cold should not be used in clients with Raynaud's phenomenon, cold hypersensitivity, cryoglobulinemia (presence in blood of a protein that forms gels at low temperatures), or paroxysmal cold hemoglobinuria (the presence of hemoglobin in the urine after local or general exposure to cold). Cold also should be avoided if it is uncomfortable to the client.[20]

A practical homemade hot pack can be made by placing a wet facecloth or small towel in a plastic freezer bag that then can be heated in a microwave oven for 1 minute. The heated pack is then wrapped in a damp towel and applied to the affected area for 15 to 20 minutes. Hot packs should not be applied to inflamed joints, because the heat may potentially cause harm by increasing the intra-articular temperature of a joint.[5,15] Localized heat also may be hazardous in conditions involving impaired arterial circulation, impaired sensation, local hemorrhage, malignancy, or inflammation.[21]

Electrical Stimulation

Analgesic electrical stimulation plays a limited role in the management of clients with RA but can be useful in the treatment of intractable regional pain. The two modalities in common use are transcutaneous electrical nerve stimulation (TENS) and interferential currents. Electrical muscle stimulation (EMS) also has been used to enhance performance in muscles inhibited by pain and swelling.

Transcutaneous Electrical Nerve Stimulation

Application of TENS results in release of endorphins in the spinal cord due to increased stimulation of large myelinated nerve fibers, which tend to override the nociceptive inputs from unmyelinated C and small myelinated delta (δ) fibers.[22,23] Altogether, 25 randomized trials of TENS have been published; of these, only 2 involved clients with RA. The first was a double-blind study involving 32 subjects allocated to receive active TENS and placebo TENS to the wrist, whose pain was stabilized with "anti-inflammatory analgesics."[24] Resting pain and gripping pain were measured with a visual analogue scale. The experimental group had a statistically significant reduction in both resting and gripping pain; however, the observation period lasted only 3 weeks, and clients were not followed-up longer. Also, sample size estimates were not given. The second trial also was double blind and involved 33 clients allocated to receive TENS and placebo TENS. No statistically significant differences were seen between the two groups. Sample size calculations were not performed.[25]

Results of the remaining 23 studies of clients without RA also conflict, with about one half showing that TENS is not better than placebo.[4] In view of this, TENS continues to be a controversial modality and its effects on clients with RA must be investigated more rigorously.

Portable TENS devices lend themselves well for home use and application by the client. To determine response to TENS, three trials are first attempted—one at rest, another during walking, and a third during normal manual activities. The pain visual analogue scale is used to determine responses under these conditions. TENS is usually applied for a period of 30 to 45 minutes. Criteria for success are 3 hours of pain relief, improved sleep, and reduced intake of pain medications.

Interferential Currents

Interferential currents are a special modification of middle-frequency currents (>1000 Hz), that tend to avoid the sensory disadvantage of lower-frequency currents such as TENS (80 to 120 Hz) by passing through the skin without being felt.[4] Interferential currents are impractical for clients with RA with multiple joint involvement, and the high cost of devices to deliver these currents (>$10,000) diminishes their importance as a therapeutic choice. More importantly, there are no randomized clinical trials assessing treatment efficacy in clients with RA. Results of an unpublished randomized trial of the efficacy of interferential current in clients with OA of the knee showed no difference between active and placebo therapy.[26]

> **The effects of TENS on clients with RA requires further investigation.**

Electrical Muscle Stimulation

EMS is usually applied to the motor point of a muscle and is used to recruit motor units that are inactive due to reflex inhibition, a consequence of joint pain and swelling in RA. This produces the higher-intensity muscle contractions that are required to effectively increase muscle strength.

A systematic review of the effects of EMS on patients with RA identified two RCTs, and only one met the study criteria.[27] This study was double blind with 15 patients with RA assigned at random to an active EMS group or a no-treatment control group. The first dorsal interosseus muscle of the hand was targeted to receive 168 hours of EMS in 70 separate sessions over a 10-week period.[28] With use of a patterned EMS signal statistically significant improvements were seen for all seven outcome variables related to specific hand functions. The other RCT was excluded from the review because of major methodological flaws.[29]

Effects of Systemic Rest

The systemic manifestations of RA, reflected by fever, weight loss, anemia, and visceral involvement, suggest that an acute episode may be rapidly relieved by a period of physical bed rest. Total bed rest is rarely advisable, because it can lead to deconditioning. Some clients also have expressed fears of becoming crippled if confined to bed. Younger clients also fear that prolonged bed rest may threaten income and job security.[30] On the other hand, hyperactive clients and those with stressful lifestyles who have systemic disease and multiple joint involvement can benefit from a short period of complete bed rest. The value of rest has been attributed to a slowing down of metabolic demand during joint use, which may reduce the level of microinfarctions of synovial villi, the source of rice bodies found in severely involved joints.[31] The prohibitive cost of hospitalization to clients, government, and third-party payers makes total bed rest unattractive in today's climate of cost constraints. Two RCTs comparing total bed rest with activity showed no significant overall anti-inflammatory effect in the bed rest groups, and the other benefits shown were marginal.[30–32] This is not to be confused with hospitalization for RA: inpatient therapy was shown to be superior to intensive outpatient therapy.[33]

Because RA can put a tremendous strain on both physical and emotional resources, bed rest for 1 to 2 hours once or twice daily may prevent fatigue and improve recuperation.[30,34] The benefits of resting specific joints using resting splints made of a variety of materials and in different shapes are discussed in Chapter 14.

> In today's climate of cost constraints imposed by governments and other health insurers, total in-hospital bed rest is unattractive because of its prohibitive cost.

Therapeutic Exercises

Muscle wasting is a common feature of clients with RA and is not due to disuse alone. The leading causes of muscle atrophy are deposition of inflammatory cells in the muscles of clients with RA (myositis); inflammation of the endothelial layer of blood vessels supplying muscle spindles, muscle fibers, and nerves of skeletal muscles (vasculitis); deposition of inflammatory cells in peripheral nerves leading to demyelination (neuropathy); reflex inhibition induced by pain and swelling; and finally disuse atrophy. Movement loss and immobility also may lead to fixed contractures of periarticular and intra-articular soft tissue structures through shortening of collagen, which also may cause loss of articular cartilage.

For a therapeutic exercise program to succeed, the factors leading to atrophy of muscle fibers, listed in the preceding paragraph, must be eliminated first. Hence, anti-inflammatory therapy in any form is at the core of exercise management. Therapeutic exercise for clients with RA serves many purposes, and usually only one purpose is achieved optimally by any specific exercise.[35] For example, exercises to increase ROM cannot be substituted for exercises designed to strengthen muscles, and these in turn are not a substitute for endurance or conditioning exercises.

> Anti-inflammatory therapy is at the basis of exercise management. Causes of muscle atrophy first must be controlled.

The main objectives of therapeutic exercises are to do the following:

- Preserve motion or restore lost motion
- Increase muscle strength, and increase endurance
- Provide cardiovascular conditioning
- Increase bone density
- Enhance a feeling of well-being
- Provide active recreation

For clients with controlled disease but residual impairment, exercise is by far the most important aspect of their therapy; however, exercise must be given at all stages of RA and should be tailored to suit the client's disease state.[2]

To date, there is strong evidence that clients with inflammatory arthritis will benefit from regular supervised exercise without aggravation of their joint symptoms.[36–43] Clients with RA also can increase their muscle strength with isometric exercise.[44] Other investigators have demonstrated that clients with RA can increase both type 1 and type 2 muscle fiber size, as well as their strength and aerobic capacity, after performing endurance training on treadmills or bicycles. This also correlated with improvements in activities of daily living.[36,39,40,45] These findings were supported by later studies using similar design and treatment maneuvers.[38,46,47] The intense but recent drive to prescribe aerobic exercise for endurance training must be tempered by other sobering effects of exercise. Excessive use of limbs affected by erosive arthritis affects the degree of joint destruction. Indeed, it has been shown that loss of limb use due to paralysis appears to confer on clients some sparing of disease effects.[48] This leaves unanswered the question whether the ameliorating effect of a unilateral neurological lesion is simply a lack-of-use phenomenon or whether the presence of fully functioning nerves is necessary for the development of arthritis.[49]

A recent systematic review was conducted to assess the effects of dynamic exercise therapy in improving ROM, muscle strength, aerobic capacity, and daily functioning in clients with RA.[50] Of 30 identified RCTs, only 6 met the review's criteria. As a result of heterogeneity of outcome measures, data could not be pooled. The results suggested that dynamic exercise therapy is effective for increasing aerobic capacity and muscle strength. The effects of exercise therapy on ADL and progression of changes on radiographs are unclear. No detrimental effects of exercise on disease activity or pain were observed.[50] Two recent RCTs not included in the above review showed significant benefits. The first study demonstrated that an intensive exercise program in clients with active RA is more effective in improving physical function and muscle strength than a conservative exercise program and did not have deleterious effects on disease activity.[51] The second RCT showed that in the short term clients with RA who received exercise therapy combined with thermal modalities to the hands had statistically significant improvement in hand pain, joint tenderness, ADL score, and ROM. All objective measures used in the study deteriorated in the no-treatment control group.[52]

For RA, four types of exercise by objective exist:

- Active mobilizing exercise to maintain or restore joint movement and the flexibility of soft tissue structures
- Strengthening exercise to maintain or restore muscle strength
- Conditioning exercise to maintain or restore endurance and aerobic capacity
- Passive techniques of joint mobilization

Mobilizing Exercise

The objectives of mobilizing exercises are to increase joint mobility and therefore relieve joint stiffness and to enhance the flexibility of soft tissue structures that may be compromised by immobility, abnormal posture, or pathological changes triggered by the inflammatory process.

Before embarking on a mobilizing regimen, a thermal modality should be applied to improve connective tissue flexibility in targeted structures. Cold is the modality of choice for actively inflamed as well as chronically inflamed joints, and moist heat may be used for stiff and damaged joints that are not actively inflamed. However, the typical client with RA may require mobilization of multiple joints, for which the local application of cold or hot packs may be inefficient. In these clients, a localized cold immersion bath for limbs, a warm shower, or a swim in a warm pool may be preferable. Some of the mobilizing exercises prescribed can be carried out in the shower or a pool heated to 85° F (29° C).

Mobilizing Techniques

Actively inflamed joints should be moved gently through the possible range by the client or with assistance from another person, following instruction by a physical therapist. Three repetitions for each joint, once or twice daily, are recommended. Because of the possibility of pain and ligamentous stretching, the limbs should be handled with extreme care. As joint inflammation subsides, the joints should continue to be moved as above, but through the full range, possibly with assistance at the end of the range, to ensure that shortened joint structures and tendons are fully stretched. Special proprioceptive neuromuscular facilitation (PNF) techniques could be applied early on for selected muscle groups, moderated by the extent and severity of the inflammation.[53] Because these involve the use of manual resistance to muscle contraction, the amount of resistance can be varied according to the client's tolerance and joint inflammation status. In clients with joint laxity, these techniques should be applied with caution. Two techniques are in common use for actively inflamed and painful joints: hold-relax and slow reversal-hold-relax.

> **Special PNF techniques should be applied with caution and moderated by the extent and severity of the inflammation.**

Hold-relax involves applying moderate manual resistance to an isometric contraction. Because no joint motion is involved, this is the technique of choice to achieve relaxation when muscle spasm is accompanied by pain.[53] For example, in a client with RA and tightness of knee flexors limiting extension range, the part may be taken passively to the limit of extension; at that point the operator applies slowly moderate manual resistance to the knee flexors, by instructing the client to hold that position, allowing no movement. The operator then instructs the client to relax the knee flexors. As tension is released, the part may be taken passively into extension to the limit of the range or limit of pain. The process is repeated again for a number of times to client tolerance, with each repetition gaining further extension. The underlying principle in hold-relax is that an isometric contraction of the flexors is followed by flexor inhibition and extensor facilitation due to the Golgi tendon organ effect.[53]

Slow reversal-hold-relax using the above example involves an isotonic contraction of knee extensors, followed *without relaxation* by an isometric contraction of the knee flexors, followed by voluntary relaxation of the flexors, and then by isotonic contraction of the extensors that moves the joint to a few more degrees of extension. Again, the maneuver is repeated several times to client tolerance. Maximal isometric resistance to the flexors is applied to their rotation component to achieve maximal voluntary relaxation and facilitation of the extensor muscle group. Because this technique involves more vigorous isotonic and isometric muscle contractions, it would be more suitable for clients whose joint inflammation is controlled but who are left with residual muscle tightness. The techniques *should not be used* on clients with joint pain or joint laxity.

Physical therapists with knowledge of PNF movement patterns should apply these techniques to selective muscle groups in their respective diagonal spiral patterns. A sensation of full muscle stretch accompanies these techniques, but their application should be pain free. Pain after their application lasting for more than 1 hour should be a warning to be

Table 9-3. Muscles and Joints Targeted for Strength Training and Stretching

Joints	Muscle Group	
	Strengthen	Stretch (ROM)
Head and neck	Extensors, flexors	All muscle groups*
Scapulo/humeral	Scapular retractors and depressors	Scapular protractors and elevators
	Shoulder flexors, abductors, and rotators	Shoulder adductors and rotators
Elbows	All muscle groups	All muscle groups
Forearm, wrist, and hands	Supinators, pronators, adductors and abductors of wrist and fingers, flexors and extensors of wrist and fingers	Supinators, pronators, wrist and finger flexors and adductors, hand intrinsics
Hips	Abductors, extensors, rotators	Flexors, rotators, and adductors
Knee	Extensors, flexors	Flexors (hamstrings, gastrocnemius)
Foot and ankle	All muscle groups	All muscle groups
Trunk	Flexors, extensors	All muscle groups

Adapted from Helewa A, Smythe HA: Physical therapy in rheumatoid arthritis. In Wolfe F, Pincus T (eds): *Rheumatoid Arthritis. Pathogenesis, Assessment, Outcome and Treatment.* New York, Marcel Dekker, 1994, pp 415–433.
*Contraindicated in subluxated atlantoaxial joints.
ROM = range of motion.

cautious, less vigorous, or to not use the technique. If a physical therapist is not readily available to apply these techniques, they can be taught in a modified format to nursing staff or other caregivers following instructions by a physical therapist.

Passive stretching techniques used by athletes in preparation for training should be applied with extreme caution on clients with RA, because they may lead to an inflammatory response in otherwise controlled joints or lead to further laxity in compromised joint structures. Muscle groups and joints targeted for mobilizing exercise are shown in Table 9-3. *Water* is an excellent medium for free active mobilizing exercises, as in regular swimming or structured group exercises. Because clients with RA may be sensitive to cold, the water temperatures should be about 85° F (25° C). Buoyancy in water diminishes joint loading by reducing the effect of gravity. Water also provides generalized relaxation and enhances pain-free motions.[54] Clients who live at home could join a biweekly YMCA or YWCA swim program or some other community pool program to help maintain their mobility and function. Unfortunately, some of these pools do not have sufficient heat and may not be accessible to disabled clients with RA. Swimming also

can be a very effective means to build endurance in the extremities. It also is a useful form of socialization for otherwise homebound individuals.

> Aquatherapy is an ideal medium for mobilizing and strengthening joints, because buoyancy in water reduces the effect of gravity and thus loading on joints. However, clients with RA require higher water temperatures than usual.

Strengthening Exercise

The objective of strengthening exercise is to restore and maintain optimal strength in muscles that support affected joints. More often than not these muscles have residual atrophy, brought on by the inflammatory process, reflex inhibition, and disuse. The ultimate objective is the recovery of function rather than the restoration of normal muscle morphology.

In planning a strengthening exercise program the following principles must be kept in mind:

- The joint condition should not be worsened by the exercise.
- The muscles should not be exercised to fatigue, and any resistance offered to isotonic or isometric contractions must be submaximal.
- Actively inflamed joints should not be put through many repetitions and movement should not be resisted.
- Muscles acting on actively inflamed joints should be exercised isometrically for both strength and endurance.
- Joint swelling and pain that exceed 1 hour in duration after exercise are indications of excessive exercise, especially if symptoms increase overnight.

The choice of a therapeutic exercise program should be related to the client's normal activities, and the client should be encouraged to keep this in mind. Therefore, in planning a program a number of questions should be asked:

- Is the object to concentrate on isolated muscle action or isolated joint movement, or is the object to encourage mass muscle action and functional multiaxial movement patterns?
- Should the exercises for a particular muscle group be isometric or isotonic?
- What starting position should be used? Should resistance be applied, and, if so, how much resistance and by what means?

Isolated Movements versus Mass Patterns

Because the ultimate object of therapeutic exercise is to restore or maintain function, functional mass movement patterns are the technique of choice. Mass movement patterns should be based on those developed by Voss et al,[53] because they confer several advantages:

- The mass movement patterns are based on observed normal activities, incorporating three-dimensional movements.
- In keeping with Beevor's axiom, the brain knows nothing of individual muscle action but knows only of movement; hence, the movement patterns, being natural, are easier to learn.
- In managing a complex and widespread joint disease such as RA, mass movement patterns, especially those performed bilaterally, are less time consuming and provide for normal and coordinated group action of muscles, as well as integrated joint mechanics.[53]

In contrast, isolated muscle work and simple joint movements take longer to learn and longer to perform. Isolated movements can be useful for specific regional impairments, for which mass movement patterns may be contraindicated because of joint damage or deformity.

Isometric versus Isotonic

The choice between these two types of muscle contractions depends on the inflammatory status of the joints on which these muscles are acting and on the objective of exercise. Isometric exercise at submaximal effort offers greater protection for inflamed or unstable rheumatoid joints. At maximal effort, a study of clients with RA showed that three maximal isometric contractions of the quadriceps muscle, in full extension and at 90 degrees of flexion, held for 6 seconds, produced a 27% increase in strength in the quadriceps of the exercised leg and 17% in the quadriceps of the contralateral limb.[44] Although isometric training has been shown to improve performance of isotonic tasks, clinically important improvements also have been noted for both types of tasks regardless of type of contraction.[55]

Isometric exercise at submaximal effort is preferred for inflamed or unstable joints in RA. In contrast, isotonic work is best for isotonic tasks, and if applied judiciously with submaximal resistance to noninflamed joints, it can enhance muscle performance and improve function. However, it must be tailored to the needs of the client with RA, taking into consideration factors related to age, severity, strength, amount of joint destruction, and the client's special functional needs.[56] One session a day is recommended, increasing the number of repetitions and resistance to tolerance.

Isometric or *isotonic* muscle work, combined with mass muscle contractions using normal patterns, may provide the greatest potential for improvements in functional performance.[53] Techniques such as isometric reversals, slow reversal, or slow reversal hold, superimposed over mass patterns using submaximal manual resistance, provide adequate facilitation, particularly in the early stages of recovery.[53] Manually resisted isometric reversal techniques can be applied in functional postures, such as sitting, standing, or a variety of ambulation stances. In the absence of joint inflammation, the resistance and the repetitions can be increased, and the use of external resistance, such as weights, weight-and-pulley systems, or elastic materials such as dental dam, can be encouraged. Self-resisted isometric exercises also can be applied by the client by using an unyielding strap or by pressing against a stable surface.

Starting Positions

A number of positions can be used, varying from lying to sitting and standing. For mass movement patterns, the lying position provides the greatest stability. Sitting and various stances in standing are ideal functional positions for enhancing the stability of upright postures.

Resisted Muscle Work

Repetitive muscle overloading results in hypertrophy and increased functional capacity, whereas lack of use produces atrophy.[57] Type II muscle fibers respond to techniques that use high resistance and a low number of repetitions. Increases in the cross-sectional area of these fibers are predominantly responsible for the observed hypertrophy.[57] In applying resistance, extreme care should be exercised. Isometric manual resistance in the subacute stage progressing to isotonic work confers many advantages over mechanical resistance. More specifically, the operator can do the following:

- Handle the limb with care, avoiding painful regions.
- Gauge and vary the amount of resistance the client can sustain throughout the range without stressing the joints.
- Gauge better the client's power output, particularly when adherence is a problem.
- Vary more readily the point where resistance is applied.
- Resist more readily opposing muscle groups during reciprocal motion or during postural stabilization.
- Apply more effectively facilitatory techniques such as pressure on the muscle belly, traction, approximation, and the stretch response.

In most situations the point of resistance should not cross a joint but preferably be applied to one joint at a time. The amount of manual resistance for isometric work should not exceed the client's ability to maintain the position, and in the subacute stage should be submaximal. Clients with acutely inflamed joints should perform free active isometric work with minimal or no outside resistance. To obtain a training effect, resistance to isotonic work must not exceed 80% of the client's maximal effort, and in all cases movement should not be impeded. *Mechanical resistance* can take the form of weights or materials with elastic properties. Weights have the disadvantage of offering constant resistance throughout the range in isotonic work, placing the muscles at a mechanical disadvantage owing to the changing angle of pull. Elastic materials such as springs, dental, or rubber dam offer greater resistance the more they are stretched, putting muscles again at a disadvantage as they shorten, due to the decreasing angle of pull and shortening of muscle fibers. Weight and elastic resistance are best suited for muscle work in the outer to middle range. Muscle groups and joints targeted for strengthening exercises are shown in Table 9-3.

Conditioning Exercise

Conditioning exercises through endurance training can have two major purposes:

- To improve the maximal aerobic capacity (i.e., to increase the maximal mechanical power output that can be maintained aerobically)
- To increase aerobic capacity (i.e., to increase the capacity to sustain a given workload for a longer time)[7]

Clients with RA often are limited in their activities by pain or fear of pain, disability, fatigue, and a belief that strenuous physical activities are to be avoided.[2] These limitations lead to lower physical work capacity, low muscle strength, and low cardiovascular capacity and endurance [58] The value of rest as a way to control disease and prevent deformities has been challenged by investigators who recommend early activity and fitness training.[37,38] This trend toward early activity also is seen in other disease categories, such as cardiovascular and respiratory diseases, as a valuable part of recovery. Early control of disease activity through (1) aggressive drug management, lessening the need for rest and joint protection techniques, (2) the increased cost of hospitalization and its debilitating effects, and (3) greater public preoccupation with physical fitness may all have contributed to that trend.[2] More important are findings that clients with RA have a low level of cardiopulmonary fitness and that conditioning exercises to improve endurance help these clients resume optimal function.[39,41,47]

For a detailed discussion of this form of training and a description of fitness assessments and training program components, the reader is referred to Chapter 13.

Manual Therapy

Techniques of manual therapy to peripheral joints, as recommended by Maitland, Kaltenborn, and others, have a very limited role to play in the management of RA. Because most joints in RA are unstable due to ligamentous laxity, accessory passive movements only increase the risk of injury. One exception might be the shoulder joint, for which grade I or II *mobilization* may be attempted, provided the joint is not *inflamed*. Manipulation techniques have *no* role to play in the management of peripheral or spinal joints in RA, because the laxity often encountered in ligaments, especially of the upper cervical joints, when subjected to a sudden manipulative thrust, could lead to *tragic consequences*. Passive mechanical traction to the *cervical spine* is rarely used in clients with RA because of ligamentous laxity and the potential danger of subluxation or dislocation of the atlantoaxial joint.

Reeducation of Gait

The mobility and ambulatory activities of clients with RA are hampered by pain, the effects of joint inflammation, and joint destruction. The restrictions are not only limited to lower limb structures but also involve all weight-bearing joints including those of the upper limbs when walking aids such as canes, crutches, or a walker are required. In preparation for gait activities, clients should have proper footwear as described in Chapter 14.

A review of the biomechanical and pathophysiological status of joints should determine whether the client should ambulate independently with aids or use a wheelchair. Acutely inflamed weight-bearing joints should not be unduly stressed and unstable destroyed joints may not provide sufficient stability to ambulate safely. Under these conditions, walking aids must be considered. For clients with severely involved joints, a walker with or without wheels may be required. Alternately, the use of aluminum forearm support crutches (to avoid weight bearing on hands and wrists) may be advisable. Clients with less involved joints may manage with canes (two are always better than one) that have contoured handles. Clients who are unable to stand may have to use motorized scooters. Further discussion of the use of walking aids and safety measures for ambulation is found in Chapter 16.

> **Therapists should ensure that acutely inflamed weight-bearing joints are not unduly stressed and that flail-destroyed joints have sufficient stability for safe ambulation.**

Techniques of rhythmic stabilization will be very helpful in the reeducation of upright posture and a sense of balance.[53] Propulsion forward, backward, or sideways can be initiated with the assistance of the physical therapist, actively by the client, or against resistance. Walking then can be progressed from parallel bars to crutches, to canes, and finally to free walking.

Posture

Clients with RA often have problems maintaining correct posture, whether in lying, sitting, standing, walking, or during the performance of a variety of activities. Incorrect postures can lead to contracture of soft tissue structures, poor balance, and increased energy expenditures; all are factors that can be detrimental to the rehabilitation outcomes for these clients.

Postural awareness and correction with mirror feedback in sitting, standing, and walking is a useful approach and increases clients' perceptions of their body position in space. Proper balance and posture can be taught by applying judiciously techniques of rhythmic stabilization in a variety of starting positions as discussed earlier.[53]

During prolonged periods of sitting and lying, special attention to correct posture and positioning is critical if contractures and deformities are to be avoided. Correct positioning must be tempered with client comfort. A physical therapist's unrealistic expectations often can lead to poor client adherence with the recommended postures. For example, insistence on maintaining a straight knee in bed if the joint is inflamed leads to extreme pain and discomfort. The joint effusion forces the knee into about 30 degrees of flexion, a position that permits the joint to hold a maximal amount of fluid. Indeed, it would be desirable for the acutely inflamed knee to be held in flexion to maintain the integrity of vulnerable and possibly lax collateral ligaments. Achievement of 0 degrees at the knee is a goal, because knee flexion contracture increases the energy cost of gait and pressures across the joint and contributes to hip flexion contractures.

Whether the client is sitting or lying, the guiding principle is the maintenance of well-supported functional positions, comfort, and frequent changes of position.

Restoration of Function

Clients with inflammatory joint disease, such as RA, have varying degrees of functional limitations compared with healthy persons. Symptoms of pain, fatigue, stiffness, and decreased muscle strength, interfere with daily activities such as dressing and grooming, cooking a meal, cleaning, shopping, work and leisure activities. Therefore, the physical, personal, familial, social, and vocational consequences of RA are extensive.[59] For that reason, occupational therapy is at the core of RA management.

Strategies to restore function are designed to help people in their ADL, overcoming barriers by maintaining or improving abilities or compensating for decreased activity in the performance of occupations.[60] The most important interventions in OT are training of skills, counseling, education about joint protection, prescription of assistive devices, provision of splints, and modifications to footwear.

A systematic review of OT for RA found "limited evidence" for the effectiveness of OT for functional ability training and relief of pain. Studies that evaluated comprehensive OT and those that evaluated instruction in joint protection interventions, also showed limited evidence for the effectiveness of these interventions on functional ability, whereas studies that evaluated splinting reported "indicative findings" (lower on the evidence scale) for effectiveness in reducing pain.[59] These results show modest progress in the past decade and are encouraging, demonstrating that OT can be an important part of treatment for clients with RA. Nonetheless, the review also showed that other components of OT management, such as skill training and advise in use of assistive devices, are under-researched.[59] For some OT strategies see Chapter 14 and for an illustration of rehabilitation management see Figure 9-1.

Psychosocial Support

Psychosocial counseling and assistance to clients with RA form the third corner of a rehabilitation strategic triangle, which includes PT and OT. Rheumatologically trained social workers and nursing staff can help clients with RA who need counseling. Social workers, in particular, assist clients in making the necessary adjustment to living with a chronic progressive condition and the effects it has upon client roles within the family structure. They also help facilitate the transition from being homebound to the workplace. They act as advocates to assist with the formalities of benefits, disability pensions, financial assistance in the purchase of special equipment, or returning to work on a part-time basis. Family or personal counseling is often needed to help clients and family cope with the deleterious effects of RA. For detailed psychosocial interventions for clients with RA and for other forms of arthritis see Chapter 15.

Physical Intimacy and Love-Making

Concerns about his or her own sexuality can weigh heavily on the mind of a client with RA. Those with a high degree of morning stiffness worried significantly more about their body image and reported significantly more problems during love-making.[61] That finding of a high frequency of sexual dysfunction also was confirmed in two other investigations.[62,63]

Clients with RA report little desire for sex and worry about whether anti-inflammatory medications will affect their libido or whether the sex act itself can cause a flare of disease. Some complain of pain during intercourse, worry about their self-image, especially the deformed appearance of their joints, worry about straying sex partners, and wonder with whom to consult about their concerns. Because fatigue, pain, and stiffness can be limiting factors during intercourse, clients must be taught that love-making does not always have to include sexual intercourse. Romance and intimacy can be just as satisfying. Although some of the concerns mentioned here are real, clients must be reassured that there are ways and means to enjoy pain-free love-making, that it can be a healing energy, and that heightened stimulation (e.g., on reaching orgasm) can in fact reduce pain as a result of endorphin surges, similar to the kind that causes a "runner's high."

The following suggestions may help some clients improve the quality of their love-making:

- Using a hot shower, a period of rest, a cocktail, and soft music to induce relaxation
- Choosing the time of day when the client is at his or her best
- Timing prescribed pain medication so that it is maximally effective during love-making
- Avoiding painful positions or excessive skin friction
- Generous use of pillows and pads to support painful joints
- Seeking painless coital positions
- Exchanging feelings and desires before, during, and after the sex act with their partners

Appendix I lists resources available to clients on the subjects of intimacy and love-making.

Management of Surgical Candidates with RA

Clients with RA with irreversible joint destruction in key joints may be suitable candidates for rheumatoid surgery. Pre- and postoperative PT and OT are of critical importance for successful surgical outcomes. Chapter 7 describes the common surgical procedures used in clients with arthritis and the criteria applied by orthopedic surgeons, rheumatologists, physical therapists, and occupational therapists to determine a candidate's suitability for a particular surgical procedure.

Clients with RA who are considered for surgery often have advanced disease with clear evidence of joint destruction, manifested by joint instability, cartilage destruction, gross limitation of movements with ankylosis, and torn and damaged soft tissue structures. The client's condition may be further complicated by intractable pain and gross limitation of function. For example, it is common for clients with severely damaged hips or knees to be confined to a wheelchair. The pain and functional limitations often lead to poor aerobic fitness and muscle wasting. Therefore, successful postoperative outcomes depend on the extent of preoperative preparation and conditioning.

Presurgical Management

At the outset, the risks and benefits of surgery are explained to the client by the surgeon, anesthetist, physical therapist, and occupational therapist, each presenting her or his own perspective. The client then can make an informed decision about proceeding with surgery, balancing the risks and benefits against his or her own personal goals. The value of presurgical physical conditioning is explained to the client, and a structured, individualized program, is offered at least 2 weeks before surgery. A three-pronged approach is at the core of presurgical management:

- Determined anti-inflammatory therapy
- General physical conditioning, and strengthening of muscles that will be directly compromised by the surgery
- Control of joint inflammation before surgery, especially weight-bearing joints, to make mobility, transfers, and ambulation easier postoperatively

General conditioning involves a modified aerobic training program, preferably in a pool. The object is to increase endurance and cardiovascular conditioning. Because RA is a systemic disease that may compromise cardiac and pulmonary function, surgical candidates must be taught preoperative breathing exercises and abdominal muscle strengthening exercises to help with coughing and expectoration. Instructions should be given in free active exercises for the lower limbs in bed to be practiced after surgery, which will prevent postsurgical venous stasis and thereby reduce the risk of a potentially fatal pulmonary embolism.

A program to strengthen muscles that are directly compromised is very important for successful surgical outcomes. If joint surgery is contemplated (e.g., for a knee replacement), isometric resisted exercises for the quadriceps and hamstring muscles will be required to strengthen muscles that may be reflexly inhibited by pain postsurgically. Familiarity with walking aids that may be needed after surgery also is required. An occupational therapist will show candidates for hand surgery the type of resting or dynamic splints that may be needed in the recovery process. Consultations with home care services will be initiated at this stage as part of discharge planning to ensure that proper support is available to the client on discharge.

Postsurgical Management

After surgery, the client with RA and the physical and occupational therapists face unique challenges owing to the articular and extra-articular manifestations of the disease. Other factors such as age, sex, adherence, type of surgery, hardware used, surgical site (i.e., upper or lower limb), surgeon's objectives, ambulatory status of the client, and his or her home or work environment influence the rehabilitation process. Also, the psychosocial implications of surgery, financial resources and the availability of care-givers at home after discharge, will have a bearing on surgical outcomes.

The articular and extra-articular manifestations of rheumatoid disease are unique challenges in postoperative rehabilitation. The overall objective is to return the client to his or her optimal level of function in the shortest possible time without compromising the surgical outcome.

Postsurgical Conditioning

The client with RA, more than any other surgical candidate, is susceptible to severe deconditioning and vascular and cardiopulmonary complications. Those confined to bed in the immediate postoperative period (e.g., clients with lower limb surgery) must begin the day after surgery, in bed, a general activity program designed to minimize muscle atrophy, joint contractures, demineralization of long bones, vascular obstructions, and chest complications. This can be accomplished by a program of general free active or resisted active exercise to the nonsurgical sites, lasting about 10 minutes, performed three times a day, for as long as the client is confined to bed. Where possible, isotonic/isometric presses taught to the clients can be a very useful and practical approach to management, because the physical therapist may not be available that often, and clients can participate in their own management at an early stage. Upon returning from the recovery ward, breathing exercises and coughing routines are very important in the first 3 days to enhance the cough reflex inhibited by the action of the general anesthetic and to clear the airways.

Another important early management objective is to prepare the client for ambulatory activities and transfers from lying to sitting to standing with assistance. This will involve trunk exercises, strengthening of antigravity muscles of the other lower limb, and strengthening of upper limbs. For clients with lower limb surgery whose upper limbs are involved, this will present a unique challenge. Clients with upper limb surgery, who require a walking aid to ambulate, will be equally challenged. Postsurgical hand splints must be checked by the occupational or physical therapist for fit, pressure points, and discoloration, as well as freedom of movement in unsplinted joints of the upper limb.

Early Local Management

Management of structures close to the surgical site will depend on the type of surgery and the surgical objectives established by the surgeon. Generally, muscle tone and joint mobility must be restored as early as permissible. Isometric setting exercises are by far the safest to perform when movements in the early stages are contraindicated. Similarly, resisted exercises to the contralateral limb or other body segments, as well as providing conditioning, will produce stimulation of muscles at the surgical site through overflow. Joint mobility in the early stages can be restored by means of active assisted exercise and the application of hold-relax PNF techniques. After the surgical wound is healed, the client may begin to exercise safely in a pool or whirlpool bath, well supported by water buoyancy.

Postsurgical Ambulation

More often than not, the client with RA will ambulate with assistance or walking aids after surgery. Initially, the client progresses from performing transfers in and out of bed or chair, followed by standing, non–weight bearing, or partial weight bearing. An excellent medium for early ambulation is a hydrotherapy pool equipped with parallel bars. Rhythmic stabilization exercises to the trunk and limbs, in sitting and standing with aids, are useful preparatory strategies that correct posture and provide clients with confidence. Ambulatory aids can range from walkers to crutches or canes, depending on the client's status. The occupational therapist must review footwear for fit and safety in candidates for lower limb surgery.

Late Postsurgical Management

The management objectives for the surgical site, after wound healing, are similar to those for postacute inflammatory disease. Specific PNF techniques can be employed using modified patterns of movement, with carefully applied manual resistance. Slow reversals combining isotonic/isometric muscle work would be the best universal techniques for building endurance, coordination, or muscle strength. Isometric reversals and hold-relax will be the techniques of choice for joint mobility. In the latter stages, mechanical resistance may be added to the program together with a home program on discharge from the hospital. Clients with hand or upper limb surgery will require special work with an occupational therapist for training in ADL and functional independence. Figure 9-1 indicates the role of surgery after inadequate response to conservative management.

Goal Setting and Contracting

To maximize the benefits of rehabilitation it is essential that the components of the proposed treatment program are acceptable to the client and relate to the client's complaints. The treatment goals should be negotiated based on what the client, physical therapist, or occupational therapist identify as important, realistic, and achievable.

The client requires sufficient information about the disease process and its potential effects to make informed choices of treatment strategies. Therapists need to understand the impact of the disease on the individual client's lifestyle and function to propose a treatment package that is likely to result in the desired outcome. The risks and benefits of the proposed treatment should be explained to the client, as well as the risks of not adhering to the treatment regimen. Both parties, where possible, should agree to time frames and agree to the factors that will indicate that goals have been achieved or require modification.

A contract may be developed acknowledging the client's responsibilities, as well as those of the therapists and other care providers. An understanding should be reached that the contract is likely to succeed, but can be renegotiated if necessary. An example of a goal-setting process is as follows.

The client identifies shoulder pain, an inability to reach the second shelf in the kitchen cupboard, and an inability to put on overhead garments. The physical therapist identifies the cause of the problem as active inflammation in the shoulder joint, reduced ROM due to soft tissue contracture, and decreased muscle strength. The physical therapist proposes ice to the shoulder as the analgesic therapy of choice, followed by isometric strengthening exercises and five repetitions of active

ROM exercises twice daily for 2 weeks. The client expresses dislike for ice treatment, states that she cannot be sure to adhere to two sessions daily, but feels confident that she can apply heat and do three repetitions of ROM exercises, twice daily, 5 days/week. The indicators that the treatment objectives have been met may be a reduction of pain by 50% and an ability to reach beyond the second shelf in the cupboard. If treatment outcomes remain unchanged the contract can be renegotiated with a view to increasing the intensity of the exercise program or change the analgesic modality to ice. These, in themselves, may be the rewards for effort expended by the client. Other rewards could be a "day off" from treatment or an outing. Although this negotiation process may seem onerous, it provides the client with an element of control in the overall management process of their disease. It focuses the intervention on areas of importance to the client and reduces the frustration inherent in imposing lengthy, complicated, unwanted, or unnecessary protocols destined for failure due to nonadherence.

Self-Efficacy

Self-efficacy (SE), the belief that one has the ability to engage in a course of action sufficient to reach a desired outcome, is one of the variables that can influence treatment outcome. Lorig et al[64] have shown that high baseline levels of SE for pain management and functional ability in clients with RA are strongly associated with low levels of pain, disability, and depression at baseline and at a 4-month follow-up assessments. The results correlated with low frequencies of observable displays of pain behavior even after controlling for demographic factors and disease severity.[65]

The Team Approach

The associations between functional loss and deformity, chronic pain and medications, self-concept, and appearance are complex.[66] Different but comprehensive strategies are needed to treat all features of the disease. The core rehabilitation team consisting of physical and occupational therapists, physicians (mostly rheumatologists), social workers, pharmacists, and nurses plays an important role in the care of clients with RA by teaching them how to evaluate and solve problems pertaining to mobility, self-care, and psychosocial function.[66] Other team members such as psychologists, orthotists, physiatrists, and orthopedic surgeons are recruited on a consultation basis to deal with complex

problems relevant to their specialty. A review of Figure 9-1 will explain the role of this team in the management of inflammatory joint disease.

Clients with work-related problems also can benefit from job or vocational counseling. Determination of the client's level of function, the ergonomics or energy requirements to perform work, and an evaluation of the work site with respect to physical barriers are all important factors to consider in job counseling.

Research Questions

In the physical management of clients with RA, there are many questions that remain unanswered. Although information on the beneficial effects of exercise and certain treatment adjuncts is available, few of the reported studies employed an RCT design, and even fewer studies have looked at the long-term benefits or risks of PT or OT. Further, the few systematic reviews and meta-analyses performed to date included a small number of RCTs with heterogeneous outcome measures, making it difficult to pool the information. Important research questions to ask are the following:

- Are the long-term outcomes of clients with RA improved after a program of conditioning exercises?
- Are the long-term outcomes of clients with RA improved after a structured, but custom-tailored, program of physical therapy or occupational therapy?
- Are the long-term outcomes of clients with RA improved with fewer joint complications (laxity, contractures, erosions, cartilage destruction) after a program of physical therapy, occupational therapy, and determined anti-inflammatory therapy?
- Do clients with RA have fewer destroyed joints when they are exposed to energy conservation and joint protection techniques?
- Are the long-term outcomes of clients with RA improved after a program of home PT or OT?
- Do PNF relaxation techniques confer greater benefits to clients with RA than passive stretching?
- Is a water aerobic training program better than recreational swimming in deconditioned clients with RA?

Case Study

Family and Clinical History.   Mrs. G. is a 45-year-old woman, divorced with three children (14, 10, and 8 years old), and works as a full-time secretary. She attends fitness classes once a week. A year ago, she described onset of foot pain, after prolonged walking, relieved by a change in footwear. Her wrists became swollen and stiff. She saw a general practitioner (GP) who diagnosed her problem as carpal tunnel syndrome. Her wrist problems improved with nonsteroidal anti-inflammatory drugs (NSAIDs) and wrist support.

Three months later, Mrs. G. complained of general fatigue, increased foot pain, bilateral knee pain, and difficulty managing stairs. Her wrists and several finger joints were painful and swollen. She had difficulties gripping objects, such as turning a water tap. She continued to work full-time, but stopped fitness classes.

At 6 months, Mrs. G. was exhausted and depressed, and additional joints were involved. She had difficulty sleeping due to pain, as well as increased difficulty with stairs and kitchen activities. She experienced morning stiffness lasting 90 minutes after waking up and moving around. She also had difficulty getting on or off a bus and doing general housework. At this time she revisited her GP, who told her she had "arthritis." NSAIDs were prescribed again and Mrs. G. took time off from work. She had a homemaker visit twice a week and was subsequently referred to a physical therapist, an occupational therapist, and a rheumatologist.

Mrs. G.'s chief complaints were painful hands, wrists, shoulders, knees, and feet; swelling of wrists, metacarpophalangeal joints, and knees. She had general difficulties with ADL, tired easily, had low-grade pyrexia, and was unable to go to work.

Initial Assessment.
- Morning stiffness: 90 minutes
- Grip strength: right (R), 142/20; left (L), 138/20
- Active joints: 25, of which 10 were effusions and no joint destruction (Figure 9-2)
- Extra-articular features; nodules: left olecranon and flexor tendon of R index finger
- Muscle strength using modified sphygmomanometer: quadriceps R, 92/20; L, 104/20; shoulder abductors R, 86/20; L, 110/20.
- ROM reduced due to pain in all affected joints.

Treatment Plan.
1. Education about disease, its effects, and its management
2. Resting and work splints for wrists, footwear modifications
3. Joint protection techniques—posture and work habits
4. Tips on how to conserve energy—general rest
5. Analgesic modalities: oil and glove routine to hands; ice to knees and wrists; warm shower AM with shoulder exercises
6. Therapeutic exercises: ROM—knees, wrists, shoulders, and hands, three repetitions, two to three times daily and gradually increase as inflammation subsides. Isometric presses to quadriceps, hip abductors, hip

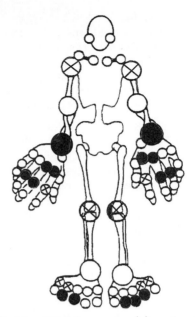

Figure 9-2. Mrs. G.'s joint count. (•), active joint; (×), active joint with effusions.

extensors, and all shoulder muscle groups, performed twice daily—increasing repetitions and intensity as inflammation subsides

Adherence. The client adhered well to her rest program, application of analgesic modalities, and exercise programs. She practiced joint protection, wore splints as required, and used a tap turner, jar opener, and so forth.

Rheumatologist. The rheumatologist prescribed disease-modifying antirheumatic drugs (DMARDs) and NSAIDS and injected local steroids to knees, wrists, and shoulder joints. Attending therapists reinforced the importance of adherence to prescribed medications.

Six weeks later, the PT and OT reassessment showed the following:
- Less fatigue
- Morning stiffness of 30 minutes
- 10 active joints with 3 effusions
- Grip strength: R, 166/20; L, 154/20
- Muscle strength: quadriceps R, 124/20; L, 140/20; shoulder abductors R, 98/20; L, 124/20
- Increased shoulder ROM
- Full L knee extension; R knee flexion contracture of 10 degrees
- Wrists: flexion R, 80 degrees; L, 90 degrees; extension R, 70 degrees; L, 80 degrees
- Ability to do some light activities in the home—climbing stairs and getting on and off chairs was easier

PT Plan Progression.

- Increase muscle strength and endurance using slow reversal techniques for upper and lower limb patterns—combination of isometric/isotonic muscle work
- Increase ROM in resistant joints by using hold-relax techniques to shoulders, wrists, and knees
- Participate in a water aerobics program in a local pool

The rheumatologist noted a decrease in inflammatory measures, but because the disease was still active, recommended adding low-dose systemic steroids to Mrs. G's drug management; however, Mrs. G. was reluctant. She returned to work part-time and was able to continue with PT at home on her own.

Six months later, Mrs. G. has been able to continue with work, uses splints, but was tired at the end of the day; her children help with house chores. She attends a pool program regularly, decreased use of analgesic modalities, and continues with exercise. She continues taking NSAIDs and DMARDS, but still has pain and swelling, especially of the hands. Her shoulder ROM is still limited.

Eight months later, Mrs. G. experienced a generalized flare of the disease as follows:

22 active joints, 8 effusions, morning stiffness for 75 minutes, grip strength: R, 148/20; L, 142/20, losing ROM in shoulders, knees swollen bilaterally, difficulty with tasks such as dressing, grocery shopping, etc., inability to go to work.

Rheumatologist. Mrs. G. agrees to use biologic agents in addition to DMARDs and was rereferred to a physical therapist, an occupational therapist, and a social worker for assistance in obtaining home help and disability benefits.

Management Goals.

- Pain relief
- Increase ROM in shoulders and knees
- Increase strength and endurance
- Restore activities of daily living

Treatment Plan.

1. Increase rest periods
2. Modify wrist splints
3. Restart analgesic modalities
4. Restart gentle ROM
5. Increase strength and endurance gradually
6. Progress to PNF techniques as inflammation subsides

Nine months later, the disease suppressant drugs gradually take hold with a substantial decrease in inflammatory activities. The active joint count was 4, with no effusions. There was morning stiffness of 20 minutes. The client continues to take a decreased dose of DMARDs and biologic agents.

The treatment program is intensified to gain full ROM, endurance, and strength, and Mrs. G. continues with pool exercises. The occupational therapist supplied new work and hand splints.

Five months later, Mrs. G. returns to work full-time, with her disease well controlled. She continues with the pool program and general conditioning exercises and continues to practice joint protection and energy conservation techniques. She is also using assistive devices and work splints. Because she was doing well on her own, she was discharged from PT and OT with instructions to seek immediate assistance if she experiences another flare-up.

Skeleton Case Study

Age: 46
Gender: Female
Occupation: Homemaker
Onset: 8 years
Stage: Acute
Severity: High
Adherence: Poor
Issues: Depression, poor family dynamics, financial difficulties

References

1. Hough AJ Jr, Sokoloff L: Pathology of rheumatoid arthritis and allied disorders. In McCarty DJ (ed): *Arthritis and Allied Conditions,* ed 11. Philadelphia, Lea & Febiger, 1989, pp 674–697.
2. Helewa A, Smythe HA: Physical therapy in rheumatoid arthritis. In Wolfe F, Pincus T (eds): *Rheumatoid Arthritis, Pathogenesis, Assessment, Outcome and Treatment.* New York, Marcel Dekker, 1994, pp 415–433.
3. Prentice WE: An electromyographic analysis of the effectiveness of heat or cold and stretching for inducing relaxation in injured muscle. *J Orthop Sports Phys Ther* 3:133–140, 1982.
4. Schlapbach P, Gerber NJ (eds): *Physiotherapy: Controlled Trials and Facts, Rheumatology,* vol 14. Basel, Karger, 1991.
5. Harris ED Jr, McCroskery PA: The influence of temperature and fibril stability on degradation of cartilage collagen by rheumatoid synovial collagenase. *N Engl J Med* 290:1–6, 1974.
6. Benson TB, Copp EP: The effects of therapeutic forms of heat or ice on the pain threshold of the normal shoulder. *Rheumatol Rehab* 13:101-104, 1974.
7. Knutsson E, Mattsson E: Effects of local cooling on monosynaptic reflexes in man. *Scand J Rehabil Med* 1:126–132, 1969.
8. Bulstrade S, Clarke A, Harrison R: A controlled trial to study the effect of ice therapy on joint inflammation in chronic arthritis. *Physiother Pract* 2:104–108, 1986.
9. Williams J, Harvey J, Tannenbaum H: Use of superficial heat versus ice for the rheumatoid arthritic shoulder: a pilot study. *Physiother Can* 38:8–13, 1986.

10. Robinson V, Brosseau L, Casimiro L, et al: Thermotherapy for treating rheumatoid arthritis (Cochrane Review). The Cochrane Library, Issue 3, Oxford, Update Software, 2002.
11. Ayling J, Marks R: Efficacy of paraffin wax baths for rheumatoid arthritic hands. *Physiotherapy* 86:190–201, 2000.
12. Dellhag B, Wollersjo I, Bjelle A: Effects of active hand exercise and wax bath treatment in rheumatoid arthritis. *Arthritis Care Res* 5:87–92, 1992.
13. Hawkes J, Care G, Dixon JS et al: Comparison of three different treatments for rheumatoid arthritis hands. *Physiother Pract* 2:155–160, 1986.
14. Hamilton DE, Bywaters EGL, Please NW: A controlled trial of various forms of physiotherapy in arthritis. *BMJ* I:542–544, 1959.
15. Oosterveld FGJ, Rasker JJ, Jacobs JWG et al: The effect of local heat and cold therapy on the intraarticular and skin surface temperature of the knee. *Arthritis Rheum* 35:146–151, 1992.
16. Casimiro L, Brosseau L, Robinson V et al: Therapeutic ultrasound for the treatment of rheumatoid arthritis (Cochrane Review). The Cochrane Library, Issue 3, Oxford, Update Software, 2002.
17. Hawkes J, Care G, Dixon JS et al: Comparison of three different treatment for rheumatoid arthritis of the hands. *Physiother Pract* 2:155–160, 1986.
18. Konrad K: Randomised, double blind. Placebo controlled study of ultrasonic treatment of the hands of rheumatoid arthritis patients. *Eur J Phys Med Rehabil* 4:155–157, 1994.
19. Olson JE, Stravino VD: A review of cryotherapy. *Phys Ther* 52:840–853, 1972.
20. Sutej PG, Hadler NM: Current principles of rehabilitation for clients with rheumatoid arthritis. *Clin Orthop* 265:116–124, 1991.
21. Lehmann JF, DeLateur BJ: Therapeutic heat. In Lehmann JF (ed): *Therapeutic Heat and Cold,* ed 3. Baltimore, Williams & Wilkins, 1982.
22. Ersek RA: Transcutaneous electrical neurostimulation: a new therapeutic modality for controlling pain. *Clin Orthop* 128:314–324, 1977.
23. Sjolund B, Terenius L, Eriksson M: Increased cerebrospinal fluid levels of endorphins after electro-acupuncture. *Acta Physiol Scand* 100:382–384, 1977.
24. Abelson K, Langley GB, Sheppeard H et al: Transcutaneous electrical nerve stimulation in rheumatoid arthritis. *NZ Med J* 96:156–158, 1983.
25. Langley GB, Sheppeard H, Johnson M et al: The analgesic effect of TENS and placebo in chronic pain clients. *Rheumatol Int* 4:119–123, 1984.
26. Young SL, Woodbury MG, Fryday-Field K et al: Efficacy of interferential current stimulation alone for pain reduction in clients with osteoarthritis of the knee: a randomized placebo control clinical trial. *Phys Ther* 71(suppl):S52, 1991.
27. Pelland L, Brosseau L, Casimiro L et al: Electrical stimulation for the treatment of rheumatoid arthritis (Cochrane Review). The Cochrane Library, Issue 3, Oxford, Update Software, 2002.
28. Oldham JA, Stanley JK: Rehabilitation of atrophied muscles in the rheumatoid arthritis hand: a comparison of two methods of electrical muscle stimulation. *J Hand Surg* 14:294–297, 1989.
29. Golin RS, Hershkowitz S, Juris PM et al: electrical stimulation effect on extensor lag and length of hospital stay after total knee arthroplasty. *Arch Phys Med Rehabil* 75:957–959, 1994.
30. Alexander GJM, Hortas C, Bacon PA: Bed rest, activity and the inflammation of rheumatoid arthritis. *Br J Rheumatol* 22:134–140, 1983.
31. Cheung HS, Ryan LM, Kozin F et al: Synovial origins of rice bodies in joint fluid. *Arthritis Rheum* 23:72–76, 1980.
32. Mills JA, Pinals RS, Ropes MW, et al: Value of bed rest in clients with rheumatoid arthritis. *N Engl J Med* 284:453–458, 1971.
33. Helewa A, Bombardier C, Goldsmith CH, et al: Cost-effectiveness of inclient and intensive outclient treatment of rheumatoid arthritis. A randomized, controlled trial. *Arthritis Rheum* 32:1505–1514, 1989.
34. Lee P, Kennedy AC, Anderson J et al: Benefits of hospitalization in rheumatoid arthritis. *Q J Med* 43:205–214, 1974.
35. Swezey RL: Rheumatoid arthritis: the role of the kinder and gentler therapies. *J Rheumatol* 17(suppl 25):8–13, 1990.
36. Nordemar R: Physical training in rheumatoid arthritis: a controlled long-term study. II. Functional capacity and general attitudes. *Scand J Rheumatol* 10:25–30, 1981.
37. Nordemar R, Ekblom B, Zachrisson L et al: Physical training in rheumatoid arthritis, a controlled long term study. I. *Scand J Rheumatol* 10:17–23, 1981.
38. Minor MA, Hewett JE, Webel RR, et al: Efficacy of physical conditioning exercise in clients with rheumatoid arthritis and osteoarthritis. *Arthritis Rheum* 32:1396–1405, 1989.
39. Ekblom B, Lovgren O, Alderin M, et al: Effect of short term physical training on clients with rheumatoid arthritis. I. *Scand J Rheumatol* 4:80–86, 1975.
40. Nordemar R, Edstrom L, Ekblom B: Changes in muscle fibre size and physical performance in clients with rheumatoid arthritis after short-term physical training. *Scand J Rheumatol* 5:70–76, 1976.
41. Ekblom B, Lovgren O, Alderin M et al: Effect of short term physical training on clients with rheumatoid arthritis. A six month follow-up study. *Scand J Rheumatol* 4:87–91, 1975.
42. Hicks JE: Exercise in clients with inflammatory arthritis and connective tissue disease. *Rheum Dis Clin North Am* 16:845–870, 1990.
43. Hsieh LF, Didenko B, Schumacher HR Jr et al: Isokinetic and isometric testing of knee musculature in clients with rheumatoid arthritis with mild knee involvement. *Arch Phys Med Rehabil* 68:294–297, 1987.
44. Machover S, Sapecky AJ: Effect of isometric exercise on the quadriceps muscle in clients with rheumatoid arthritis. *Arch Phys Med Rehabil* 47:737–741, 1966.
45. Nordemar R, Berg U, Ekblom B et al: Changes in muscle fibre size and physical performance in clients with

rheumatoid arthritis after 7 months physical training. *Scand J Rheumatol* 5:233–238, 1976.

46. Perlman SG, Connell KJ, Clark A, et al: Dance-based aerobic exercise for rheumatoid arthritis. *Arthritis Care Res* 3:29–35, 1990.

47. Stenstrom CH, Minor MA: Evidence for the benefit of aerobic and strengthening exercise in rheumatoid arthritis. *Arthritis Care Res* 49:428–434, 2003.

48. Bland JH, Eddy WM: Hemiplegia and rheumatoid hemiarthritis. *Arthritis Rheum* 11:72–80, 1968.

49. Vignos PJ: Physiotherapy in rheumatoid arthritis. *J Rheumatol* 8:173, 1981.

50. Van den Ende CH, Vliet Vlieland TPM, Munneke M et al: Dynamic exercise therapy for treating rheumatoid arthritis (Cochrane Review). The Cochrane Library, Issue 3, Oxford, Update Software, 2002.

51. Van den Ende CH, Breedveld FC, le Cessie S et al: Effect of intensive exercise on patients with active rheumatoid arthritis: a randomized controlled trial. *Ann Rheum Dis* 59:615–621, 2001.

52. Buljina AI, Taljanovic MS, Avdic DM et al: Physical and exercise therapy for treatment of the rheumatoid hand. *Arthritis Care Res* 45:392–397, 2001.

53. Voss DE, Ionta MK, Myers BJ (eds): *Proprioceptive Neuromuscular Facilitation—Patterns and Techniques*, ed 3. Philadelphia, Harper & Row, 1985.

54. Gerber LH, Hicks JE: Exercise in rheumatic disease. In Basmajian JV, Wolf SL (eds): *Therapeutic Exercise*, ed 5. Baltimore, Williams & Wilkins, 1990.

55. DeLateur B, Lehmann J, Stonebridge J et al: Isotonic versus isometric exercise: a double-shift transfer-of-training study. *Arch Phys Med Rehabil* 53:212–217, 1972.

56. Semble EL, Loeser RF, Wise CM: Therapeutic exercise for rheumatoid arthritis and osteoarthritis. *Semin Arthritis Rheum* 20:32–40, 1990.

57. Galloway MT, Jobe P: The role of exercise in the treatment of inflammatory arthritis. *Bull Rheum Dis* 42:1–4, 1993.

58. Ekblom B, Lovgren O, Alderin M et al: Physical performance in clients with rheumatoid arthritis. *Scand J Rheumatol* 3:121–125, 1974.

59. Steultjens EMJ, Dekker J, Bouter LM et al: Occupational therapy for rheumatoid arthritis: a systematic review. *Arthritis Care Res* 47:672-685, 2002.

60. Lindquist B, Unsworth C: Occupational therapy-reflections on the state of the art. *WFOT Bull* 39:26-30, 1999.

61. Gutweniget S, Kopp M, Muire E et al: Body image of women with RA. *Clin Exp Rheumatol* 17:413–417, 1999.

62. Blake DJ, Maisiak R, Alarcon G et al: Sexual quality of life of patients with arthritis compared to arthritis-free controls. *J Rheumatol* 14:570–576, 1987.

63. Blake DJ, Maisiak R, Kaplan A, et al: Sexual dysfunction among patients with arthritis. *Clin Rheumatol* 7:50–60, 1988.

64. Lorig K, Chastain RL, Ung E et al: Development and evaluation of a scale to measure perceived self-efficacy in people with arthritis. *Arthritis Rheum* 32:37–44, 1989.

65. Beuscher KL, Johnston JA, Parker JC et al: Relationship of self-efficacy to pain behaviour. *J Rheumatol* 18:968–972, 1991.

66. Gerber L: Rehabilitation of clients with rheumatic diseases. In Schumacher HR (ed): *Primer on the Rheumatic Diseases*, ed 10. Atlanta, Arthritis Foundation, 1993, pp 314–319.

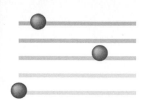

CHAPTER 10

Management of Persons with Ankylosing Spondylitis

Barbara Stokes, Dip, PT

This chapter will focus on the role of rehabilitation in the management of ankylosing spondylitis (AS), a condition that has an unpredictable course but usually has a favorable outcome with appropriate management.

The etiology, diagnostic criteria, disease characteristics, and medical management are discussed in Chapter 4. Rehabilitation management can be an important adjunct to anti-inflammatory medication.

In a Cochrane review of physical therapy (PT) interventions for AS,[1] 5 of 21 studies met the review criteria; of these 2 were follow-up studies and were therefore excluded. In the three remaining randomized, controlled trials,[2-4] therapeutic exercise was the main intervention whether delivered in the hospital, outpatient facilities, or the home. The results of these trials demonstrated short-term beneficial effects on spinal mobility, posture, and function. The results of

PHYSICAL REHABILITATION IN ARTHRITIS, Joan M. Walker, PhD, PT, and Antoine Helewa, MSc(Clin Epid), PT, Elsevier Inc. © 2004.

the two follow-up studies[5,6] indicated that these effects were sustained at 8 and 9 months, respectively.

Spa therapy, an intensive combination of PT interventions including hydrotherapy and exercise lasting up to 3 weeks, can be offered to individuals or groups. Spa therapy has been shown to be effective in improving function, global well-being, lessening the pain and the duration of morning stiffness.[7] This form of treatment is generally administered in hospitals in Europe.

Most clients report high satisfaction with exercise programs supervised by a physical therapist. Hidding et al[3] suggested that group physical therapy has the advantages of mutual encouragement, reciprocal motivation, exchange of experiences, and socialization.

It is therefore not surprising that many physical therapists find it gratifying to treat people with AS. Clients are usually young, are otherwise healthy, and generally acknowledge that they feel better after exercise. AS also can be a challenge because of the slowly progressive nature of the condition. This may

Table 10-1. Differential Diagnosis Between Ankylosing Spondylitis and Low Back Pain

Ankylosing Spondylitis	Other Low Back Disorders
Slow onset	Sudden onset
Worse with rest, improves with exercise	Better with rest, worse with activity
Sacroiliitis on radiograph	Negative radiograph
Positive family history (HLA B27-positive)	Negative family history

require ongoing monitoring and treatment to prevent or reduce the postural changes and slow loss of function that can occur. Clients with AS should consider exercising as a part of their regular routine. Depending upon personal preferences, level of disease activity, and the severity of symptoms, clients with AS may choose unsupervised, recreational activities or supervised individual PT, attend group PT sessions, or choose pool exercise programs.

> **The PT must educate and motivate.**

The current health care environment in North America does not allow for intensive inpatient therapy or spa therapy, nor, in most cases, does it provide for outpatient physical therapy over many months. Education and self-management strategies are critical to the success of the treatment program. The responsibility for monitoring posture and for exercising regularly must rest with the client. The physical therapist plays a major role as an educator and motivator.

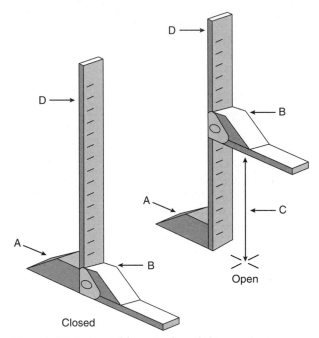

Figure 10-1. Portable spinal mobility scale in open and closed position. *A*, Fixed stop; *B*, spring loaded, sliding stop; *C*, extension to sliding stop; *D*, fixed scale.

Assessment

History of the Disorder

In contrast to common low back disorders, AS distinguishes itself clinically by a history of insidious onset of low back pain and stiffness lasting more than 3 months, unrelieved by rest, and improved by exercise. It is not unusual in clinical practice to receive a referral that states simply, "low back pain." Given such an inadequate diagnosis, the PT needs to obtain a detailed history of the complaint from the client and to be alert to the possibility of a missed diagnosis, especially in relatively young adults, 20 to 40 years of age. Table 10-1 highlights the differences between AS and other low back disorders.

Physical Assessment

Physical examination of the spine is covered in detail in Chapter 5. Of particular note in the client with AS is the characteristic posture seen caused by loss of lumbar lordosis, increased thoracic kyphosis, and the compensatory extension of the cervical spine (see Figure 4-11). These changes, however, are not always obvious, especially in the early stages of the disease, and a slight flattening of the lumbar spine may be overlooked. Therefore, it is important to carry out specific measurements of spinal mobility to establish

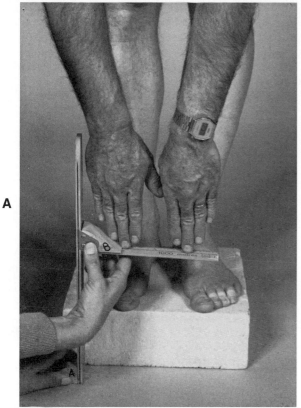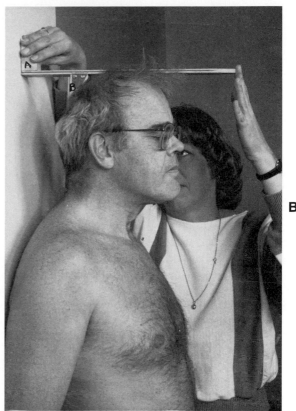

Figure 10-2. *A*, Portable spinal mobility scale used to measure standing, finger-to-floor distance. *B*, Portable spinal mobility scale used to measure occiput to wall distance. (From Stokes BA, Helewa A, Goldsmith CH et al: Reliability of spinal mobility measurements in ankylosing spondylitis patients. *Physiother Can* 40:338–344, 1988.)

a baseline and to monitor treatment effect or disease progression. Measurement techniques should be standardized, applied consistently, and preferably be performed at the same time of day, before exercise.

Two indices that measure physical impairment in AS are the Bath Ankylosing Spondylitis Disease Activity Index (BASDAI) and the Bath Ankylosing Spondylitis Metrology Index (BASMI). The BASDAI measures fatigue, spinal pain, joint pain and swelling, tenderness, and morning stiffness. It is self-administered, uses a visual analogue scale, is fast and simple to apply, and is reproducible and responsive.[8] The BASMI has been shown to be reproducible and responsive to treatment effects. It is an index that measures spinal mobility, combining cervical extension, lumbar flexion, cervical rotation, lumbar side flexion, and intermalleolar distance.[9]

There are a number of valid techniques available for measuring spinal mobility.[10–12] Of these, perhaps the simplest overall measure of spinal mobility is the finger-to-floor technique, which is valid, reliable, and reproducible. In a validation study carried out before the trial of home PT discussed earlier, a portable spinal mobility scale (Figures 10-1 and 10-2) was found to be superior to a flexible measuring tape in terms of reliability and reproducibility and was recommended for clinical practice.[13] The device also was useful for measuring occiput-to-wall distance. Range of motion of the cervical spine can be measured with a flexible tape and the distances recorded as follows:

- Flexion-extension—base of chin to sternal notch in full flexion and then full extension
- Rotation—cleft of chin to lateral edge of acromion process in full rotation to right and left

- Lateral flexion—tragus to lateral edge of acromion process in full lateral flexion to right and left
- Occiput-to-wall—base of occiput to wall with client in standing, heels, buttocks, and shoulders against the wall (use of the portable spinal mobility scale for occiput-to-wall distance is recommended)

The three 10 cm segment test used to measure ROM of the lumbar spine in the sagittal plane is described in Chapter 5. Also known as the Smythe test or modified Schober test, it is useful for establishing baseline measures and for follow-up, but it may be difficult to do with clients who have established limitation of hip flexion or who are unable to lie prone.

Chest expansion also should be monitored because of the potential for diminished movement in costovertebral joints and the effect on vital capacity. This is easily done by placing the measuring tape around the client's chest at the level of the xiphisternum, asking the client to exhale completely and then breathe in deeply, and recording the difference in the measurements.

Peripheral joint involvement may be present, and for this reason an active joint count (see Chapter 5) is appropriate, as well as measurement of range of motion in any affected peripheral joints. Particular attention should be paid to the shoulders and to the hip joints, because these joints may be involved, owing either to active synovitis or to soft tissue contractures.

Some clients may have pain and tenderness at the entheses (sites where tendon attaches to bone). The attachment of the Tendo Achilles to the calcaneus, the site where the patellar tendon attaches to the tibial tubercle, and the upper medial and lateral borders of the patella are common sites, as well as costochondral junctions. Isometric muscle strength can be measured using the modified sphygmomanometer where there is evidence of muscle weakness (see Chapter 5). An example of a single-page physical assessment form is illustrated in Figure 10-3.

Functional Assessment

The functional losses associated with AS differ from those of clients with arthritis affecting mainly peripheral joints. It is therefore important to recognize these differences when assessing function. Several functional assessment questionnaires specific to AS have been reported.[14,15] In a review of 27 clinical trials dealing with the Bath Ankylosing Spondylitis Functional Index (BASFI) and the Dougados Functional Index (DFI), both were shown to be valid and reliable; how-

ever, the BASFI had better responsiveness than the DFI in PT trials,[16] is fast and simple to administer, and can be useful to monitor treatment outcomes. (See Appendix II for the BASFI.)

Common functional activities that the client with AS may have problems with are the following:

- Body transfers
- Dressing
- Ambulation
- Work activities
- Bending/lifting/carrying
- Activities with high repetition or requiring endurance
- Sleeping
- Driving
- Love-making and intimacy

> **Functional assessment and questionnaires specific to AS are available and are useful in monitoring treatment outcome.**

Difficulties with body transfers usually relate to problems with rolling in the lying position, or when rising from the floor. Other activities involving rotational movements of the spine may be difficult to perform. Inability to reach the feet may result in difficulties with dressing. Ambulation may be affected by loss of rotational movements or arm-swing or hip involvement. Work activities involving static positions or bending/lifting/carrying can pose problems due to pain or stiffness. Loss of respiratory function, pain, and limitation of movement all result in diminished endurance. An occupational therapist can be very helpful in working with the client to identify solutions to functional difficulties either through the provision of assistive devices or finding alternative means of performing certain tasks.

Psychosocial Issues

Because this disorder commonly affects young people, it is often important to explore, with clients, their current work situation and any difficulties that they are experiencing or that may be foreseen. In this way, planning may be undertaken to avoid future problems. Clients in all age groups may have needs relating to career, sexuality, and family planning, as well as fears about future functional losses. Early identification will allow these to be addressed either through provision of disease education or through appropriate counseling. A social worker (SW) can be of great

Patient's Name: _____   Date: _____

Posture (as observed in standing)	Yes	No
hyperextension of cervical spine	___	___
thoracic kyphosis	___	___
diminished lumbar curve	___	___

A.M. Stiffness

_____ Hr _____ Min

Chest expansion

_____ cm

ACTIVE JOINTS

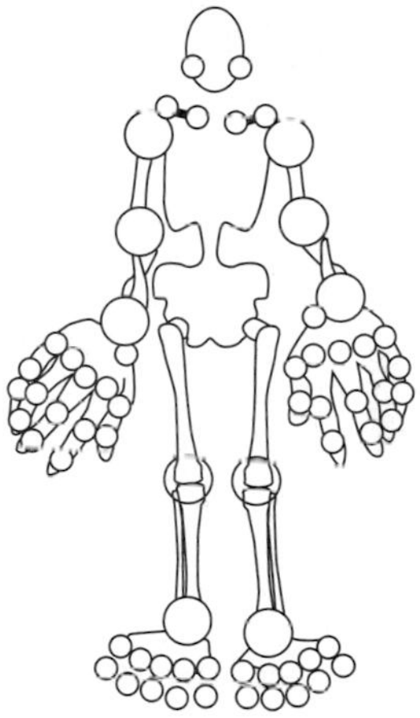

● = active joints
If range is limited, indicate loss in degrees adjacent to affected joint.

RANGE OF MOTION (in cm)
CERVICAL SPINE   R   L

	R	L
Flex. (chin-sternal notch)	___	___
Ext. (chin-sternal notch)	___	___
Rot. (chin-acromion process)	___	___
Lat. flex. (tragus-acromion process	___	___
Occiput to wall	_____	

THORACOLUMBAR SPINE

Flex. (fingertip-floor)   _____

Smythe Test
      - upper   _____
      - mid   _____
      - lower   _____

Side flex. (stride sitting   R   L
fingertip to floor)   ___   ___

MUSCLE TESTING*

Muscle Group	R	L	Muscle Group	R	L
_____	___	___	_____	___	___
_____	___	___	_____	___	___
_____	___	___	_____	___	___
_____	___	___	_____	___	___

ADDITIONAL COMMENTS _____

_____

_____

* using modified sphygmomanometer

Figure 10-3. Physical assessment form for ankylosing spondylitis.

assistance in helping clients and their families come to terms with the uncertain prognosis and the emotional impact of a chronic disease (see also Chapter 15).

Love-Making and Intimacy

Sexual functioning may be affected by pain and limited spinal mobility as well as by hip joint involvement. Pain control, open communication, and positioning are key issues that may be addressed on an individual basis. The medications used to treat AS generally do not have side effects that negatively affect sexual desire nor sexual function. Therapists may suggest to clients that they take their pain medication so that it has its maximum effect at the time of love-making. They should first take a warm shower or bath and use pillows to ensure comfort. Because most people with AS report that their symptoms improve with exercise, sexual activity may, in fact, relieve pain and stiffness.

Clients with low back and hip involvement may experience difficulty with standard positions for intercourse. The physical therapist can work with the client to identify alternative positions that are comfortable for sexual activity. The partner may experience apprehension about causing pain and may refrain from initiating intimacy. Encouraging candor between partners and suggesting measures to reduce pain, to promote relaxation, and to find mutually satisfying techniques are recommended in an excellent, illustrated brochure, "A Guide to Intimacy," available from the Arthritis Foundation in the United States and The Arthritis Society in Canada. The social worker plays a role in assisting couples to communicate effectively and to find solutions.

Pregnancy may be a concern in women with AS. The use of nonsteroidal anti-inflammatory drugs (NSAIDs) after 30 weeks' gestation may cause problems in the baby.[17] A flare of AS after the client discontinues medication may require PT intervention. If the disease has resulted in loss of range of motion of the hips, a cesarean section may be required. If the neck and jaw are affected, intubation may be difficult. However, most women do well through pregnancy and labor. They need to be reassured that the AS has no effect on the pregnancy with proper medical supervision and that they can look forward to a healthy pregnancy and normal delivery.

Elements of Management

An algorithm for management of AS is shown in Figure 10-4. This algorithm outlines the comprehensive evaluation, management, and follow-up of clients with this condition, incorporates the therapeutic measures that may be undertaken as well as indicates the need for periodic reassessment and adjustment of the management plan.

The aims of treatment include educating the client and family members; maintaining or improving spinal mobility, posture, and function; as well as encouraging adherence to a management plan over a potentially long time.

Aims of Management

The aims of management for AS are the following:

- Provide disease education
- Decrease pain
- Increase mobility
- Maintain/increase respiratory function
- Improve posture
- Increase strength and endurance
- Adapt/improve activities of daily living
- Improve function and quality of life

Education

An understanding of the disease process, the importance of self-monitoring and regular exercise, and the role of drug therapy should form the basis of any proposed management program. The program should be tailored to the specific needs of each client. Clients also may wish to have access to information about alternative therapies. Therapists should be well informed about these therapies. Most have little evidence to support their use, and clients should be encouraged to discuss these products either with their pharmacist or physician and should be cautious about concurrent administration with prescription medicines.

Because disease progression and its effects on posture and spinal mobility tend to be insidious, emphasis should be placed on teaching the client to self-monitor any losses of range of motion or postural changes. Most clients should be taught the principles of proper posture in standing, sitting, and lying during work and leisure activities. It is useful to demonstrate the normal curves of the spine using a model or good illustrations.

Self-help groups in Canada and the United States provide good educational materials that explain the disease process and medical treatment and outline strategies to manage the condition. Audio- and videotapes as well as printed materials are available from these organizations at low cost. These resources are useful adjuncts to the individualized education provided by the physical therapist, occupational therapist, or social worker (see Appendix I).

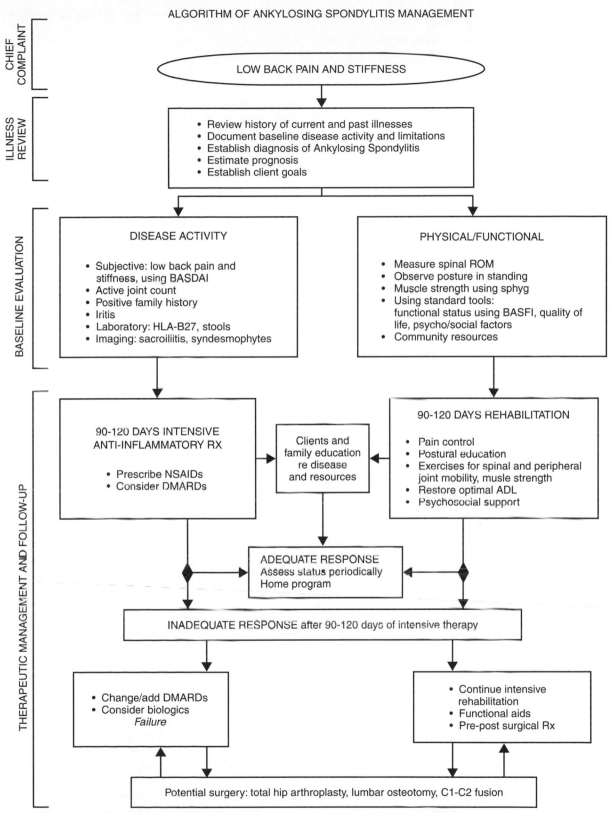

Figure 10-4. Management algorithm for clients with ankylosing spondylitis. ADL = activities of daily living; BASDAI = Bath Ankylosing Spondylitis Disease Activity Index; BASFI = Bath Ankylosing Spondylitis Functional Index; DMARDs = disease-modifying antirheumatic drugs; ESR = erythrocyte sedimentation rate; NSAIDs = nonsteroidal anti-inflammatory drugs; ROM = range of motion.

Table 10-2. Indications for Proprioceptive Neuromuscular Facilitation Techniques

Indication	Technique
Acute pain/spasm affecting mobility	Hold-relax or rhythmic stabilizations
Chronic or no pain but limited mobility	Contract-relax or slow reversals followed by free active exercise
Decreased rib cage expansion	Slow reversals, using bilateral upper limb patterns with deep breathing to enhance chest expansion. Resisted rib cage expansion with or without the stretch reflex
Poor postural habits	Rhythmic stabilizations
Limitations of strength	Slow reversals with maximal resistance: repeated contractions
Decreased endurance	Low resistance slow reversals

Pain Management

In the active or uncontrolled phase of AS, clients may experience acute pain that affects sleep, function, mobility, and emotions. The cause of the pain may be inflammation in the sacroiliac joints, the apophyseal joints, or the surrounding soft tissues. Acute muscle spasm may be present.

Pain relief may be achieved through the use of anti-inflammatory drugs to control the inflammation. Analgesic medications, as well as the application of simple modalities such as hot or cold packs, may provide sufficient short-term relief to improve sleep and function. When used in preparation for therapeutic exercise, they can relieve pain and spasm, therefore improving exercise outcomes. Transcutaneous electrical nerve stimulation (TENS) applied regionally for 30 to 45 minutes may help with pain relief, but evidence of its effectiveness is lacking. Use of ultrasound or other electrotherapeutic modalities is not warranted because of cost and a lack of studies reporting their use in AS. Relief of acute muscle spasm can be achieved by using proprioceptive neuromuscular facilitation (PNF) techniques of hold-relax or contract-relax, as outlined in Table 10-2.[18]

Mobility

Reduced spinal mobility may be due to a number of factors. Acute pain and muscle spasm may be the primary cause, as may soft tissue contracture and ankylosis of certain areas of the spine. Large peripheral joints may be affected by enthesopathy, soft tissue contracture, or ankylosis. The exercise techniques selected should be based on the assessed causes of the limitation. Although there is no scientific evidence that exercise prevents ankylosis, there are data to show that exercise improves mobility, posture, and function.[2–7,19,20] Emphasis should be placed on maintenance or improvement of mobility, because it is related both to the relief of pain and stiffness, as well as to improvements in function. Because the disease is progressive in nature, it is critical for clients to be able to monitor their mobility and to regularly carry out a self-administered program of stretching and free active exercise.

Clients should be taught to have at least 5 minutes of warm-up before exercising, by applying a hot pack or preferably by taking a warm shower followed by light arm movement or brisk walking to prepare the muscles for exercise. It also is advisable for clients to perform the exercises at the time of day when they are the least stiff or tired.

Target areas for stretching are the suboccipital muscles, pectoral girdle muscles, hamstrings, hip flexors, and spinal rotators. The modified PNF techniques outlined in Table 10-2 will assist in selection of appropriate manually applied techniques. Manually applied exercises that may be used in the hands-on component of the treatment program are shown in Figure 10-5.

Clients with peripheral joint involvement may not be able to tolerate forces exerted across inflamed joints (e.g., resistance at the ankle with the knee in extension). There also may be permanent restrictions for areas of the spine. In these cases, traditional holds involved in PNF techniques may need to be adapted to the client's condition by applying the resistance closer to the fulcrum. However, the patterns of movement and basic procedure will remain unchanged.

At the beginning of the course of treatment, these techniques are emphasized and augmented by a self-administered program of free active exercise designed to increase mobility, strength, and endurance. Gradually,

Region	Starting	Patterns	Technique
1. Neck	Sitting, head in desired range. Back supported.	Flexion and rotation to right and extension and rotation to left. Same for contralateral side. 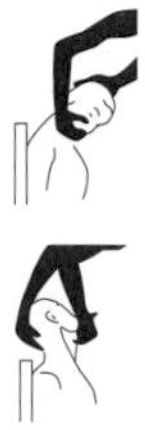	Rhythmic stabilization and hold relax
2. Neck and upper trunk	Sitting, head and upper trunk in desired range.	Flexion and rotation to right of neck and upper trunk. Same for contralateral side.	Rhythmic stabilization Slow reversal
3. Trunk	Stride standing.	Upper trunk rotation to right, lower trunk rotation to left. Same for contralateral side. Also side to side. 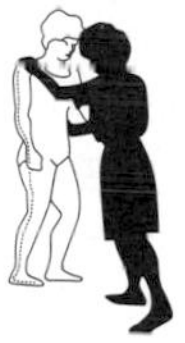	Rhythmic stabilization
4. Lower trunk	Crook lying to bridging.	Lower trunk rotation left to right and right to left. Same for contralateral sides. Also side to side. 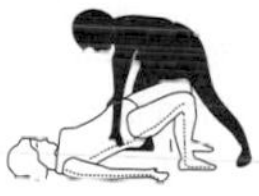	Rhythmic stabilization
	Crook lying.	Anterior to posterior pelvic tilting.	Slow reversals

Figure 10-5. Recommended neck and trunk patterns and techniques using proprioceptive neuromuscular facilitation. (Adapted from Voss DE, Ionta MK, Myers BJ: *Proprioceptive Neuromuscular Facilitation,* ed 3. Philadelphia, JB Lippincott, 1985, pp 33, 163, 188.)

the self-administered component of the program should be increased over several weeks and the hands-on PT component correspondingly decreased. The use of orthopedic mobilization and manipulation techniques is ill advised in AS because of the inflammatory nature of the disease, the involvement of ligaments and tendon insertions, and the potential to aggravate already inflamed tissues. Some clients may seek chiropractic treatment before diagnosis, considering their symptoms to be mechanical low back pain. Part of the therapist's responsibility is to educate the client and caution against treatments that could be harmful.

Respiratory Function

Pain due to inflammation of the costochondral joints or costovertebral joints may inhibit deep breathing. Clients may find applications of heat or the use of pain medication helpful. They should be encouraged to practice deep breathing, with emphasis on full rib cage expansion. Use of a towel or the hands helps to provide resistance to expansion and can assist in pulling the lower ribs down and toward the midline on expiration. Towel pressure on the chest wall can then slowly be released to permit the rib cage to rise on full inspiration (Figure 10-6). Clients should be educated about the increased risks of respiratory infections, encouraged to cease smoking and to maintain their respiratory function through regular exercise.

> **The practice of deep-breathing exercises, with emphasis on full rib cage expansion should be encouraged.**

Strength and Endurance

Improvement of strength and endurance may be addressed through both the therapist-applied PNF exercise techniques and the self-administered exercise program by increasing resistance using weights or elastic resistance material as tolerated, increasing repetitions, or increasing speed. Major muscle groups to which strengthening exercise should be directed include back extensors, shoulder retractors, hip extensors, and other postural muscles. If no peripheral joint involvement is present, strengthening of the muscles of the upper and lower extremities can be carried out using exercise equipment in fitness facilities. If peripheral joints are affected, the exercises may need to be adapted or the affected joint protected by use of a splint. For example, if the wrist is affected, a wrist splint may supply adequate support. Weight-training equipment may be used for specific muscle groups but should initially be performed under super-

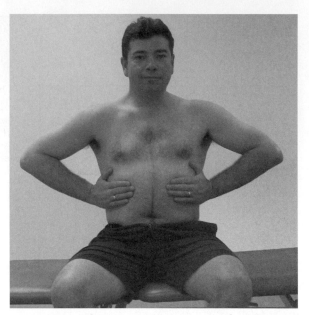

Figure 10-6. Rib cage expansion, manual resistance.

vision to ensure safety and maintenance of an erect posture. Equipment that puts strain on the back and neck should be avoided. Brisk walking and cycling (with upright handlebars) are examples of aerobic forms of exercise that can be safely and enjoyably performed.

Exercise in water offers a number of advantages and is an enjoyable means of promoting relaxation, by stretching through the assistance of buoyancy and support to joints. Muscles may be strengthened through the resistance offered by the water or the use of flotation devices. Exercise in water also has the advantage of providing cardiovascular conditioning and can improve endurance.

> **AS is progressive. It is critical that clients learn to monitor their mobility and regularly self-administer their exercise program.**

Posture

As mentioned earlier in this chapter, education plays an important role in the management of AS. Clients who are well educated about the importance of maintaining correct posture and about the functions of the spine will be able to monitor the changes that may take place as a result of the disease process or the treatment program.

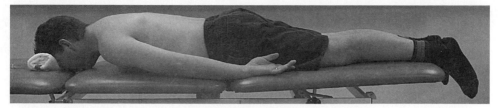

Figure 10-7. Positioning in prone lying. Note the rolled towel under the forehead.

Clients can be instructed in basic assessment techniques, such as checking postural alignment by attempting to touch the occipital protuberance to the wall while standing with the heels, buttocks, and shoulders against the wall and maintaining their chin parallel to the floor. A simple means of monitoring postural change is for clients to measure their height on a regular basis. They should be taught to avoid positions that encourage a stooped posture, such as slouching in chairs, and cautioned against maintaining a fixed position that encourages spinal flexion for prolonged periods. While working at a desk, clients should stop and check their posture from time to time or perform some simple stretching exercises. Working at a drafting table may facilitate movement and help to maintain an upright posture for some clients.

Attention should be paid to sleeping positions and advice given about the use of pillows or neck supports during sleep. In some instructional materials clients are advised to sleep on a firm mattress with one small flat pillow. For a client with established neck deformities, this is extremely difficult. The important thing is to have the client achieve as much extension as possible by providing adequate support to the painful or restricted areas. This may require the addition of pillows or rolled towels to provide adequate support. If the client can gain some relaxation, the amount of support may be decreased.

Prone lying for a period of 15 minutes or more, performed on a daily basis, is often required. Again, if the client can tolerate this position, it may be helpful in maintaining hip extension, but if the client cannot lie flat in the prone position, adaptations may be necessary. A pillow may be placed under the abdomen, or to compensate for the inability to turn the head to the side, a rolled towel placed under the forehead allows the client to be more comfortable (Figure 10-7). Lying supine at the end of a bed with the buttocks on the edge and the hips extended can be substituted when the client is unable to lie prone. If, despite determined anti-inflammatory therapy, exercise, and posture training, complete ankylosis occurs, maintenance of the upright posture and avoidance of flexion is essential.

Maintaining normal, reciprocal arm swing while walking and encouragement of rotational movements of the lower spine and pelvis should be taught, because many clients tend to lose the reciprocal patterns of normal gait. PNF techniques of resisted walking can enhance the mobility of arm swing and pelvic rotation.

> **Mobility in spinal and pelvic rotation is essential.**

Assistive Devices

This group of clients rarely requires assistive devices because they usually maintain good function of the distal extremities. The provision of assistive devices is indicated only if the client's motion is restricted or safety is a concern. For activities involving reaching the floor or the feet, reaching implements, such as grabbers, dressing sticks, or long-handled shoehorns are helpful. If postural changes have affected the client's ability to maintain balance because of displacement of the center of mass of the trunk, prevention of falls is important.[21] The use of railings, grab bars, and safety mats should be considered, as well as walking aids. Another area of concern is the client's inability to turn his or her head to back up a car or safely make a lane change. Many automotive supply stores carry a range of wider rear-view mirrors, which not only make driving simpler for the client but also are safer. A booklet, "Car Driving with Ankylosing Spondylitis" contains helpful information and is available from the National Ankylosing Spondylitis Society of Great Britain (see Appendix I). An occupational therapist can work with the client to solve problems and recommend appropriate devices or activity modification. Chapter 14 contains other suggestions that may apply to the population with AS.

Work/Leisure Activities

Some clients may benefit from a workplace assessment, particularly if they report difficulty with seating, desk height, placement of computer screens and keyboards, or angle of work surfaces. Many clients find it difficult to maintain a static posture and some simply cannot meet the physical demands of their job. An on-site assessment by an occupational therapist may lead to identification of opportunities for changes in the physical environment or the adaptation of tasks to accommodate the client's need. Older age at onset, lower educational level, longer disease duration, greater physical impairment, and jobs requiring more physical activity have been reported as significant risk factors for permanent work disability,[22,23] so vocational counseling may be indicated and job retraining may be facilitated with input from the social worker. The social worker may recommend referral to an appropriate agency.

PT intervention can result in clients reporting a decrease in pain and stiffness and a corresponding increase in their functional ability and in their sense of general well-being. It is appropriate at this stage to explore with the client recreational activities that they had previously enjoyed and may have abandoned due to pain, restriction, or fear of injury.

Some of the educational materials designed for clients contain excellent suggestions and guidelines, as well as being tailored to clients with varying degrees of involvement and severity (see Appendix I). Clients should be advised to avoid rough contact sports and encouraged to participate in activities that involve free active movement, contain rotational movements, and increased cardiovascular fitness, such as archery, walking, swimming (especially the backstroke or breast-stroke), and cross-country skiing. These activities do not replace the therapeutic exercise program but provide a recreational and social benefit for overall well-being.

By following the formal exercise program and improving posture and fitness levels, many clients are able to remain active. Once convinced that they feel better after exercise, they are encouraged to participate in recreational activities and to maintain their fitness level.

Surgical Intervention

The common surgical procedure required is total hip replacement. In a follow-up of 340 individuals studied after 14 years, 85% of clients considered the outcome "very good" in terms of pain, function, and satisfaction.[24] Advanced postural deformities may be an indication for osteotomy of the lumbar spine, which has a high risk. Spinal fusion may be necessary in instances of painful pseudoarthrosis (see also Chapter 7).

Whatever the surgical procedure, the treatment team members should present to the client the risks and benefits of the surgery. The physical therapist should emphasize the importance of physical conditioning before surgery. A preoperative treatment program should be offered that is individualized and focuses on strengthening of the muscles likely to be affected by the surgery, training in transfers, and use of mobility devices.

Because clients with AS may have decreased chest expansion and compromised respiratory function due to their disease, it is especially important to incorporate deep breathing and coughing exercises into the program so that the client is fully prepared to carry out these exercises after surgery. An active exercise program to reduce the risk of circulatory complications should be implemented and the muscle-strengthening components reintroduced and increased as tolerated.

Discharge Planning

For clients with chronic, progressive diseases that may require many lifestyle changes and that place demands upon the individual, it is vital that the overall plan of management be acceptable to them. The treatment program must be realistic and relevant to the individual. The exercise scheme should be short and simple, and although it may cause discomfort, this discomfort should not result in an increase in pain. If these criteria are not met, clients will become discouraged and disinterested and will discontinue this important aspect of the management of their condition.

The overall goal in the provision of physical and occupational therapy to clients with AS is to enable the individual to manage her or his disease through a variable, usually progressive course, maintaining independence and function. The client's ability to self-manage AS is facilitated by a thorough understanding of the disease and its effects and of the options for treatment that exist. Most clients are able to adhere to the management program for short periods, but some may require a "refresher course" or they may experience exacerbations and new symptoms, requiring modification of the management program. Santos et al[25] analyzed the demographic and clinical variables in clients with AS that might influence adherence to exercise. They found that adherence was associated with rheumatologist follow-up, belief in the benefits of exercise, and a higher educational level. Consistency rather than quantity of exercise was deemed important.

Before discharge, clients should be made aware of community resources for pool programs and fitness classes. They also should be told what symptoms require medical intervention and when to seek other kinds of assistance, such as information on transportation or job retraining. Encouragement should be given for clients to continue self-monitoring and to request regular PT checks to avoid future problems. They may wish to establish a series of regular assessments with the physical therapist, on an ongoing basis (e.g., every 3 months). In summary, the overall prognosis for these clients is favorable and the key to successful management of AS is the intelligent application and commitment to therapeutic exercise (see Figure 10-4).

Research Questions

Although evidence is accumulating that exercise is effective in the treatment of AS, there is a need to determine which exercise forms are most beneficial and which have better long-term outcomes. There also is a need to investigate the use of other PT modalities, such as manual therapy, electrophysical agents, and educational programs, as well as therapeutic inventions of other involved health professionals.

- Is group therapeutic exercise more effective than individually delivered exercise?
- What are the effects of spinal mobility techniques on function?
- Are the modified, manually applied techniques of PNF more effective than free active home exercise in AS?
- Are the outcomes of early PT (or OT) management of clients with AS better than with late management?
- What factors enhance the client's adherence for wearing splints and/or orthotics or for using recommended assistive devices?

Case Studies

The first case study illustrates the early success of PT intervention for AS in a well-motivated client with good family support who adhered to the suggested treatment program. The second case study describes a more complex situation in a client with severe and progressive disease and a challenging lifestyle.

Case Study 1

Mr. D.C. is a 46-year-old married man, with a family of two, who works as a human resources officer. His symptoms began at age 15 with low back pain onset and stiffness after a session of gymnastics. He did not see a physician at that time, and over the next 10 years he noticed a decrease in his ability to do gymnastics and experienced episodic stiffness of his lower back. He attended fitness classes and felt better after exercise, but after 6 months, he noticed pain in his mid back and a decreased ability to do the fitness exercises. He occasionally took aspirin or pain relievers for his symptoms. At age 30, he went to a sports medicine clinic where his symptoms were diagnosed as mechanical strain. He was referred to PT for strengthening of his abdominal muscles and given some postural training.

Over the next 3 years the back pain progressed, and he eventually had radiographs taken that showed evidence of sacroiliitis. He was referred to a rheumatologist, and a diagnosis of AS was established. He was treated with indomethacin and naproxen, which provided good relief of pain, but he stated that he was always aware of stiffness in his mid and low back that prevented him from gardening and recreational sailing.

Mr. D.C. was referred to The Arthritis Society for home PT when he complained to his rheumatologist about his increasing stiffness and reduced function. When the physical therapist visited, he stated that he had no other history of illness, but the family history indicated that both his mother and an aunt had low back pain.

Functional assessment. His sleep was disturbed by back discomfort, he tired easily, and he noticed shortness of breath on exertion. He had difficulty with dressing activities, such as tying shoelaces and bending to put on shorts or trousers. He had difficulty getting in and out of the car and turning his head while driving. He reported increased pain and stiffness after sitting at his desk to read or write for any longer than a brief period. His ability to sail his boat had decreased because of a lack of mobility and agility. He was feeling depressed about his loss of energy and inability to carry out recreational activities with his family. His wife stated that he was irritable and tired at the end of each day and that they were discouraged and worried about the future.

Physical assessment.
- Slight thoracic kyphosis and flattening of the lumbar curve
- Decreased cervical rotation to right (R) and left (L)
- Decreased lateral cervical flexion to R and L
- Fingertip to floor distance: 23.5 cm
- Decreased side flexion in stride sitting of 13 cm R and 14.5 cm L (fingertip to floor)
- Pain and spasm in the thoracolumbar region

Management goals. Reduce the level of pain Mr. D.C. was experiencing, and to improve his ability to perform dressing activities, body transfers, and tolerance for working at his desk. He also wanted information about the disease and managing fatigue. The physical therapist spent time with Mr. D.C. and his wife, explaining the nature of AS, its treatment, and the value of exercise in this condition. A referral was made to The Arthritis Society's social worker to provide supportive counseling to the couple.

Management program.
- Provision of educational materials, booklets, and an audiotape
- Application of heat to the affected areas, neck, and back in the form of either hot packs for severe back pain or a warm shower preceding Mr. D.C.'s exercise routine
- Setting up of a daily exercise program to include modified PNF techniques followed by free active exercise designed to improve mobility of the spine
- Twice weekly visits from the physical therapist for the first 3 weeks to monitor and progress the exercise routine and instruction of Mr. D.C.'s wife in the application of resistance to various patterns of movement
- Mr. D.C. was instructed in the use of hold-relax techniques and how to self-administer these in his work setting to relieve the muscle spasm in his mid to low back
- Provision of posture correction and advice for positioning of his work surface and the value of taking regular breaks to stretch and relieve stiffness

The frequency of the physical therapist's visits was decreased from twice weekly to once every 2 weeks over 4 months.

After 4 months, Mr. D.C. and his wife reported high satisfaction with the program. His functional ability had improved. He dressed with no difficulty, found body transfers much easier, and was able to tolerate working at his desk for longer periods by performing the rhythmic stabilizations with help from his wife or a co-worker and by taking periodic exercise breaks. He and his wife had resumed gardening and sailing activities together and reported that his mood was much improved. Supportive counseling and restoration of mobility and function had alleviated their distress.

Physical assessment.
- Less thoracic kyphosis
- Improved cervical rotation
- Improved lateral cervical flexion
- Finger to floor distance: 11 cm
- Improved side flexion in stride sitting, ability to touch the floor
- Only occasional mild pain and stiffness in thoracolumbar region

Discharged.   The client was provided assurance that he would be seen again should the need arise. Six weeks after discharge, he telephoned to inquire about joining the local AS self-help group to enhance his compliance with exercise and to provide encouragement to others.

Case Study 2

Ms. A.K. is a divorced, 34-year-old mother of an 11-year-old boy. She works as a social worker for a children's agency. She has a 15-year history of low back pain and stiffness and an 11-year history of intermittent neck pain and stiffness associated with a gradual loss of mobility of her lower spine and cervical spine.

Initially, her low back pain was diagnosed as mechanical low back strain and treated with rest and analgesics. Over the next 4 years, she noticed difficulty turning her head when driving and had difficulty with bending to put on shoes or to pick up objects from the floor. She remained relatively active, working part time and cycling and swimming regularly. After the birth of her son, she experienced increasing low back pain and stiffness, pain in her neck, and occasional pain in her shoulders. She related this to the increased physical demands of caring for an infant and took analgesics and used hot baths for relief. In 1986, she was divorced and went back to work fulltime. She saw her family physician regularly and was advised that her back pain was probably chronic and that she should get more rest and take aspirin as necessary.

One year later, Ms. A.K's low back pain flared, her neck became very painful and stiff, and she had difficulty sleeping as a result of the pain. Her family physician referred her to a rheumatologist. Radiographs showed bilateral sacroiliitis, and she was found to have a positive HLA-B27 antigen. The diagnosis of AS was confirmed, naproxen 500 mg/day was prescribed, and the client was referred to The Arthritis Society for home PT.

Physical assessment.
- Morning stiffness: 45 minutes
- Posture in standing: increased cervical lordosis, thoracic kyphosis, flattened lumbar curve
- Occiput to wall distance: 6 cm
- Cervical rotation reduced to R and L
- Fingertip to floor distance: 12 cm
- Side flexion in stride sitting: 8 cm R, 7 cm L (fingertip to floor)

Functional assessment.   Ms. A.K. had difficulty with household activities, such as vacuuming, reaching into low cupboards, cleaning the bathroom, and hanging laundry. Her work involved driving, and she was experiencing difficulty with backing the car and with lane changes. Getting in and out of the car was difficult, and she found that sitting for long periods increased her pain.

Management goals.

- Learn more about disease and management strategies
- Relief of pain
- Improve mobility and function
- Maintain independence

Management program.

Disease education with emphasis on the importance of exercise and posture training

Advice regarding sleeping position, positioning of the car seat, use of a back support in the car and at work, and purchase of a wide rear-view mirror

An exercise program designed to relieve muscle spasm and improve mobility of her lower spine and her neck using modified PNF techniques

Stretching and mobilizing exercises for the shoulder girdle and hip flexors

A self-administered exercise routine for upper and lower spine, hips, and shoulders to be performed daily

Because of the client's reluctance to take time off from work, it was not possible for her to receive the hands-on component of the treatment program, as she was able to see the physical therapist only once every 2 weeks. Over the next year, she performed the exercises "when she had time and when she wasn't too tired."

At the end of that year, she experienced another flare, saw the rheumatologist, and agreed to take 1 month off from work. Her medication was changed to indomethacin 150 mg/day with good results. She was referred again to The Arthritis Society.

Physical assessment.

- Morning stiffness: 60 minutes
- Increased postural changes
- Occiput to wall distance: 8 cm
- Cervical rotation to R and L
- Fingertip to floor distance: 16 cm
- Side flexion in stride sitting: 8 cm R, 7.5 cm L

She was seen by the physical therapist, who visited twice weekly over the next month. It was agreed that Ms. A.K. would perform her exercise routine daily after a warm shower and that she would think about how exercise could be incorporated into her schedule when she returned to work.

Ms. A.K. was alarmed by the results of the physical assessment and concerned about the deterioration of the spinal mobility measures and also very worried about the loss of function that was occurring. She reported increasing difficulty with activities that required stooping or bending, difficulty with dressing activities, and inability to participate in recreational activities. One incident that frightened her significantly occurred when she was returning home one evening and dropped the keys to her house. She was unable to pick them up, and after many tries resorted to waking a neighbor. The threatened loss of independence had an influence on her willingness to incorporate an exercise routine into her life. A referral was made to the occupational therapist who visited Mrs. A.K. at home and made suggestions about the use of assistive devices and adaptations to the household and to the manner in which tasks were performed. She also suggested adaptations to the car seating and the purchase of wide mirrors for the car.

After the month off from work and an increased number of visits from the physical therapist, Ms. A.K. had improvement in all measures of spinal mobility and had regained some of her dressing skills. The improvement was sufficient to motivate her to rise earlier in the morning to do her exercises before work and join the local pool exercise program. She negotiated with her employer for some space where she could lie down for breaks twice a day. On these breaks, she could do a few exercises and could spend some time lying prone. The physical therapist visited Ms. A.K. monthly to monitor progress and increase the scope of the exercise program.

Physical assessment.

- Morning stiffness: 20 minutes
- Improved posture in standing
- Occiput to wall distance: 4 cm
- Cervical rotation improved by 3 cm bilaterally
- Fingertip to floor distance: 9 cm
- Side flexion in stride sitting: 6 cm R, 7 cm L

Functionally, Ms. A.K. still found heavy household activity such as vacuuming very difficult, but she was able to perform dressing activities with greater ease. She could reach into cupboards and had little difficulty with stockings or shoes. She had purchased a folding reacher that she kept in her handbag. She then could retrieve her house keys and had no worry about returning home from the pool program and being unable to enter her home! Her tolerance of driving improved with the addition of a back support and purchase of wide mirrors.

Comment. Often young and busy people will ignore the insidious onset of the limitations of spinal mobility with unfortunate consequences. This client learned the value of exercise after a setback. Today, 3 years after the last PT visit, she still attends the pool program and continues to work and care for her son. *The moral of this case history is "do your exercises"!*

Skeleton Case Study

Age: 27
Gender: Male
Occupation: Auto mechanic
Onset: 4 years
Stage: Acute
Severity: Medium
Adherence: Medium
Issues: Pain, stiffness, limited work tolerance, future plans

References

1. Dagfinrud H, Hagen K: Physiotherapy interventions for ankylosing spondylitis (Cochrane Review). The Cochrane Library, Issue 3, Oxford, Update Software, 2002.
2. Kraag G, Stokes B, Groh J et al: The effects of comprehensive home physiotherapy and supervision on patients with ankylosing spondylitis—a randomized controlled trial. *J Rheumatol* 17:228–233, 1990.
3. Hidding A, van der Linden S, Boers M et al: Is group physical therapy superior to individualized therapy in ankylosing spondylitis? *Arthritis Care Res* 6:117–125, 1993.
4. Helliwell P, Abbott CA, Chamberlain MA: A randomized trial of three different physiotherapy regimes in ankylosing spondylitis. *Physiotherapy* 82(2):85–90, 1996.
5. Kraag G, Stokes B, Groh J et al: The effects of comprehensive home physiotherapy and supervision on patients with ankylosing spondylitis—an 8-month followup. *J Rheumatol* 21:261–263, 1994.
6. Hidding A, van der Linden S, Gielen X et al: Continuation of group physical therapy is necessary in ankylosing spondylitis. *Arthritis Care Res* 7:90–96, 1994.
7. Van Tubergen A, Landewe R, Van Der Heude D et al: Combined spa-exercise therapy is effective in patients with ankylosing spondylitis: a randomized controlled trial. *Arthritis Care Res* 45:430–438, 2001.
8. Garrett S, Jenkinson T, Kennedy LG et al: A new approach to defining disease status in ankylosing spondylitis: the Bath ankylosing spondylitis disease activity index. *J Rheumatol* 21:2286–2291, 1994.
9. Jenkinson TR, Mallorie PA, Whitelock HC et al: Defining spinal mobility in ankylosing spondylitis (AS). The Bath AS Metrology Index. *J Rheumatol* 21:1694–1698, 1994.
10. Frost M, Stuckey S, Smalley LA et al: Reliability of measuring trunk motions in centimeters. *Phys Ther* 62:1431–1437, 1982.
11. Miller M, Lee P, Smythe HA et al: Measurement of spinal mobility in the sagittal plane: new skin contraction technique compared with established methods. *J Rheumatol* 11:507–511, 1984.
12. Pile KD, Laurent MR, Salmond CE et al: Clinical assessment of ankylosing spondylitis: a study of observer variation in spinal measurements. *Br J Rheumatol* 30:29–34, 1991.
13. Stokes BA, Helewa A, Goldsmith CH et al: Reliability of spinal mobility measurements in ankylosing spondylitis patients. *Physiother Can* 40:338–344, 1988.
14. Calin A, Garrett S, Whitelock H et al: A new approach to defining functional ability in ankylosing spondylitis: the development of the Bath Functional Assessment Index. *J Rheumatol* 21:2281–2285, 1994.
15. Dougados M, Gueguen A, Nakache JP et al: Evaluation of a functional index and an articular index in ankylosing spondylitis. *J Rheumatol* 15:302–307, 1988.
16. Ruof G, Stucki G: Comparison of the Dougados Functional Index and the Bath Ankylosing Spondylitis Functional Index. A literature review. *J Rheumatol* 26:955–960, 1999.
17. Guidelines for monitoring drug therapy in rheumatoid arthritis. American College of Rheumatology Ad Hoc Committee on Clinical Guidelines. *Arthritis Rheum* 39:723–731, 1996.
18. Voss DE, Ionta MK, Myers BJ: *Proprioceptive Neuromuscular Facilitation,* ed 3. Philadelphia, JB Lippincott, 1985.
19. Sweeney S, Taylor G, Calin A: The effect of a home based exercise intervention package on outcome in ankylosing spondylitis: A randomized controlled trial. *J Rheumatol* 29:763–766, 2002.
20. Viitanen JV, Suni J, Kautiainen H et al: Effect of physiotherapy on spinal mobility in ankylosing spondylitis. *Scand J Rheumatol* 21:38–41, 1992.
21. Bot SDM, Caspers M, Van Royen BJ et al: Biomechanical analysis of posture in patients with spinal kyphosis due to ankylosing spondylitis: a pilot study. *Rheumatology* 38:441–443, 1999.
22. Ward MM, Kuzis S: Risk factors for work disability in patients with ankylosing spondylitis. *J Rheumatol* 28:315–321, 2001.
23. Barlow JH, Wright CC, Williams B et al: Work disability among people with ankylosing spondylitis. *Arthritis Care Res* 45:424–429, 2001.
24. Sweeney S, Gupta R, Taylor G et al: Total hip arthroplasty in ankylosing spondylitis: outcome in 340 patients. *J Rheumatol* 28:1862–1866, 2001.
25. Santos H, Brophy S, Calin A: Exercise in ankylosing spondylitis: how much is optimum? *Rheumatology* 25:2156–2160, 1998.

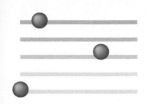

CHAPTER 11

Management of Persons with Osteoarthritis

Carolee Moncur, PhD, PT

The demographics, etiology, pathophysiology, and assessment of persons with osteoarthritis (OA) have been introduced elsewhere in this textbook. It is important to recall this information, because OA is a common condition for which, in consultation with the client, a realistic and feasible treatment plan is necessary. Often persons with OA report having been told that nothing can be done for them and they will have to learn to live with the condition and take analgesics. Although much of the rationale for physical therapy (PT) in OA is based on tradition and anecdotal data, this does not preclude the existence of sound alternatives to remedy some individual complaints and symptoms and to empower clients to manage their arthritis with lifestyle changes. For example,

PHYSICAL REHABILITATION IN ARTHRITIS, Joan M. Walker, PhD, PT, and Antoine Helewa, MSc(Clin Epid), PT, Elsevier Inc. © 2004.

data generated by Felson et al[1] demonstrated that the greatest risk factor in development of OA of the knee is obesity, the prevention of which may require changing eating and exercise habits.

Process of Clinical Decision Making

There are several ways to approach the design and implementation of a plan of care for the client with OA; however, I will outline the process of clinical decision making that I find is in keeping with the "Guide to Physical Therapist Practice" published by the American Physical Therapy Association (APTA).[2] The process is depicted in Figure 11-1 and contains the elements of patient/client management leading to optimal outcomes.[3–16] I have integrated the five elements of examination, evaluation, diagnosis, prognosis, and intervention as they apply to OA (osteoarthrosis and

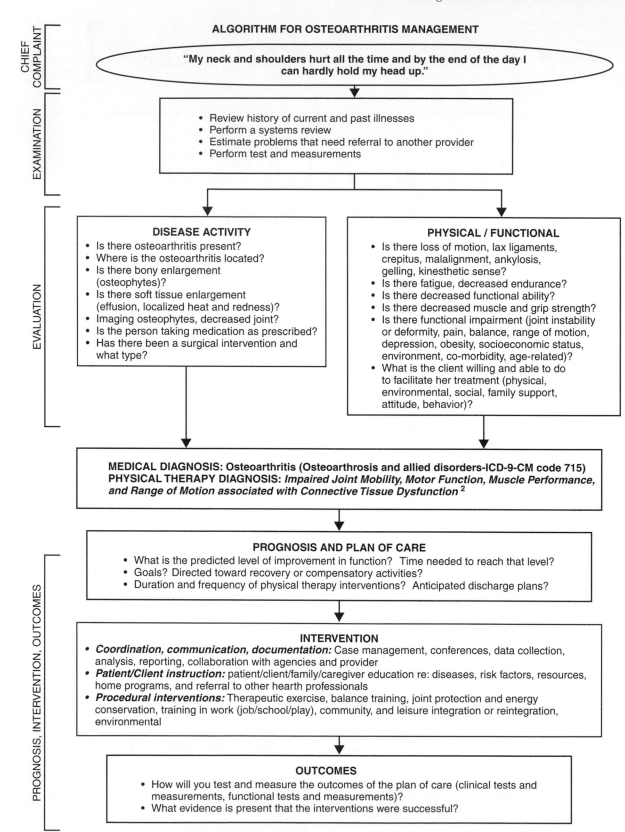

Figure 11-1. Algorithm for osteoarthritis management.

allied disorders—ICD-9-CM code 715).[17] For the remainder of this chapter, I intend to provide the reader with the current rationale for the finished plan of care including both evidence-based and anecdotal data.

Elements of Treatment Planning

Having reviewed Figure 11-1 carefully to determine how to proceed, consider the case of Mrs. G., who is a 73-year-old widow, slightly obese by 35 kg (77 lb), who has been referred for PT with a diagnosis of cervical spondylosis[18] at the level of C5–C7. Her chief complaint is "My neck and shoulders hurt all the time and by the end of the day I can hardly hold my head up." Using information from Chapter 5, an examination can be performed as outlined in the Figure 11-1. Upon evaluation it will be determined that OA is present, located in the cervical spine, and there are joint changes as revealed by her radiographs.

The evaluation process has revealed that the client has pain in a radicular pattern over C5–C7, particularly at the extreme ends of rotation of the head to the left and right. This clinical sign may be due to osteophyte production in either the facet joints or at the edges of the vertebral body. Furthermore, she demonstrates the following characteristics:

- Decreases in all neck movements
- Decreased strength in the neck muscles and abductors of the glenohumeral joint
- Complaints of fatigue and decreased endurance when holding her head in one position for an extended period of time
- Difficulty sleeping due to night pain
- Audible joint crepitus as she rotates her head right and left
- Forward head posture with a slight kyphosis of the thoracic spine
- Point tenderness in the trapezius muscle in the suboccipital and suprascapular regions
- Difficulty in looking over her right shoulder when she is backing her car out of the garage
- Discouragement because she is unable to work at her computer for more than 10 minutes because of neck pain (during her history she reported that she is an avid genealogist and wears glasses with trifocal lenses)

This information will help formulate the answer to the question: *Is there functional impairment?* It is important to determine Mrs. G.'s beliefs about her spondylosis and her expectations of and preferences for treatment. Mrs. G. agrees that she has functional impairment because she is less able to do the important things in her life.

It appears that Mrs. G. does not have joint instability, decreased balance, comorbid conditions such as heart disease, or concerns about her socio-economic status. However, she does demonstrate the following characteristics:

- Joint deformity (forward head posture and kyphosis)
- Decreased range of motion of the neck and right shoulder joint
- Gelling and stiffness due to loss of range of motion
- Occasional pain in her neck and down her arms
- No paresthesias
- Obesity
- Age-related changes
- Trifocal lenses
- Decreased muscle strength that could be due to disuse, aging, and/or protective responses to pain stimuli
- Concerns about her avocation, driving her car, and working at her computer

Given all of this information, the answer to *Is her functional impairment due to osteoarthritis?* is Yes. To formulate the plan of care the next question is: *What is Mrs. G. willing and able to do for her treatment?* In the *physical area*, Mrs. G. is willing to do neck and shoulder exercises at least once daily and is willing to begin a walking program 3 to 5 days/week, gradually working toward a 30- to 45-minute period of steady walking. She does not believe she can be successful in making significant changes in her eating habits. Mrs. G. will use a cervical pillow during sleeping hours to support her head and neck.

In the *environmental area*, Mrs. G. is willing to modify her computer station so that her monitor screen is at eye level. She can place her typing materials to avoid always turning her head to one side. She is willing to purchase a pair of glasses that has the lenses she needs to work at the computer so that she does not have to hyperextend her neck. She also is willing to pace her work so that she does not sit in front of the computer for long periods of time without standing and moving her head.

In the *social area*, Mrs. G. is a socially active woman with her friends and family. She has agreed, however, to take better control of her time so that she intersperses periods of rest with her social activities.

In the *family support* area, Mrs. G. has excellent family support. She has four grown children who with their spouses and children are responsive to her needs. Her need for approval from all of them does place increased stress and demand on her as a baby-sitter, confidante, and visitor. She notes that she has more problems with her neck when she has had "a lot of company."

In *attitude and behavior*, Mrs. G. is a self-assured older adult in many respects. She appears to be determined to stay independent and not become a burden on her family. She needs to have honest answers and a rationale for why she should follow the therapist's advice. As a result of the above information, Mrs. G. and her physical therapist can create a contract between them. This contract can serve as an instrument of motivation and as an outcome measure of her successes or setbacks during treatment.

The preferred medical diagnosis for Mrs. G. is osteoarthritis and allied disorders (ICD-9-CM code 715).[17] In the United States, physical therapists complete the examination and evaluation and make a PT diagnosis to define the prognosis and appropriate interventions for clients such as Mrs. G. The PT diagnosis indicated by the APTA Guide[2] is *impaired joint mobility, motor function, muscle performance,* and *range of motion associated with connective tissue dysfunction.*

Prognosis and Plan of Care

The next decisions the physical therapist must make are related to the prognosis and the plan of care for Mrs. G. Given the results of her examination and evaluation, Mrs. G. has a good prognosis for managing her osteoarthritis. She should be able to achieve the goals for improved function and decreased pain in 3 months. Some of the activities she will need to learn will be compensatory in nature for her to completely reach the mutually established goals. An important question is: *What are you willing and able to do to facilitate Mrs. G.'s treatment plan in terms of prevention, soft tissue care, handling techniques, and exercises?*

Interventions

As I consider my plan of care for Mrs. G., I will include the following components to help us achieve the goals we have established: coordination, communication, and documentation processes; patient/client instruction; and procedural interventions. As I plan which procedural interventions I will select, apply, or modify as required for Mrs. G.'s plan of care, I like to organize the interventions into four categories: prevention, soft tissue care, handling techniques, and exercises. These categories are derived from the art of PT practice and making observations about what occurs as I plan for the care of Mrs. G. Therefore, for this discussion, the categories will be defined as follows.

Prevention

Prevention is the component of the plan of care that addresses how the person with arthritis might prevent further injury to the joints and prevent further decreases in mobility and activities of daily living (ADL).

Soft Tissue Care

Soft tissue care is the component of the plan of care that focuses on relieving symptoms, such as muscle tightness, pain, trigger points, tenderness, and swelling. This is not an all-inclusive listing, because other soft tissue problems might be identified.

Handling Techniques

Handling techniques are those measures therapists do by direct hand contact with the client, such as posture training, joint mobilization, facilitation techniques, and therapeutic exercises.

Exercise

This component of the plan comprises activities that require the client to perform exercises to improve his or her quality of life, mobility, and general health. Initial guidance from the therapist may be given; however, it is the responsibility of the client to accomplish the exercise program as prescribed.

Accepting the rationale that most of the plan of care will fall into one or more of these categories, the plan of care for Mrs. G. will become more specific. To implement the plan of care, let us give consideration by category and activity to what Mrs. G. might do for her cervical spondylosis. Each category is presented in tabular form. Table 11-1 depicts activities and choices that might be used in the category of prevention, Table 11-2 outlines some alternatives for soft tissue care, Table 11-3 describes options for handling techniques, and Table 11-4 outlines activities that might fall under exercises accomplished by the client. The activities suggested are not meant to be the only alternatives to treat Mrs. G. but rather to demonstrate a way of planning. Some activities overlap categories. The purpose of the overlap is to demonstrate the importance of addressing Mrs. G.'s plan of care more completely.

After the PT interventions are established, it then becomes important to ensure that Mrs. G. adheres to her program. Although it is outside the scope of this chapter to discuss techniques that enhance adherence, there is ample literature on the subject from which to obtain ideas.[19–25] First and foremost, the therapist must focus on Mrs. G.'s most important goal and see it through. In Mrs. G.'s case, she wants to be able to continue driving her car and to continue with her genealogy work on the computer.

Table 11-1. Treatment Implementation: Prevention Component in Osteoarthritis

Joint Protection	Energy Conservation	Environmental Adaptations	Home Program
Cervical collar	Short rest periods	Modify computer station	Relaxation techniques
Cervical pillow for sleep	Pace activities	Change glasses	Gentle exercise program
High-backed chair for head rest	Relaxation techniques	Modify telephone use	Modify sitting and sleeping postures

Table 11-2. Treatment Implementation: Soft Tissue Care in Osteoarthritis

Pain Management	Home Program
Heat or ice as tolerated	Moist heating pad
Ultrasound?	Cervical pillow for night
TENS	TENS
Acupressure	Resting/relaxation techniques
Gentle stretching	Isometric exercises progressing to isotonic strengthening exercises
Isometric exercises	Gentle range of motion exercises
Resting/relaxation techniques	
Cervical collar	
Intermittent gentle traction in supine position	
Massage techniques	

TENS = transcutaneous nerve stimulation.

Table 11-3. Treatment Implementation: Handling Techniques in Osteoarthritis

Therapeutic Exercises	Mobilization	Home Program
Range of motion exercises for head, neck and shoulders	Gentle distraction and stretching	Short version of range of motion, stretching, and strengthening exercises
Stretching exercises	Posture training	Walking program 3 times a week for 30 minutes for 10 weeks
Strengthening exercises		
Aerobic exercises for general body conditioning		

Suppose the goals mutually agreed upon that are directly related to PT have been achieved, but Mrs. G. does not seem to understand the importance of relaxation techniques as a method of stress management. Although you were trained to use these methods, teaching relaxation techniques was never your strength and might be better done by another provider. Now I ask: *Is there another provider who can teach Mrs. G. relaxation techniques? Is such a provider accessible to Mrs. G.?* Answering this question requires consultation

Table 11-4. Treatment Implementation: Exercise Component in Osteoarthritis

Ambulation	Functional Training	Therapeutic Exercises	Home Program
Suggest good walking shoes and changes in gait deviations	Brisk walking	Gentle range of motion, isometric, and strengthening exercises on a daily basis	Exercises for head, neck and shoulders
Discuss falls Prevention	Rest periods		Relaxation techniques Walking program

Table 11-5. Two Main Categories of Outcome Measures: Clinical Tests and Functional Tests and Measurements

Clinical Tests and Measurements	Functional Tests and Measurements
Range of motion in degrees or percentage of gain or loss	Pain free range of motion in rotation while backing car out of driveway.
Muscle test scores	Increased length of walking time.
Visual analogue scales	Increased tolerance for sitting at the computer measured in time or self-report.
Decreased use of TENS	Decreased fatigue as measured by self-report.
Scores on standardized functional assessment tools (Western Ontario and McMaster Index, Arthritis Impact Measurement Survey, Arthritis Impact Measurement Survey 2, Health Assessment Questionnaire, Sickness Index Profile, Functional Status Index, Short Form-36)	

TENS = transcutaneous nerve stimulation.

with more experienced colleagues, including the client's physician, to find a suitable individual, such as a clinical psychologist or health educator. The Arthritis Society or Arthritis Foundation might provide the client with a listing of individuals who specialize in instruction in biofeedback or relaxation techniques.

Outcome

Suppose Mrs. G. is cooperative in most respects and is achieving the mutual goals established early in the planning phase of her care. The next question is: "How will you measure the outcome of Mrs. G.'s treatment?" For a capsule view of the answer to this question, Table 11-5[3–16] depicts the options. From the data collected before and after treatment, the therapist should systematically review the measures in relation to the important variables for the client. The therapist can then develop objective data to report to the client, family, and insurance payers.

Literature Review Related to the Plan of Care

The foregoing process of creating a plan of care has been based on both anecdotal information and literature pertinent to OA. There are some treatment issues that have been investigated and reported in the literature related to PT in OA, some issues that have been decided based entirely on clinical experience, and still some issues that need to be investigated. I will review the literature with the client as a treatment team member. Topics reviewed include cooperation and adherence issues, prevention measures, soft tissue care, handling techniques, exercise, and outcome measures that could be utilized to assess client progress and the plan of care. Because conditioning exercise is addressed in Chapter 13, the discussion on this subject will be a selective review.

The Client as a Worker

Wiener[26] has postulated that the client is the central worker in his or her care and that as such presents to the physical therapist, or any other provider, untrained, unpaid, and often unacknowledged for the important role ahead of them. When a chronic illness such as OA intrudes upon the life of untrained clients, it demarcates quickly what they might have perceived they were in the past from what they perceive themselves to be now that they have OA. The change in perception of the body's ability to perform activities, its appearance, and its physiological function can change the inner core of beliefs the person possesses. Accommodating to these changes is *work* for the client, along with all the other day-to-day complexities that could arise from having OA. Living, coping with OA, and everyday work must be integrated by the client, as well as completing the *work* of cooperating with a treatment regimen.[26] These are important concepts to recognize during treatment planning and implementation.

Unfortunately, in our Western society, we equate the worth of work with the amount of pay received or vice versa. Our client, as a worker, is unpaid.[26] As therapists it is important that we value and dignify the effort the client is making to complete the work that goes with having OA, such as emotional work, living life, balancing treatment options, pacing activities, and coping with disability if it is present. Recall that just because we are unable to see the work the client is doing does not mean that he or she is not making an honest effort.[27] The client is the one who does the bulk of the work to manage a chronic illness, not the physical or occupational therapist. An important professional role that all members of the health care team can play is to acknowledge and honestly praise clients for the work they are doing to contribute to their care.

Ross et al[28] discussed the role of expectations and preferences in health care satisfaction of persons with arthritis. Expectations are what people *expect* from care and preferences are what people *want* from care.[28] These authors suggested that expectations and preferences are different constructs and have different mechanisms for influencing client satisfaction with care. It has been demonstrated that an association exists between arthritis experience, when measured by duration of joint discomfort, number of affected joints, and number of treatments or procedures; physical functioning and depression; and expectations.[28] Lower expectation of care occurred in patients with greater disease experience, lower physical functioning, and greater depression. The implication of these findings for either the physical or occupational therapist is that clients who have longstanding arthritis and low expectations from treatment may experience dissatisfaction with therapy regardless of the quality of care given. Thus, it is important for the therapist to try to ascertain what the expectations of the client might be.

> The client's expectations and preferences should be considered in planning and implementation of care.

No one has identified the preferences of client care wanted by a person with arthritis.[28] Persons with arthritis may represent a distinct subgroup of individuals seeking care who differ in important ways from others seeking care with respect to the value they place on health care.[28] Although the ultimate satisfaction with care of persons with arthritis may not differ, their preferences for specific attributes of care could differ.[28] For example, the person with OA may realize that there are certain limits to the success that might be achieved from care and shift his or her priority to having a valuable relationship with the provider. The intent is to maintain a good relationship with the provider and to have support and advice through the sometimes variable course of OA.[28] In other words, the person with OA may come to value the interaction with the physical or occupational therapist rather than an emphasis on efficiency and access to care (although these are indeed important). The conclusion to draw from this information is that the client's expectations and preferences are important considerations when a plan of care is devised and implemented.

Prevention

From data obtained by cross-sectional survey the incidence of OA has been reported to be higher in persons who consistently overuse certain joints, who are obese,[1] and who sustain a traumatic injury to a joint.[29] This information is useful during treatment planning related to joint protection and energy conservation techniques. In a study using a control group, Brown et al[30] investigated the energy required by patients with OA of the hip to walk before and after a total hip arthroplasty. The difference in energy consumption before surgery was 56% of the predicted maximum capacity. One year after total hip arthroplasty the customary walking speed increased from 41 m/min (50% of normal) to 55 m/min (67% of normal) and the oxygen cost decreased, although not within limits established for equivalent persons without OA. Gussoni et al[31] measured the energy costs of walking in 12 patients with hip joint impairments and 10 subjects without impairments of similar age and body size. Their data revealed that patients' energy costs increased up to 50% above that of the healthy subjects during level treadmill walking and up to 70% during walking on a 5% incline.

The addition of *assistive devices*, such as a cane or crutches, can have a dramatic impact on the energy requirements, provided the upper extremities can tolerate their use.[32] Data were generated from physiological measurements in individuals with rheumatoid arthritis (RA), who were candidates for total joint arthroplasty, as they used crutches, canes, or walkers. These data revealed that the use of these devices influences gait parameters, heart rate, and oxygen uptake.[32] Individuals who did not require assistive devices had the highest velocity of 45 m/min and had the highest oxygen uptake of 11.0 ml/kg/min. Those requiring bilateral crutches or a walker had the slowest velocities of 26 and 21 m/min, respectively. Oxygen consumption was the lowest in those requiring a walker. Considering the slow velocity of gait by individuals with a walker, the oxygen costs were considered high by the researchers. The highest heart rate was found in persons using both arms with bilateral crutches or a walker and lowest in individuals using one cane or a crutch. Caution must be exercised when these results are applied to persons with OA. We do not know from these data the extent of involvement of the upper extremities of the client with RA, which could influence the weight-bearing ability of the client with the assistive devices. These individuals were candidates for total joint replacements who were seen preoperatively, and probably only surgery would make a difference in their functional capacity. No mention was made about how the initial use of the assistive device contributed to lessening the pain the clients experienced. This example is offered to emphasize the fact that when an assistive device is added to help a person walk, the energy costs may increase, although pain decreases.

> **When only one hip is involved, the cane should be used on the opposite side and loads carried on the same side.**

Clients with unilateral hip disease should use a cane on the opposite side and carry loads on the same side. Joint protection principles originated as intuitive thought; however, Neumann[33] completed a biomechanical analysis of the use of a cane as a method of hip joint protection. Although therapists have routinely suggested that clients place the cane in the hand opposite to the hip with arthritis, the results from this study explain biomechanically why use of the cane in this way is important. In addition, the results of this study suggest that clients with unilateral hip disease should carry loads *on the side* of the hip with arthritis so a cane can be used on the opposite side.[33]

Use of *knee bracing* for single compartment OA of the knee has become a treatment option to provide pain relief. Self et al[34] investigated the use of a valgus loading brace designed for persons with medial compartment OA to determine the varus moments at the knee during level gait. Five individuals with medial compartment OA wore an instrumented valgus-loading knee brace while lower limb kinematic and force data were gathered. Each subject was instructed to walk across the force plate with and without the brace. After analyzing the data, the authors reported that the largest varus loading moments at the knee occurred during the stance phase of gait. The results of this study demonstrated that the use of a medial compartment-unloading brace reduced the varus moments at the knee during stance. These findings may have clinical relevance because they show reduction of pain during the walking cycle for persons with medial compartment disease.[34]

Cervical collars are commonly suggested for use in OA of the cervical spine. Based upon anecdotal experience, the rationale for their use is to immobilize and rest the joints of the neck, provide protection and heat, and provide weight release.[35,36] Spondylosis causes pain and occasionally radicular symptoms that move into the neck and arm. Selection of a collar is made based upon the goals to be achieved by use of the collar. Johnson et al[37] compared the effectiveness of a soft cervical collar, a Philadelphia collar, a four-poster brace, a cervicothoracic brace, a Somi brace, and a halo device with a plastic body vest in limiting neck motion in healthy subjects. The results of their investigation indicated what might be expected. The halo device limited the greatest amount of motion (96% of flexion and extension of the neck) and the soft cervical collar limited the least amount (26% of flexion and extension). Rotation was poorly controlled by all of the collars with the exception of the halo device.

What this suggests is that the physical therapist and client must be realistic about the use of a cervical

Table 11-6. Factors to Consider in the Use of Thermal Agents in Osteoarthritis

Factors	Conditions
1. Inflammatory versus noninflammatory polyarthritis	**Osteoarthrosis:** Use a deeper heating technique such as diathermy.
2. Acute versus chronic inflammation	**Inflamed:** Use cold and/or electrical stimulation to reduce pain and inflammation.
3. Loss of range of motion	**Joint capsule shortening or musculotendinous contracture:** Use deep heat with slow, gentle stretch; use cold applications cautiously.
4. Position for treatment	**Joints should be positioned to decrease pain or to decrease the chance of pain occurring during treatment.**
5. Joints involved	**Multiple joints involved:** Use hydrotherapy in the form of Hubbard tank or swimming pool.
6. Clinic versus home care	Select **practical methods** the client can easily use at home safely.
7. Precautions/contraindications	Some **medical or comorbid conditions or co-morbidity** existing with the OA in the client may preclude the use of thermal agents.
8. Preconceived notions	Some **clients have varied experiences** with the use of heat, cold, or home remedies. They may need to be reeducated about the use of these modalities.

Data from Lehman.[46]

collar. If the goal is to provide an analgesic effect on the painful joints of the neck by resting them or assisting them biomechanically, then a soft collar may be a suitable choice. If, on the other hand, there are neurological warnings of an active destructive process, use of a more rigid collar, such as a Philadelphia collar or a cervicothoracic brace, may be indicated. A neck support should be used to reinforce and protect damaged joints rather than as a corrective measure for a postural deviation in the neck. Biomechanical derangement of facet joints due to OA may be aggravated by the use of an externally applied corrective force from a brace or collar through contact on the mandible, occiput, and thorax. Using a cervical collar for joint protection during sleep also can be recommended to the client.

Other joint protection and energy conservation techniques might include taking elevators rather than stairs, riding in a golf cart rather than walking, limiting the number of times stairs are used, using high stools rather than standing at work stations, and pacing activities so that light tasks (e.g., sweeping) are mixed with heavy tasks (e.g., digging).[38] Additional measures for joint protection are given in Chapter 14. Often,

clients fail to realize that the more physically fit they are, the more efficient the body becomes in terms of joint protection and energy conservation. Various authors have demonstrated that individuals with OA can improve their fitness level without worsening their arthritis.[39-44]

Soft Tissue Care

Use of thermal agents in treating OA is common; however, deciding which thermal agent to use is not always straightforward. Michlovitz[45] suggested several guidelines based on anecdotal and objective data that may be used to reach a decision. These guidelines are listed in Table 11-6. The author recommended that acute symptoms in OA might be treated with cold, electrical stimulation, or superficial heat, whereas chronic manifestations respond better to conversion heat, such as ultrasound or diathermy, superficial heat, or cold application.

The literature on the efficacy of ultrasound in treatment of OA contains mixed reviews. Lehman et al[46] reported increases in the range of motion of the shoulder with the use of ultrasound and exercise compared with the use of microwave diathermy and exercise. Other researchers suggested that there is no statistically significant difference, based on data from a placebo-control trial, in the range of motion achieved in persons with OA of the knee who received sham versus actual treatment with ultrasound and exercise.[47] Falconer et al[48] published a systematic review of the literature on the use of ultrasound and pain relief and concluded that although persons with OA may experience pain relief, we, as clinicians, cannot be confident that ultrasound caused this improvement. Placebo effects and experimenter expectancy bias may have contaminated the results. Further well-designed clinical trials on the use of ultrasound in OA must be completed.

Treatment of OA with other modalities including low-level laser therapy (classes I, II, and III)[49] and transcutaneous nerve stimulation (TENS)[50] has been reported. Brosseau et al[49] concluded from a systematic review of the literature on low-level laser therapy that for OA the results are conflicting and trials are not well controlled. They recommended the need for randomized, controlled clinical trials focusing on wavelength used, treatment duration, dosage, and site of application over nerves instead of joints. Osiri et al[50] systematically reviewed the literature related to the use of TENS in treatment of OA of the knee. They concluded that TENS and acupuncture-like TENS were more effective than a placebo for control of pain.

Sheon et al[51] suggested that, based on their clinical experience, the use of medications may be the least important form of treatment of soft tissue disorders accompanying OA. Gentle stretching exercises, joint distraction in the form of manual or mechanical traction, and avoidance of aggravating factors on the joint often provide more sustained benefit. Soft tissue techniques were particularly useful in the treatment of painful musculoskeletal conditions and impaired function. Danneskiold-Samsoe et al[52] investigated the effects of massage on myofascial pain and determined that 21 of 26 patients improved symptomatically with a concurrent decline in muscle tension. Using measurable biochemical parameters, they determined that a gradual decline occurred in plasma myoglobin concentration after each massage session.

Several investigators reported their results from studies of the effects of heat and exercise versus exercise alone for increasing range of motion in arthritis.[53–55] The results of these randomized, controlled trials suggested that heat and exercise together produce no more range of motion in patients with RA or OA of the hips and knees or in patients after total knee arthroplasty (TKA) than exercise alone. Hecht et al[56]

noted that cold and exercise produced no greater increase in the range of motion of patients after TKA than exercise alone. Chamberlain et al[53] indicated that short-wave diathermy and exercise produced no difference in muscular endurance in a group of patients with OA of the knee compared with a group receiving exercise alone. Before one concludes, however, that heat and cold add little to exercise regimens for improving strength, pain, range of motion, and endurance, it is important to ask at least one crucial question: *Are there other variables that are affected by use of heat and cold?* Swezey[57] noted that the placebo phenomenon should not be discounted when therapeutic modalities are used for arthritis management. Little is known about the action of these agents in OA; hence, there exists a need for further clinical investigations to demonstrate their efficacy.

Handling Techniques

Placing the hands upon a client to guide their exercises, reeducate muscle, direct body movements, or mobilize soft tissues is a characteristic essential to the profession of PT. The extent to which sophisticated mobilization techniques may be used depends upon the interest and ability of the therapist and the status of the client to receive these techniques. It is not the purpose of this chapter to teach the basics of manual therapy, but rather to suggest that the person with OA who experiences, hypomobility, pain, disability, and decreased range of motion might benefit from the proper use of mobilization to reverse these conditions. Various authors have described joint mobilization as an attempt to improve joint mobility or decrease pain by using selected grades of accessory movements.[58–61] The rationale they provide for the use of accessory movements suggests that these techniques could be useful in persons with OA (Table 11-7). Gentle distraction of the joint and stretching of the capsular tissues can be useful to increase mobility. Other authors also have described guidelines based on empirical data for manual techniques that could be used in the treatment of OA.[60–62]

Connective tissue massage,[63] proprioceptive neuromuscular facilitation techniques, resisted exercises, and stretching exercises should be applied with a complete understanding of the status of the joint, the musculature, and the tolerance of the client for any of these measures. Nothing will turn the client away from care quicker than the use of excessive force on painful joints. The application of therapeutic techniques used judiciously will enhance the client's ability to reach established treatment goals.

Table 11-7. Rationale for the Use of Accessory Movements in Joint Mobilization for Osteoarthritis[58-62]

1. Used when primary resistance is encountered from the ligament and capsule of the joint and there is minimal muscular resistance
2. Can be done in any part of the physiological range of motion
3. Can be done in any direction (posteriorly, caudally, or anteriorly)
4. Causes less pain per degree of range of motion gained
5. Used for tight articular structures
6. Safe method because it uses short- lever arm techniques

Data from Barak et al,[58] Cyriax,[59] McKenzie,[60] Mennell,[61] and Kessler.[62]

General Exercise

Considerable progress has been made in understanding of the effects of exercise on OA, particularly that of aerobic conditioning.[64–69] It is important to monitor how the client does his or her exercise program. There are some individuals who believe that more exercise may be better; therefore, the client should be cautioned to avoid doing too much or too little of their home program. Unfortunately, the client is often the only person who can determine what his or her level of tolerance for exercise will be. A walking program might be given to a person with OA, provided that the lower extremity joints will tolerate walking. The same program could be done in a swimming pool. The reader is referred to Chapter 13 for in-depth guidelines and the scientific rationale for proceeding with an exercise program for people with OA.

How the client exercises is critical in terms of protecting the joint from further damage. Consideration should be given to mechanical factors such as movements produced around the joint, the duration of the exercise, and the status of joint structures. In a healthy knee, these forces may be easily tolerated; however, in an eburnated, painful knee joint, loading with excessive resistance will only exacerbate the problem. In an elderly, sedentary individual, lifting the weight of the leg when the knee is painful may be a maximum effort. *Nothing will interfere with client adherence more than providing treatment that causes more harm than good.* Thus, it is important to have the client begin joint protection activities early in the course of treatment in the form of carefully planned exercise, taking into account his or her age and physical status. Sanders[67] suggested that low-intensity exercises of short duration, with minimal repetitions and frequent sessions per day, may be the only way for the client to achieve initial success. Intensity was defined by the author as the percentage of the maximal

capacity a person should exercise, duration as the length of time the person can do continuous exercise, and frequency as the number of workout periods per day or week.

Consideration should be given to the aerobic capacity of the person; however, age, medications taken, physical status, and a willingness to adhere to the program are important factors. Low intensity for a 60-year-old person who has been inactive may be 50% to 60% of the maximal heart rate. Short duration may be 5 to 10 minutes of continuous work. Minimal repetitions may be from 5 to 10 completed 2 to 3 times daily.

Although minimal guidelines have been described by the American College of Sports Medicine (ACSM) for increasing the capacity of the client to exercise, they are only guidelines.[68] Westby[69] published a systematic review of the literature that describes aerobic fitness activities and provides suggestions for exercise prescription for individuals with arthritis.

Physical Therapy Considerations Related to Sexuality

It is not outside the scope of practice for a physical therapist to be asked by a person with OA, particularly one who has painful hips or knees, how he or she might best achieve pain-free sexual activity. The guidance given will need to be driven by client need and the clinical judgment of the therapist, because no guidelines supported by research data have been stated in the literature. The Arthritis Foundation[70] and Arthritis Society have published helpful literature on sexual intimacy to assist the individual with arthritis (see Appendix I). Persons with back, hip, or knee pain may need to modify the positions they assume to have sexual intercourse. This will require cooperation of both partners for the experience to be satisfying. The therapist can teach the person with

OA what his or her physical limitations might be and then suggest positioning for sexual activity to reduce pain and increase satisfaction. If there are complex issues that fall outside the scope of PT practice, the therapist should not hesitate to refer the client to a clinical psychologist or to an individual qualified to give sexual counseling.

Physical Therapy Considerations for the Client Undergoing Surgery

Selection of Treatment Procedures

Whereas PT measures may be used to provide relief of pain and restoration of function, there may be a time when the client will need surgical intervention to restore joint function. The single major advance in the relief of pain of OA and restoration of a knee or hip severely damaged from OA has been total joint replacement. Although there are surgical options other than joint replacement, particularly in younger clients, older clients may be encouraged to have an arthroplasty when their quality of life is being measurably affected and severe deterioration of the joint surfaces has occurred. Although surgeons and physical therapists consider rehabilitation to be imperative after a total joint arthroplasty, there are few published studies that describe the ideal PT program for clients.[71] Surgeons usually refer their clients for PT based upon their experience that active participation of the client in a postoperative exercise program will improve muscle strength, increase motion, and educate the client in proper protection of the operated joint.

PT after total joint arthroplasty appears to be based largely on local custom and surgeon preference. Figgie[72] suggested that patients with a hip arthroplasty should not be discharged from the hospital until they are ambulatory with a walking aid and can manage stairs independently. After TKA, the client should be able to bend the knee to 90 degrees and to maneuver up and down stairs before leaving the hospital. Little information describing the rehabilitation process undertaken by physical therapists has been published; however, there seems to be some consistent aspects of a plan of care that therapists should consider. For example, if there is an opportunity to conduct a preoperative evaluation of the client and the joint slated for surgery, some of the elements that should be determined are range of motion, muscle strength, muscular imbalances, gait deviations, age, mental status, living arrangements, and family and social support networks. The client should be made aware of the goals of PT management and what he or she might expect after surgery.

Postoperative Rehabilitation Procedures

Kampa et al[73] and others[74,75] suggested guidelines, based on their clinical experience, for postoperative rehabilitation that are important for a physical therapist to consider. A summary of the customary programs is found in Tables 11-8 and 11-9. Postoperative rehabilitation will be influenced by the age, cognitive status, muscular strength, general health, type of prosthesis used (cemented versus cementless), surgical approach, and cooperative behavior of the client. The foregoing parameters, as well as the surgeon's preference for bearing weight on the prosthesis, will influence the weight-bearing status of the client.

> Research has shown that *touchdown weight bearing*, performed correctly, generates less acetabular stress than full, partial, or non–weight bearing with the knee extended.

In recent years, several authors have completed clinical trials with clients who had total joint arthroplasty that have enhanced our understanding of rehabilitation practices for these clients. Barrett et al[76] and Stauffer et al[77] reported that clients with OA of the knee demonstrate diminished position sense compared with healthy subjects of various ages. Furthermore, Barrett et al[76] determined that clients with TKAs exhibit greater accuracy in position sense compared with subjects who have OA in their knees ($p < .02$). These authors compared position sense accuracy in clients having semiconstrained knee replacements with that in those who received constrained prostheses. Test results favored the clients with the semiconstrained knee, although statistical significance was not achieved. It was concluded that the TKA probably restores joint alignment and "joint space height," contributing to improved position sense; however, recovery did not reach the accuracy of age-matched subjects with healthy knees. These data are important to consider when a PT regimen is planned either preoperatively or postoperatively. The therapist could reasonably expect that postoperative joint position sense will improve in clients with a TKA.

In a case-control study, Jevsevar et al[78] compared locomotor activities in 15 subjects (19 knees) with knee arthroplasties (KA group), and 11 control subjects (22 knees). All subjects were analyzed kinematically and kinetically while walking barefoot, climbing and descending stairs, and rising from a chair. Using sophisticated gait analysis equipment, the investigators showed that although the KA group had an excellent result when assessed clinically, this group demonstrated

Table 11-8. Physical Therapy Protocol for Total Hip Arthroplasty

Status and Time	Activity
Preoperative:	
1 month before prior to admission	1. Attendance in class on total hip arthroplasty 2. Evaluation of range of motion, strength, limb length, pain, gait patterns 3. Review of precautions and postoperative exercise plan 4. Fitting of walker and instruct in use
Postoperative:	
Day 1	1. Supine bed exercises 2. Bed-to-chair transfers
Day 2	1. Supine bed exercises: isometric and ankle pumping exercises 2. Active-assistive range of motion 3. Assisted walker/crutch ambulation dependent upon weight-bearing status
Days 3–5	1. Supine bed exercises 2. Sitting bed exercises 3. Bathroom transfers 4. Gait training on level surfaces
Day 6 to discharge	1. Progressive strengthening program 2. Ambulation training with walker 3. Discharge planning 4. Home program instruction and future
4–6 weeks	1. Home exercise program 2. Crutch walking: full weight bearing with cemented prosthesis 3. Crutch walking: partial weight bearing with cementless prosthesis 4. Stationary bicycle with no resistance precautions
7–12 weeks	1. Continuation of exercises: strengthening, balance, proprioception activities 2. Gradually begin walking without use of crutches if local custom permits 3. Increase in time on the stationary bicycle with slight resistance
12–24 weeks	1. Continuation of exercises 2. Maintain flexion of knee at 110 degrees and extension to 0 degrees 3. Walking program for 15–20 minutes 4. Stationary bicycle for 20–30 minutes with slight resistance

functional performance decrements, particularly in knee torque and angular velocity during locomotion compared with the healthy control subjects.

A combination of factors could account for these results, such as severity of preoperative OA, scar tissue formation after surgery, and concurrent OA of the hip. Because clients with a TKA will need to compensate for any loss of range of motion in the knee by increasing hip motion, severe OA of the hip should be addressed before a TKA is done. The investigators recommended that exercise programs for rehabilitation should be selected to address knee angular velocity and torque during gait and ADL. They further con-

cluded that locomotor ADL demand relatively slow loaded angular velocities and low knee torques, also important when planning exercise protocols.[78]

Quantification of Contact Pressures at the Hip

Strickland et al[79] and Givens-Heiss et al[80] reported data derived from a single client who underwent the implantation of a right instrumented hip endoprosthesis designed to quantify contact pressures on the acetabular cartilage. The prosthesis instrumentation has been described elsewhere.[81,82] The prosthesis was designed to transmit acetabular cartilage pressure data via 10

Table 11-9. Physical Therapy Protocol for Total Knee Arthroplasty[75]

Status and Time	Activity
Preoperative: 1–2 months	1. Instruction in range of motion exercises 2. Restoration of or improvement in functional strength of the knee 3. Instruction in and/or fitting with continuous passive motion machine to acquaint client 4. Instruction in deep breathing exercises
Postoperative: 24 hours	1. Check on continuous passive motion machine or complete manual passive motion 2. Deep breathing and coughing exercises 3. Exercises for circulation and range of motion within a pain-free range
Day 2	1. Gentle mobility of patella 2. Bed-to-chair transfers 3. Ambulation with walker with assistance if this is local custom
Days 3–5	1. Range of motion exercises 2. Gentle strengthening exercises 3. Ambulation training with walker
Day 6 to discharge	1. Reinforce bed exercises 2. Reinforce postoperative precautions 3. Gait training 4. Stair climbing 5. Discharge planning 6. Home exercise and ADL program
First clinic visit: 2–3 weeks after surgery	1. Review home program 2. Add standing hip abductor exercises 3. Supine iliotibial band stretches 4. Walker/crutch ambulation review
Second clinic visit: At 6 weeks	1. Review exercise program 2. Side lying hip abduction 3. Supine iliotibial band stretches 4. Cane ambulation (cemented prosthesis) 5. Progressive weight bearing with walker/crutches (uncemented prosthesis)
Third clinic visit: At 12 weeks	1. Review entire exercise program 2. Begin cane ambulation with uncemented prosthesis

*ADL = activities of daily living.

different transducers to a computer where it could be stored and analyzed. Although data are reported only for a single client, the results are revealing about the effect of various exercises and activities upon the hip joint. During the period immediately after surgery, the client was asked to complete several non–weight-bearing activities, because it is a common belief that these activities require reduced contact on the joint surfaces while the client is lying supine, namely, isometric quadriceps setting, isometric gluteus maximus setting, active hip flexion, and active hip abduction. Measured in megapascals (MPa), active hip flexion produced the greatest amount of acetabular pressure (4.79 MPa), and isometric quadriceps contraction with the knee in extension produced the lowest. The next highest peak pressure on the acetabular cartilage was obtained during isometric gluteus maximus contraction (4.65 MPa).

Researchers have reported that *touchdown weight bearing*, when performed correctly, generates less acetabular stress than partial weight bearing, full weight bearing, or non–weight bearing with the knee extended.[79–82] Weight-bearing activities included stepping exercises with both right and left legs (weight shifting) and standing up from a chair. When all activities were placed in order of pressure produced, the pressures on the acetabulum occurred in the following ascending order: isometric quadriceps setting (3.44 MPa), stepping right, active abduction exercise, stepping left, standing up, isometric gluteus maximus exercises, and active hip flexion (4.79 MPa). Although these results cannot be extrapolated to other clients with an endoprosthesis, they do point out that exercises we ask clients to do are not benign activities. We could be asking the client to complete exercises that are producing higher femoroacetabular pressures than those required by weight-shifting and standing-up activities. More studies must be completed before these results are generalizable to all clients with total hip replacements.

Measurement of Other Parameters

In a subsequent study of the postacute phase after surgery in this same patient,[82] other rehabilitation parameters were measured including full weight-bearing free speed walking, partial weight-bearing (13.6 kg) ambulation with crutches, touchdown weight-bearing (4.5 kg) ambulation with crutches, non–weight-bearing ambulation with crutches (swing to or through gait), maximal voluntary isometric abduction exercise with resistance, and straight leg raising. These were evaluated to determine in vivo pressures on the acetabular cartilage. Study results showed that aided gait can reduce the stress on the acetabular cartilage. Partial weight-bearing, touchdown weight-bearing, and non–weight-bearing ambulation, however, did not always follow a hierarchical relationship based on the degree of prescribed weight bearing. The authors suggested that exercises such as straight leg raising and gravity-reduced abduction that do not produce high muscle forces could be favored over resisted isometric exercise to reduce acetabular contact pressures. There might be, however, lower muscle strength gains than expected from resisted exercises.

To generalize these findings, further research is needed on a larger sample of clients. These studies are a good start for determining what actually happens when a person with an endoprosthesis exercises and ambulates.

During rehabilitation, the physical therapist should consider other health care providers who can assist in improving the client's progress and quality of life. For example, the occupational therapist could recommend joint protection aids for use during ADL at home and in the workplace (see Chapter 14). A social worker could be involved in helping the client with financial concerns and with obtaining short- and long-term disability payments or special parking permits. A therapeutic recreational therapist may assist in enabling clients to return to former sport and recreational activities, such as golf.

Outcome Measures

Objective treatment outcomes are needed in all spheres of PT, as regulators and health services payees demand more cost-effective services. You will recall from Figure 11-1 that outcome measures were divided into two major categories: clinical tests and measurements and functional tests and measurements (see Appendix II).

Clinical Tests and Measurements

These tests are not necessarily unique to the assessment of a person with arthritis but rather are generic measures used in other orthopedic entities. Unique to these tests is the rheumatological slant in their interpretation. For example, in the rheumatology literature, scores related to joint pain on motion, joint tenderness, or joint swelling are usually reported on a scale from 0 to 3, with 3 being the most severe situation.[83] The score may appear as an examiner's score or as a self-report score by the client. The Visual Analogue Scale (VAS)[84–86] is commonly used to determine by client report how well she or he is doing in terms of pain, tolerance for the disease, fatigue, sleep, and any other factors known only by the client. It is important to ask the client for his or her assessment in terms of "today," because memory of past experiences can be deceiving.

Walking is a complex task that can identify important clinical information about the person with OA. The outcomes of walking are particularly relevant because decreases in walking speed and changes in stride length can be observed.[87,88] Fransen et al[89] has assessed the reliability of measurements of quantitative gait variables at two self-selected walking speeds in persons with OA of the knee. They reported that quantitative gait analysis and self-reported physical function data provided reliable baseline measurements in the 41 persons they assessed. Furthermore, gait at a *fast* self-selected walking speed provided more reliable measurements than did gait at normal self-selected walking speed.

Manual or any other forms of muscle testing can have spurious results when there is joint pain, instability, or deformity. Having the client perform functional tests, such as the "get-up and go test"[15] and timing how long it takes the client to do this activity will give more realistic information about the status of the involved lower extremity. Balance tests while the client is standing on the lower extremity, in the absence of central nervous system disease, will inform the therapist about the status of the ligaments, muscles, and mechanoreceptors of the joints in the kinetic chain.[16] It is well known that strength and balance decline with age[90] and with OA of the knee.[91,92] The presence of strength decline and joint impairment of the knee and ankle contribute to the potential for falls.[93] The data from these studies readily support the need for physical therapists to recommend preventive and rehabilitative programs that incorporate both strength and balance exercises.

In OA, pain can be referred to other sites that may or may not be involved with the disease. OA of the hip can cause referred pain to the groin and to the knee, OA of the lumbar spine can cause pain referred to the hip and knee, and OA of the shoulder may refer pain to the lateral humerus. The pain referral patterns identified during the initial evaluation and throughout the course of treatment may diminish as the client's condition improves.

Functional Tests and Measurements

Several standardized assessment questionnaires have been developed to assess the abilities of the client with OA (for specific tests see Appendix II and Chapter 17). Each of these instruments has strengths and weaknesses.

The Western Ontario and McMaster Universities (WOMAC)[3] Index has been validated by Bellamy et al[3] for specific measurement of clients with OA in clinical trials. The WOMAC Index asks the client to report information in three dimensions: pain, stiffness, and physical function. It is a useful tool to use before and after treatment to measure the perception of the client about their treatment. McConnell et al[94] recently reported their conclusions on the utility and measurement properties of the WOMAC when using

it to evaluate therapeutic interventions. They stated that the WOMAC is well suited to measure outcomes in total knee or hip arthroplasties. Nilsdotter et al[95] compared the Functional Assessment System (FAS),[96] the WOMAC,[3] and the Medical Outcomes Study 36-Item Short Form (SF-36) (in persons with OA scheduled for total hip replacement). They determined that the WOMAC[3] and the SF-36[10,11] were more responsive measures of pain and function than range of motion, performance tests, and observer-administered questions (FAS) after total hip replacement.

The following measurement scales mentioned were validated on rheumatoid arthritis clients; therefore, the generalizability of these tests to the measurement of outcomes in OA must be considered. The Arthritis Impact Measurement Scale (AIMS)[4] was developed for use as a research tool to collect a wide variety of information from clients about their arthritis, general health, and socioeconomic well-being. Although it is an invaluable data-collecting instrument, it is not easily administered in a busy clinic. The authors of this instrument have created a shorter version of this instrument called the AIMS2,[5] which could be used by clinicians.

The Health Assessment Questionnaire (HAQ)[6] is a widely used self-report tool given to clients to determine their opinion of their functional abilities. It is easily filled out and could be used as a pre- and post-treatment test if client report is what is wanted. Another functional assessment tool is the Functional Status Index.[9] This tool is available in both an interview and self-report form. The Sickness Impact Profile[7,8] is well known for assessing clients' perceptions of how their illness affects their life.

A generic health-related quality-of-life measure, the SF-36, has been reported by various authors[10–12] for use as a measure of disease-specific pain, physical function, quality of life, mobility, and so forth before and after a total knee or hip replacement. Comparisons made between the AIMS2 and the SF-36 suggest that the two should be used together to gain important information regarding the status of the client, because these two instruments complement each other.[10]

A considerable body of literature published on PT demonstrates the importance and use of measurement scales that are reliable and valid. For example, testing at the same time of the day, by the same observer, and in the same environment will enhance the reliability of the measurement. Careful selection of the instrument to be used to evaluate the client is critical if the test is to be valid. As therapists, if we are to make any statement about treatment efficacy, the accuracy and precision of instruments must be carefully considered.

Future Challenges and Implications

It is well known that the prevalence of OA increases with age. Physical therapists should expect to treat more older adults during the 21st century. A major challenge for therapists, when creating a treatment plan, is to understand changes that are due to the aging musculoskeletal system and distinguish them from changes that are produced by OA or problems that may be due to comorbid conditions, such as osteoporosis. Clients who maintain an appropriate weight, engage in a moderate exercise program, and adopt other healthy lifestyles often do well. A second challenge is for therapists to resist the temptation to tell clients that they will have to live with their arthritis. A final challenge is to create a mutually agreed upon plan of care that clients will willingly follow and work to take care of themselves.

Research Questions

A challenge to PT researchers will be to validate treatment methods and suggest improved ways of delivery of care. For example, to what extent do the modalities we use to treat OA make a difference on the outcomes of treatment? What are the most effective ways to deliver PT or OT services to persons with OA? How do we measure outcomes to indicate whether PT or OT has increased the quality of life of the client? To what extent does PT or OT intervention deter disability and enhance a return to the workforce by persons with OA? To what extent are alternative forms of medicine or therapies being used by the client and how are these affecting PT management? To what extent does deficit joint position sense in OA affect PT management?

Because a cure for OA is not imminent, our attitudes and practices as therapists should maximize the quality of life experienced by our clients. This question remains to be answered: *What are our preconceived notions about persons with OA and do these attitudes influence treatment and outcome measures?* These are some issues that current and future researchers might investigate.

Skeleton Case Study

Age: 71 years
Gender: Male
Diagnosis: OA of right knee (medial compartment > lateral compartment)
Occupation: Retired rancher
Onset: 10 years ago
Stage: Chronic, stage II radiographs, functional class 3
Severity: Moderate to severe, crepitus, bony tenderness and enlargement, stiffness for <30 minutes
Adherence: Moderate
Pharmacological management: Naproxen 400 mg qid, status post closed tidal joint lavage
Ethnic group: North American white

References

1. Felson DT, Anderson JJ, Naimark A et al: Obesity and knee osteoarthritis: the Framingham Study. *Ann Intern Med* 109:18–24, 1988.
2. American Physical Therapy Association: Guide to Physical Therapist Practice, ed 2. *Phys Ther* 81:9–744, 2001.
3. Bellamy N, Buchanan WW, Goldsmith CH et al: Validation study of WOMAC: a health status instrument for measuring clinically important patients relevant, outcomes to antirheumatic drug therapy in patients with OA of the hip or knee. *J Rheumatol* 15:1833–1840, 1988.
4. Meenan RF: The AIMS approach in health status measurement: conceptual background and measurement properties. *J Rheumatol* 9:785–788, 1982.
5. Meenan RF, Mason JH, Anderson JJ et al: AIMS2: the content and properties of a revised and expanded Arthritis Impact Measurement Health Status Questionnaire. *Arthritis Rheum* 35:1–10, 1992.
6. Fries JF, Spitz P, Kraines RG et al: Measurement of patient outcome in arthritis. *Arthritis Rheum* 23:137–145, 1980.
7. Bergner M, Bobbitt RA, Pollard WE et al: The Sickness Impact Profile: validation of a health status measure. *Med Care* 14:56–67, 1976.
8. Pollard WE, Bobbitt RA, Bergner M et al: The Sickness Impact Profile: reliability of a health status measure. *Med Care* 14:146–155, 1976.
9. Jette AM: Functional Status Index: reliability of a chronic disease evaluation instrument. *Arch Phys Med Rehabil* 61:395–401, 1980.
10. Chewning B, Bell C, Nowlin N et al: A comparison of AIMS2 and SF-36 health quality of life measures. *Arthritis Rheum* 37(suppl):S225, 1994.
11. Bombardier C, Melfi CA, Paul J et al: Comparison of a generic and a disease-specific measure of pain and physical function after knee replacement surgery. *Arthritis Rheum* 37(suppl):S225, 1994.
12. Stucki G, Liang MH, Phillips C et al: The Short Form-36 is preferable to the SIP as a generic health status measure in patients undergoing elective total hip arthroplasty. *Arthritis Care Res* 8:174–181, 1995.
13. Moll JMH, Wright V: Normal range of spinal mobility: an objective clinical study. *Ann Rheum Dis* 30:381–386, 1971.
14. Tinetti ME: Performance-oriented assessment of mobility problems in elderly patients. *J Am Geriatr Soc* 34:119–126, 1986.

15. Mathias S, Nayak USL, Isaacs B: Balance in elderly patients: the "get-up and go" test. *Arch Phys Med Rehabil* 67:387–389, 1986.
16. Berg KO, Maki BE, Williams JI et al: Clinical and laboratory measures of postural balance in an elderly population. *Arch Phys Med Rehabil* 73:1073–1080, 1992.
17. World Health Organization: 715. Osteoarthrosis and allied disorders. *International Classification of Diseases*, ed 9 revision. Clinical Modification (ICD-9-CM 2001), vols 1 and 3. Chicago, American Medical Association, 2000.
18. Mathews JA: Neck pain. In Klippel JH, Dieppe PA (eds): *Rheumatology*. St Louis, Mosby Yearbook, 1994, pp 5.1–5.14.
19. Dunbar J, Dunning EJ, Dwyer K: Compliance measurement with arthritis regimen. *Arthritis Care Res* 2:S8–S16, 1989.
20. Ross FM: Patient compliance—whose responsibility? *Soc Sci Med* 32:89–94, 1991.
21. Sluijs EM, Knibbe J: Patient compliance with exercise: Different theoretical approaches to short-term and long-term compliance. *Patient Educ Couns* 17:191–204, 1991.
22. Sluijs EM, Kok GJ, van der Zee J: Correlates of exercise compliance in physical therapy. *Phys Ther* 73:771–782, 1993.
23. Parker JC, Bradley LA, DeVellis R et al: Biopsychosocial contributions to the management of arthritis disability. *Arthritis Rheum* 36:885–889, 1993.
24. Jensen GM, Lorish C: Physical therapists' approach to home exercise programs: identification of routine beliefs and behaviors. *Phys Ther* 72:S72, 1992.
25. Dexter PA: Joint exercises in elderly persons with symptomatic osteoarthritis of the hip or knee: performance patterns, medical support patterns, and the relationship between exercising and medical care. *Arthritis Care Res* 5:36–41, 1992.
26. Wiener C: Untrained, unpaid, and unacknowledged: the patient as a worker. *Arthritis Care Res* 2:16–21, 1989.
27. Daniels A: Invisible work. *Soc Probl* 34:403–415, 1987.
28. Ross CK, Sinacore JM, Stiers W et al: The role and expectations and preferences in health care satisfaction of patients with arthritis. *Arthritis Care Res* 3:92–98, 1990.
29. Mankin HJ: The reaction of articular cartilage to injury and osteoarthritis. *N Engl J Med* 291:1335–1340, 1974.
30. Brown MB, Hislop HJ, Waters RL et al: Walking efficiency before and after total hip replacement. *Phys Ther* 60:1259–1263, 1980.
31. Gussoni M, Margonato V, Ventura R et al: Energy cost of walking with hip joint impairment. *Phys Ther* 70:295–301, 1990.
32. Waters RL: Energy expenditure. In Perry J (ed): *Gait Analysis: Normal and Pathological Function*. Thorofare, NJ, Slack Publishers, 1992, pp 444–481.
33. Neumann DA: Biomechanical analysis of selected principles of hip joint protection. *Arthritis Care Res* 2:146–155, 1989.
34. Self BP, Greenwald RM, Pflaster DS: A biomechanical analysis of a medial unloading brace for osteoarthritis in the knee. *Arthritis Care Res* 13:191–197, 2000.
35. Hart DL: Spinal mobility: Braces and corsets. In Gould JA (ed): *Orthopedic and Sports Physical Therapy*, ed 2. St Louis, CV Mosby, 1990, pp 272–280.
36. Krämer J: The treatment of cervical syndrome. In Krämer J (ed): *Intervertebral Disc Diseases: Causes, Diagnosis, Treatment and Prophylaxis*. Chicago, Year Book Publishers, 1981, pp 85–102.
37. Johnson RM, Hart DL, Simmons EF et al: Cervical orthoses: a study comparing their effectiveness in restricting cervical motion in normal subjects. *J Bone Joint Surg Am* 59:332–339, 1977.
38. Cordery J, Rocchi M: Joint protection and fatigue management. In Melvin JL, Jensen G (eds): *Rheumatologic Rehabilitation: Assessment and Management*, vol 1. Bethesda, MD, The American Occupational Therapy Association, 1998, pp 279–322.
39. Peterson MGE, Kovar-Toledano PA, Otis JC et al: Effects of a walking program on gait characteristics in patients with osteoarthritis. *Arthritis Care Res* 6:11–16, 1993.
40. Kovar PA, Allegrante JP, MacKenzie CR et al: Supervised fitness walking in patients with osteoarthritis of the knee: a randomized, controlled trial. *Ann Intern Med* 116:529–534, 1992.
41. Minor MA, Hewett JE, Webel RR et al: Efficacy of physical conditioning exercise in patients with rheumatoid arthritis and osteoarthritis. *Arthritis Rheum* 32:1396–1405, 1989.
42. Price LG, Hewett JE, Kay DR et al: Five-minute walking test of aerobic fitness for people with arthritis. *Arthritis Care Res* 1:33–37, 1988.
43. Minor MA, Hewett JE, Webel RR et al: Exercise tolerance and disease related measures in patients with rheumatoid arthritis and osteoarthritis. *J Rheumatol* 15:905–911, 1988.
44. Beals CA, Lampman RM, Banwell BF et al: Measurement of exercise tolerance in patients with rheumatoid arthritis and osteoarthritis. *J Rheumatol* 12:458–461, 1985.
45. Michlovitz SL: Use of heat and cold in the management of rheumatic diseases. In Michlovitz SL (ed): *Thermal Agents in Rehabilitation*, vol I. Philadelphia, FA Davis Co, 1986, pp 277–294.
46. Lehman JF: Therapeutic hot and cold. In Lehman JF (ed): *Therapeutic Heat and Cold*. Baltimore, Williams & Wilkins, 1982, pp 404–602.
47. Welch V, Brosseau L, Peterson J et al: Therapeutic ultrasound for osteoarthritis of the knee (Cochrane review). The Cochrane Library, Issue 1, Oxford, Update Software, 2002. (www.cochranelibrary.com; info@cochranelibrary.com).
48. Falconer J, Hayes KW, Chang RW: Therapeutic ultrasound in the treatment of musculoskeletal conditions. *Arthritis Care Res* 3:85–91, 1990.
49. Brosseau L, Welch V, Wells G, et al: Low level laser therapy (classes I, II and III) for treating osteoarthritis (Cochrane review). The Cochrane Library, Issue 1, Oxford, Update Software, 2002. (www.cochranelibrary.com; info@cochranelibrary.com).

50. Osiri M, Welch V, Brosseau L et al: Transcutaneous electrical nerve stimulation for knee osteoarthritis (Cochrane review). The Cochrane Library, Issue 1, Oxford, Update Software, 2002. (www.cochranelibrary. com; info@cochranelibrary.com).

51. Sheon RP, Moskowitz RW, Goldberg VM: Introduction: an overview of diagnosis and management. In Sheon RP, Moskowitz RW, Goldberg VM (eds): *Soft Tissue Rheumatic Pain: Recognition, Management, Prevention,* ed 3. Baltimore, MD, Williams & Wilkins, 1996, pp 1–17.

52. Danneskiold-Samsoe B, Christiansen E, Andersen RB: Myofascial pain and the role of myoglobin. *Scand J Rheumatol* 15:174–178, 1986.

53. Chamberlain MA, Care G, Harfield B: Physiotherapy in osteoarthrosis of the knee: a controlled trial of hospital versus home exercises. *Int Rehabil Med* 4:104–106, 1982.

54. Falconer J, Hayes KW, Chang RW: Effect of ultrasound on mobility in osteoarthritis of the knee: a randomized clinical trial. *Arthritis Care Res* 5:29–35, 1992.

55. Green J, McKenna F, Redfern EJ et al: Home exercises are as effective as outpatient hydrotherapy for osteoarthritis of the hip. *Br J Rheumatol* 32:812–815, 1993.

56. Hecht PJ, Bachmann S, Booth RE et al: Effects of thermal therapy on rehabilitation after total knee arthroplasty. *Clin Orthop* 178:198–201, 1983.

57. Swezey RL: Therapeutic modalities for pain relief. In Swezey RL (ed): *Arthritis. Rational Therapy and Rehabilitation.* Philadelphia, WB Saunders, 1978, pp 1–17.

58. Barak T, Rosen ER, Sofer R: Basic concepts of orthopedic manual therapy. In Gould JA (ed): *Orthopedic and Sports Physical Therapy,* ed 2. St Louis, CV Mosby, 1990, pp 195–211.

59. Cyriax J: *Textbook of Orthopedic Medicine. Treatment by Manipulation, Massage and Injection,* vol 2. Baltimore, Williams & Wilkins, 1974.

60. McKenzie RA: *Mechanical Diagnosis and Therapy.* Waikanae, New Zealand, Spinal Publications, 1981.

61. Mennell J: *Joint Pain Diagnosis and Treatment Using Manipulative Techniques.* New York, Little, Brown & Co, 1964, p 178.

62. Kessler RM: Arthrology. In Hertling D, Kessler RM (eds). *Management of Common Musculoskeletal Disorders: Physical Therapy Principles and Methods,* ed 2. Philadelphia, Harper & Row, 1983, pp 33–38.

63. Travell JG, Simons DG: Apropos of all muscles. In Travell JG, Simons DG (eds): *Myofascial Pain and Dysfunction: The Trigger Point Manual,* vol I. Baltimore, Williams & Wilkins, 1983, pp 86–88.

64. Burckhardt CS, Clark SR, Nelson DL: Assessing physical fitness of women with rheumatic disease. *Arthritis Care Res* 1:38–44, 1988.

65. Lankhorst GJ, Van de Stadt RJ, von der Korst JK et al: Relationship of isometric knee extension torque and functional variables in osteoarthrosis of the knee. *Scand J Rehabil Med* 14:7–10, 1982.

66. Liberson WT: Brief isometric exercises. In Basmajian J (ed): *Therapeutic Exercise,* ed 4. Baltimore, Williams & Wilkins, 1984, pp 236–256.

67. Sanders B: Exercise and rehabilitation concepts. In Malone TR, McPoil TG, Nitz AJ (eds): *Orthopedic and Sports Physical Therapy,* ed 3. St Louis, CV Mosby, 1996, pp 211–224.

68. American College of Sports Medicine: *Guidelines for Graded Exercise Testing and Exercise Prescription,* ed 2. Philadelphia, Lea & Febiger, 1980, p 151.

69. Westby MD: A health professional's guide to exercise prescription for people with arthritis: a review of aerobic fitness activities. *Arthritis Care Res* 45:501–511, 2001.

70. Arthritis Foundation: *The Arthritis Foundation's Guide to Intimacy with Arthritis.* http://www.arthritis.org/resources, accessed 2/28/03.

71. Sledge CB: Introduction to surgical management. In Kelley WN, Harris ED, Ruddy S et al (eds): *Textbook of Rheumatology,* ed 4, vol 2. Philadelphia, WB Saunders Co, 1993, pp 1745–1751.

72. Figgie MP: Introduction to the surgical treatment of rheumatic diseases. In Klippel JH, Dieppe JA (eds): *Rheumatology.* St Louis, CV Mosby, 1994, pp 8.20.1–8.20.6.

73. Kampa K: Hip injuries: a rehabilitation perspective. In Lewis CB, Knortz KA (eds): *Orthopedic Assessment and Treatment of the Geriatric Patient.* St Louis, CV Mosby, 1993, pp 243–262.

74. Knortz KA: Knee injuries: a rehabilitation perspective. In Lewis CB, Knortz KA (eds): *Orthopedic Assessment and Treatment of the Geriatric Patient.* St Louis, CV Mosby, 1993, pp 301–322.

75. Nelson KA, Rasmussen T: *Total Knee Replacement.* Salt Lake City, Intermountain Health Care, 1985, pp 1–20.

76. Barrett DS, Cobb AG, Bentley G: Joint proprioception in normal, osteoarthritic and replaced knees. *J Bone Joint Surg Br* 73-B:53–56, 1991.

77. Stauffer RN, Chao FYS, Gryöry AN: Biomechanical gait analysis of the diseased knee joint. *Clin Orthop* 126:246–255, 1977.

78. Jevsevar DS, Riley PO, Hodge AW et al: Knee kinematics and kinetics during locomotor activities of daily living in subjects with knee arthroplasty and in healthy control subjects. *Phys Ther* 73:229–239, 1993.

79. Strickland EM, Fares M, Krebs DE et al: In vivo acetabular contact pressures during rehabilitation. Part I. Acute phase. *Phys Ther* 72:691–699, 1992.

80. Givens-Heiss DL, Krebs DE, Riley PO et al: In vivo acetabular contact pressures during rehabilitation. Part II. Postacute phase. *Phys Ther* 72:700–710, 1992.

81. Mann RW, Burgess RG: An instrumented endoprosthesis for measuring pressure on acetabular cartilage in vivo. In *Proceedings of the Workshop on Implantable Telemetry in Orthopaedics.* Berlin, Federal Republic of Germany, 1990, pp 1–13.

82. Krebs DE, Elbaum L, Riley PO et al: Exercise and gait effects on in vivo hip contact pressures. *Phys Ther* 71:301–309, 1991.

83. American Rheumatism Association: Joint examination. In *Dictionary of the Rheumatic Diseases.* New York, Contact Associates International, 1982, pp 75–80.

84. Dixon JS, Bird HA: Reproducibility along a 10 cm. vertical visual analogue scale. *Ann Rheum Dis* 40:87–89, 1981.

85. Scott J, Huskisson EC: Vertical or horizontal visual analogue scales. *Ann Rheum Dis* 38:560, 1979.

86. Langley GB, Sheppard H: The visual analog scale: Its use in pain measurement. *Rheum Int* 5:145–148, 1985.

87. Blin O, Pailhous J, Lafforgue P, Serratrice G: Quantitative analysis of walking patients with knee osteorthritis: a method of assessing the effective of non-steroidal anti-inflammatory treatment. *Ann Rheum Dis* 4:990–993, 1990.

88. Kroll M, Otis J, Sculco T et al: The relationship of stride characteristics to pain before and after total knee arthroplasty. *Clin Orthop* 239:191–195, 1989.

89. Fransen M, Crosbie J, Edmonds J: Reliability of gait measurements in people with osteoarthritis of the knee. *Phys Ther* 77:944–953, 1997.

90. Rogers MA, Evans WJ: Changes in skeletal muscle with aging: effects of exercise training. *Exerc Sport Sci Rev* 21:65–102, 1993.

91. Fisher NM, Pendergast DR, Gresham GE, Calkins E: Muscle rehabilitation: its effect on muscular and functional performance of patients with knee osteoarthritis. *Arch Phys Med Rehabil* 72:367–374, 1991.

92. Messier SP, Loeser RF, Hoover JL et al: Osteoarthritis of the knee: effects on gait, strength, and flexibility. *Arch Phys Med Rehabil* 73:29–36, 1992.

93. Messier SP, Glasser JL, Ettinger WH Jr et al: Declines in strength and balance in older adults with chronic knee pain: A 30-month longitudinal, observational study. *Arthritis Care Res* 47:141–148, 2002.

94. McConnell S, Kolopack P, Davis AM: The Western Ontario and McMaster Universities Osteoarthritis Index (WOMAC): a review of its utility and measurement properties. *Arthritis Care Res* 45:453–461, 2001.

95. Nilsdotter AK, Roos EM, Westerlund JP, et al: Comparative responsiveness of measures of pain and function after total hip replacement. *Arthritis Care Res* 45:258–262, 2001.

96. Öberg U, Öberg B, Öberg T: Validity and reliability of a new assessment of lower-extremity dysfunction. *Phys Ther* 74:861–871, 1994.

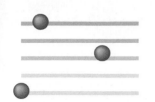

CHAPTER 12

Management of Persons with Chronic Muscle Pain Syndromes

Roger A. Scudds, PhD, PT,
Rhonda J. Scudds, PhD, PT, and
Katherine Harman, PhD, MSc, BSc(PT)

Muscle tissue as a source of pain is especially familiar to physical therapists, and the focus of much of our work is with muscle pain that resolves. However, the presence of pain that is resistant to treatment presents a difficult clinical challenge. Pain is a complex multidimensional experience with sensory, affective, and cognitive components.[1] This description is very important to remember for any pain state but is particularly relevant when chronic muscle pain syndromes (CMPSs) are considered, in which any one of these three components can lead to or promote the maintenance of chronic pain. Adequate management of CMPSs for optimal treatment and outcome will require that each of the three factors is addressed. In this chapter we present background information about chronic pain, guidelines for differentiating myofascial pain from fibromyalgia, and current management of CMPSs with an emphasis on evidence that demonstrates efficacy.

PHYSICAL REHABILITATION IN ARTHRITIS, Joan M. Walker, PhD, PT, and Antoine Helewa, MSc(Clin Epid), PT, Elsevier Inc. © 2004.

Chronic Muscle Pain Syndrome

A standard definition of chronic pain is "pain that persists for a period of more than 6 months".[2] However, a more practical way to conceptualize chronic pain perhaps, is to define it as "pain that outlasts the expected resolution of tissue damage."[3] In either view the result is the same: pain that has been experienced for a significant period of time will affect the person's lifestyle, personality, relationships, and work capacity. When pain becomes so dominant that it affects all interactions between an individual and his or her environment, then the person can be said to have a chronic pain syndrome (CPS).[4] The challenges of chronic pain are not only the impact it has on day-to-day life but also the difficulty in understanding its cause and effect. Whereas people with CPS experience high levels of pain, physical disability, and psychological distress, these may have no direct relationship with the original cause of the pain. These are key considerations in CPS and must be understood by both health professionals and clients for successful management.

Most health care professionals base their interventions on objective physical findings that are related to the cause of the symptoms, from which treatment plans are developed. However, with CMPSs, goals planned in this manner may not be achievable because, by the time muscle pain becomes chronic, the objective findings may no longer relate to the original cause. This is because strong, noxious stimulation results in the sensitization of the central nervous system, which then responds to subsequent stimulation (noxious and non-noxious) in a hypersensitive manner.[5] This heightened response leads to other symptoms and behaviors that health professionals might not expect to see in connection with the original condition, posing a diagnostic and treatment challenge to the client and the clinician. This may lead to frustration, mistrust, and wasted effort for both parties, as well as a temptation for the health care provider to believe that there is nothing to treat. Adopting this position only leads the person with a CMPS to seek second opinions and alternative therapies in search of a cure. Simple pain reduction should not be the aim of treatment, rather it should be rehabilitation in its truest sense, whereby the clinician helps the person with a CMPS to maximize her or his abilities in the presence of physical, psychological, and social challenges. The two main presentations of chronic muscle pain are fibromyalgia and myofascial pain, and these two conditions will be presented below from the perspective of their different clinical presentation.

History

Muscular rheumatism is the term originally used to describe chronic muscle pain conditions of which fibromyalgia (originally fibrositis) and myofascial pain are two subsets. It was through efforts to relieve pain by massage that the palpable bands of myofascial pain and the classic tender points of fibromyalgia were first described.[6] The two sets of symptoms have been challenges for diagnosis and description ever since, but a body of knowledge has slowly evolved that clearly differentiates the two conditions.

Fibromyalgia

Clinical Presentation

Fibromyalgia is a common condition that has a reported prevalence of 2% to 3.3%, with a higher number of women presenting with the condition than men (ratio of 3.4:0.5).[7,8] The common clinical presentation of fibromyalgia is a gradual onset of symptoms in mid-life; however, there also is often an initial traumatic (physical or psychological) event.[9] As described in Chapter 4, the principal presentation is widespread pain, but other common symptoms include fatigue, sleep difficulties, paresthesia, and a swollen feeling in the extremities. In addition, because comorbid conditions include headache, chronic fatigue syndrome, environmental sensitivity, and irritable bowel syndrome, these findings have stimulated research into the implications of the immune system on fibromyalgia.[7,10] Another clinical presentation of note is the lack of joint swelling and usually the presence of normal range of motion (ROM) and neurological function.[11] Indeed, many people with fibromyalgia appear normal, and yet their pain significantly disables them. As with other chronic pain conditions, concomitant psychological challenges associated with fibromyalgia have been identified.[12] The most common problems are increases in anxiety, depression, and hypochondriasis. The clinical finding that is the most striking and that also forms the criteria for diagnosis is the existence of tender points.[13] In everyone, these tender points are more sensitive than other points in the body, but they are much more sensitive in people with fibromyalgia than in healthy control subjects and in people with rheumatoid arthritis (RA).[14] This sensitivity is believed to be a reflection of an impaired pain modulation system.[15] However, it has been shown that the tender point sensitivity returns toward normal values after successful treatment.[16] (See Chapters 4 and 5 for more in-depth coverage.) Fibromyalgia also is diagnosed in

Table 12-1. The American College of Rheumatology 1990 Criteria for the Classification of Fibromyalgia

History of widespread pain.
  Definition. Pain is considered widespread when all of the following are present: pain in both sides of the body, pain above and below the waist. In addition, axial skeletal pain (cervical spine, anterior chest, thoracic spine or low back) must be present. Low back pain is considered lower segment pain.
Pain in 11 of 18 tender points on digital palpation.
  Definition. Pain, on digital palpation, must be present in at least 11 of the following 18 tender point sites:
  Occiput: at the suboccipital muscle insertions
  Low cervical: at the anterior aspects of the intertransverse spaces at C5–C7
  Trapezius: at the midpoint of the upper border
  Supraspinatus: at origin, above the scapula spine near the medial border
  Second rib: upper lateral aspects of the second costochondral junction
  Lateral epicondyle: 2 cm distal to the epicondyles
  Gluteal: in upper outer quadrants of buttocks in anterior fold of muscle
  Greater trochanter: posterior to the trochanteric prominence
  Knee: at the medial fat pad proximal to the joint line
Digital palpation should be performed with an approximate force of 4 kg. A tender point has to be painful at palpation not just "tender."

Adapted from Wolfe F, Smythe HA, Yunas MB, et al: The American College of Rheumatology 1990 Criteria for the Classification of Fibromyalgia. Report of the Multicenter Criteria Committee. *Arthritis Rheum* 33:160–172, 1990.

children and adolescents, with a clinical presentation much the same as that in adults.[17]

Current Diagnostic Criteria

In 1990, a multicenter study established the criteria for the diagnosis of fibromyalgia.[7] The American College of Rheumatology adopted these criteria, which are shown in Table 12-1. These criteria were shown to have a sensitivity of 88.4% and a specificity of 81.1% for distinguishing fibromyalgia from other rheumatic conditions, such as RA, osteoarthritis (OA), and other arthralgia syndromes. The major signs of fibromyalgia are chronic, generalized pain with the addition of extreme tenderness to digital pressure at predefined tender points throughout the body. These points are shown in Figure 12-1.

It should be emphasized that although people with fibromyalgia have exquisite tenderness at these tender points they are unlikely to be aware of that tenderness until specifically examined. People with fibromyalgia complain of "pain all over," not at specific points. This is one reason why the points are so useful in the diagnosis of fibromyalgia in the person who has not been educated previously about their significance.

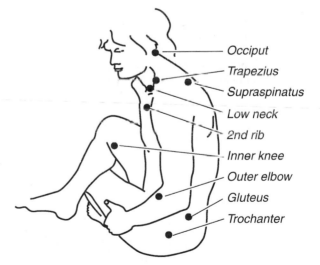

Figure 12-1. The tender points in the American College of Rheumatology criteria set. Scoring: 0 (none) to 4 (client untouchable; withdraws without palpation).

The diagnostic criteria do not include the many other distressing symptoms that often are associated with fibromyalgia, such as sleep disturbance, chronic fatigue, peripheral vascular changes, and irritable bowel syndrome; these require separate assessment.[17]

Theories on Etiology

The cause of fibromyalgia is unknown; however, research has focused on muscle metabolism, sleep disturbance, and neurochemical changes, as well as consideration of psychological factors. Study results suggest that people with fibromyalgia have abnormalities in muscle energy metabolism, local muscle hypoxia, and reductions in high-energy phosphate levels.[18,19] Along with the chronic pain of fibromyalgia, people experience physical deconditioning. Although muscle changes consistent with deconditioning are found with almost the same frequency in sedentary control subjects, they may contribute to findings of decreased physical performance[20] and muscle fatigue in those with fibromyalgia. Recent evidence has shown that afferent input from damaged muscles is very effective in producing neuroplastic changes,[21] such as hyperexcitability in sensory neurons in the spinal cord.[22] Theoretically, this might lead to the secondary hyperalgesia and subsequent spontaneous pain that is seen in fibromyalgia.

Moldofsky[23,24] conducted several sleep studies that led to the hypothesis that fibromyalgia was the result of a delta-rhythm sleep disorder; however, this causal hypothesis has not been supported.[25,26] In addition, the presence of the sleep disorder in healthy persons and its absence in a significant number of people with fibromyalgia has negated its interpretation as related to the pathophysiology of fibromyalgia.[25,27] Serotonin, a neurochemical involved in the modulation of sleep, mood, and pain, has been implicated in fibromyalgia. In addition, serotonin is involved with stress, which has been identified as being an important component to the genesis of fibromyalgia.[28] Thus, pharmacological manipulation of serotonin has been a focus of medical management of the condition.[15,29]

The widespread pain that is experienced by people with fibromyalgia has prompted the hypothesis that central systemic processes may be involved in its genesis or maintenance.[30] Apart from serotonin, the most salient finding to date has been elevated substance P (SP) levels in the cerebrospinal fluid (CSF) of individuals with fibromyalgia.[31] Correlations have been demonstrated between CSF SP and delta-rhythm sleep abnormalities.[30] The production of CSF SP can be enhanced by ongoing peripheral pain,[32] elevated levels of CSF nerve growth factor, or CSF dynorphin.[33]

Each of these factors may, in part, account for the symptoms of fibromyalgia. It also has been suggested that deficiencies in the inhibition of pain might result from low spinal Met-enkephalin levels[34] or serotonin levels,[35] both of which have been demonstrated in fibromyalgia. Abnormal brain blood flow also has been found in fibromyalgia, and this has been associated with altered levels of brain SP.[36] Interestingly, it has been suggested that changes in intestinal motility, autonomic neural function, and other fibromyalgia symptoms could relate to a central neurotransmitter imbalance.[30]

Finally, a relatively recent study found a genetic link in fibromyalgia and proposed that there may be a fibromyalgia-associated gene on chromosome 6.[37] If this hypothesis proves to be true, it would be important in identifying the cause of fibromyalgia. At present, however, the etiology of fibromyalgia is still unclear.

Myofascial Trigger Point Pain Syndrome

Clinical Presentation

Although fibromyalgia has been clearly aligned with rheumatology, the regional pain condition of myofascial trigger point pain syndrome (MTPS) also is encountered in people with arthritis. Incidence and prevalence studies of myofascial trigger point pain are lacking, owing to the absence of a clear diagnostic classification system; however, it is considered to be a very common condition with equal representation in men and women.[38] An individual with MTPS will present with pain that has a *regional* representation. That is, the pain will be confined to a body region (e.g., lumbar, shoulder, or neck). The pain complaint is most often described as a dull ache that can range in its presentation from constant to intermittent, with clear aggravating factors. The regional area of pain can have one defined focus or, in more complex presentations, involve a more widespread area. In association with the pain, other symptoms often encountered are restricted range of motion, muscle weakness, postural discomfort, numbness or paresthesia, and peripheral hypothermia. Trigger points are sensitive parts of muscle that, when stimulated with sufficient pressure, will result in pain referred in a pattern that is stereotypic to the muscle containing the trigger point(s). Trigger points do not fall in the same anatomical locations as the tender points of fibromyalgia, but overlap significantly with acupuncture points[39] and are highly associated with motor endplates.[40]

These nondermatomal patterns have been mapped,[41,42] assisting in diagnosis, as well as in determining the source of the pain (i.e., the muscle where the trigger point is located). *Active trigger points* will produce symptoms spontaneously. Such symptoms could be pain but also could be numbness, dysesthesia, or autonomic signs, such as coldness. Often the trigger point may not be actively referring symptoms but becomes activated after trauma, strain, injury, or digital compression or with faulty posture. These points are known as *latent trigger points*. The restricted range of motion and muscle weakness are related to the muscle(s) where the trigger point lies. In addition, directly associated with the trigger point is a physical finding called a *taut band*. This is described as a rope-like firmness within the muscle that can be rolled under palpating fingers.

Although often classed as a chronic muscle pain syndrome, MTPS is unlike other CMPSs because it has an obvious acute phase in which it is responsive to specific interventions, such as injection with lidocaine, spray and stretch techniques and dry needling. However, similar to other pain conditions, it can become long-standing with other associated perpetuating factors, making it resistant to treatment. Examination should include muscle imbalance, such as asymmetry of muscle strength and length, the presence of postural deviation, and ergonomic factors both at home and at work.

Current Diagnostic Criteria

The identification of a trigger point is central to the diagnosis. The currently accepted criteria for MPS are shown in Table 12-2. Most authors agree that the required criteria for MPS are the presence of trigger points, a taut palpable band that lies along the length of the muscle, and an associated pattern of referred pain from the trigger point.

Theories on Etiology

Explanations for the cause of MPS usually point to trauma of muscle or joint in the area where the trigger points and taut bands develop. Postural alignment also is identified as causing the development of MPS; this can be due to structural or habitual patterns that result in lengthened and weakened muscles opposing shortened muscles. Trigger points present in muscle are believed to cause local shortening, furthering the effect of the muscle imbalance. In addition, electromyographic studies have demonstrated that muscles with trigger points are hyper-responsive, show impaired relaxation, and are more easily fatigued.[40] The physiological explanation for trigger points continues to be aggressively researched, with investigation of increased activity at the motor endplate being the theory for which the most convincing evidence exists.[43] Morphological examinations have revealed sarcomeres that are markedly contracted (called *contraction knots*) and dysfunctional motor endplates.[22]

Differentiation between Fibromyalgia and Myofascial Pain and Other Chronic Muscle Pain States

When the clinician assesses a person who has had pain for a long period of time, history taking and examination require careful attention (see the algorithm of management in Figure 12-2). Thus, what may seem to be a simple occurrence of lateral epicondylalgia, anterior chest pain, or a cervical facet joint syndrome may in fact be part of the syndrome in which the person has tenderness over multiple fibromyalgia tender points. After the clinical presentations of the pain conditions described earlier are understood, their differentiation is not so difficult. However, there is often confusion because of the terms that are used to describe the points in both conditions: *trigger points* in MPS and *tender points* in fibromyalgia. Keep in mind that the differential diagnosis of fibromyalgia is one of exclusion. Apart from the diagnostic criteria of chronic widespread pain (on both sides of the body, above and below the waistline) and the presence of tenderness in at least 11 of the 18 fibromyalgia tender

---

Table 12-2. Diagnostic Criteria for Myofascial Pain Syndrome

Trigger point—one or more
Local tenderness
Muscle feels tense
Referred pain pattern—either spontaneous or on activation
Local twitch response

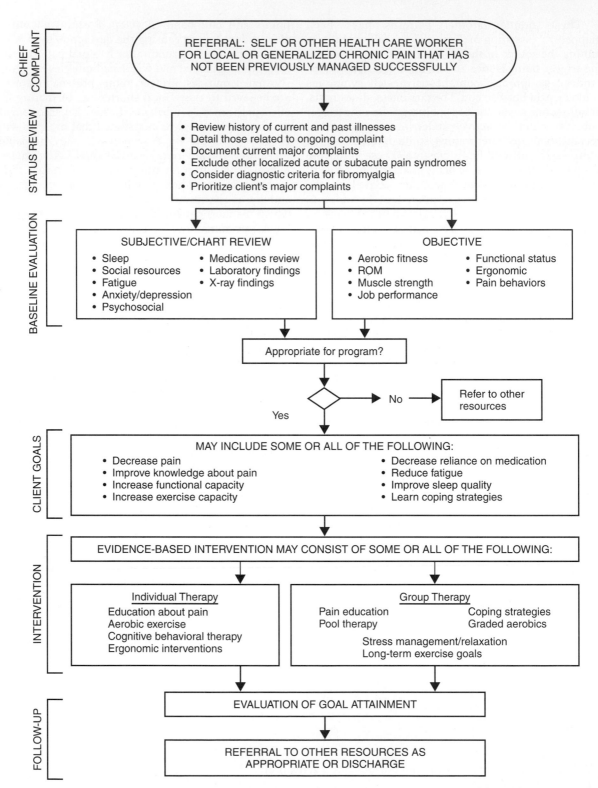

Figure 12-2. Management algorithm for clients with chronic muscle pain syndromes. ROM = range of motion.

Table 12-3. Differences between Fibromyalgia and Myofascial Pain That Assist in Diagnosis

	Fibromyalgia	Myofascial Pain
Cardinal signs	Tender points	Trigger points, taut bands, stereotypic pain referral pattern
Location	Widespread	Regional/local
Nature	Diffuse	Aching
Sensitivity	Responds to weather	
Aggravation factors	Weather, fatigue, exercise, cold	Movement, resisted exercise, sustained postures
Associated symptoms	Irritable bowel syndrome, environmental sensitivity, headache, sleep disturbance	Peripheral hypothermia, restricted range of motion, muscle weakness, numbness, paresthesia
Incidence	Females > males	Females = males

points, there are currently no other routine confirmatory tests that will point to the diagnosis of fibromyalgia. The key concept to remember about MPSs is that pain is generally constrained within a specific site, such as back pain or neck pain. A difficulty can arise when the two conditions coexist in the same individual.[11] Prolonged unresolved pain in one area may lead to secondary changes in another area with a subsequent reduction in pain threshold. Therefore, it is the whole pattern that is important.

There are many points of comparison that assist in the differential diagnosis of the two muscle pain conditions. Table 12-3 presents a comparison of these two entities.

It is important to remember that fibromyalgia in particular and all CMPSs in general can masquerade as other acute pain syndromes. Regrettably, most clinicians do not actively seek out CMPSs but rather look for acute pain syndromes. This may be expected, however, because entry-level physiotherapists lack adequate education in chronic pain.[45] Management must be directed to each possible component of the pain: sensory, affective, and cognitive.

> For legal purposes, use objective tender point assessment and quantitative point counts.

Management of Chronic Muscle Pain Syndromes

When any muscle pain condition becomes chronic, there is much more to deal with than the original cause. Irrespective of the diagnosis—fibromyalgia, myofascial pain, or other muscle pain conditions—there are sensory, affective, and cognitive aspects that must be part of the management program.

Precise management guidelines for most CPMSs and fibromyalgia are limited because of a lack of understanding of their basic pathophysiology. Treatment is based largely on symptom patterns, as well as on the phenomena that are expressed as part of the syndrome, such as physical deconditioning and psychological disturbance. Masi and Yunus[16] suggested that the most effective management approach is a personalized, comprehensive, client-involved program in which the multifactorial nature of the condition is recognized and dealt with in a multidimensional manner.

Medication

As in most pain syndromes, medication is an important part of management of CMPSs. It should be noted, however, that medications may reduce but do not abolish symptoms. Further, the long-term efficacy in these treatments is unknown. The common medications used in chronic pain are analgesics and antidepressants. Reductions in pain and improvements in sleep are the common benefits of medication, but these benefits have not been validated in long-term controlled studies. Clients with chronic pain are at risk of becoming dependent on pain medications, especially after several years of use. In these instances, weaning a client off medications should be one of the aims of management. (See also Chapters 4 and 6.)

> Clients need to recognize their everyday activities as abilities rather than disabilities.

Behavior Modification and Education

Possibly the most influential aspects of any program is education of clients about their illness and modifying their behavior to maximize their coping strategies. Often clients with CMPSs take an "all or nothing" approach to life, overvolunteering for tasks in their lives and thus actively, if unconsciously, contribute to their exhaustion. These clients need to learn how to say "no" to reduce their tendency to become overburdened. It is also important for clients to recognize that although they may voice their inability to do anything at all they actually achieve a fair amount in their daily lives. For example, getting children off to school and taking public transport or driving to their clinical appointments are personal achievements. On the other hand, when an individual realizes that pain is experienced with almost everything that she or he does, then a natural response is to stop doing things that evoke pain. This behavioral response to chronic pain is problematic because the simple avoidance of activity triggers a serious cascade of negative effects. The cardiovascular and musculoskeletal systems become unfit. This deconditioning then becomes a secondary effect that must be addressed in rehabilitation. The avoidance behavior is difficult to reverse, because there are strong psychological obstacles to overcome. Many rehabilitation programs help clients by teaching them that even though they may experience some pain or discomfort as they engage in exercise, this pain will not make them worse but will in fact contribute to their recovery. Therapists can modify a client's behavior by validating what they achieve in their everyday lives and getting the client to see daily functioning as an ability rather than as a disability.

Clients also should be encouraged to participate in social activities, to be an active, contributing member of the group, and to give rather than always receive to reduce the tendency to become isolated and self-centered. Participation in a support group and encouragement to share coping strategies, for example, can support the reaching out and giving aspect that also enhances a client's sense of self-worth. For further detail of coping strategies see Chapter 15.

Physical Rehabilitation Intervention

Exercise

Although pain relief is an important management goal in CMPSs, exercise techniques that will restore symmetry in joint range of motion and improve muscle strength, aerobic capacity, as well as functional activities also are essential. Although not the focus of the program, any lessening of a client's pain will benefit their participation and adherence with a prescribed exercise program. Many clients with CMPSs experience musculoskeletal pain during and after exercise, and this is a major impediment to adherence with an exercise program. The mere presence of pain, however, is not a contraindication to exercise.[47] An additional benefit of exercise is the reduction of fatigue.[48] Aerobic exercise appears to improve the symptoms of fibromyalgia.

McCain et al[49] first demonstrated the efficacy of cardiovascular fitness training in the treatment of a group of subjects with fibromyalgia compared with a group who received only stretching exercise. People with fibromyalgia who had completed cardiovascular fitness training demonstrated increased cardiovascular fitness, improved client and physician global scores, and an increased tender point pain threshold (a measure of fibromyalgia tenderness), whereas the stretching group received lesser benefits from their program. An important point in this research was the ability of subjects who showed improvement to achieve an aerobic threshold during exercise.

In a recent randomized, controlled (RCT) study,[50] 50 of 132 clients with fibromyalgia were randomly assigned to either an aerobic exercise group or a flexibility and relaxation group. Those in the exercise group, with prescribed aerobic exercise, had significantly better outcomes than those who took part in the relaxation and stretching group. Apart from deconditioning, it has been shown that, although people with fibromyalgia may have the same exercise capacity as other people, their perceived exertion while doing the same amount of work was greater.[51] Despite the favorable effects of cardiovascular training, many clients experience worsening of symptoms immediately after exercise.[52] This is not surprising because with CMPSs many people experience pain for a long period of time with consequent deconditioning of muscle and stiffening of joints. These symptoms should not be a deterrent to aerobic exercise. Proper guidance in the gradual increase of exercise intensity is essential.

Although group exercise sessions are popular, individual prescription combined with education on the benefits of exercise and constant encouragement may yield the best results as the person with a CMPS goes through the inevitable ups and downs of the condition.[53,54] Interestingly, Oliver and Cronan[54] demonstrated that exercise self-efficacy, or the perception of one's ability to perform exercise, was a strong predictor of future exercise participation in people with fibromyalgia. In a recent critical review of the subject, it was concluded that there was moderate strength to support the use of aerobic exercise in fibromyalgia but that more RCTs were needed.[55] For further detail on aerobic programs see Chapter 13.

> The presence of pain, stiffness, and weakness should not be regarded as a deterrent to exercise.

Postural Reeducation

Attention should always be paid, where possible, to correction of any muscle imbalances, asymmetry of muscle action, or range of motion or postural deviations. The use of proprioceptive neuromuscular facilitation techniques, such as contract-relax, and repeated contractions may be used to gain end range, and the client should be taught stretching exercises to maintain gained range (see also Chapter 10).

Ergonomic Factors

Faulty work habits and postures either at home or at work should be given attention. A therapist (occupational or physical) may visit the work site to determine if any changes made there, such as desk height, chair style, computer set-up, or general working arrangement, may contribute to improvement in the client's condition and attitude. Specific attention should be given to the client's sleeping arrangements, the quality of the mattress (to avoid the princess and the pea syndrome), and special neck support pillow(s), as well as the posture adopted during sleep to ensure that the neck is fully supported, not twisted, and pressure from the arm and shoulder is relieved.

Other Modalities

Few treatments have been subject to RCTs. However, methods such as acupuncture, aromatherapy, cold, heat, magnetic therapy, manipulation, massage, music therapy, and transcutaneous electrical nerve stimulation (TENS) have all been used with anecdotal claims for success. People with fibromyalgia have been shown to have a preference for passive treatments but will claim to respond to many treatments

initially.[56] It would seem that most modalities will produce a temporary reduction in the pain, but this is seldom long-lasting and might possibly be attributed to a placebo effect.

Modalities, such as heat, cold, laser,[57] electrical stimuli and massage, acupuncture, and manual therapy, are beneficial in terms of achieving muscle relaxation, improved circulation, and pain relief. A survey of fibromyalgia support groups in Canada found that hydrotherapy was the first choice of therapy,[47] but that hot packs, TENS, and relaxation also were highly preferred treatments.[57]

Acupuncture also may be of use in fibromyalgia. A Consensus Statement from the National Institutes of Health[56] stated that there was promising evidence to support the use of acupuncture in fibromyalgia but that controlled clinical trials should be carried out to demonstrate its efficacy. A recent review of the treatment concluded that the limited amount of high-quality evidence that was available suggests that real acupuncture is more effective than sham acupuncture in the management of fibromyalgia.[58] However, the authors point out that few trials are available. Deluze et al[59] used electroacupuncture and sham acupuncture in a controlled trial in their clients with fibromyalgia. They found that more than 75% of clients showed either "satisfactory improvement" or "complete improvement" of their symptoms after the trial. These authors did not provide long-term follow-up data. In a long-term manual acupuncture study over a 6-month period, Sandberg et al[60] reported that fibromyalgia symptoms gradually became markedly diminished and remained low at follow-up. The authors reported that sleep patterns were an important predictor of a successful outcome.

Treatment for MPS is focused on the shortened muscle. To relax or deactivate a trigger point, dry needling[61] and injections with anesthetic agents have been used; these two approaches produced equivalent pain reduction.[62] Non-invasive techniques also are used, such as massage, ultrasound, and cold laser, but these are most often combined with stretching or exercise. A trigger point compression massage with sustained stretches was compared with a active range of motion program for myofascial trigger points in neck and upper back pain. This controlled study revealed that a 5-day home program reduced pain intensity in the massage and stretch group compared with an active range of motion group.[63] An RCT of ultrasound, massage, and exercise to treat neck and shoulder myofascial trigger point syndrome revealed that the ultrasound was not effective, but the massage and exercise resulted in significant improvements in the symptoms.[64]

> Clients need to recognize and accept the fact that active coping strategies will be more efficacious in the long term than any passive therapy, such as heat, TENS, or acupuncture. Therapists should minimize a client's dependence on passive therapies.

Hydrotherapy

Aquatic therapy, the performance of exercise in a pool with moderately warm water, has gained in popularity in the last decade as a method of managing the symptoms of CMPSs. Such programs usually involve a group of people and one therapist. An individual session lasts up to 1 hour, sessions are held two to three times per week, and a series of sessions is spread over a 3- to 6-month period; however no data exist to determine the most efficacious frequency and duration of a program. Aquatic therapy is popular with both the individual and the clinician because it combines the elements of aerobic exercise, relaxation, resisted exercise, and social support from the group. Studies have looked at the effectiveness of pool therapy,[65,66] and investigators concluded that pool therapy could improve outcomes ranging from physical fitness and pain to depression and fatigue. In common with most global management strategies for CMPSs, most pool therapy programs also include an educational element in the overall management of the person. Thus, it is difficult to evaluate the effects of pool therapy alone. A promising outcome is that the beneficial effects of pool therapy were still present at the end of a 6-month follow-up period.[66] It is possible that these results have been achieved because of the relatively long course of therapy that affords the person with fibromyalgia the time to learn new positive skills and behaviors.

Recreational versus Therapeutic Pool Programs Clients, however, may become fixated on the warmhot water component of pool therapy as being the main contributing factor to the improvement of their condition rather than the active exercise component performed in water. Therefore, clients should be encouraged to attend recreational pool programs in their community, rather than regularly attend a pool program in the clinical setting. Because of initial deconditioning, programs, such as those offered by the YWCA or YMCA for people with arthritis, should initially be used with the client progressing to more aerobic programs. Caution also should be exercised because the use of heat, especially at the temperature of spa pools, can be exhausting to individuals who already complain of excessive fatigue.

Sleep Disturbance Interventions

As has been noted, the clinical problem list of clients with chronic muscle pain can be lengthy, and the interactions among the main problems of pain, mood, and sleep disturbance are well documented.[67,68] Interventions targeting sleep disturbance can result in an attenuation of some symptoms but can also provide more rest for the individual, thus improving their capacity to cope with other issues.

A key concept to the understanding of sleep interventions is that people who develop sleep disturbances often have poor sleep habits and think about their sleep disturbance in a manner that contributes to anxiety about sleep, perpetuating the problem. Sleep disturbance takes the form of three main presentations:

- Difficulty with sleep onset (falling asleep)
- Fragmentation of the sleep period
- Early awakenings without being able to fall asleep again

Often a combination of these three presentations contributes to the problem. There are three approaches that are commonly used to address these problems: sleep hygiene, stimulus control, and sleep restriction protocol. These will be presented in order of increasing difficulty to achieve.

Sleep Hygiene   Sleep behavior has a tendency to be ritualistic; that is, people often follow a pattern of activity before falling asleep, and if they have difficulty in falling or staying asleep, certain activities promote the problem. Table 12-4 provides a list of the common problems that occur and that are relatively easy to correct. Bringing these hygiene rules to the client's attention may provide quick remediation of some bad habits that have been learned. For example, an individual who has trouble falling asleep, lies awake worrying about it, stares at the clock for 1 hour, and

Table 12-4. Sleep Hygiene Approach

Avoid daytime napping
Reduce time in bed
Avoid trying to sleep
Avoid clock watching
Avoid late-night exercise
Avoid tobacco, alcohol, caffeine
Establish a regular wake-up time

Table 12-5. Stimulus Control Therapy

1. Go to bed only when sleepy.
2. Use bed only for sleeping and sex.
3. If unable to sleep, move to another room. Stay up until really sleepy. The goal is to associate bed with falling asleep quickly.
4. Awaken at the same time every morning, regardless of total sleep time.
5. Do not nap.
6. Repeat no. 3 as often as necessary.

From Bootzin RR, Perlis ML: Nonpharmacologic treatments of insomnia. *J Clin Psychiatry* 53(suppl):37–41, 1992.

then finally gets up and has a cigarette has engaged in several activities that will not help with falling asleep.

Stimulus Control After clinical research identified the principal factors that cause arousal and association of wakefulness when a person tries to sleep, a set of stimulus control rules was developed.[69] These can be described and explained to the client (Table 12-5).

Sleep Restriction Protocol This is a more difficult route to take and requires one-on-one coaching. In essence, the individual undergoes sleep deprivation in an effort to realign their biological clock and consolidate their sleep/wake cycle. Difficulties with this approach include excessive daytime fatigue and also a potential danger if an individual must operate machinery or drive. However, it has been used in the population with chronic pain with good results.[70,71]

It is quite normal for persons to have temporary periods of sleep disturbance, but the presence of pain is a stress that often results in persistence of the problem. Good results can be obtained from educating clients on the rules of sleep hygiene and stimulus control therapy and helping them to make the decisions necessary to change their behavior.

Biopsychosocial Therapies

It is usual for clients with CMPSs to experience emotional distress as a result of their constant battle with chronic pain and fatigue. Often, these individuals benefit from psychosocial counseling.[72] Through discussion and problem-solving with clients, specific suggestions on coping strategies and pain management techniques can assist in setting realistic treatment goals. Various measures, such as biofeedback[73] and cognitive behavioral therapies,[28] have been found to be successful in promoting stress reduction, which in turn decreases CMPS symptoms. Extensive work with people who have arthritis has shown that

adequate knowledge of the condition can enhance clients' abilities to improve self-efficacy and to develop coping skills.[74] Self-efficacy also was shown to improve in people with fibromyalgia after they attended a 6-week educational program.[75] Hypnotherapy also has shown promising results in a controlled study.[76]

Multidisciplinary Approach

Neilson and Weir[77] provided an excellent summary of the biopsychosocial approaches to the management of chronic pain that emphasized the physiological, psychological, and social determinants of health. This places the individual and that person's needs at the center of management of the condition. In the biopsychosocial approach the three determinants of health are always presumed to play a role. Thus, although individual therapies, e.g., stress reduction and biofeedback, may be used, the person with CMPS or fibromyalgia would be better served in the context of a multidisciplinary therapy program. In this context, the whole team that includes nurses, physicians, psychologists, occupational and physical therapists evaluate the person. The management program is designed to most suit the dominant manifestations of CMPS in that person at that time. The program assumes that pain is a multidimensional experience and that only through management of all the components of pain will the most successful management result. Some components, e.g., physical, psychological, or social, will receive more emphasis between people and within an individual over time. The key is to reveal the interacting factors, such as mood, sleep, and pain, that can together result in a perpetuation of the symptoms. However, the goal is always to maximize the person's abilities, while increasing exercise and work capacity, improving psychological and social adjustment, and reducing dependency on medication. A recent qualitative study[78] described some of the themes that were derived from people with fibromyalgia in their description of themselves; some of these eloquently speak to the nature of the problem:

- Pain, the constant presence
- Fatigue, the invisible foe
- Sleep, the impossible dream
- Longing for a normal life
- Seeking a diagnosis
- Living within boundaries

These personal statements offer a window into the experience that people with fibromyalgia have. Even for those treatment studies in which improvements in fibromyalgia symptoms have been demonstrated, complete relief of pain is rare. This is to be expected with a chronic pain syndrome. However, the combination of medication, physical methods of pain relief, and exercise, together with education and coping strategies, offers the client hope.

> Listen to the client. Together, work out reasonable and achievable goals. Do not dwell on the pain because it is only part of the picture.

Research Questions

The management of persons with chronic muscle pain syndromes and specifically fibromyalgia remains largely unexplored. Although information is available on the beneficial effects of exercise and other physical pain-relieving modalities, very few of the studies used a randomized clinical trial design, their results tended to be borderline, and even fewer of these studies looked at the long-term benefits or risks of these management approaches. The same critique can be stated for psychosocial approaches, such as biofeedback, self-efficacy, counseling, and cognitive behavioral therapies. The paucity of systematic or meta-analytic reviews of these therapies is telling and is largely due to the small number of well-designed trials published to date. Some areas for research are the following:

- Are the outcomes of clients with fibromyalgia (or CMPSs) improved in the long term after a community-based program of conditioning exercise?
- Are the outcomes of clients with fibromyalgia (or CMPSs) improved in the long term after a program of group hydrotherapy?
- In clients with fibromyalgia, what are the effects of a multidisciplinary management program on quality of sleep, pain, and activities of daily living?

Summary

Optimal management of CMPSs demands that the three components of pain—sensory, affective, and cognitive—are addressed because any one of these components can lead to or promote chronic pain. Diagnosis is not easy; other causes must be eliminated and this process can be highly frustrating and depressing to the person with CMPS. Successful management requires the active participation of the client and use of active coping strategies that enable the person to maximize their abilities in the presence of physical, physiological, and social challenges. When the multifactorial nature of CMPS is recognized and managed in a multidimensional manner, therapy can be effective.

Case Study

Mrs. M., a 42-year-old, woman presents with a history of neck and back pain over a period of 3 years. She is divorced, is raising two now teenaged sons, and lives in a house that has a mortgage. She works as a bank manager but is finding it increasingly difficult to cope with the job stress in an uncertain market and uncertain times, as well as with her pain. She has previously been seen by physicians, a chiropractor, a massage therapist, and physical therapists and recently was referred to a psychiatrist. Her pain comes and goes but is always present to some extent and sometimes gets so bad that she "hurts all over." She complains of a very broken sleep pattern and because of constant pain and fatigue is short tempered with both her sons and the staff and clients at work. The use of prescription analgesics, muscle relaxants, and hypnotics gave only some relief.

Assessment.   The objective examination revealed average range of motion in the cervical and lumbar spine with some tightness at the end of range. She demonstrated a poking chin, a hyperextended neck posture, and a slight, correctable kyphosis. Muscles of her shoulder girdle and neck feel tight on palpation. Muscle strength is normal but on testing she tired quickly and reported low endurance to exercise, both specific and general. She did not complain of referred pain. On closer examination, 12 of 18 fibromyalgia tender points tested positive to pressure, therefore fulfilling the criteria for fibromyalgia. She has no other radiological or serological abnormalities and no environmental sensitivities. She did not want to undertake a sleep study at this time.

Multidisciplinary Team Management.   Initial treatment consisted of education about fibromyalgia and chronic pain in general. She was willing to participate in a weekly fibromyalgia support group. Mrs. M. was given a prescription for low-dose amitriptyline and encouraged to gradually reduce usage of all other medications, both prescription and over-the-counter. Mrs. M. proved to be receptive to most of the suggestions for managing her condition and was a regular participant in prescribed activities.

The occupational therapist made a work site visit to recommend changes to her work environment, specifically an optimal arrangement of her computer work area and a change in the chair. She agreed to have her eyes tested to determine whether she needed glasses when using the computer.

Mrs. M. agreed to an aerobic exercise program of general and specific exercises performed to music at home. This individually designed program was to increase both in intensity and repetitions. For 6 weeks she also attended a twice weekly group pool program of specific exercises and distance swimming at her local YWCA to improve her exercise tolerance.

The psychologist worked with her on coping skills, with special emphasis on coping with her teenaged sons and resolving staffing problems at the bank.

Assessment Six Months Later. Mrs. M. still has pain; however, she is no longer looking for a cure for her pain. Her posture has improved, and she now wears glasses when using the computer. Because she enjoys swimming, she regularly swims for exercise. She has not continued with her home exercise program, but she has taken up Tai Chi, which she says has been very useful. She no longer takes any medication and has stopped seeing her psychologist. Her relations with her sons have improved; she sleeps well, is happier and more active, and is working well. Mrs. M has realistic expectations of what she can do and an improved attitude to cope with things she cannot change. She will be followed annually.

Skeleton Case Study

Age: 32
Gender: Female
Occupation: Postmistress
Onset: 5 years
Severity: 15 tender sites
Adherence: Poor
Issues: Depression, poor sleep patterns, threat of job loss

References

1. Melzack R, Casey KL: Sensory, motivational and central control determinants of pain: a new conceptual model. In Kenshalo D (ed): *The Skin Senses*. Springfield, IL, Charles C Thomas, 1968, pp 423–443.

2. Turk DC, Rudy TE: IASP taxonomy of chronic pain syndromes: preliminary assessment of reliability. *Pain* 30:177–189, 1987.

3. Vasudevan SV: Impairments, disability, and functional capacity assessment. In Turk DC, Metzack R (eds): *Handbook of Pain Assessment*. New York, Guilford Press, 1992, pp 100–108.

4. Black RG: Evaluation of the pain patient. *J Disabil* 1:85–97, 1990.

5. Balfour W: *Observations with Cases Illustrative of New Simple and Expeditious Mode of Curing Rheumatism and Sprains*. Edinburgh, Adam Black, 1816. Cited in *Myofascial Pain and Fibromyalgia Syndromes: A Clinical Guide to Diagnosis and Management*. Edinburgh, Churchill Livingstone, 2001.

6. Wolfe F, Smythe HA, Yunus MB et al: The American College of Rheumatology 1990 Criteria for the Classification of Fibromyalgia. Report of the Multicenter Criteria Committee. *Arthritis Rheum* 33:160–172, 1990.

7. White K, Speechly M, Harth M et al: The London fibromyalgia epidemiology study: the prevalence of fibromyalgia syndrome in London, Ontario. *J Rheumatol* 26:1570–1576, 1999.

8. Waynolis GW, Perkins RH: Post-traumatic fibromyalgia. *Am J Phys Med Rehabil* 73:404–412, 1994.

9. Yunus M, Masi A, Aldag J: A controlled study of primary fibromyalgia syndrome: clinical features and association with other functional syndromes. *J Rheumatol* 19(suppl):62–71, 1989.

10. Yunus M, Masi A, Calabro J et al: Primary fibromyalgia (fibrositis): clinical study of 50 patients with matched normal controls. *Semin Arthritis Rheum* 11:151–171, 1981.

11. Bradley LA: Fibromyalgia: a model for chronic pain. *J Musculoskeletal Pain* 6:19–28, 1998.

12. Tunks EH, Crook J, Norman G et al: Tender points in fibromyalgia. *Pain* 14:563–569, 1988.

13. Scudds RA, Rollman GB, Harth M et al: Pain perception and personality measures as discriminators in the classification of fibrositis. *J Rheumatol* 14:563–569, 1987.

14. Lautenbacher S, Rollman GB: Possible deficiencies of pain modulation in fibromyalgia. *Pain* 13.189–196, 1997.

15. Scudds RA, McCain GA, Rollman GB et al: Improvements in pain responsiveness in patients with fibrositis after successful treatment with amitriptyline. *J Rheumatol* 19(suppl):98–103, 1989.

16. Buskila D, Press J, Gedalia A et al: Assessment of non-articular tenderness and prevalence of fibromyalgia in children. *J Rheumatol* 20:368–370, 1993.

17. Wolfe F, Ross K, Anderson J et al: The prevalence and characteristics of fibromyalgia in the general population. *Arthritis Rheum* 38:19–28, 1995.

18. Eisingerj P, Plantamura A, Ayavou T: Glycolysis abnormalities in fibromyalgia. *J Am Coll Nutr* 13:144–148, 1994.

19. Simms WR, Roy SH, Hrovat M et al: Lack of association between fibromyalgia syndrome and abnormalities in

muscle energy metabolism. *Arthritis Rheum* 37:794–800, 1994.

20. Mannerkorpi K, Burckhardt CS, Bjelle A: Physical performance characteristics of women with fibromyalgia. *Arthritis Care Res* 7:123–129, 1994.

21. Mengshoel AM, Saugan E, Forre O et al: Muscle fatigue in early fibromyalgia. *J Rheumatol* 22:143–150, 1995.

22. Mense S, Simons DB, Russell IJ (eds): *Muscle Pain: Understanding Its Nature, Diagnosis and Treatment.* Philadelphia, Lippincott Williams & Wilkins, 2001.

23. Moldofsky H, Scarisbrick P, England R et al: Musculo-skeletal symptoms and non-REM sleep disturbance in patients with 'fibrositis syndrome' and healthy subjects. *Psychosom Med* 37:431–451, 1975.

24. Moldofsky H, Scarisbrick P: Induction of neurasthenic musculoskeletal pain syndrome by selective sleep state deprivation. *Psychosom Med* 38:35–44, 1976.

25. Pivik RT, Harman K: A reconceptualization of EEG alpha activity as an index of arousal during sleep: all alpha activity is not equal. *J Sleep Res* 4:131–137, 1995.

26. Older SA, Battafarano CL, Danning JA et al: The effects of delta-wave sleep interruption on pain thresholds and fibromyalgia-like symptoms in healthy subjects. *J Rheumatol* 25:1180–1186, 1998.

27. Rains JC, Penzien DB: Sleep and chronic pain: challenges to the α-EEG sleep pattern as pain specific sleep anomaly. *J Psychosom Res* 5:77–83, 2003.

28. Bradley LA: Cognitive-behavioral therapy for primary fibromyalgia. *J Rheumatol* 16(suppl 10):131–136, 1989.

29. Carette S, Bell MJ, Reynolds WJ et al: Comparison of amitriptyline, cyclobenzaprine and placebo in the treatment of fibromyalgia. *Arthritis Rheum* 37:32–40, 1994.

30. Russell IJ: Neurochemical pathogenesis of fibromyalgia syndrome. *J Musculoskeletal* 7:183–191, 1999.

31. Vaeroy H, Helle R, Forre O et al: Elevated CSF levels of substance P and high incidence of Raynaud's pheno-menon in patients with fibromyalgia: new features for diagnosis. *Pain* 32:231–236, 1988.

32. Nyberg F, Liu Z, Lind C et al: Enhanced levels of substance P in patients with painful arthroses [abstract]. *J Musculoskeletal Pain* 3(suppl 1):2, 1995.

33. Vanderah TW, Laughlin T, Lashbrook JM et al: Single intrathecal injections of dynorphin A or des-tyr-dynorphins produce long-lasting allodynia in rats: blockade by MK-801 but not naloxone. *Pain* 68:275–281, 1996.

34. Welin M, Bragee, B, Nyberg F et al: Elevated substance P levels are contrasted by a decrease in met-enkephalin in patients with fibromyalgia [abstract]. *J Musculoskeletal Pain* 3(suppl 1):4, 1996.

35. Kang Y-K, Russell IJ, Vipriao GA et al: Low urinary 5-hydroxyindole acetic acid in fibromyalgia syndrome: evidence in support of a serotonin-deficiency patho-genesis. *Myalgia* 1:14–21, 1998.

36. Bradley LA, Alberts KR, Alarcon GS et al: Abnormal brain cerebral regional blood flow and CSF levels of patients and non-patients with fibromyalgia (abstract). *J Musculoskeletal Pain* 3(suppl 1):S212, 1998.

37. Yunus MB, Khan KK, Rawlings JR et al: Analysis of multicase families with fibromyalgia syndrome. *J Rheumatol* 26:408–412, 1999.

38. McCain G: Fibromyalgia and myofascial pain syndromes. In Wall PD, Melzack, R (eds): *Textbook of Pain.* Edinburgh, Churchill Livingstone, chapter 26, 1994.

39. Melzack R, Stillwell D, Fox E: Trigger points and acupuncture points for pain: correlations and impli-cations. *Pain* 3:3–23, 1977.

40. Simons D, Mense S: Understanding and measurement of muscle tone related to clinical muscle pain. *Pain* 75:1–17, 1998.

41. Simons DG, Travell JG, Simons LS: *Myofascial Pain and Dysfunction: The Trigger Point Manual,* vol 1: *Upper Half of the Body,* 2nd ed. Baltimore, Williams & Wilkins, 1999.

42. Travell JG, Simons D: *Myofascial Pain and Dysfunction: The Trigger Point Manual,* vol 2, *Lower Half of the Body,* Baltimore, Williams & Wilkins, 1992.

43. Gerwin R: Differential diagnosis of myofascial pain syndrome and fibromyalgia. *J Musculoskeletal Pain* 7:209–215, 1999.

44. Bengtsson A, Henriksson K, Jorfeldt L: Primary fibromyalgia—a clinical and laboratory examination of 55 patients. *Scand J Rheumatol* 15:340–347, 1986.

45. Scudds RJ, Scudds RA, Simmonds MJ: Pain in the physical therapy curriculum: a faculty survey. *Physiother Theory Pract* 17:239–256, 2001.

46. Masi AT, Yunus MB: Fibromyalgia—which is the best treatment? A personalized comprehensive, ambulatory, patient-involved management programme. *Baillieres Clin Rheumatol* 4:333–370, 1990.

47. Rosen NB: Physical medicine and rehabilitation approaches to the management of myofascial pain and fibromyalgia syndromes. *Baillieres Clin Rheumatol* 8:881–916, 1994.

48. Guymer EK, Clauw DJ: Treatment of fatigue in fibromyalgia. *Rheum Dis Clin North Am* 28:367–378, 2002.

49. McCain GA, Bell DA, Mai FMS et al: A controlled study of the effects of a supervised cardiovascular fitness training program on the manifestations of primary fibromyalgia. *Arthritis Rheum* 31:1135–1141, 1988.

50. Richards SC, Scott DL: Prescribed exercise in people with fibromyalgia: parallel group randomized controlled trial. *BMJ* 325:185, 2002.

51. Nichols DS, Glenn TM: Effects of aerobic exercise on pain perception, affect, and level of disability in individuals with fibromyalgia. *Phys Ther* 74:327–332, 1994.

52. Burckhart CS: Nonpharmacologic management strategies in fibromyalgia. *Rheum Dis Clin North Am* 28:291–304, 2002.

53. Jones KD, Clark SR: Individualizing the exercise prescription for persons with fibromyalgia. *Rheum Dis Clin North Am* 28:419–436, 2002.

54. Oliver K, Cronan T: Predictors of exercise behaviors among fibromyalgia patients. *Prev Med* 35:383–389, 2002.

55. Sim J, Adams N: Systematic review of randomized clinical trials for non-pharmacological interventions for fibromyalgia. *Clin J Pain* 18:324–336, 2002.

56. National Institutes of Health: *Consensus Statement on Acupuncture*. Washington, DC, National Institutes of Health, vol 15, no 5, 1997.

57. Scudds RA, Charron J, Santilli D et al: A survey of people with fibromyalgia on the perceived usefulness of physical therapy (abstract). *Physiother Can* 48:7, 1996.

58. Berman BM, Ezzo J, Hadhazy V et al: Is acupuncture effective in the treatment of fibromyalgia? *J Fam Pract* 48:213–218, 1999.

59. Deluze C, Bosia L, Zirbs A et al: Electroacupuncture in fibromyalgia: results of a controlled trial. *BMJ* 305:1249–1253, 1992.

60. Sandberg M, Lundeberg T, Gerdle B: Manual acupuncture in fibromyalgia: a long-term pilot study. *J Musculoskeletal Pain* 3:39–58, 1999.

61. Gunn CC, Milbrandt WE, Little AS et al: Dry needling of muscle motor points for chronic low-back pain: a randomized clinical trial with long term follow-up. *Spine* 5:279–291, 1980.

62. Jaeger B, Skootsky S: Double blind, controlled study of different myofascial trigger point injection techniques. *Pain* 4(suppl):S292, 1987.

63. Hanten WP, Olson SL, Butts NL et al: Effectiveness of a home program of ischemic pressure followed by sustained stretch for treatment of myofascial trigger points. *Phys Ther* 80:997–1003, 2000.

64. Gam AN, Warming S, Larsen LH et al: Treatment of myofascial trigger-points with ultrasound combined with massage and exercise—a randomised controlled trial. *Pain* 77:73–79, 1998.

65. Mannerkorpi K, Nyberg B, Ahlmen M et al: Pool exercise combined with an education program for patients with fibromyalgia syndrome: a prospective randomized study. *J Rheumatol* 27:2473–2481, 2000.

66. Jentoft ES, Kvalvik AG, Mengshoel AM: Effects of pool-based and land-based aerobic exercise on women with fibromyalgia/chronic widespread muscle pain. *Arthritis Rheum* 45:42–47, 2001.

67. Harman K, Pivik RT, D'Eon JL et al: Sleep in depressed and nondepressed participants with chronic low back pain: electroencephalographic and behavioural findings. *Sleep* 25:775–783, 2002.

68. Nicassio PM, Moxham E, Schuman C et al: The contribution of pain, reported sleep quality, and depressive symptoms to fatigue in fibromyalgia. *Pain* 100:217–279, 2002.

69. Bootzin RR, Perlis ML: Nonpharmacologic treatments of insomnia. *J Clin Psychiatry* 53(suppl):37–41, 1992.

70. Morin CM, Kowatch RA, Wade JB: Behavioral management of sleep disturbances secondary to chronic pain. *J Behav Ther Exp Psychiatry* 20:295–302, 1989.

71. Morin CM, Kowatch RA, O'Shanick G: Sleep restriction for the inpatient treatment of insomnia. *Sleep* 13:183–186, 1990.

72. Goldenberg DI, Kaplan KH, Nadeau MG et al: A controlled study of a stress-reduction, cognitive-behavioral treatment program in fibromyalgia. *J Musculoskeletal Pain* 2:53–66, 1994.

73. Ferraccioli G, Ghirelli I, Scita F et al: EMG-biofeedback training in fibromyalgia syndrome. *J Rheumatol* 14:820–825, 1987.

74. Lorig K, Konkol L, Gonzalez V: Arthritis patient education: a review of the literature. *Patient Educ Counseling* 10:207–252, 1987.

75. Burckhardt CS, Mannerkorpi Y, Hedenberg L et al: A randomized, controlled clinical trial of education and physical training for women with fibromyalgia. *J Rheumatol* 21:714–720, 1994.

76. Haanen HCM, Hoenderdos HTW, Van Romunde LKJ et al: Controlled trial of hypnotherapy in the treatment of refractory fibromyalgia. *J Rheumatol* 18:72–75, 1991.

77. Neilson WR, Weir R: Biopsychosocial approaches to the treatment of chronic pain. *Clin J Pain* 17(Suppl):114–127, 2001.

78. Sturge-Jacobs M: The experience of living with fibromyalgia: confronting an invisible disability. *Sch Inq Nurs Pract* 16:19–31, 2002.

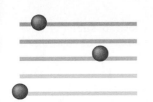

CHAPTER 13

Health and Physical Fitness for the Client with Multiple Joint Involvement

Marian A. Minor, PhD, PT

Prolonged inactivity and poor fitness are clearly associated with increased mortality and morbidity. Inactivity is an independent risk factor in all causes of mortality. Inactivity is as important as smoking, obesity, and elevated cholesterol levels in increasing the likelihood of coronary artery disease, arteriosclerosis, hypertension, diabetes, and some types of cancer.[1] Whether inactivity is due to a self-selected

PHYSICAL REHABILITATION IN ARTHRITIS, Joan M. Walker, PhD, PT, and Antoine Helewa, MSc(Clin Epid), PT, Elsevier Inc. © 2004.

sedentary lifestyle or to the diagnosis of arthritis, the threat to health and longevity is similar and clear. In addition, for the person with multiple joint involvement, the consequences of prolonged inactivity add dramatically to the problems of pain, stiffness, loss of motion, weakness, functional limitation, and disability.

The purpose of this chapter is to provide information relevant to exercise, physical fitness, and health for the person with multiple joint involvement. The impact of inactivity and the benefits and feasibility of increased physical activity and exercise for the person with arthritis will be described. The role of the health professional in promoting successful exercise behaviors will be discussed, as well as methods of appropriate physical fitness assessment and exercise prescription. The discussion of exercise program implementation will include program content and structure.

Inactivity and Exercise in Arthritis

The presence of arthritis can create serious health problems in ways other than as direct consequences of the disease and side effects of therapy. Arthritis is the primary cause for limitation in physical activity in adults. Of persons older than 65 years of age, 12% report limitation in physical activity due to arthritis.[2] Heart disease is a close second. Persons with a diagnosis of rheumatoid arthritis (RA) have reported that one of the first adaptations they make is to give up leisure and recreational activities, a primary source of physical activity for adults. In addition to the threat of prolonged inactivity to general health, inactivity produces many of the same signs and symptoms traditionally attributed to the arthritis disease process, namely, muscle weakness and atrophy, decreased flexibility, cardiovascular deficit, fatigue, osteoporosis, depression, and lowered pain threshold (see Chapter 3).

It is well documented that many persons with arthritis are deconditioned and less fit than their peers without arthritis. Marked cardiovascular deficits, elevated energy expenditure, muscle weakness, and functional limitations have been reported. Figure 13-1[3] displays measurements of fitness and functional tasks in persons with RA and osteoarthritis (OA). Are people with arthritis in poor physical condition because of the disease process itself? Do we think to ourselves, "Of course she's in bad shape, she has arthritis"? In recent years, this widespread assumption has been challenged by both persons with arthritis and arthritis health professionals who have engaged in studies of the efficacy of conditioning exercise programs to improve health and fitness.

A growing number of well-controlled, randomized trials of exercise in arthritis provide convincing evidence of the safety and benefits of exercise for many people with arthritis. Reviews of this literature, both narrative and systematic, consistently report positive findings and add credence to the importance and feasibility of exercise for this population. In RA, evidence supports the use of both aerobic and resistance exercise in both early and later stages of the disease for persons with American College of Rheumatology functional class I to III who have low to moderate disease activity and whose medication usage is stable. Most of the research subjects have been female, and the exercise has been in supervised and group settings. Reported interventions have varied in duration from 1 to 24 months with intensity progressed to conditioning levels. Results show improvements in aerobic capacity and muscle function with no increase in pain or joint damage.[4,5] Exercise research in OA has most often included people with OA of the knee and hip. Controlled trials of both moderate intensity aerobic and muscle conditioning exercise report improvements in aerobic capacity, strength, and proprioception as well as decreased pain.[6,7] Lower extremity conditioning using a combination of supervised instruction and a home exercise program has been used effectively in OA of the knee.

Similar exercise modalities have been studied in both RA and OA. Walking, stationary bicycle riding, low impact aerobic dance, and water exercise appear to be safe and effective for improving aerobic fitness. Muscular fitness has improved in programs using elastic bands, functional exercise, and resistive equipment. Exercise frequency, duration, and intensity used in the studies to date are consistent with current guidelines for fitness and health in the general population. Most interventions occur 2 to 4 times a week for 20 to 60 minutes and progress to a level of 60% to 80% of maximal capacity. The findings of these studies, the majority of which were randomized, controlled trials, demonstrate that many people who were deconditioned when they began to exercise were able to exercise at levels necessary to produce a training effect and made significant gains in fitness, health status, and function.

Role of the Health Professional in Exercise Adoption and Maintenance

The person with arthritis can exercise to maintain or improve health and physical fitness. Information to guide development of successful exercise programs is now becoming available to both health professionals and persons with arthritis. Knowledge itself, however, is not sufficient to ensure adoption and maintenance of safe and healthy exercise behaviors.

Beliefs and Barriers

Positive beliefs about the usefulness of exercise and minimal barriers to the performance of exercise are necessary for a person to adopt and maintain new exercise behaviors. The health professional must believe that exercise for health and fitness is

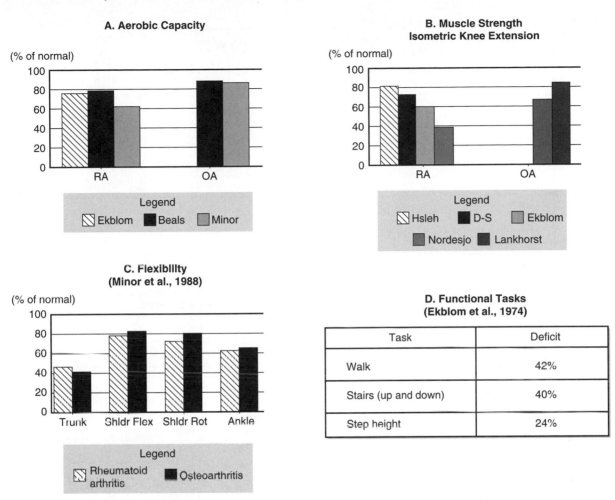

A. Aerobic Capacity

(% of normal)

Legend: Ekblom, Beals, Minor

**B. Muscle Strength
Isometric Knee Extension**

(% of normal)

Legend: Hsleh, D-S, Ekblom, Nordesjo, Lankhorst

**C. Flexibility
(Minor et al., 1988)**

(% of normal)

Trunk, Shldr Flex, Shldr Rot, Ankle

Legend: Rheumatoid arthritis, Osteoarthritis

**D. Functional Tasks
(Ekblom et al., 1974)**

Task	Deficit
Walk	42%
Stairs (up and down)	40%
Step height	24%

Figure 13-1. Comparative physical function in arthritis. Measurements of (*A*) aerobic capacity, (*B*) muscle strength, (*C*) flexibility, and (*D*) functional performance of persons with rheumatoid arthritis (RA) and osteoarthritis (OA) compared with control subjects or published norms. Results are expressed as a percentage of normal (100%) of each measurement. Shldr Flex = shoulder flexion; Shldr Rot = medial and lateral shoulder rotation; Ankle = dorsiflexion. (From Minor MA: Physical activity and management of arthritis. *Ann Behav Med* 13[3]:117–123, 1991. With permission.)

important and feasible and be willing to explore the beliefs of the client in the process of making exercise recommendations. In addition, work and home roles and responsibilities, socioeconomic considerations, and client preference and experiences must be considered to reduce as many barriers as possible.

Self-Efficacy for Exercise

One of the most important factors in the willingness to adopt and subsequently maintain new behavior is a positive belief in the ability to perform that behavior—

self-efficacy. This is particularly true in exercise and affects both adoption and maintenance. Self-efficacy for a particular activity can change; it increases with successful experiences, positive role models, peer support, and positive interpretation of sensations surrounding the activity.[8]

The health professional plays a key role in helping the person with arthritis build self-efficacy for exercise. Setting realistic goals, recalling previously successful experiences, offering peer groups, and designing periodic assessments to reinforce the efficacy of the exercise are only a few strategies that can be used to

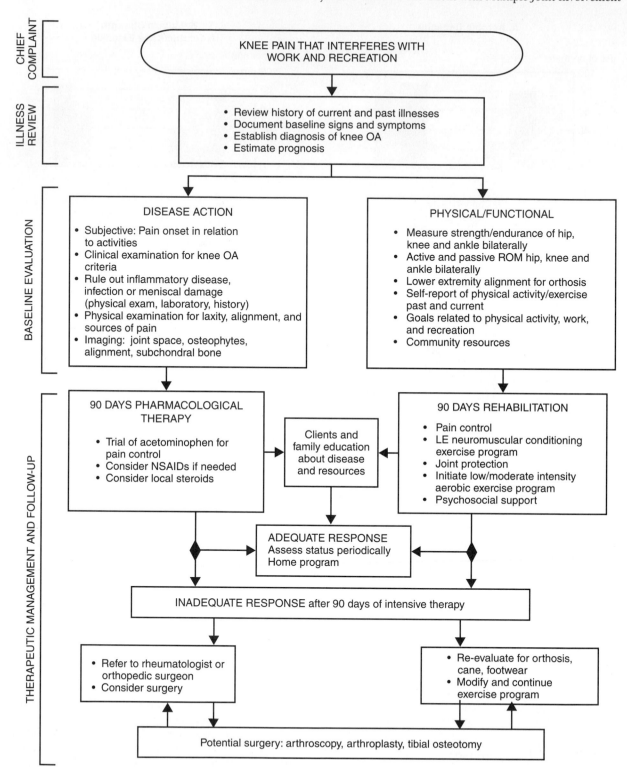

Figure 13-2. Algorithm for management of knee pain that interferes with work and recreation. OA = osteoarthritis; ROM = range of motion; NSAIDs = nonsteroidal anti-inflammatory drugs; LE = lupus erythematosus.

build self-efficacy for exercise. Figure 13-2 presents an algorithm for an overall management plan using the knee as an example.

Physical Activity and Exercise

It is important to recognize the distinction between exercise training to improve physical fitness and adequate levels of physical activity to achieve general health benefits. Physical activity can be defined as "any bodily movement produced by skeletal muscles that results in energy expenditure." Adequate levels of regular physical activity are necessary for general health, a reduction in risk for a number of diseases, and reduced levels of dysfunction and disability in arthritis.

Early investigators in the field of exercise science often studied healthy, athletic young men. The focus was generally to improve competitive performance in persons who were already fit. Therefore, much of the information about prescribing exercise to improve fitness indicated that fairly intense exercise regimens were needed. Recent epidemiological studies of health risk factors and prospective studies in less fit populations reveal important findings relevant to the health and fitness of persons with musculoskeletal impairments and limitations in mobility.

It is not necessary for a person to participate in an intense, highly regimented exercise program or attain a high level of athletic fitness to improve health status. Even persons with low fitness levels who engage in relatively moderate physical activity on a regular basis are at significantly less risk for a number of degenerative and potentially fatal conditions. Furthermore, adequate levels of physical activity improve health status even in the presence of other risk factors.[9] The accumulation of 30 minutes of moderate intensity physical activity on most days of the week is necessary for health maintenance and is sufficient to significantly reduce the probability of cardiovascular illness.[10] Such a routine would be comparable to a comfortable but somewhat brisk walk, bicycle ride, or swim or performance of household tasks, such as mowing the yard or raking leaves. Public health initiatives in many countries are now focused on increasing the levels of physical activity in the population to reduce morbidity and mortality related to inactivity. Most people with arthritis can be included in these programs.

Exercise, a subset of physical activity, is defined as "planned, structured, and repetitive bodily movement done to improve or maintain one or more components of physical fitness." For the person with arthritis, exercise may be prescribed by a health professional or undertaken as a self-directed project; it may be supervised in a clinical setting or be done in a home program or a community-based setting. Exercise may be therapeutic or recreational or a combination of both. However, the basic tenet is that exercise is tied to specific components of physical fitness and requires assessment and prescription to reach specific goals.

Persons with arthritis are a heterogeneous population, ranging widely in age, disease severity, impairments, function, goals, and interests. Some are interested in and capable of performing exercise programs with a goal of improving physical fitness. Others may need instruction and support to participate in cardiovascular or pulmonary rehabilitation programs. Others may not be candidates for fitness training programs but can be educated and encouraged to adopt appropriate exercise habits to improve or maintain health and reduce the risk of inactivity-related illness (Table 13-1).

The purpose of this chapter is to provide the therapist with the knowledge and skills to recommend appropriate physical activity or exercise to achieve both arthritis-specific and general health or fitness objectives for the person with multiple joint involvement. The concept of physical fitness will be used to organize the discussion.

Physical Fitness Assessment

Physical fitness is a useful concept in the assessment and recommendation of exercise for all persons. Physical fitness has five components: cardiovascular status, muscle strength, muscle endurance, flexibility, and body composition. A comprehensive exercise evaluation should consider current capacity and needs in all five areas. An effective and safe exercise prescription incorporates the current status and abilities of the individual in a training program that supplies physiological overload to produce adaptation.

Assessment of physical fitness and exercise status, in addition to disease-related considerations, is the foundation for the prescription of safe and effective exercise for the person with arthritis. Assessment also provides a baseline to measure progress and monitor for harm. The multidimensional, holistic concept of physical fitness is particularly appropriate for assessment and exercise recommendation for persons with

Table 13-1. Physical Activity for Health

Exercise mode

Full body physical activity incorporated into daily tasks (walking, stair climbing, house or yard work)

Frequency

On most days of the week

Duration

Accumulate 30 minutes per exercise day

Intensity

Moderate intensity; 50%–70% of age-predicted maximal heart rate

Self-monitoring strategies

Scale of perceived exertion: 3–5 (0–10 scale); 11–12 (0–20 scale)
Talk Test: able to converse comfortably during activity

Physical Activity and Health: A Report of the Surgeon General. Atlanta, GA, US Department of Health and Human Services, Centers for Disease Control and Prevention, National Center for Chronic Disease Prevention and Health Promotion, 1996, p 33.

arthritis (see also Figure 13-2). Physical fitness involves a comprehensive look at musculoskeletal and cardiovascular function. This comprehensive yet categorical perspective allows specificity and grading of the exercise program as required by current need and changes in disease status. Physical fitness also provides a popular health- and wellness-oriented framework into which therapeutic exercise can be incorporated. This can be especially important for the acceptance and adoption of healthy exercise behaviors by the person with arthritis.

Assessment measures should be chosen to meet client and professional needs. There are a variety of assessments of the components of fitness that have been standardized and allow comparison to age- and gender-matched peers without arthritis.[11,12] Other measures, such as grip strength, 13.5 m (50 feet) walking time, isokinetic knee extension, and aerobic capacity have been used in arthritis and exercise research and reported in the scientific literature.[13] These measures have proven valid and safe for persons with arthritis. A comprehensive test of physical fitness must include assessment of all five components.

Cardiovascular Assessment

Cardiovascular fitness or aerobic capacity is primarily a function of the body's ability to transport and use oxygen to sustain physical exertion. Good cardiovascular fitness requires an efficient heart, healthy pulmonary and vascular systems, and aerobically conditioned muscle.

Cardiovascular assessment before exercise is performed for two reasons: *to identify contraindications to exercise* and *to assess current aerobic fitness.* Information to guide exercise intensity can be obtained by self-report or by a submaximal test of exercise performance. The assessment of current fitness by these means, however, does not supply information about possible cardiovascular disease. Safety for increased activity must be addressed before exercise testing. The Physical Activity Readiness Questionnaire (PAR-Q) (Figure 13-3)[14] is often used for initial screening in nonmedical settings before exercise testing or beginning an exercise program.

The American College of Sports Medicine (ACSM) recommends that risk factors, symptoms, and the intensity of the exercise to be performed should be considered in determining the need for a physician-supervised exercise stress test.[15] Guidelines for exercise testing recommendations appear in Table 13-2.

For persons with systemic inflammatory disease and the potential for cardiovascular or pulmonary involvement, a careful history and medical review are necessary before any marked increase in physical activity is prescribed. The choice of a submaximal or symptom-limited stress test, with or without physician supervision or gas exchange analysis, should be based on medical considerations and institutional policy.

Physical Activity Readiness
Questionnaire - PAR-Q
(revised 1994)

PAR - Q & YOU

(A Questionnaire for People Aged 15 to 69)

Regular physical activity is fun and healthy, and increasingly more people are starting to become more active every day. Being more active is very safe for most people. However, some people should check with their doctor before they start becoming much more physically active.

If you are planning to become much more physically active than you are now, start by answering the seven questions in the box below. If you are between the ages of 15 and 69, the PAR-Q will tell you if you should check with your doctor before you start. If you are over 69 years of age, and you are not used to being very active, check with your doctor.

Common sense is your best guide when you answer these questions. Please read the questions carefully and answer each one honestly: check YES or NO.

YES	NO		
☐	☐	1.	Has your doctor ever said that you have a heart condition <u>and</u> that you should only do physical activity recommended by a doctor?
☐	☐	2.	Do you feel pain in your chest when you do physical activity?
☐	☐	3.	In the past month, have you had chest pain when you were not doing physical activity?
☐	☐	4.	Do you lose your balance because of dizziness or do you ever lose consciousness?
☐	☐	5.	Do you have a bone or joint problem that could be made worse by a change in your physical activity?
☐	☐	6.	Is your doctor currently prescribing drugs (for example, water pills) for your blood pressure or heart condition?
☐	☐	7.	Do you know of <u>any other reason</u> why you should not do physical activity?

If

you

answered

YES to one or more questions

Talk with your doctor by phone or in person BEFORE you start becoming much more physically active or BEFORE you have a fitness appraisal. Tell your doctor about the PAR-Q and which questions you answered YES.

- You may be able to do any activity you want — as long as you start slowly and build up gradually. Or, you may need to restrict your activities to those which are safe for you. Talk with your doctor about the kinds of activities you wish to participate in and follow his/her advice.
- Find out which community programs are safe and helpful for you.

NO to all questions

If you answered NO honestly to <u>all</u> PAR-Q questions, you can be reasonably sure that you can:

- start becoming much more physically active — begin slowly and build up gradually. This is the safest and easiest way to go.
- take part in a fitness appraisal — this is an excellent way to determine your basic fitness so that you can plan the best way for you to live actively.

DELAY BECOMING MUCH MORE ACTIVE:
- if you are not feeling well because of a temporary illness such as a cold or a fever — wait until you feel better, or
- if you are or may be pregnant — talk to your doctor before you start becoming more active.

Please note: If your health changes so that you then answer YES to any of the above questions, tell your fitness or health professional. Ask whether you should change your physical activity plan.

<u>Informed Use of the PAR-Q:</u> The Canadian Society for Exercise Physiology, Health Canada, and their agents assume no liability for persons who undertake physical activity, and if in doubt after completing this questionnaire, consult your doctor prior to physical activity.

You are encouraged to copy the PAR-Q but only if you use the entire form

NOTE: If the PAR-Q is being given to a person before he or she participates in a physical activity program or a fitness appraisal, this section may be used for legal or administrative purposes.

I have read, understood and completed this questionnaire. Any questions I had were answered to my full satisfaction.

NAME _____

SIGNATURE _____   DATE _____

SIGNATURE OF PARENT _____   WITNESS _____
or GUARDIAN (for participants under the age of majority)

continued on other side...

Supported by: ◆ Health Canada Santé Canada

Figure 13-3. Physical Activity Readiness Questionnaire (PAR-Q) (revised 1994), for people aged 15 to 69. (From *Canadian Standardized Test of Fitness Operations Manual*, 3rd ed. Fitness Canada, Canadian Society for Exercise Physiology, Gloucester, 1986; revised 1994, With permission.) *Illustration continued on opposite page*

PAR - Q & YOU

Physical Activity Readiness
Questionnaire - PAR-Q
(revised 1994)

...continued from other side

We know that being physically active provides benefits for all of us. Not being physically active is recognized by the Heart and Stroke Foundation of Canada as one of the four modifiable primary risk factors for coronary heart disease (along with high blood pressure, high blood cholesterol, and smoking). People are physically active for many reasons — play, work, competition, health, creativity, enjoying the outdoors, being with friends. There are also as many ways of being active as there are reasons. What we choose to do depends on our own abilities and desires. No matter what the reason or type of activity, physical activity can improve our well-being and quality of life. Well-being can also be enhanced by integrating physical activity with enjoyable healthy eating and positive self and body image. Together, all three equal VITALITY. So take a fresh approach to living. Check out the VITALITY tips below!

Active Living:

- accumulate 30 minutes or more of moderate physical activity most days of the week
- take the stairs instead of an elevator
- get off the bus early and walk home
- join friends in a sport activity
- take the dog for a walk with the family
- follow a fitness program

Healthy Eating:

- follow Canada's Food Guide to Healthy Eating
- enjoy a variety of foods
- emphasize cereals, breads, other grain products, vegetables and fruit
- choose lower-fat dairy products, leaner meats and foods prepared with little or no fat
- achieve and maintain a healthy body weight by enjoying regular physical activity and healthy eating
- limit salt, alcohol and caffeine
- don't give up foods you enjoy — aim for moderation and variety

Positive Self and Body Image:

- accept who you are and how you look
- remember, a healthy weight range is one that is realistic for your own body make-up (body fat levels should neither be too high nor too low)
- try a new challenge
- compliment yourself
- reflect positively on your abilities
- laugh a lot

Enjoy eating well, being active and feeling good about yourself. That's VITALITY®

FITNESS AND HEALTH PROFESSIONALS MAY BE INTERESTED IN THE INFORMATION BELOW.

The following companion forms are available for doctors' use by contacting the Canadian Society for Exercise Physiology (address below):

The **Physical Activity Readiness Medical Examination (PARmed-X)** - to be used by doctors with people who answer YES to one or more questions on the PAR-Q.

The **Physical Activity Readiness Medical Examination for Pregnancy (PARmed-X for PREGNANCY)** - to be used by doctors with pregnant patients who wish to become more active.

References:
Arraix, G.A., Wigle, D.T., Mao, Y. (1992). Risk Assessment of Physical Activity and Physical Fitness in the Canada Health Survey Follow-Up Study. **J. Clin. Epidemiol.** 45:4 419-428.
Mottola, M., Wolfe, L.A. (1994). Active Living and Pregnancy, In: A. Quinney, L. Gauvin, T. Wall (eds.), **Toward Active Living: Proceedings of the International Conference on Physical Activity, Fitness and Health**. Champaign, IL: Human Kinetics.
PAR-Q Validation Report, British Columbia Ministry of Health, 1978.
Thomas, S., Reading, J., Shephard, R.J. (1992). Revision of the Physical Activity Readiness Questionnaire (PAR-Q). **Can. J. Spt. Sci.** 17:4 338-345.

To order multiple printed copies of the PAR-Q, please contact the

Canadian Society for Exercise Physiology
1600 James Naismith Dr., Suite 311
Gloucester, Ontario CANADA K1B 5N4
Tel. (613) 748-5768 FAX: (613) 748-5763

The original PAR-Q was developed by the British Columbia Ministry of Health. It has been revised by an Expert Advisory Committee assembled by the Canadian Society for Exercise Physiology and Fitness Canada (1994).

Disponible en français sous le titre «Questionnaire sur l'aptitude à l'activité physique - Q-AAP (revisé 1994)».

Supported by: Health   Santé
Canada   Canada

Figure 13-3. *Continued*

Table 13-2. Recommendations for Exercise Testing and Participation (ACSM)

- Screen for risk factors and symptoms before exercise testing or participation with a valid tool, such as the Physical Activity Readiness Questionnaire (PAR-Q).
- *A person with no known cardiovascular, pulmonary, or metabolic disease and without symptoms of disease can begin a MODERATE exercise program or perform submaximal exercise testing without a medical examination or physician supervised testing.*
- A medical examination and physician supervised exercise testing before initiating exercise is recommended for the following
  - A person with known cardiovascular, pulmonary, or metabolic disease or with one or more of the following signs/symptoms: suspected ischemic pain; shortness of breath or unusual fatigue with usual activity; heart rate irregularities or murmur; intermittent claudication or ankle edema
  - Men > 45 years and women > 55 years or with two or more risk factors (see below) before participation in vigorous exercise

Risk Factors

Sedentary lifestyle	Does not accumulate at least 30 minutes a day of moderate physical activity as recommended in the US Surgeon General's Report
Obesity	Body mass index > 30 kg/m^2 or waist girth > 100 cm
Family history	Heart disease in first-degree relative before age 55 in men and 65 in women
Cigarette smoking	Current smoker or within past 6 months
Hypertension	Blood pressure > 140 mm Hg systolic or > 90 mm Hg diastolic or on medication
Blood glucose	Fasting blood glucose > 110 mg/dl confirmed on 2 occasions
Cholesterol	Total serum cholesterol > 200 mg/dl or high-density lipoprotein (HDL) < 35 mg/dl or receiving medication

Data from *ACSM's Guidelines for Exercise Testing and Prescription*, 6th ed. Philadelphia, Lippincott Williams & Wilkins, 2000, pp 22–27.

Aerobic Capacity

Aerobic capacity can be assessed by a variety of methods. Self-reports of intensity, duration, and frequency of current physical activity can be useful. Submaximal clinical and field tests of exercise performance estimate aerobic fitness by comparing the intensity of the exercise (speed or distance traveled or workload achieved) and the heart rate response. Results can be expressed as levels of fitness or by rate of oxygen consumption (in milliliters per kilogram per minute). Choice of an assessment measure should be based on the following considerations: need to compare to normative data, research or clinical use of data, current ability, and joint status of the client. Follow-up testing to evaluate effectiveness of the exercise program will provide the most meaningful information if the assessment mode matches the training mode (e.g., bicycle exercise/bicycle ergometer; walking exercise/treadmill, or walking field test).

Muscle Strength

Muscular strength is the force generated by muscular contraction. Strength can be improved and measured by isometric, isotonic, or isokinetic methods. Muscle strength is associated with strength in tendons and ligaments, as well as with increased muscle mass. To achieve functional gains, muscle strengthening programs must consider the principle of specificity of training. Therapeutic assessment of muscle strength is traditionally performed by a manual muscle test, by determination of a maximum load (one repetition maximum [1RM]), or with a dynamometer to quantify torque and work. Fitness assessments of muscle strength also have been developed for use in field settings and are generally performance based. Grip strength and pull-ups are examples of these tests. When performing muscle strength assessment (type, speed, and range of contraction), the clinician should consider the following: muscle groups that will be trained, muscle groups that could be expected to improve as a result of the general exercise routine, and muscle strength important to function. Dynamometers may be as elaborate as those used for isokinetic testing or as simple as a hand-held dynamometer to quantify isometric muscle strength. (See Chapter 5 for isometric muscle testing using a sphygomanometer.)

Muscle Endurance

Muscle endurance is the capacity of muscle to sustain force over time. Endurance measurements and training in all type of contractions can be either aerobic or anaerobic. Muscle endurance is associated with the ability to sustain a level of performance and is closely related to functional ability and strength. Endurance is tested easily with timed repetition tests of submaximal muscular effort (sit-ups, leg extensions) or functional tasks (sit to stand, toe raises). Using this strategy, a greater number of repetitions accomplished within the time period represent improved muscle endurance. Endurance testing also is possible on most of the computerized muscle testing and rehabilitation equipment. Meaningful measures of muscle endurance are those that simulate functional needs and are specific to the muscle groups responsible for the performance.

Flexibility

Flexibility is the component of fitness measured by the active range of motion of the spine and extremities. Flexibility, affected by joint structure and by peri-articular tissue extensibility, is a measure particularly relevant for persons with arthritis. Disease processes, inactivity, and pain converge to produce decreased joint range of motion, stiffness, and general inflexibility. Goniometry of selected joints and field tests, such as the sit-and-reach test (Canadian Standardized Test of Fitness), are useful for exercise prescription and baseline information. Progress in client-selected functional tasks that are limited by lack of flexibility also may be used to assess progress (reaching over head, kneeling, putting on shoes).

> **Meaningful measures of muscle endurance should simulate functional needs and be specific to the muscle groups responsible for the performance.**

Body Composition

Body composition is the proportion (percentage) of lean to fat body mass. Body composition is a better gauge of health and fitness than is weight. Although definitions of obesity vary, 20% and 30% body fat are considered upper limits of body fat for men and women, respectively. Weight management programs that include dietary and exercise changes can influence levels of body fat successfully. Exercise programs that increase muscle mass, stimulate fat oxidation, and/or increase energy expenditure can reduce the percentage of body fat.

Body composition can be assessed adequately by measurement of skin folds and use of appropriate tabled norms or formulae.[16,17] Computerized bio-electrical impedance methods also are available. Calculation of waist/hip girth ratio can be used to assess body fat distribution. Fat deposits in chest and abdomen are associated with greater risk for cardiovascular disease. A waist/hip girth ratio greater than 0.9 is considered a health risk (measurement of waist circumference divided by hip circumference).

Assessment Tools

Selecting appropriate measurement tools to measure physical fitness in persons with multiple joint involvement requires a consideration of physical ability and disease status. See the 'Additional Readings' at the end of the chapter for measurement tools from which to choose.

Exercise Program Components

A comprehensive fitness program has three parts: a warm-up, an aerobic exercise period, and a cool-down. Within this framework it is possible to include exercises to improve or maintain flexibility, range of motion, muscle strength and endurance, and cardiovascular fitness and health. Specific therapeutic goals and disease-related considerations for disease activity, joint protection, progressive grading, and self-management strategies also are easily accommodated.

This compartmentalized approach to the exercise prescription gives the health professional and the person with arthritis an easily individualized and modifiable exercise program. For example, an extremely deconditioned person may require an initial program to increase flexibility and strength to prepare for more vigorous and weight-bearing activities. In this case, the health professional and client design an appropriate flexibility and strengthening program with goals to increase strength and flexibility, improve function, manage pain, and prepare for the addition of an aerobic component. When the client is able to perform 8 to 10 repetitions of these exercises within a 15-minute period, the client will be able to add a short aerobic component, such as 5 minutes of walking or stationary bicycling, gradually progressing to 20 to 30 minutes. A brief cool-down follows this more vigorous activity. If a disease flare occurs or there is increased joint pain, the client can reduce aerobic activity and perform only the warm-up routine until the acute episode subsides. In this way, the exercise habit is maintained, and the client gains the knowledge and experience to self-manage exercise and activity.

Warm-Up or Preaerobic Component

This component provides a neuromuscular and cardiovascular warm-up and is essential to the exercise routine. During this time, exercises are done for range of motion, for flexibility, and to prepare the body for more vigorous activity. This warm-up is needed for exercise safety by all exercisers and is particularly important for the person with arthritis. The warm-up routine can be designed to incorporate individualized range of motion and endurance exercises and may serve as an initial home exercise program.

The warm-up can be progressed in number of exercises and repetitions to include 12 to 15 exercises performed at 5 to 10 repetitions each. It is extremely important to include pelvic stabilization and trunk rotation exercises in the warm-up to minimize the chances for low back pain with the increased activity. The goal can be 15 minutes of continuous low-intensity exercise, which is an indication of readiness to proceed to an aerobic stimulus activity.

Aerobic Exercise

The aerobic exercise component provides the stimulus for adaptation and training of cardiovascular efficiency, muscular endurance, and activity tolerance. This dynamic, repetitive exercise requiring the use of large muscle groups also appears to benefit general health, emotional status, weight management, self-concept, and fatigue.

The aerobic component can be designed to meet individual needs and variations in disease activity. Experience with and availability of a variety of aerobic activities give the exerciser freedom to alternate modes. A prescription of exercises with flexible intensity, duration, and frequency that the client understands and can adjust to meet daily needs promotes self-management skills and appropriate activity levels.

The utilization of *interval training techniques* (i.e., alternate bouts of brisk and low-intensity activity) and *additive bouts of exercise* (i.e., add four 5-minute exercise bouts during the day for 20 minutes of exercise) enable even the most deconditioned and sedentary person to safely engage in health-promoting physical activity.[18] Alternating exercise intensity within an exercise session or performing several short sessions during the course of the day also provides the person who has vulnerable joints and fluctuating disease activity with a method to establish a health-promoting exercise program.

Exercise success and maintenance appear to be enhanced by using time rather than distance as the aerobic exercise goal. For example, 20 minutes of walking, biking, or swimming is easier to maintain successfully than a set mileage or number of laps. Using alternate forms of exercise that vary weight bearing and joints involved also fosters maintenance of the exercise habit. Stationary bicycle riding is a good alternate for walking on days when knees are sore; a walk may be a better choice of exercise than swimming on a day when hands, wrists, and shoulders are painful. These strategies are particularly useful to the person with arthritis who has "good and bad days" and needs to regulate, but not omit, exercise.

Cool-Down Component

When the client is performing 10 minutes or more of aerobic activity at an intensity of 70% or more of age-predicted heart rate (moderate intensity), a 3- to 5-minute cool-down period is necessary. During this time, exertion is reduced to a low intensity and gentle calisthenics or stretching of exercised muscles is performed. The goal of the cool-down period is to allow the cardiovascular response to safely adjust to less demand and to gently stretch muscle to minimize the possibility of delayed-onset muscle soreness.

As with the warm-up routine, low-intensity cool-down activities can be designed and used in a daily program that provides general as well as therapeutic benefit. The warm-up and cool-down may be combined to form a 25- to 30-minute exercise routine for flexibility, strength, and pain management without the more intense aerobic period. These routines can be used on days when aerobic exercise is not done.

Resistance Training

Recommendations for physical fitness for the general population now include guidelines for muscle strengthening. Maintaining muscle mass and strength is an important part of good health and fitness.

Appropriate resistance training in persons with RA and OA can result in muscle strengthening, improved function and independence, and increased lean body mass without increased joint pain or disease activity.

Knowledge of the disease process, biomechanics, and joint protection principles must form the foundation for any resistance program for the client with joint involvement. Research confirms the safety and benefit of resistive exercise. A whole body/circuit resistance type of program targeting 8 to 10 major muscle groups has produced improvements in both RA and OA. In OA of the knee, lower extremity muscle training using elastic bands, free weights, and functional exercise has produced improvements in neuromuscular activity, function, and pain.

Exercise Prescription

The exercise prescription derives from the physiological principles of overload and specificity of training. The *overload principle* states that a physiological stress greater than that to which the organ or organ system normally is subjected is necessary to produce physiological adaptation and increased capacity. The exertion required to overload the cardiac function of a 70-year-old woman who has been inactive for the last 10 years will be much less than that required to produce improved cardiovascular fitness in a 25-year-old recreational athlete. *Specificity of training* means that gains in capacity and performance are greatest when the training activities correspond closely to the desired outcome. If you want to swim faster you must train by swimming fast. If you want to improve walking speed you must include faster walking in the training program. Physiological overload and specificity of training are addressed in the exercise prescription through recommendations for (1) modes of exercise, (2) intensity, (3) duration, and (4) frequency. Manipulation of these variables in accordance with results of a fitness assessment and personal exercise goals produces an individualized exercise prescription. For the person with arthritis, this prescription also takes into account disease-related needs and may incorporate therapeutic objectives and recreational exercise.

> Education of the client for *self-management* is important so that he or she can adjust the exercise routine as needed for changes in disease activity, pain, weather, exercise resource availability, schedule conflicts, and personal interests.

Exercise success and maintenance may be enhanced by using time rather than distance as the aerobic exercise goal. Exercise recommendations for the person with arthritis must include education about response to joint inflammation and adaptation of physical activity to reduce joint stress. For example, swimming or stationary bicycling may be substituted for walking when there is knee, hip, or ankle inflammation. Graded progression of return to vigorous or resistive exercise after immobilization is necessary to protect weakened cartilage, bone, and periarticular structures.

The client must be educated for self-management so he or she can adjust the exercise routine as needed for changes in disease activity, pain, weather, availability of exercise resources, schedule conflicts, and interests. The concept of physical fitness and the prescription of distinct components of the exercise program are particularly useful in helping the individual understand how to wisely select and modify activities.

Arthritis-Related Considerations

As a group, people with arthritis tend to be at high risk for undetected coronary disease, osteoporosis, and musculoskeletal injuries. Effects of disease, consequences of therapy, and long periods of inactivity contribute to the problem list.

Extra-articular Manifestations

Extra-articular manifestations of systemic inflammatory diseases should be assessed and considered in the exercise prescription. Systemic involvement requires that a careful history and physical examination precede any conditioning exercise program. Pericarditis, nephritis, and vasculitis *preclude* vigorous activity. Pulmonary fibrosis may limit ventilation and safe exertion at high intensity. Signs of active, systemic disease should be heeded and the initiation of more vigorous exercise delayed awaiting effective medical control. Cardiovascular and pulmonary complications may limit exercise capacity, particularly in persons with diseases that have a major systemic component, such as systemic sclerosis, systemic lupus erythematosus (SLE), and RA. The seronegative spondyloarthropathies (ankylosing spondylitis [AS] and psoriatic arthritis) may be associated with heart involvement and conduction defects. In general, the limitations do not interfere except during high-intensity exercise. However, elderly, deconditioned, and biomechanically inefficient people expend considerably more energy than younger, fit, and agile people to accomplish the same task. In a deconditioned or biomechanically inefficient person, walking at a slow speed (less than 2 mph) requires significantly greater exertion than might be expected.

Articular Manifestations

Articular manifestations of arthritis should be considered in terms of active inflammation and joint integrity. Inflamed joints are particularly vulnerable to injury. Synovial tissue ischemia, increased intra-articular temperature and pressure, and the presence of immune complexes are associated with joint inflammation. Painful, swollen joints need to be protected from deforming forces and unnecessary stress. Acute joint inflammation should be controlled before conditioning exercise. This may require a course of drug therapy and/or joint aspiration. There is some evidence that knee joint effusion may be reduced by increased synovial circulation that occurs during active motion such as walking or cycling.[16] For a disease flare in one or a few joints, it is often possible to alternate modes of exercise so that the exercise habit is maintained and joints are protected. For example, a painful and swollen knee may be protected by a change from a 30-minute walking routine to exercise on a stationary bicycle with no resistance. Although the effects of repetitive, active exercise appear to be health promoting for the joint, current knowledge does not support vigorous activity in the presence of active inflammation.

> **Control of inflammatory disease processes and joint swelling should be achieved *before* a conditioning exercise program.**

Joints with loss of joint space, damaged cartilage, laxity or tightness in the periarticular tissue, chronic effusion, or malalignment are susceptible to activity-related injury. Joint pain and swelling after activity should be treated as an "overuse" or athletic injury. Preventive steps should be taken to strengthen the joint in preparation for a return to activity. If joint integrity or stability is not amenable to change, activity modifications can decrease the amount of joint stress incurred. A clinical knowledge of biomechanics is essential. For example, intra-articular pressure in the hip can be reduced up to 50% by use of a cane in the contralateral hand during ambulation,[17] biomechanical stress at the knee joint increases with faster walking speed particularly for people with genu varus, and stair climbing produces the greatest hip joint pressures of any locomotor activity.[19]

Intensity

Intensity is determined by the exertion or effort expended during exercise. The recommendation for intensity is based on the pre-exercise fitness assessment. Persons who are deconditioned or who have not exercised for 3 months or more should begin at a low intensity. In persons with low initial aerobic capacity, intensity of 50% to 60% maximal heart rate (MHR) is both safe and adequate to produce a training effect. For persons with average levels of fitness, intensity of 60% to 80% MHR will be appropriate and probably well tolerated. Intensity of exercise is related to the individual and also can be described in terms of the exerciser's ability to maintain the activity (Table 13-3).

Intensity during aerobic exercise sessions most often is monitored by heart rate response or self-report of perceived exertion. It is useful to prescribe an exercise range with a lower intensity as the threshold for training and the higher intensity as the "not to exceed" level. Individuals can learn to regulate activity successfully within the range, modifying exertion as desired.

Table 13-3. Definitions of Relative Exercise Intensity

Moderate Exercise
Well within current capacity
Sustainable comfortably for 45 minutes with gradual initiation and progression
45%–60% maximal VO_2 = 50%–70% maximal heart rate
Vigorous Exercise
>60% maximal VO_2 = >70% maximal heart rate
Substantial cardiorespiratory challenge
Data from *ACSM's Guidelines for Exercise Testing and Prescription*, 6th ed. Philadelphia, Lippincott Williams & Wilkins, 2000, pp 22–27.

Heart rate response may not be an appropriate measure of intensity if the person is taking medications to regulate heart rate or has a pacemaker or if the economy of effort is poor then heart rate is not a meaningful indicator of actual energy expenditure. For these reasons, it is often desirable to prescribe and teach exercise intensity regulation with the rating of perceived exertion scale. For some persons, the simple "talk test" may be the most useful way to make sure that exercise intensity does not exceed a moderate level. The talk test only requires that the person be able to speak normally and converse while exercising. If the exerciser is short of breath, or cannot speak in comfortable sentences, the exercise is too intense and effort should be decreased.

The weight or resistance determines intensity of strengthening or resistive exercise and the number of repetitions performed. The combination of resistance and repetitions also determines the exercise effect in terms of producing increased strength or improved endurance. High resistance and low repetition exercise promotes strength and hypertrophy. Low to moderate resistance and high repetition exercise promotes muscular endurance. Achievement of 50% to 80% 1RM for 8 to 12 repetitions has been used to prescribe intensity in strength training in arthritis.

High-intensity exercise is clearly associated with increased injury and relapse. For the person with arthritis, maintaining intensity at a safe and satisfying level is a challenge for both the exerciser and the health professional. It is often the younger client who presents the greatest challenge. Balancing joint health, intensity, and socially desirable activities is necessary to produce age-appropriate, enjoyable, and safe exercise opportunities.

Duration

Duration of the exercise session is highly variable and can be manipulated with intensity to provide the desired exercise stimulus. The duration of the aerobic portion of the exercise period probably needs to be at least 30 minutes of continuous activity at a level of intensity above normal daily activity to produce changes in cardiovascular fitness. Minimal requirements for health, however, suggest that an accumulation of 30 minutes of moderate intensity activity on most days of the week may provide significant health benefits (see Table 13-1).

Two modifications in duration may provide particular benefit to persons with arthritis who are unable to comfortably exercise for 30 continuous minutes. The first modification is *interval training*. This method incorporates alternate bouts of high- and low-intensity exercise during the exercise session. For example, the runner may alternate 30 seconds of sprinting with 30 seconds of jogging. This scheme delays fatigue and allows a greater total exertion and work over a period of time than a continuous high-intensity activity. For the person with arthritis who may not be able to sustain a continuous 20-minute brisk walk without knee swelling and fatigue, a regimen of slow and brisk walking could be combined as follows: slow walk 5 minutes/brisk walk 3 minutes; slow walk 3 minutes/brisk walk 3 minutes; slow walk 3 minutes/brisk walk 3 minutes; slow walk 5 minutes; for a total of 25 minutes of continuous activity. If tolerated, a gradual increase in the periods of brisk walking provides a conditioning period and a safe progression to longer duration and greater intensity. A second modification of the duration component is the use of *additive bouts* of exercise. Performing several short bouts of exercise throughout the day may increase the total duration of exercise. If a person is unable to perform 30 minutes of continuous walking, he or she may wish to walk for 10 minutes in the morning, 10 minutes after lunch, and 10 minutes in the afternoon. Additive bouts of exercise appear to be sufficient to fulfill the requirements for exercise for health but probably do not provide the stimulus necessary for improving cardiovascular fitness. Some persons who initially use additive bouts of exercise, however, can lengthen and combine these short bouts as endurance and strength improve, and eventually perform a longer continuous session. Other persons may continue to obtain the health-related benefits of regular activity in the form of several short sessions during the day.

Frequency

Frequency of exercise depends on the exercise goal, intensity, and mode of exercise. A frequency of 3 to 4 times a week for a moderate aerobic stimulus appears to produce optimal results in terms of cardiovascular benefit with a minimal risk of injury or fatigue. A frequency of 5 to 6 days per week is safe and effective when the intensity is lower. Similarly, resistance training to improve strength should be performed no more often than 2 to 3 days a week to allow the muscle time to repair and adapt.

Stretching and Flexibility

Stretching and flexibility exercises are most effective when performed at least once daily. Flexibility exercise performed in the morning may reduce morning stiffness and pain in preparation for the day's activities. Flexibility exercise performed in the afternoon, when

Table 13-4. Exercise Tips for the New Exerciser

Walking

- Start on flat, level surface. Use cane if helpful.
- Stretch out heel cord and calf muscles before and after.
- Warm-up and cool-down with a stroll.
- Choose a comfortable pace. Sing or talk as you go along.
- If knees get sore, walk more slowly and swing your arms to get the briskness you want.
- Wear supportive shoes with good soles. Athletic (shock absorbing) insoles can help increase comfort and reduce shock on feet, knees, hips, and spine.

Swimming

- Swim only with lifeguard present.
- Vary strokes for comfort and overall conditioning.
- Use mask and snorkel if head turning is a problem.
- Begin and end at a slower pace.
- If water is cool, finish up with a warm shower or soak.

Water Aerobics

- Protect your feet with water shoes or slippers.
- Do not get chilled. Take a warm shower or bath afterward.
- Wear tights, T-shirt, and disposable latex gloves to retain body heat in the water.

- Use flotation device to add buoyancy if knees and hips are painful.
- Regulate exercise intensity by changing the speed, arc of movement, and length of lever arm. Going more slowly, through a smaller arc, or with flexed elbows or knees lessens your exertion and joint stress.

Bicycle (outdoors or stationary)

- Start and end with no resistance or on flat ground.
- Pedal with ball of your foot.
- Make sure seat height allows your knee to be comfortably straight at the bottom of the pedal stroke.
- Don't lean on or over handlebars.
- Feet should be able to swivel freely within pedal straps.
- Keep speed of pedaling at or below 60 rpm. Use gears if applicable to protect knees.

Low-Impact Aerobic Dance

- Wear shoes and exercise on a hard floor or firm carpet.
- Do not bounce, lunge, or do low squats.
- Control your movements. Do not move too fast at the outer range of your movements.
- Change movements frequently if you start to feel muscle fatigue or joint soreness.
- Avoid prolonged exercise with arms, especially with arms above shoulder level.

motion may be greatest, can maintain or increase range with a minimum of pain and stretching. Flexibility exercise performed in the evening may significantly reduce morning stiffness in people with RA.[18]

Exercise Choices

The choice of exercise modalities depends upon client preference, exercise goals, musculoskeletal impairment, and available resources. It is wise to help the client identify and learn to be comfortable in performing at least two activities that require rhythmic, repetitive muscular work of large muscle groups. These activities should vary in requirements for weight bearing and joints used to perform the activity. Other considerations might be activities for both indoors and outdoors, for

changes in weather, and for solitary or group exercise. Table 13-4 presents exercise tips for the *new exerciser*.

Disease-Specific Considerations in Aerobic Exercise

Osteoarthritis

Although the origins of OA may be in bone as well as cartilage, protection of articular cartilage and joint structures is the basis of OA management and a key consideration in exercise. Cartilage health requires motion and the mechanical action of repetitive loading and unloading (rest) for nutrition and stimulation of normal remodeling. Hyaline cartilage failure can be caused by either excessive loading of normal cartilage or by physiological loading of abnormal cartilage. Hyaline cartilage also atrophies with prolonged periods of non–weight bearing or immobilization (see Chapter 3).

The therapeutic exercise regimen should supply regular, moderate loading and motion to the joint with OA to promote nutrition and normal remodeling without undue stress. This can be achieved by altering duration and/or intensity of joint loading and mode of exercise. It has been suggested that continual weight bearing should last no longer than a maximum of 2 to 4 hours, followed by at least 1 hour of non–weight bearing to allow the cartilage to decompress.[20]

Muscular strength and endurance are important for joint protection, particularly at the knee. The major mechanism within the body for absorbing the shock of impulsive loading occurs through reflex controlled neuromuscular mechanisms and eccentric contraction (active lengthening of muscle while maintaining tension). Weakness, fatigue, and unskilled motion interfere with this mechanism and increase the risk of injury.

There is evidence that a person with genu varus and/or pronounced joint space narrowing of the medial tibiofemoral compartment may have increased knee joint stress with faster walking[21] and may not respond as well to an exercise program.[22] The clinical response to this situation is to mechanically improve alignment when possible and monitor walking speed. Of course, initiation of exercise before disease consequences are severe should be encouraged.

Furthermore, joint stability and alignment are improved by strong and extensible ligaments, tendons, and muscles that cross joints. Exercise to improve muscle strength and endurance is mandatory when the knee joint is involved.

Stretching exercises that include the knee should be carefully selected. Joint laxity is common. If this is the case, further stretching of posterior structures (hamstring stretching), rotation with a fixed foot, or pressure on medial and lateral joint structures is contraindicated. Many popular fitness routines contain such exercises (i.e., long sitting stretches, hurdler's stretch, lunges).

OA in one joint is a multijoint problem. Assessment of strength, range of motion, and functional performance at the hip, knee, and ankle bilaterally should be performed and deficits should be addressed in the exercise program (see Figure 13-2). Generally, weakness, stiffness, and pain in one knee are associated with limited motion and strength in the contralateral knee, hips, and ankles.

> Osteoarthritis in one joint is a multijoint problem. Strength and range of motion deficits also appear in unaffected adjacent and contralateral joints.

Rheumatoid Arthritis

In RA, three areas in which synovitis, pain, and instability often occur and are overlooked in exercise planning are hands and wrists, feet, and cervical spine. Activities that require a tight grasp, vigorous repetitive motion, or weight bearing by hands and wrists may be contraindicated in a person with active or chronic hand and wrist involvement. Often, activities can be adapted to protect these vulnerable joints: upright rather than racing style handlebars on bicycles, weight bearing on forearms rather than on hands and wrists during mat and calisthenic exercises, adapting aquatic exercises to avoid the need to grip the side of the pool or exercise equipment.

Foot

Hindfoot instability, clinically expressed as calcaneal valgus, often is associated with collapse of the medial longitudinal arch, midfoot and metatarsal subluxation and pain, and digit deformities. Involvement of foot and ankle can occur quite early in the disease process and severely limit daily activities and the ability to bear weight. Foot and ankle symptoms often are overlooked and undertreated. Early attention to hindfoot position and stability and support and maintenance of mid- and forefoot alignment is essential. Semirigid and rigid orthoses that supply biomechanical correction or support can significantly decrease foot, ankle, and knee pain and protect joints (see Chapter 14).

Spine

Cervical spine involvement is seen in 40% to 80% of people with RA. These joints are the second most commonly involved joints in RA. Subluxation and erosions may occur, leading to possible nerve root and/or spinal cord compression. Excessive motion, upper extremity or occipitally radiating pain, and tenderness to pressure over involved vertebrae are early signs of cervical spine disease and require diagnosis and appropriate management. Exercise should be designed to maintain adequate flexibility (but not hypermobility) in the cervical region and muscular strength and endurance to promote proper head and upper body posture. Isometric exercise and proper head and upper body posture, during activity and rest, help improve tone and strength of periarticular structures and reduce mechanical impingement of cord or nerve roots (see Chapter 14).

Extreme flexion or extension or any position that places pressure on the base of the skull or cervical spine should be avoided (i.e., plough position or extreme bridging). Neck pain may be a problem in curl-ups for abdominal strengthening. This difficulty also may occur in OA of the cervical spine. It is possible to perform abdominal strengthening and keep the head and neck supported by maintaining a pelvic tilt against resistance provided by weight of the lower extremities (leg raises from supine).

Ankylosing Spondylitis and Psoriatic Arthritis

These seronegative spondyloarthropathies are characterized by inflammatory involvement of the spine, ribs, sacroiliac, peripheral joints, and enthesopathies. Exercise-related management includes particular attention to range of motion, flexibility, posture, and chest expansion. Enthesopathies may cause pain and stiffness and at the same time make the site of ligament insertion vulnerable to injury during exercise. Gentle, static stretching performed daily to prevent tightness and contracture is safer and more effective than remedial stretching.

In AS, special attention must be paid to maintenance of good posture, strengthening hip and back extensors, and maintenance of ventilatory function. A properly prescribed and performed exercise program is extremely effective for preserving function in clients with this disease. Some time spent prone daily helps to avoid hip and trunk flexion contractures. Low-impact activities, good musculoskeletal and cardiovascular fitness, and good shoes with shock-absorbing insoles can help clients maintain an active lifestyle. Swimming, with mask and snorkel to reduce the need for cervical rotation, has proved to be an extremely effective and well-accepted form of fitness exercise for people with AS. (See also Chapter 10.)

Systemic Lupus Erythematosus

Exercise-related issues are fatigue, often compounded by inactivity and deconditioning; intermittent arthralgias and myalgias; systemic deficits that may affect activity choice; and protection from overexposure to the sun. Regular moderate activity has been shown to decrease fatigue and improve mood in women with SLE.[23] Use of corticosteroids to control disease activity increases the risk of osteoporosis, stress fractures, and avascular necrosis of the femoral head. *Complaints of pain in back or lower extremities should be considered as serious.* People at risk for these problems should engage in low-impact activities and carefully increase exercise duration in conjunction with general muscle strengthening when disease is under control. (See also Chapter 9.)

Fibromyalgia

Attention to proper posture and conditioning exercise regimens may be useful in managing this disorder. Regular participation in dynamic, low to moderate intensity exercise is known to enhance slow wave sleep, aerobically condition muscle, reduce exercise-induced muscle microtrauma, raise pain threshold, and promote muscular relaxation. (See also Chapter 12.)

Sample Exercise Program

Client

A 55-year-old woman college student has had RA for 25 years. Her medical management consists of oral methotrexate and a biological response modifier, entanercept. She has limited motion and pain of all upper extremity joints with chronic effusions in elbows, wrists, and metacarpophalangeal joints. There is knee, midfoot, and forefoot pain with some swelling and loss of motion in both knees. Knee and foot pain is aggravated by weight-bearing activities. Her gait is slow with limited motion in knees and ankles. In standing, she demonstrates a forward head, rounded shoulders, mild kyphosis, and slight flexion at hips and knees. (Also review Figure 13-2.)

Exercise Goals

Her exercise goals are to (1) improve general flexibility, strength, and endurance; (2) improve posture; and (3) develop exercise habits for maintenance of physical fitness through life.

Exercise Plan

Phase I: Daily Preaerobic Conditioning Program
Flexibility exercises with emphasis on hands and wrists, shoulders, hips, knees, ankles, and spine and strengthening exercises (gravity resisted and with elastic bands) for hip, knee, ankle, trunk extensors, and posterior shoulder girdle are prescribed. She is to start with 3 to 5 repetitions of 12 exercises and increase repetitions to 15. She may continue to build to a 30-minute regimen if desired, and may add an aerobic component when 15 minutes of exercise is well tolerated.

Phase II: Aerobic Component

Add 3 times a week alternating aerobic activities as desired:

1. Ride a stationary bicycle starting with 5 to 10 minutes of pedaling at 50 to 0 rpm with no resistance. This may be performed in two or three bouts per day. Gradually increase resistance and speed as tolerated, always beginning with a 5-minute warm-up. Use additive bouts to reach the goal of 30 minutes per exercise day.
2. Initiate a walking program with 5 to 10 minutes of walking at a comfortable pace, in supportive shoes, and on level ground. Regulate speed and distance to avoid postexercise knee pain and swelling. Use additive bouts of walking to reach the goal of 30 minutes per exercise day.

Phase III: Total Physical Fitness Program

1. Perform daily flexibility routine of 10 to 20 minutes.
2. Perform aerobic exercise of choice 3 to 4 times per week. Also explore swimming, water aerobics, walking, and outdoor bicycling as alternate forms of aerobic activity.
3. Add resistive exercise component of 8 to 12 exercises, progressing to 10 to 15 repetitions, 2 or 3 times a week. Use free weights, elastic bands, or equipment. Use wrist weights or equipment that does not require gripping to avoid hand and wrist stress.

Research Questions

Exercise Physiology and Therapeutic Effects

Does joint swelling in RA respond differently to similar aerobic exercise done on land or in the water?

Exercise Response

What characteristics of persons with knee OA (joint space width, lower extremity alignment, pain, duration of disease, strength, obesity etc.) predict a positive response to an aerobic walking program?

Therapeutic Benefits of Exercise

Is there a difference in exercise outcomes for a person with RA (pain, stiffness, function, global self assessment) related to aerobic exercise performed in the morning or afternoon?

Osteoarthritis Case Study

Mrs. C. is a 68-year-old woman whose bilateral knee pain has increased over the past 6 months. She is 5 feet 2 inches (1.57 m) tall and weighs 180 pounds (67.2 kg). She has type II diabetes, hypertension, and hypercholesterolemia for which she takes prescribed medication. She has the diagnosis of fibromyalgia, largely because of her complaints of generalized muscle pain, fatigue, and poor sleep. She decided not to continue taking the prescribed sleeping medication because it makes her feel groggy in the morning. She lives with her daughter's family, takes care of the two young grandchildren and helps with housework during the day while the parents are at work. She has had intermittent knee pain and stiffness for the past 5 years and has treated her symptoms with over-the-counter medications including aspirin, acetaminophen, and nonsteroidal anti-inflammatory drugs. She also has used topical agents and a number of alternative therapies since her muscular pain began last year. She recently visited her primary care physician because the increased pain and stiffness has made it extremely difficult for her to continue her work in the home. She is having trouble getting up and down from seating, using stairs, getting in and out of the car, taking care of the children, or walking for more than 10 minutes at a time. Radiographs show bilateral joint space narrowing, more in the medial compartments, and greater on the right. There is evidence of bony sclerosis and osteophytes. Joint alignment is good on the left, but there is slight genu varum on the right. Her physician has suggested a course of conservative measures at this time and has referred her to rehabilitation. Mrs. C. and her doctor have agreed to discuss surgical options if she is not satisfied with her knee in 3 to 6 months.

History and examination. Weakness and loss of motion in knees, hips, and ankles bilaterally; an antalgic and slow gait; left knee pain of 7 while walking and 9 for stairs, and right knee pain at 6 for all activities (visual analogue scale, 0 to 10 rating). She responds painfully to pressure applied to tender points in her back and hips. She says that she no longer goes out to shop, visit, or eat out with the family because she hurts, is slow, tires quickly, and requires help to get in and out of the car and up curbs and steps. She admits to feeling low and blue much of the time. Her knee pain is usually relieved by rest and wakes her up only occasionally at night. Her muscle pain is constant. She is wearing house slippers and shows marked pronation on the right. Her goals are to have less pain, sleep better, and be able to stay active and continue her role in the family. She has heard about glucosamine and chondroitin sulfate and magnets to sleep on. She asks about their effectiveness and safety.

Questions. What are her major impairments and functional limitations?

What assessment/evaluation would be useful for developing exercise recommendations?

What should be recommended in terms of therapeutic exercise?

What would you recommend for physical activity for health/fitness?

Skeleton Case Study

Age: 73
Gender: Male
Occupation: Retired postman, Master golfer
Diagnosis: OA left hip and obesity
Severity of OA: Moderate
Height, weight: 6 feet, 315 lbs
Issues: Pain on exertion, decreasing tolerance for gardening, stairs and inclines, competing as a Master golfer.

References

1. Blair SN, Kohl HW, Paffenbarger RS et al: Physical fitness and all-cause mortality. a prospective study of healthy men and women. *JAMA* 262:2395–2401, 1989.
2. Yelin EH, Felts WR: A summary of the impact of musculoskeletal conditions in the United States. *Arthritis Rheum* 33:750–755, 1990.
3. Minor MA: Physical activity and management of arthritis. *Ann Behav Med* 13:117–124, 1991
4. Van den Ende CHM, Vilet Vlieland TPM, Munneke M et al: Dynamic exercise therapy in rheumatoid arthritis: a systematic review. *Br J Rheumatol* 37:677–687, 1998.
5. Stenstrom CH, Minor MA: Evidence for the benefit of strengthening and aerobic exercise in rheumatoid arthritis. *Arthritis Care Res* 49:428–434, 2003.
6. van Baar ME, Assendelft WJJ, Dekker J et al: Effectiveness of exercise therapy in patients with osteoarthritis of the hip or knee: a systematic review of randomized clinical trials. *Arthritis Rheum* 43:1361–1369, 1999.
7. Baker K, McAlindon T: Exercise for knee osteoarthritis. *Curr Opinion Rheumatol* 12:456–463, 2000.
8. Holman H, Mazonson P, Lorig K: Health education for self-management has significant early and sustained benefits in chronic arthritis. *Trans Assoc Am Physicians* 102:204–208, 1989.
9. Blair SN, Kohl HW, Barlow CE et al: Changes in physical fitness and all-cause mortality: a prospective study of healthy and unhealthy men. *JAMA* 273:1093–1098, 1995
10. U.S. Department of Health and Human Services: Physical Activity and Health: A Report of the Surgeon General. 1996. Available at http://www.cdc.gov/nccdphp/sgr/sgr.htm. Accessed March 13, 2001.
11. Cole B, Finch E, Gowland C et al: In Basmajian J (ed): *Physical Rehabilitation Outcome Measures,* 2nd ed. Toronto, Ontario, Canadian Physiotherapy Association, 2002.
12. Minor MA, Kay DR: Arthritis. In Durstine JL, Moore GE (eds): *ACSM's Exercise Management for Persons with Chronic Diseases and Disabilitites,* 2nd ed. Champaign, IL, Human Kinetics, 2003.
13. Stenstrom CH, Nisell R: Assessment of disease consequences in rheumatoid arthritis: a survey of methods. *Arthritis Care Res,* 10:135–150, 1997.
14. *Canadian Standardized Test of Fitness Operations Manual.* 3rd ed, Gloucester, Fitness Canada, 1986, revised 1994.
15. *ACSM's Guidelines for Exercise Testing and Prescription.* 6th ed, Philadelphia, Lippincott Williams & Wilkins, 2000, pp. 22–27.
16. James MJ, Cleland LG, Gaffney RD et al: Effect of exercise on 99Tc-DTPA clearance from knees with effusions. *J Rheumatol* 21:501–504, 1994.
17. Neumann DA: Biomechanical analysis of selected principles of hip joint protection. *Arthritis Care Res* 2:146–155, 1989.
18. Byers PH: Effect of exercise on morning stiffness and mobility in patients with rheumatoid arthritis. *Res Nursing Health* 8:275–281, 1985.
19. Tackson SJ, Krebs DE, Harris BA: Acetabular pressures during hip arthritis exercises. *Arthritis Care Res* 10:308–319, 1997.
20. Bland JH: Joint, muscle and cartilage physiology as related to exercise. *Arthritis Care Res* 1:99–108, 1988.
21. Sharma L, Hurwitz DE, Thonar EJ et al: Knee adduction moment, serum hyaluronan level, and disease severity in medial tibiofemoral osteoarthritis. *Arthritis Rheum* 41:1233–1240, 1998.
22. Fransen M, Crosbie J, Edmonds J: Physical therapy is effective for patients with osteoarthritis of the knee: a randomized controlled clinical trial. *J Rheumatol* 28:156–164, 2001.
23. Robb-Nicholson LC, DaHroy L, Eaton H et al: Effects of aerobic conditioning in lupus fatigue: a pilot study. *Br J Rheumatol* 28:500-505, 1989.

Additional Readings

Sources of Fitness Measurement Tools

Cole B, Finch E, Gowland C et al: In Basmajian J (ed): *Physical Rehabilitation Outcome Measures,* 2nd ed. Toronto, Ontario, Canadian Physiotherapy Association, 2002.

Minor MA, Kay DR: Arthritis. Durstine JL, Moore GE (eds): *ACSM's Exercise Management for Persons with Chronic Diseases and Disabilitites,* 2nd ed. Champaign, IL, Human Kinetics, 2003.

Neiman DC: *Fitness and Sports Medicine.* Palo Alto, CA, Bull Publishing Company, 1990.

Pollock ML, Wilmore JH: *Exercise in Health and Disease,* 2nd ed. Philadelphia, WB Saunders, 1990.

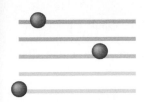

CHAPTER 14

Splinting, Orthotics and Lifestyle Factors

Susan L. Street, MScOT(C), OTRegNS

Overview

Rheumatic diseases can have a significant and often debilitating effect on a person's ability to perform and engage in everyday activities and occupations. Arthritis is one of the most common diseases encountered in occupational therapy (OT) practice today. Clients with arthritis may face unique challenges that require intervention to enable optimal occupational functioning in their daily tasks and routines. The first two sections of this chapter describe the role and use of hand splints, foot orthoses, and appropriate footwear for clients with arthritis. The third section describes some of the lifestyle and occupational

PHYSICAL REHABILITATION IN ARTHRITIS, Joan M. Walker, PhD, PT, and Antoine Helewa, MSc(Clin Epid), PT, Elsevier Inc. © 2004.

performance factors that must be considered in the day-to-day management of arthritis. Clients can and should be actively involved in all stages of planning, goal-setting, and the overall implementation of their treatment programs in the process of learning to safely and effectively manage their arthritis. The principles outlined in this chapter may be adapted and incorporated into an individual's daily life and occupations and may help to foster a greater sense of personal control over her or his disease.

Splinting and Orthotics

Rheumatoid arthritis (RA) affects the peripheral joints of the hand, wrist, and foot in 90% of clients. Most deformities of these joints are caused by inflammation and proliferation of the synovial tissue in the joints. In turn, this causes destruction of cartilage, erosion of bone, ligamentous laxity, muscle and tendon imbalance, and possibly tendon rupture. The end result may include subluxation, instability, or complete dislocation of joints.[1]

Splints and *orthotics* are synonymous terms that refer to externally applied devices that position, protect, support, mobilize, or immobilize various parts of the body, especially joints, and also may serve to promote joint function. In 1992, the American Society of Hand Therapists (ASHT)[2] established a standardized splint classification system and determined that the two terms may be used interchangeably; therefore, a splint and/or orthotic may be defined as "a flexible or rigid appliance used for the prevention of movement of a joint or for the fixation of displaced or moveable (body) parts." Other commonly used terms (pertaining to splints and orthotics) include *brace* and *support*. In more technical terms, a *splint* refers to a temporary device that is part of a treatment program; alternatively, an *orthosis/orthotic* refers to a more permanent device that replaces or substitutes for loss of muscle function or provides optimal positioning. For the purpose of this chapter, splints will be discussed in the context of hand splinting, and orthotics will refer to foot orthoses.

> **The two terms "splint" and "orthotic" are interchangeable.**

In current OT practice, splints and orthotics are generally used to maintain, enhance, and/or prevent motion. The ASHT Splint Classification System classifies splints according to their (1) function and (2) the number of joints they secondarily affect.[2] For clients with arthritis and other rheumatic diseases, splints and orthotics serve a variety of purposes; for example, in the management of the hand with rheumatic disease, splints are often used to stabilize joints, provide optimal positioning, reduce pain, prevent deformity, and maintain or improve overall function, thus enabling clients to better engage in their daily occupations.[3,4]

Early historical evidence of splint and orthotic use dates back to the papyrus splint in the 6th century B.C. During World War II, hand splinting became an important part of physical rehabilitation. The poliomyelitis epidemics of the 20th century greatly contributed to the evolution and subsequent development of specialized hand splints, braces, and foot/lower limb orthotics.[5] Improved biomechanical designs and the introduction of strong, lightweight low-temperature materials that are able to be custom molded yet are resistant to wear have provided the client with a wide array of splinting and orthotic options. Although there is a consensus among rehabilitation professionals that splinting may play an important role in pain relief, joint protection, edema management, and promoting functional performance, few randomized controlled studies or clinical control trials have accurately measured or determined the efficacy of splinting interventions for the client with arthritis who is not a candidate for surgery.[4,6–9]

Assessment and Evaluation

Upon first contact with a client, a detailed initial assessment and systematic evaluation of the wrist, hand, and foot joints must be completed. Because the course of arthritis is variable for each client, subsequent reassessments and regular follow-up sessions are often necessary to monitor changes in the client's condition and her or his occupational function. A comprehensive evaluation is essential before the clinician establishes goals for any splinting or orthotics program and should include the following key components:

1. **Client Interview and Subjective Assessment:** Obtain a clear and detailed history of the disease including onset, medical intervention to date, duration of symptoms, occupational history, impact on functional and occupational performance (person-environment-occupation, physical, psychosocial, cultural, spiritual, emotional). In addition to a semistructured client interview, the use of the highly standardized Canadian Occupational Performance Measure (COPM) would help to systematically identify areas of occupational functioning that are important to the client in addition to those that are potentially compromised or at risk for decline.[10,11] Subjective assessment of pain, fatigue, joint stiffness, coping skills, and social support should be included, in addition to other information regarding duration, intensity, "triggers," and activities/situations that worsen or improve symptoms.

2. **Objective Evaluation and Measurements:** Observation skills are essential to augmenting objective measurements. These measurements should include an assessment of various components such as functional joint range of motion (ROM), deformities, sensation, muscle strength, endurance, stiffness, and joint integrity/laxity; observation of specific functional abilities and occupational performance (e.g., ability to perform personal care skills and instrumental

activities of daily living [ADL]); and environmental analyses as appropriate. Completion of a standardized foot or hand assessment is highly recommended if possible (e.g., Arthritis Hand Function Test).[12]

3. **Visual Assessment, Inspection, and Analysis:** Signs of articular and nonarticular involvement can be identified through close observation of joint alignment, skin coloration, edema, and ligamentous and tendon integrity. Such indicators should be addressed and reassessed throughout the splinting process.

4. **Setting Client Goals and Treatment Goals:** A collaborative, client-centered approach should be taken in identifying and setting realistic, individualized treatment goals in splinting programs. Depending on the degree of severity, the disease process, and the client's progress, these goals may require frequent reassessment and revision throughout the duration of the splinting program.

The chapter Appendix provides an example of a *foot assessment form;* other details are presented in Chapter 5.

Purposes of Splinting and Orthotics

Splints and orthotic devices serve a variety of purposes for the client with arthritis. Although splinting is considered to be an important treatment component, it is seldom used alone. Instead it is usually integrated and combined with other interventions and modalities in the general treatment plan. Splinting serves many key functions[3,4,7]:

- Provide symptom relief and reduce pain.
- Prevent deformity.
- Decrease inflammation.
- Rest and support function.
- Correct deformity.
- Protect structures and promote proper healing postoperatively.
- Assist in maximizing functional use of the hand.
- Protect and improve joint stability and alignment.
- Maintain tissue length.
- Limit motion after nerve, tendon, or bone-ligament injury or repair.

The indications for which therapists use splints vary greatly, and the evidence in the literature to support the benefits of splints is controversial. Most therapists, however, agree that splinting does play an important role in the overall management of arthritis and other rheumatic diseases.

> **Splinting should be integrated with other interventions in the management plan.**

Basic Types of Splints and Orthotics

Only common types of hand splints and foot orthoses recommended for clients with arthritis will be described in this chapter. Note that specific details concerning dynamic hand splinting protocols and postsurgical splinting guidelines are well beyond the scope of this chapter and therefore are not discussed. Further reading on these topics is provided in the Additional Readings section at the end of this chapter.

Given their professional training, education, and clinical backgrounds, occupational therapists, certified hand therapists, and certified orthotists are generally considered to be "experts" in the design and fabrication of specialized, custom splints and orthotics, most of which are not available from commercial stores. However, therapists must remain abreast of current splinting techniques and materials because they frequently change. The ASHT classifies hand splints in one of three categories[2]:

1. Immobilization (static)
2. Mobilization (dynamic)
3. Restrictive

Static (restrictive or immobilization) splints are designed to provide support to areas of the body and have no movable components.[13] The purpose of a static splint is essentially threefold: to immobilize and rest a joint (or several joints), to prevent further deformity, and to prevent soft tissue contractures. By maintaining stretch on soft tissues to increase range of motion and correct joint alignment, static splints can prevent further deformity. Static splints also may provide support for ligamentous injuries and joint laxity and can prevent soft tissue contractures by holding joints in their most functional positions. Dynamic (mobilization) splints may serve a variety of functions depending on the client's condition. These splints tend to be highly specialized and may help to correct an existing deformity, provide controlled motion, aid in joint alignment and wound healing, and substitute for loss of neuromotor function.[14]

Hand Splints

Resting Hand Splint

The static splint most associated with arthritis is the resting hand splint (Figure 14-1), also referred to as a

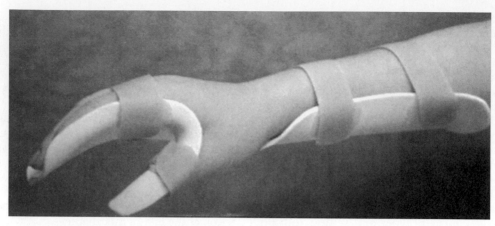

Figure 14-1. Custom thermoplastic resting hand splint with the hand in a functional (midpoint) position: this static splint assists in pain relief, reduction of inflammation, and proper joint positioning. (From Coppard BM, Lohman H [eds]: *Introduction to Splinting: A Critical-Thinking and Problem-Solving Approach.* St Louis, Mosby-Year Book, 1996, p 14. With permission.)

static wrist-hand orthosis. This splint plays an essential role in the treatment of acute wrist-hand synovitis. It helps to relieve pain, reduce inflammation, and properly position joints.[7,15] Fabrication of resting splints requires a custom-molded fit. Low-temperature thermoplastics are the preferred materials of choice because they are durable, easy to work with, relatively inexpensive, also they can be adjusted and remolded.

Zoeckler and Nicholas[15] found that 63% of the clients in their study received "moderate" to "great" relief from pain and morning stiffness through the use of night resting splints. These investigators also determined that splints should be worn consistently at night when active inflammation is present in the hand joints.[15] Biddulph[16] conducted a similar study of 22 clients with arthritis who wore a static wrist-hand orthosis for 10 days.[16] This author reported a 24% improvement in clients' grip strength, a reduction in pain, and an improvement in their ability to perform ADL.[16]

The underlying pathologic changes of arthritis must be taken into consideration when the hand is positioned in a resting splint. Every joint has a *maximum loose-packed position,* or *resting position,* in which the joint capsule is most relaxed and the greatest amount of joint play is possible. The maximum loose-packed position is often adopted by inflamed joints because the capsule is then able to accommodate the most fluid. This position is often used for prolonged immobilization in casts or splints, to avoid damaging the joint when inflammation is present. There may be circumstances in which it is difficult or impractical to use the maximum loose-packed position. When an

actual resting position is chosen for an inflamed joint, it is important to balance the need for the "loosest" position possible with correction for deformity.[17]

Suggested functional (midpoint) positions of the resting hand splint (Figure 14-1) include the wrist in neutral to 10 degrees of extension (as tolerated by the client), the metacarpophalangeal (MCP) joints at 20 to 30 degrees of flexion, and the proximal interphalangeal (IP) joints in a gentle relaxed flexion (10 degrees).[3,7,14] The palmar arches should be maintained at all times. When the thumb is involved, it may be positioned midway between palmar and radial abduction for greater comfort.[3,18] The design of the resting splint should assist in reduction of median nerve compression in the carpal tunnel. Based on biomechanical principles, the forearm trough of the resting hand splint should extend proximally two thirds the length of the forearm and distally to just beyond the MCP joints, allowing the IP joints to flex. Sometimes full finger support is given (see Figure 14-1). The width of the splint should be one half the circumference of the forearm. If both thumbs are involved, the most affected joint should be supported in a thumb trough that extends $\frac{1}{2}$ inch beyond the end of the thumb, with a pincer grasp allowed on the less affected hand. Splint straps (usually made of Velcro) may need to be padded, trimmed, and/or adapted to ensure a client's independence in the safe application and removal of the splint.[19]

Wearing schedules for resting hand splints vary depending on the diagnostic condition, disease status, physician order, and splint purpose. Clients with arthritis often wear resting splints at night. If a client has bilateral resting hand splints, she/he may choose to alternate splints each night. This may facilitate a client's ability to tolerate bilateral splints and probably improve adherence with her or his wearing schedule.[14]

Wrist Cock-up Splint

A *static wrist orthosis*, commonly referred to as a wrist-cock-up splint, wrist immobilization splint, or work splint, is often prescribed for a painful wrist to improve overall hand function. This splint maintains the wrist in a functional position (neutral or slightly extended) and helps relieve pain by supporting and immobilizing the wrist joint while allowing full MCP flexion and thumb mobility (Figure 14-2).

These splints are usually worn during the day to reduce wrist stress when the client performs daily occupations and heavier activities. Static wrist cock-up splints, which permit some degree of wrist movement, have been shown to improve the client's grip strength at pain onset.[7] A minor design drawback of this splint is that it may interfere with fine motor tasks requiring active wrist flexion/extension, a full palmar grasp, or fine manual manipulation.[8,20,21]

A rigid wrist orthosis worn continually can create compensatory stress on the MCP joints. If a client has acute wrist synovitis and active MCP synovitis, this increased stress can aggravate MCP joint inflammation.[22] Education of the client is necessary to enable her or him to develop an on/off wearing schedule for the static wrist splint, typically using it for heavier activities but not for less stressful tasks. This will allow the client to protect the wrist joint without compromising the MCP joints. A wrist cock-up splint should ideally hold the wrist between 0 and 10 degrees of extension to stabilize the wrist yet allow full mobility of MCP, proximal interphalangeal (PIP), and distal interphalangeal (DIP) joints, as well as the carpometacarpal (CMC) joint of the thumb. The volar support in the palm should not exceed the dorsal palmar crease, and the thenar eminence must be cleared and kept free to permit full excursion of the thumb.[7,23] Therapists also can use these splints as the base for fabricating dynamic hand/wrist splints.

Prefabricated static wrist splints (Figure 14-3) with a removable metal support bar are commercially available and may be an option for daily activities that contribute to wrist pain.[8,21,24] The metal support bar can be removed to allow a minimal amount of wrist motion as necessary; in turn, this bar may help to decrease the force placed on the MCP joints. Neoprene wrist splints also provide alternative lightweight support while allowing some degree of movement.

Given its neutral thermal (warmth) properties, neoprene may serve a dual purpose in providing some pain relief. There are many different types of prefabricated wrist orthoses available on the market through medical and health supply companies and large drugstore chains. Careful fitting and overall comfort of prefabricated splints is an important challenge, especially because many of these splints may not conform to all client limbs, given the normal

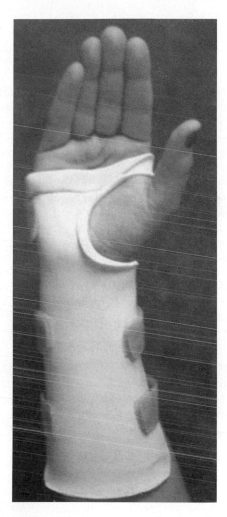

Figure 14-2. Static wrist cock-up splint: this immobilization splint maintains the wrist in a functional (neutral) position and helps to relieve joint pain through wrist immobilization and joint support. (From Coppard BM, Lohman H [eds]: *Introduction to Splinting: A Critical-Thinking and Problem-Solving Approach.* St. Louis, Mosby-Year Book, 1996, p 69. With permission.)

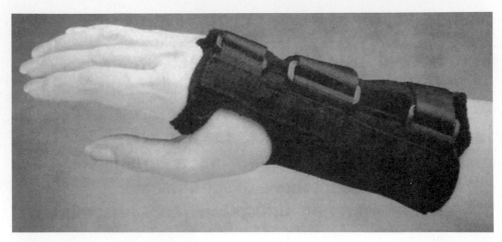

Figure 14-3. Prefabricated wrist splint: Comfort Cool D-ring wrist splint. (From Trombly CA, Radomski MV [eds]: *Occupational Therapy for Physical Dysfunction*, 5th ed. Philadephia, Lippincott Williams & Wilkins, 2002, p 321. With permission.)

variability in size and shape. As a result, commercial off-the-shelf splints cannot provide the exact form fit of custom-made splints and, thus, one size *does* not fit all. Comparisons have been made between various commercially made wrist splints in clients with arthritis, specifically in terms of comfort, fit, function, and overall satisfaction. To date, however, there have been few, if any, studies that have compared custom-made static wrist splints with prefabricated static wrist splints with regard to cost, adherence, and overall efficacy.[8,21]

> **One size does not fit all. Over-the-counter splints cannot provide an exact fit.**

Thumb Splint

As with most actively inflamed joints, the thumb may develop a variety of joint deformities with any or all of the thumb joints becoming involved to a lesser or greater degree. Specifically, in RA, the CMC joint is particularly affected. Management of the arthritic thumb is generally based on the occupational and functional needs of the client as well as on the pattern and severity of deformity. When used early on in the disease process, splinting can help to reduce pain, slow deformity, and enhance function by stabilizing the thumb joints involved during hand use.[25] Splinting is typically used as a conservative treatment measure; however, it also may be used in postoperative management.

One of the most commonly prescribed thumb splints for clients with arthritis is the *thumb immobilization splint* or *thumb spica splint* (Figure 14-4). This splint is also known as the *thumb gauntlet splint* and the *short or long-opponens splint,*[2] and its primary purpose is to protect, stabilize, rest, position, and immobilize one or all of the thumb joints while the other digits are allowed to remain free for movement. One splinting method involves immobilizing the thumb in a long forearm/wrist-based thumb spica splint that places the CMC joint in slight flexion and palmar abduction (as tolerated) to enable opposition to the middle and index fingers, the wrist in 20 to 30 degrees of extension, and the MCP joint in neutral to 5 degrees of flexion. This splint is particularly useful for clients with arthritis or those who have de Quervain's tenosynovitis (tendinitis) whose thumb joints are inflamed, painful, and require mechanical stabilization and support while they perform their daily occupations and activities.

Modifications of this splint may include a hand-based, short thumb spica splint that stabilizes the MCP and CMC joints in the thumb post (near the web space) but does not incorporate the wrist and an even shorter thumb spica splint that stabilizes only the CMC joint.[26] Depending on the severity of the deformity, the therapist will usually fabricate a splint that provides optimal support, allows for maximal function, and is least restrictive in terms of movement. Whereas custom made thermoplastic splints provide more precise and rigid support and immobilization, a variety of prefabricated thumb splints also may be useful because

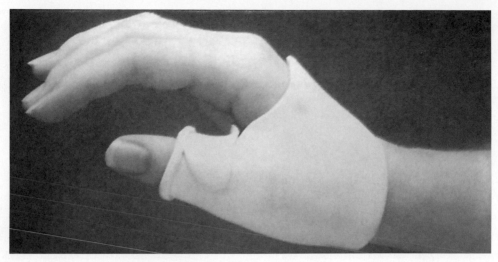

Figure 14-4. Custom thermoplastic short thumb spica splint. (From Trombly CA, Radomski MV [eds]: *Occupational Therapy for Physical Dysfunction,* ed 5. Philadephia, Lippincott Williams & Wilkins, 2002, p 322. With permission.)

they tend to give softer, more lightweight support. However, Melvin[27] cautions that many commercially available, prefabricated CMC and MCP stabilization splints have been found to be ineffective because they tend to fit client's hands and thumbs poorly and therefore cannot serve their proper splinting function.

Finger Splint

Static and dynamic splints often are indicated when reducible deformities (e.g., swan-neck or boutonnière) occur in the fingers (see Figure 3-8). Splints that apply force to the damaged rheumatoid joint may help correct the contractures caused by connective tissue shortening. "Prolonged passive stretch at moderate tension on a contracted joint may elongate tight soft tissues."[28]

Three-point pressure or a figure-of-eight splint will apply pressure to the PIP joint in either flexion or extension in an effort to reduce or prevent further joint contracture.[9] This type of splinting, however, does not resolve the predisposing condition, such as chronic synovitis, nor can it correct deformity caused by eroded cartilage or bony changes. These splints are designed to facilitate the client's use of a joint for specific hand functions by positioning the affected joint in a mechanically advantageous position in the presence of joint damage.[28]

For a swan-neck deformity, a PIP *double-ring flexion splint* could be fabricated. This splint (also referred to

as the *ring splint*) is designed to prevent the hyper-extension of the PIP joint (Figure 14-5A). Fingertip prehension is increased and, as a result, there may be improvement in grip strength, thumb and finger opposition, function in ADL, and cosmesis. For a boutonnière deformity a PIP *double-ring extension splint* could be fabricated (Figure 14-5B). This splint is designed to prevent further flexion of the PIP joint. The design of this splint will not enhance fingertip prehension, but it does assist in maintaining both flexion and extension in that joint.

These types of double-ring splints can be fabricated from different types of materials. The use of low-temperature thermoplastic splints, custom fitted by a therapist, is often indicated because of their low cost and easy accessibility. When required, permanent custom-fabricated silver rings may be used. Precise measurements by a health professional are sent to a company that fabricates the permanent silver ring splints (see Appendix I). The benefits of the silver ring splints are their slim fit that allows several to be worn on each hand, the cosmetic appeal of the jewelry-like look, and the ease of removal. Silver ring custom-fitted orthoses provide an aesthetic option for long-term management of swan-neck and boutonnière deformities.[3] Although a drawback to this type of splint is the increased cost, many insurance companies provide some coverage for such devices. Insurance coverage, however, varies across insurance carriers and the type of policy held; thus, clients should consult

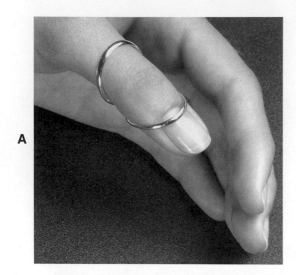
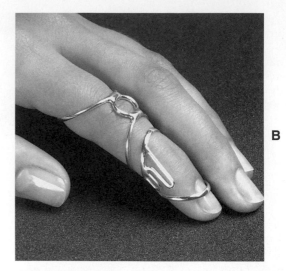

Figure 14-5. *A*, A double silver ring splint (Siris swan neck) blocks hyperextension of the IP joint of the thumb. By stabilizing the joint, power and prehension are improved. *B*, Double-ring splints (Siris boutonnière and lateral support) can stabilize and correct more complicated deformity. (Courtesy of the Silver Ring Splint Company, Charlottesville, VA.)

their insurance broker and/or policy directly for specific details about the coverage provided by their plan.

Dynamic Hand Splinting

Dynamic splinting is very specialized and must be performed by only those therapists with a high degree of experience, in-depth knowledge, and expert splinting skills. One common type of dynamic splint that is fabricated for clients with advanced MCP joint arthritis is a *postsurgical wrist-MCP* orthosis, which is used after MCP joint implant arthroplasty. This splint supports the wrist and controls the positioning and alignment of the fingers, while allowing some controlled and limited active MCP flexion. The overall splinting goal is to apply controlled low-amplitude force over a prolonged period to influence the organization and synthesis of new scar tissue forming in and around the joint capsule, which is referred to as the encapsulation process.[3,22,29]

Dynamic splinting is a highly specialized approach that is generally performed after a surgical procedure. This type of splinting is usually carried out by an occupational therapist or certified hand therapist. A therapist's involvement in this type of complex splinting often depends on her or his training and experience, as well as the types of surgical intervention being performed at the health facility or clinic. (See Additional Readings for more comprehensive resources on dynamic hand splinting.)

Education and Adherence

The principles of client education should be applied when clients are taught about their individual splinting program. In general, clients who learn and understand the purposes of splint care, as well as the directions, precautions, and expectations for splint use, will tend to have better adherence to splinting programs.[30] Limited research concerning client motivation and adherence issues with splint provision exists in the literature. A variety of factors may have an impact on motivation and adherence with a given treatment regimen or protocol; these include external factors such as socioeconomic status, culture, and family support, as well as internal factors such as the client's knowledge, locus of control, beliefs, perceptions, and attitudes towards her or his condition.[31,32] Comfort and proper fit of a splint are other factors that will increase adherence of wearing splints. It is important that a therapist with expert splinting skills, clinical experience, and knowledge of proper joint positioning in arthritis be able to fabricate these types of orthoses. Adherence may be improved when the client can apply and remove the splint(s) independently. The type of strapping used and the ability to engage in functional activities are also of utmost importance.

In a recent study adherence to splinting protocols varied greatly, ranging from 25% to almost 83%.[25] In an earlier study, Belcon et al[33] had estimated that about 50% of patients with arthritis do not comply with their treatment regimen, regardless of the nature of the intervention. These authors reviewed 19 reported studies to assess the adherence to medications, physical therapy, and splint prescription. They observed drug adherence to range from 16% to 84%, physical therapy from 39% to 65%, and splint use from 25% to 65%. Studies of splint adherence have shown that use of resting hand splints is less than optimal.[34-36] In a study designed to identify psychological factors related to adherence or non-adherence of splint use in clients with RA, Moon et al[34] reported that only one third of clients actually complied with the splint protocol ($n = 46$).

Feinberg and Brandt[35] demonstrated that the health care provider's attitude and behavior can influence client adherence with splint wearing. Forty subjects were randomly assigned to a standard treatment group or to a adherence-enhancing group. The experimental therapy consisted of the use of learning principles, sharing of expectations, and use of a positive affective tone and behavior by the therapist; additionally, clients were encouraged to assume responsibility for their care. Results showed that the experimental group wore their resting hand splints more often and had better disease outcomes as exhibited by a shorter duration of morning stiffness ($p = .01$).[35]

Using a client-centered, evidence-based approach, the therapist can positively influence the client's motivation and adherence with wearing her or his splint. It is essential that the therapist view the client as a whole individual with a unique occupational history and lifestyle that exists well beyond the clinical environment. In tandem with client cooperation is the importance of providing on-going client education about the medical and functional benefits of wearing splints.[32] Taking into consideration the clients' perspectives about how splints may affect their lifestyles and occupations, therapists should clearly communicate the type of splint required while providing a clear rationale for wearing the splint. Adherence to appropriate splint use is thought to improve when the client is shown how the splint works, when splinting goals are explained, and when a daily record of wearing time, amount of morning stiffness, grip strength, and number of painful joints are accurately recorded. This type of self-assessment may encourage the client to monitor her or his own progress while experiencing first-hand the benefits of

using the splint(s). As a result, the client may become a more active, willing participant in the implementation of a recommended treatment regimen. Therapists also should convey the information that success with splints involves an equally shared responsibility between themselves and their clients in the overall treatment plan.

> Use of various strategies to enhance adherence is critical if splints are to perform their desired function.

Foot Orthoses

Pathomechanics

Clinical involvement of the foot and ankle may be more common in clients with RA than in those with osteoarthritis (OA). With the exception of OA, few data are available on the prevalence of foot and ankle involvement in most rheumatologic disease. When assessing and treating the ankle and foot, the clinician should recognize that they comprise a *closed chain* system in which each segment is related to and dependent on the others. A loss of mobility and function at any one joint can create a domino effect that sets into motion a series of adaptations and compensatory changes that may affect most or all of the other articulations in the foot and ankle.[37] Thus, controlling the alignment of the foot and ankle with well-designed orthotic devices and proper fitting, supportive footwear may prevent painful complications in the future and further reduce unwanted joint deviations and compensatory motions.

When evaluating and managing a client's arthritic condition, the clinician needs to know whether her or his condition is reactive (e.g., active inflammation and synovitis, acute RA flare-up) or nonreactive (e.g., remitting phase in which there is no acute inflammation). This will help to determine the choice of treatment options including those that are designed to accommodate, stabilize, or realign a *nonreactive* joint and those designed to support, protect, and rest an inflamed *reactive* joint. Once a reactive structure has been treated and subsequently becomes nonreactive, the client then can be fitted with the appropriate foot orthotics and footwear and be given exercises to enable them to resume their daily activities and occupations.

For clients with arthritis, pain is a common reason for prescribing foot orthoses. Examples of foot disorders that may develop in clients with arthritis include metatarsalgia, heel pain syndrome, subtalar joint pronation, severe pes planus (low arch), hallux valgus, and plantar fasciitis.[38] Valgus deformity of the hind-foot is particularly common in clients with RA.[38,39] Changes in the forefoot associated with disease progression are another common complaint and have been discussed in detail in the literature.[39,40] Some studies have shown that as the duration of a rheumatic disease (such as RA) increases, hindfoot deformities become a greater determinant of disability.[40] Also, any alteration, restriction, or malalignment of the subtalar joint may pose significant implications for posture, gait, and overall foot function.[5,37-39,41,42]

The ankle and foot are best described as a triplanar joint mechanism that may demonstrate up to 6 degrees of "freedom" of movement at any one joint; in other words, it translates along and rotates about each of the three axes of motion. The term *triplanar* also indicates that motion occurs in all three planes: sagittal, transverse, and frontal.[43] The soft tissues and bony infrastructure of the foot and ankle are important determinants of lower extremity function in that they comprise what is known as the *foot type*. There are three primary foot types: (1) pes cavus (high arch), (2) (pes planus (low arch), and (3) rectus (normal arch). Each foot type has a distinctly unique biomechanical function and, as with most triplanar joints, each type has a predisposition to exhibit greater motion in one of the three planes.[44] In a healthy gait, the line of weight bearing begins in the lateral aspect of the heel and advances medially toward the forefoot. During this stage, the head of the talus locks into the navicular cavity and the midtarsal joints become rigid. As the foot moves into toe-off phase, forces pass through the plantar surfaces of the medial metatarsal heads and the hallux, creating maximal load and stress on the plantar soft tissues.[45] Possible causes of valgus deformity of the hindfoot include cartilaginous changes in the subtalar and midtarsal joints, laxity of joint capsules and ligaments due to chronic inflammation and swelling, rupture of the tibialis posterior tendon, equinus contracture of the ankle, and calf muscles weakness.[41] Keenan et al[39] suggested that severe hindfoot valgus can result from exaggerated pronation forces on the weakened and inflamed subtalar joint. These increased stresses may be caused by alterations in posture and gait due to symmetrical muscular weakness and compensatory efforts of the client to minimize pain. The authors reported that clients with valgus deformities of the hindfoot also experienced greater forefoot pain.[39]

In clients with RA, the foot tends to be everted during weight bearing while the axes of motion in the talonavicular and calcaneocuboid joints are more parallel than normal, which, in turn, causes an unlocking of the midtarsal and subtalar joints.[46] This prevents early heel rise in the stance phase of gait and decreases pressure over the painful metatarsal heads.[39] It is quite common for clients with severe forefoot pain to walk with their lower extremities in an exaggerated position of lateral rotation because it shortens the lever arm of the foot and further decreases the pressure and shearing stress on the metatarsal heads. This "abnormal" gait pattern results from a combination of a delayed heel rise, decreased stride length, and a slow gait velocity.[39] Also, weakened lower extremity muscles are less efficient and may result in a "shuffling" gait that often characterizes the functional mobility impairment of these clients.

Spiegel and Spiegel[40] observed that there was very little hindfoot pronation in clients during the early stages of the disease, but that as time went on the valgus deformity became more marked. The effect of time on the development of hindfoot valgus deformity indicates that this is probably an acquired deformity in clients with RA, which raises the possibility that early intervention and preventative measures may be effective.[39]

Pain in the forefoot or in the ball of the foot (*metatarsalgia*) often results from repeated stress to the soft tissues. As IP joint ligaments become stretched by inflammation, the weight-bearing stresses during stance cause extension of the toes. The metatarsal (MT) heads begin to drop and their fat pads are forced forward, leaving the bony heads unprotected. This results in painful callosities. The MT heads will begin to erode, leaving sharp bony spicules that produce the sensation of "walking on marbles."[47] The forefoot splays due to weak intrinsic muscles with lax and ineffective collateral ligaments.

As RA progresses, toe deformities often develop. Hallux valgus (bunions), a lateral deviation of the first ray, occurs as the result of ligamentous laxity and joint instability. As the forefoot abducts, weight bearing encourages lateral angulation and flattening of the longitudinal and transverse arches of the foot. Improperly fitting footwear will aggravate the resultant deformity.[48] A *rigid hammer toe* is a fixed osseous deviation (dislocation) of the MTP joint that often occurs as a result of extreme joint malalignment. There is a loss of balance between the flexors and extensors of the toes, resulting in hyperextension at the MTP joints, flexion at the PIP joints, and extension at the DIP joints. As a result, clients tend to develop thick, painful calluses over the second and third heads of the PIP joints.[49] *Claw toes* often develop due to weakness of the intrinsic muscles of the foot and extreme tightness and/or shortening of the extensor tendons. The toe joints become fixed in flexion and the tips of the toes tend to rub against the ground or shoe, creating painful calluses.[49]

Assessment

A comprehensive biomechanical examination of the foot and lower extremity must be performed before the most appropriate treatment and management strategies are selected[43] (see Appendix for a sample foot assessment). During this evaluation, it is important to assess the biomechanical integrity (including stability, presence/absence of deformity, and skeletal alignment) of the foot and ankle joints, as well as the available ROM in these structures. To understand, identify, and treat changes in joint structure and the subsequent compensatory patterns associated with mild to severe foot deformity is highly challenging. A detailed assessment requires careful observation and analysis of the entire lower extremity (not only the foot and ankle) while the client is at rest or standing and during all phases of gait. This process should include firm, but gentle, palpation of the proximal and distal lower extremity to determine areas of joint pain or tenderness, to check muscle tone, and to locate areas of fluid build-up or edema.

It is vital to conduct a close visual inspection for signs of the following:

- Arch flattening
- Excessive callusing
- Limited active and passive ROM
- Joint hypermobility
- Excessive postural compensation
- Limping
- First ray or MTP subluxation
- Skin discoloration
- Rigid or guarded gait patterns
- Tenosynovitis
- Excessive forefoot or hindfoot valgus[50]
- Erythema
- Ankle equinus (insufficient dorsiflexion)
- Triplanar deformities and joint malalignments of the foot (in all three planes)
- Pain elicited by forefoot pronation (valgus) and supination (varus) positions
- The presence of "ankle pain" (which often proves to be midtarsal or subtalar joint pain)

A complete joint count of any and/or all active and damaged joints should be conducted to determine the inflammatory status of the ankle, subtalar, midtarsal, and metatarsal joints. Active and passive ROM should be also assessed at the ankle, subtalar, and midtarsal joints. The transverse and longitudinal arches of the foot should be assessed for height and flexibility during midstance. The integrity and thickness of the skin also must be evaluated in addition to the presence (or absence) of calluses, nailbed changes, fungal in-fections, and any other notable skin surface changes. If deformities and alignment issues are detected early in the disease process, conservative treatment strategies such as footwear recommendations, fabrication of custom orthotic devices, and foot care education are more likely to be successfully implemented and may help to prevent the development of future problems and complications associated with rheumatic disease.[43]

Conservative Management

Because many studies indicate that forefoot and hind-foot valgus foot deformities in arthritis are usually acquired over time, early preventive measures are of prime importance. The key objectives in the conservative management of arthritis include pain relief and comfort, proper foot/joint alignment, maintenance/ improvement of function, and prevention of further deformity and/or disability. Part of the goal is to improve function by controlling the structural abnormalities (specifically hindfoot pronation) when possible, thereby preventing the loss of the longitudinal and transverse arches. Client education is also essential with an emphasis on the importance of pain relief, good foot care, supportive and well-fitting footwear, and the correct use of orthotics (as required) to maintain proper alignment.[43,51]

Footwear Considerations

Most individuals with arthritis encounter some form of foot problem during the course of their lives. Clients with RA tend to have more problems with their forefoot than rearfoot. Repeated bouts of inflammation can severely damage the connective tissues of the foot, resulting in joint deformity, malalignment, or mechanical problems. Clients whose feet are affected in this way often require footwear that is wide enough to accommodate joint changes (e.g., bunion, hammer toe), has a deep toe box, is made of soft supportive material that will not irritate the toes, arch, or heel, and can accommodate removable, custom-made orthoses. Foot orthotics take up more space inside the shoe and should always be worn when trying on new footwear to ensure the best fit. Proper shoe sizing (including adequate forefoot width, instep/arch height, heel depth and width, and toe box depth) in addition to supportive, well-fitting footwear with a nonslip sole design is essential to the successful clinical management of arthritis in the foot.[38,43]

Although there are many varieties of shoes on the market from which the client may choose, few are made to accommodate the significant joint changes and deformities associated with arthritis. Overall foot comfort can be achieved by preventing the development of shearing forces, stress, or irritation against the surface of the foot and ankle. Shoes must be able to protect areas of deformity while supporting areas of instability. Here is a quick reference checklist of the main characteristics to look for when purchasing footwear:

- Adequate forefoot width (measure the broadest part of forefoot) to prevent pinching
- Deep, flexible toe box to allow room for toe movement and accommodate deformities
- Shock-absorbing sole with a nonslip tread design for better grip and stability
- Relatively flat sole/low heel to decrease stress on the MT heads
- Padded collar to help prevent irritation around the ankle area
- Removable insole that can be replaced with a more supportive, custom-made orthosis (as required)
- Firm heel counter to provide support and to keep the heel bone vertical, resisting the tendency to roll the ankle or foot inward during weight bearing
- Lace-up style to provide a snug fit that can be easily adjusted to accommodate swelling; for a client with limited hand function, use Velcro straps or elastic laces
- Supportive shank (usually metal or plastic) to reinforce the sole of the shoe, provide arch support, and prevent unwanted bending of the mid-sole

High-end running shoes (Figure 14-6) can often accommodate the foot needs of clients with RA; however, these specialty shoes must be tried on before purchase to ensure a proper fit. These shoes are usually available in most adult sizes (some also come in children's sizes), and many makes and models also come in specific widths (e.g., narrow "AA" to extra wide "EE") for a better fit. As previously mentioned, running (or walking) shoes, like other footwear, should have (1) a wide, soft toe box that is rounded, (2) adequate forefoot width, (3) a removable insole, and (4) a shock-absorbing outer sole.

Sandals, such as Birkenstock, Clarks, Dexter Shoes, or NAOT brands (Figure 14-7A), may be an alterative to bulky sneakers (especially for indoor wear), provided the footbed is wide enough, arch support is adequate, and a heel cup is present to control excessive hindfoot motion.

Extra depth shoes may be required for the more involved arthritic foot (Figure 14-7B). These shoes are usually very wide and extra deep to accommodate a variety of bony deformities in addition to the client's orthoses. The upper of this shoe is often made of soft leather, such as deerskin, to decrease pressure on bony or protruding structures.

Some modifications often can be made to the heel, shank, or sole area of a shoe, depending on the foot problem and may require the addition (or removal) of metatarsal pads, longitudinal arch supports, medial or lateral posts, or wedges. These components, when used appropriately, can provide additional support and alignment to bones and joint structures during gait

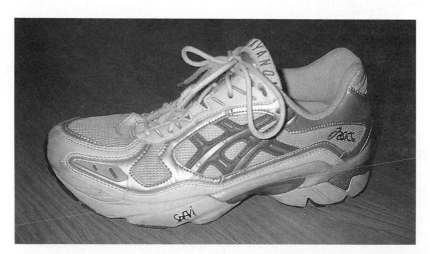

Figure 14-6. Supportive lace-up running shoes. Running or walking shoes should have (1) a wide, soft rounded toe box, (2) adequate forefoot width and heel counter support, (3) a removable insole, and (4) a shock-absorbing outer sole.

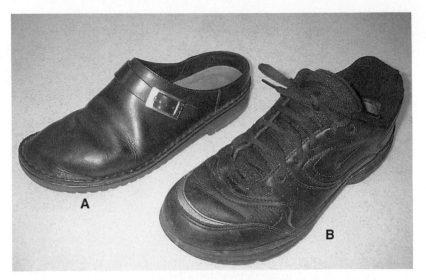

Figure 14-7. *A*, Leather slip-on sandal/clog with covered-in toe box and buckle adjustment. It also has a suede-lined, removable cork footbed with a deep heel counter that provides increased foot support, a wide rounded toe box, and a slight wedge heel. *B*, Extra-depth walking shoe with leather upper, extra wide forefoot, deep heel counter, and removable insole.

and may help to dissipate weight-bearing stresses from painful areas of the foot.

Orthosis Management

Properly adjusted and well-balanced foot orthotics are devices that work to correct malalignments of the body by reducing or eliminating abnormal gait patterns and postures associated with soft tissue and bony deformities that result from rheumatic disease. By controlling excessive or unwanted motion at certain joints, orthotics also may help to reduce the pain and symptomatic stress experienced by the client in her or his lower extremity.

Foot orthotics are generally classified in one of three categories: (1) flexible, (2) rigid, or (3) semirigid. The type of orthotics used with a given client is chosen on the basis of the client's clinical presentation and her or his individual needs. For clients who require general support and accommodative protection for bony deformities, a flexible orthosis will tend to be the best choice. Clients who require a high degree of biomechanical control, support, and joint realignment would benefit from a rigid orthosis. For those who would like to maintain some degree of movement but also need better foot alignment with some increased stability, a semirigid orthotic (Figure 14-8) would be most appropriate.[38,40,43]

> **Extra depth shoes are needed for clients with severe foot deformities.**

The key goals of orthotic intervention and management should include the following:

- Reduce pain
- Control motion (elimination of excessive, unwanted movement)
- Accommodate fixed deformities
- Realign joints via positional correction
- Limit or reduce the progression of current deformities
- Increase shock absorption and overall comfort
- Allow for biomechanical off-loading of forefoot (especially plantar-flexed metatarsal heads)
- Redistribute force and stress from high to low pressure areas
- Reduce shearing stress and abnormal shoe wear
- Provide stability to inflamed or unstable joints (especially important for clients with RA)

Orthotics are made from a variety of different materials including flexible closed-cell Plastazote, neoprene, and PPT foam (a polyurethane material) as well as more rigid materials such as leather, cork, fiberglass, high-temperature thermoplastics, and

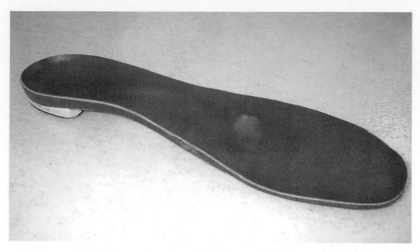

Figure 14-8. Customized semi-rigid foot orthotic. Orthotic modifications may include a deep heel cup, slight heel elevation (heel wedge), a cut-out to accommodate a bony prominence, neutral subtalar frontal plane posting (when possible), and extended flanges for greater transverse plane stability.

acrylics.[5,38,43] The orthotic prescription should include a top cover that provides some cushioning to protect and accommodate tender, inflamed, or irritated areas, and dissipate excessive forces that affect the MT heads.

When less control of the hindfoot is required, the orthotics may be fabricated from low-temperature thermoplastics, polyurethanes, or closed-cell neoprene rubber, which provide soft cushioning and gentle support. Orthotics may be fabricated by a variety of individuals, depending on their clinical expertise, background training, and scope of practice. In Canada, orthotics are typically made by a registered/licensed occupational therapist, a certified orthotist, a certified pedorthist, or a Doctor of Podiatric Medicine (DPM).

Orthotics are intended to unload the metatarsal heads during the initial to midstance phase of gait, provide shock absorption, and reduce friction under the MT heads during terminal stance. Some custom orthotics are made from a negative-cast plaster mold of the client's foot and tend to be more expensive than the temporary, off-the-shelf products. Heel pain due to plantar fasciitis, heel spurs, or rheumatoid nodules also can be a common problem. Rubber or silicone-gel heel cups have been used to alleviate painful heel syndrome. The aim of heel cups is to support the hindfoot and long arch while providing some cushioning and pain relief over the tender area(s). These products are generally available from health supply companies and large drugstore chains. Custom-made shoes are another option that may help to reduce pain and improve stability and support during ambulation for clients with severe RA foot changes. The upper, lining, and insole of the shoe are made of soft material that tends to conform to these structural changes by distributing the pressure over the entire sole of the foot. Shoemakers who specialize in making these shoes for clients with arthritis should be consulted.[42] Many health insurance plans may provide limited coverage for the cost of certain custom-made orthoses, shoes, and braces. Clients are encouraged to consult their insurance company for specific details.

Summary

Hand splints and foot orthotics are only one component of a comprehensive arthritis management program. Splinting programs will be most effective when combined with anti-inflammatory therapy and a customized exercise program, in addition to client education about joint protection and energy conservation, the proper use of the orthotics, pain reduction techniques, and maintenance of functional range of motion and muscle strength. Orthoses, therefore, must be evaluated and reassessed within both the context of the client and as an overall program. When it is not possible to eradicate all symptoms, the outcome measure(s) should directly reflect the client's goals and expectations within the limitations and constraints of a realistic prognosis.

Lifestyle and Occupational Factors

Arthritis can have a profound effect on a person's ability to engage in their daily activities, occupations, and life roles. Because of the chronic and often progressive nature of the disease, treatment and rehabilitation tend to occur over an extended period of time (often months and years).[3,4] In addition to the deleterious impact of arthritis on daily living tasks such as eating, bathing, dressing, personal hygiene, walking, and meal preparation, leisure and work (both paid and unpaid) activities are often interrupted.[52,53] In 1994, Katz[53] conducted a study in which 80% of respondents with RA reported or identified a loss of valued activities, including leisure activities. Some of the activities reported as being most often disrupted included walking, participation in sports, housework, crafts, gardening, shopping, and socializing.[52–54]

Arthritis-related impairments differ from person to person and may include:

- Pain of varying intensity, duration, and location
- Muscle weakness
- Joint swelling (extra- or intra-articular)
- Joint deformity
- Decreased ROM
- Joint instability
- Stiffness (especially in the morning)
- Fatigue
- Other systemic involvement

The concepts of joint protection and energy conservation have evolved from clinical observations that support the notion that trauma exacerbates inflammatory arthritis and that fatigue may be reduced by careful use of the joints and muscle. Joint damage, deformity, and inflammation are often responsible for inducing pain, whereas the excess energy a client may use during the performance of her or his daily routine can be a primary source of fatigue and weakness. However, there has been little systematic study of the effectiveness of these programs and techniques or of the effectiveness of occupational therapy intervention despite its longstanding role and application in the management of clients with arthritis. Many of the studies to date have demonstrated some effectiveness of occupational therapy intervention in educating clients but have not shown that this leads to long-term functional improvement or behavioral change.[51,55–57]

This section will specifically address (1) the role and use of assistive devices and (2) the principles and techniques of energy conservation and joint protection that can be used by clients with arthritis in facilitating and maximizing their functional abilities, occupational performance, and daily routines. Whenever possible, the client's functional challenges and limitations should be minimized via the use of alternative strategies and techniques. Many clients, however, may prefer to carry out an activity or occupation through a modified approach that does not include the use of additional equipment or assistive devices. Given the daily challenges faced by individuals with arthritis, alternative methods that include the principles of joint protection and energy conservation can be practically used to guide and enhance their occupational performance and functional abilities.[57,58] Through the use of ongoing client education, therapeutic intervention, as well as alternative and adaptive strategies, and with the proper support systems in place, clients with arthritis can develop a sense of personal control and empowerment in learning to effectively manage their disease.

Assistive Devices

Assistive devices are an important component of a larger area known as assistive technologies. These devices include those items, product systems, and/or pieces of equipment that may be customized or adapted, acquired via individual or commercial means, and are used to improve, maintain, or increase an individual's occupational performance and functional abilities in their day-to-day activities and routines.[59] Assistive devices are often recommended by rehabilitation professionals to reduce pain and joint stress, improve safety, increase functional independence, compensate for muscle weakness, and overcome joint limitations. Ideally, these items should be easy to use, lightweight, durable, and suitable for the client's own needs and preferences.

Examples of some commonly available assistive devices include the following:

- **Self-care** (e.g., long-handle shoe horn [Figure 14-9]; raised toilet seat [Figure 14-10]; grab bars in the bathtub)
- **Meal preparation** (e.g., double-finger [rifle] mug [Figure 14-11]; rocker knife [Figure 14-12]; built-up grips on cooking and eating utensils [Figure 14-13]; adapted lid-opener [Figure 14-14])
- **Home maintenance** (e.g., long-handled dustpan, built-up grips on hand tools)
- **Work and school** (e.g., computer forearm rests [Figure 14-15]; work bench tool organizer [Figure 14-16 and 14-17])
- **Leisure** (e.g., adapted gardening tools; book holder)

The use of assistive devices has greatly increased in the last 25 years due to an aging population, the

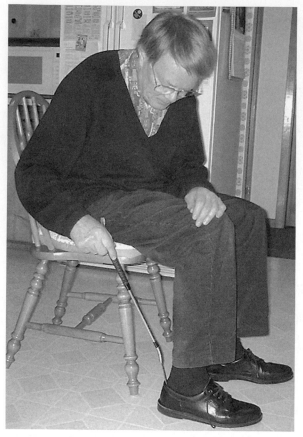

Figure 14-9. Long-handled shoe horn. To assist with donning shoes.

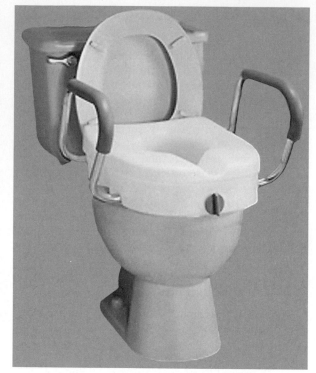

Figure 14-10. Raised toilet seat with arms.

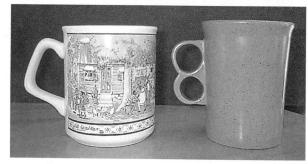

Figure 14-11. Mugs. *Left*, Regular mug. *Right*, Double-finger (rifle) mug that reduces thumb and finger joint stress by distributing the load across the index and middle fingers, as well as being much lighter.

rapid growth of universal design and access, and a growing interest in occupational ergonomics.[54,60–62] Most items are readily available to the general public through the retail sector, large chain pharmacies and drugstores, commercial sales, and other specialty shops (see Resources in Appendix I). For clients with arthritis, assistive devices can be particularly valuable for improving and/or maintaining a level of functional independence on an interim or long-term basis. A variety of physical, psychosocial, emotional, environmental, and financial factors must be taken into consideration when one prescribes or recommends the use of assistive devices, and clients should be provided an opportunity to try the device(s) before purchase to ensure it meets their needs.[62] As an educational component, it is useful to instruct clients about specific joint protection principles when they are looking for devices and products that create the least amount of joint stress. However, despite the recommendations of a qualified health care professional (e.g., occupational therapist, physiotherapist) for a given device, there is no guarantee that the client will adhere to its prescribed use.

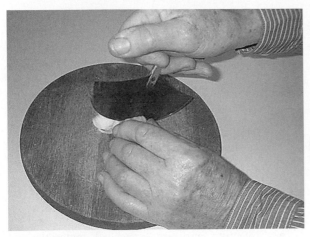

Figure 14-12. Short rocker knife.

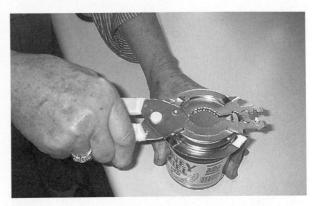

Figure 14-14. Adapted (three-size) lid-opener. Note the ulnar deviation stress on the metacarpophalangeal joints. This activity may aggravate or promote the typical deformity, ulnar deviation.

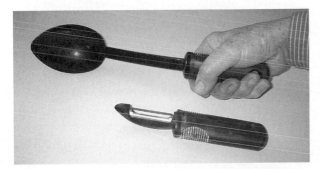

Figure 14-13. Built-up grips on cooking utensils. Handles on any utensil or tool can be enlarged by applying grip wrapping, rubber or foam, to name a few options.

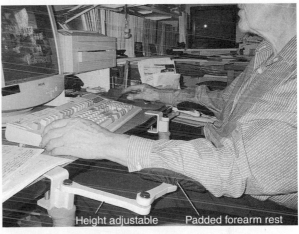

Figure 14-15. Ergonomic computer forearm rests. These height-adjustable, freely swinging arm rests promote a relaxed shoulder posture and permit easy access to the keyboard, mouse, and adjacent materials. (Available from North Coast Medical, www.ncmedical.com.)

Energy Conservation Techniques

Conserving energy and reducing the amount of effort needed to carry out daily activities is an important consideration for clients with rheumatic disease who may fatigue easily and feel exhausted after a period of exertion. Limited endurance and fatigue may pose challenges to clients' successfully performing daily tasks and occupations because these activities often require additional time throughout the day or week to accommodate a client's activity tolerance and energy levels.[57,58] Energy-saving strategies are numerous and involve planning, prioritizing, and delegating tasks. Clients should plan ahead to ensure that all necessary daily activities can be adequately managed, including rest, exercise, and leisure. Clients are encouraged to plan and organize their week in terms of essential home, child care, and work activities.

> **Clients must recognize that pain occurring during an activity is a red flag.**

Successful management of fatigue involves new ways of organizing priorities, time, tasks, and rest periods. To combat and control the effects of fatigue and low energy levels, the therapist should teach the client how to analyze her or his daily activities to determine activities that predispose the client to develop increased pain and fatigue.[57] Clients with inflammatory arthritis must learn to pace themselves and understand the physical demands of a task.

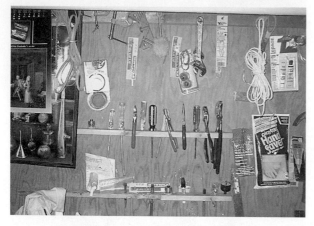

Figure 14-16. Work bench organizer.

Reducing or eliminating stressful body movements and excessive motion may help to conserve energy. By using energy-saving techniques, clients may discover they can accomplish more by using less energy, thereby improving the quality of their lives. Modifications for scheduling and performing activities may include the following:

- Prioritizing and planning the most important activities and tasks
- Performing tasks while seated whenever possible
- Preventing excessive reaching, gripping, or bending using built-up grips or extensions
- Modifying handles of tools and utensils
- Collecting and organizing all materials and supplies in one area before commencing a project
- Limiting the number of trips up and down stairs
- Taking frequent rest breaks throughout the day and especially when performing activities

For more energy-saving suggestions see Table 14-1.

Principles of Joint Protection

Occupational therapists use a variety of joint protection principles and techniques to help clients with arthritis

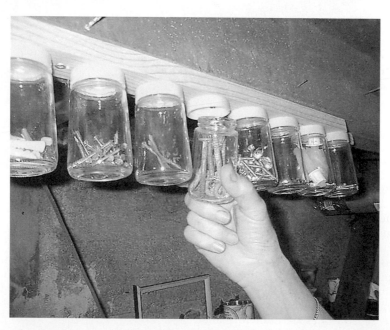

Figure 14-17. Work tool organizer or work area organizer for small objects. Because the lids are fixed, opening jars becomes easier and can be done with one hand. The eye-level location also encourages shoulder motion.

Table 14-1. Common Daily Energy-Saving Strategies

- **Limit the amount of work and delegate tasks.**

When possible, avoid excess fatigue by assigning heavier household tasks to other family members or a housekeeper (e.g., vacuuming, cleaning).

- **Avoid/reduce task demands and repetition and eliminate unnecessary tasks.**

Do smaller loads of laundry throughout the week; air-dry dishes; drip-dry clothing to limit the need for ironing.

- **Use efficient methods to simplify work.**

Organize your work areas and spaces efficiently. Store frequently used items close at hand to avoid reaching. Meal preparation can be simplified when enough food is prepared for three or four meals. A microwave oven can heat food quickly. Using frozen foods and freezing meals for future use is also helpful for decreasing time and energy used in meal preparation. Avoid standing for long periods and try to sit when doing a task (e.g., ironing). Use a utility or grocery cart on wheels to transport items.

- **Use proper body positions, postures, and equipment.**

Assistive devices can eliminate excessive bending, reaching, and stooping (e.g., long-handled reacher). Adjust your work height and use tools that are task-appropriate. Keep ergonomic principles in mind both at home and work, and watch your posture—do not put yourself at risk when lifting, carrying, or transporting objects.

- **Pace yourself and balance daily routines with frequent rest breaks.**

To avoid fatigue, pace yourself and do not rush! Frequent rest periods of 5 to 10 minutes throughout the day can replenish energy reserves and enhance functional endurance during activity. A moderate work pace consumes the least amount of energy. Clients should learn to work at a consistent and relaxed pace, using smooth movements.

- **Plan ahead.**

Schedule activities such as homemaking, shopping, appointments, and other energy-consuming tasks throughout the week. Prioritize the most important tasks, perform them early in the day before fatigue becomes a problem, and give yourself enough time to do what you need to do.

---

reduce their pain levels, minimize the degree and severity of deformity, and maintain their functional status. There are four primary goals of joint protection[57,58]:

- To reduce localized swelling and inflammation
- To reduce loading through damaged and vulnerable joints
- To relieve joint pain during activity
- To help the client develop effective strategies for preserving joint function, structure, and integrity

The principles outlined in this section follow the revised guidelines for joint protection as described by Cordery and Rocchi.[57] The therapist must clearly and carefully instruct the client about the appropriate use and application of these educational principles to facilitate carryover of learning and behavioral change. Adoption of these new behaviors, even if only for the short term, may be improved by using collaborative problem-solving and experiential learning approaches. These new behaviors also may be fostered by focusing on tasks that are familiar and important to the client and by setting realistic, achievable goals that provide the client with opportunities for mastery and success.

Some of the key principles of joint protection include the following:

1. **Respect pain:** Individuals with arthritis and other rheumatic diseases often learn to live with some level of pain in their day-to-day lives. Clients must learn how to recognize and distinguish between what is a "usual" amount

(and type) of pain and what is "not a usual" amount (and type) of pain, generally caused by overuse or misuse of a muscle or joint. If pain intensity and duration increase or acute inflammation develops, the activity thought to be the root cause should be changed, stopped, and/or avoided; strategies to reduce or eliminate joint stress also should be incorporated.

2. **Balance work and rest:** Fatigue plays a significant role for clients with arthritis. Individuals with specific forms of arthritis such as RA usually require more rest and must learn to find a balance between activities and rest to accomplish their desired activities. Pacing activities and planning ahead can prevent exhaustion and limit further injury and joint damage.

3. **Maintain muscle strength and joint ROM:** This may be achieved by using each joint to its maximum available strength and ROM during daily activities and occupations. Balanced strength around unstable joints can reduce the chance of injury to the joint capsule, cartilage, and ligaments, preventing further deformity. Joint position and adequate ROM are essential for optimal muscle functioning. For example, when sweeping, ironing, or mopping, clients should keep their backs straight while using long, smooth stroking movements, gently bending the arms as much as possible.

4. **Use each joint in its most stable and functional plane:** The most stable functional plane for joint movement is one in which the muscle provides resistance to the motion.[57] However, joint inflammation, synovitis, and bony outgrowths (e.g., osteophytes) can contribute to joint instability, deformity, and ligamentous laxity. To prevent these problems, clients should avoid using quick, rapid joint movements.

5. **Avoid positions of deformity:** Positions of comfort (e.g., flexion) can often promote the development of contractures and joint deformities during acute flare-ups in the fingers, wrists, elbows, knees, and hips. Soft tissue shortening may lead to contractures if muscles and joints are not stretched and moved through range or remain fixed in a resting position of flexion for long periods.

6. **Use the largest and strongest joints available for the job:** Force applied to larger joints is more easily and efficiently dispersed than when it is applied to smaller joints that are often more vulnerable to stress, damage, and deformity. Joint stress can be significantly reduced when a mechanical advantage is applied to the correct movement and safe handling of objects. Examples may include lifting objects while keeping the back straight and using the legs, knees, and hips instead of bending at the waist; using both arms to lift an object, keeping it close to the body; and sliding objects with both arms rather than carrying them.

7. **Avoid staying in one position:** It is important for people with arthritis to avoid awkward, static, and prolonged postures both at work and home, because they can lead to increased joint stiffness, pain, and fatigue. Clients should be encouraged to frequently change their positions throughout the day, alternating between standing and sitting, if possible (e.g., this is especially important for clients who sit for long periods at computers and other workstations).

8. **Reduce the force:** Strong resistive motions can be dangerous and painful to already damaged joints. Avoiding tight hand grasps and awkward and repetitive joint positions, and using lightweight, built-up handles on utensils and tools can help to reduce excessive stress and compression forces.

Long-term and outcomes research on the effectiveness of these techniques are limited, and such studies are difficult to carry out in a clinical setting. However, some short-term studies have revealed important information about the potential uses and benefits of joint protection and energy conservation programs. Outcomes of a 3-week joint protection education program for women with RA indicated that 95% of clients showed a significant increase in ability to perform ADL after the intervention.[63] In an observational assessment of joint protection techniques used by individuals with RA, increased use of hand joint protection was reported in clients who compensated for decreased grip strength and hand joint pain.[64] Although these studies provide an initial basis for evaluating energy conservation and joint protection programs, future research involving randomized controlled clinical trials is required to further assess, evaluate, and validate their potential benefits and long-term implications for clients with arthritis.

Conclusion

Arthritis is a serious and complex disease that requires a client-centered, team-based approach to treatment. It is vital for therapists to work closely with clients in helping them to become actively involved in their own treatment and learn to take responsibility for the long-term management of their arthritis. Incorporation of the principles and techniques outlined in this chapter will enable clients to participate more fully in their daily occupations, gain control over their disease, and enhance their quality of life.

Research Questions

1. What role does formal client education play in adherence to occupational therapy protocols recommended for clients with arthritis?
2. For clients with Osteoarthritis and Rheumatoid Arthritis, how is splinting used to improve, maintain, and/or restore occupational functioning and performance?
3. What is the impact of chronic arthritis on occupational engagement and do gender differences exist?

Case Study

Client Information. Ms. H. is a single, left-handed 46-year-old elementary schoolteacher with a 3-year history of rheumatoid arthritis; she has been followed by a rheumatologist since her initial diagnosis and is currently taking anti-inflammatory medication. She teaches grade 5 full-time and lives alone in a large, single-level two-bedroom condominium. Her chief complaint is bilateral wrist pain, worse in her dominant left hand.

An initial interview reveals that Ms. H. has increased pain and fatigue after working a full day at school. Her daily teaching schedule requires 3 hours in total spent writing on the blackboard. During the day, she opens and closes the heavy entrance doors of the school at least three or four times. Ms. H. carries a heavy briefcase and drives her four-door Toyota Camry sedan to and from work each day. She usually brings her lunch to school but finds it increasingly difficult to prepare it before she leaves the house because of morning stiffness. The pain and discomfort often decrease or subside during the weekend when she engages in relatively few active tasks such as cooking or housecleaning. She enjoys having friends over, and they often end up doing the cooking; her housekeeping tasks also have not been kept up over the last few weeks. Her wrist pain is usually eliminated during vacations and in the summer when she is not teaching. Other problems include the following:

1. Increased fatigue from prolonged standing at work
2. Bilateral wrist pain with mild inflammation (greater in the left wrist)

3. Mild to moderate pain in the balls of both feet (worse at the end of the day)
4. Difficulty doing heavy housework (e.g., vacuuming and cleaning the two bathrooms).

On evaluation, both wrists and MCP joints show mild inflammation, left (L) > right (R); there are no other notable pain complaints in other joints. Ms. H.'s grip strength is R = 140 mm Hg and L = 125 mm Hg. She reports 30 to 45 minutes of morning stiffness, but this has gradually improved with the use of anti-inflammatory medication. Her sensation is intact bilaterally with a normal distribution. There is minimal limitation of both active and passive ROM of the wrists, shoulders, and ankles attributed to pain. Some other functional limitations include the following: difficulty lifting heavy objects such as pots and pans, writing on the blackboard or preparing vegetables, and with heavy housework.

Goals of Treatment. Ms. H. was referred to occupational therapy to address the following problems:

- Fatigue from prolonged activity and standing at work
- Bilateral wrist pain (L > R), which is starting to interfere with her teaching (writing on the blackboard), as well as her ability to perform meal preparation and housework tasks
- Mild foot pain from prolonged standing at work

Goals were discussed with Ms. H. and mutually agreed upon. The goal list for Ms. H. includes the following:

1. Explore the use of bilateral hand splints during activities to improve function and reduce pain.
2. Explore alternative methods of writing on the blackboard.
3. Discuss alternative joint protection and energy conservation strategies to prevent fatigue at work; discuss these same principles to prevent wrist pain during housekeeping and meal preparation activities at home.
4. Provide Ms. H. with information and education about the selection of proper-fitting, comfortable footwear; discuss her options for dealing with on-going foot pain, including suggestions for custom-made foot orthotics.

Treatment Strategies. The occupational therapist recommended a 6-week outpatient program for Ms. H. and included the following treatment plan:

1. Bilateral custom work splints were provided to support the wrists, decrease pain, and increase strength in both wrists on activity. Bilateral resting splints were also fabricated for night wear as needed to place the joints of the wrist and fingers in a loose-packed position while providing proper positioning

and thereby reduce the amount and duration of morning stiffness. Wearing schedules and general care principles for both sets of splints were explained in detail and provided to the client in writing. Splint use gradually decreased over time as her joints became less inflamed and as function and pain improved. After 3 months, Ms. H. began to use a soft neoprene wrist splint for "flexible" support, neutral thermal warmth, and increased comfort when she wrote on the blackboard or marked papers.

2. Alternative methods of writing on the blackboard were tried, including the use of an overhead projector, markers, and transparencies and a large handled chalk-holder to limit prolonged tight pinch and decrease intercarpal pressure.

3. A foot assessment was completed and Ms. H. was provided with a prescription for custom-made flexible orthotics and supportive footwear (high-quality running shoes with good cushioning and support). When she purchased the appropriate running shoes, her custom-made, flexible orthotics were fitted into her new running shoes. This provided relief of pain in the balls of her feet and increased her tolerance for walking and standing.

4. Energy conservation and joint protection techniques that emphasized self-analysis and reflection of each activity were reviewed, taught, and practiced with Ms. H. when the therapist conducted a home assessment during the second week. Emphasis was placed on working out a balance between rest and activity. The therapist also discussed the use of alternative methods for doing important tasks without creating excessive stress on her hands and wrists. Other options for carrying loads in her briefcase were explored: suggestions included keeping the loads light while using a padded shoulder strap on the briefcase; using a backpack with padded shoulder straps; or using a luggage roller on wheels. Because her financial situation was very stable, Ms. H. decided to hire a housekeeper to do heavier housework tasks such as seasonal cleaning, laundry, vacuuming, cleaning the bathrooms, and some bulk meal preparation once a week. A hand-held shower head/brush was suggested to facilitate safety in the shower and to further protect Ms. H.'s upper extremity joints when showering. Ms. H. was provided with foam grips for some of her cooking utensils including a paring knife and vegetable peeler; the therapist also suggested use of an electric can opener and an adapted jar opener to reduce the stress on her hand joints and wrists.

5. Without the heavier tasks to complete, Ms. H. was able to prioritize her most important tasks (both at home and work) and began to pace herself better throughout her daily activities, giving more time to her early morning and after-work routines. As a result, Ms. H. was able to engage in more of her own interests and hobbies, started to fit them into her regular weekly schedule. After consulting with her rheumatologist, Ms. H enrolled in a beginning Tai Chi program once a week at the local YMCA and joined a walking club with some of her friends. She also has started cooking for herself more regularly and is able to do so with minimal hand discomfort.

At the 3-month follow-up, Ms. H. was wearing her resting splint primarily for her left hand at night and only used the work splints as needed. The inflammation in her right hand had dissipated completely and only slight swelling was noticed in her left hand and wrist. No further joint changes were noted. Grip strength had improved bilaterally (R = 210 mm Hg; L = 200 mm Hg), and morning stiffness had decreased to 10 to 20 minutes. Ms. H. reported that she had increased energy and could walk for 1.5 hours without foot discomfort. Improved hand function and endurance enabled her to vary her presentation styles—she would write on the blackboard using the adapted chalk holder for 1 hour and then switch to overhead transparencies for the remaining time. To avoid prolonged periods of standing, Ms. H. also began to use a high stool with a padded seat and backrest and a circular foot rest around the stool legs and base of support.

This case study demonstrates the importance and value of custom-made hand splints and foot orthotics, in addition to the proper use of client education strategies and energy conservation with joint protection techniques for clients learning to effectively manage their arthritis in a safe and responsible manner.

References

1. Hunter JM, Mackin EJ, Callahan AD (eds): *Rehabilitation of the Hand*, ed 4. St Louis, Mosby-Year Book, 1995.
2. American Society of Hand Therapists: *Splint Classification System*. Garner, NC, American Society of Hand Therapists, 1992.
3. Melvin JL: Orthotic treatment for arthritis of the hand. In *Rheumatic Disease in the Adult and Child: Occupational Therapy and Rehabilitation*, ed 3. Philadelphia, FA Davis, 1989, pp 379–418.
4. Phillips C: Management of patients with rheumatoid arthritis. In Hunter JM, Mackin EJ, Callahan AD (eds): *Rehabilitation of the Hand,* ed 4. St Louis, Mosby-Year Book, 1995, pp 1345–1350.
5. Shurr DG, Michael JW: Prosthetics and Orthotics, ed 2. Upper Saddle River, NJ, Pearson Education, 2002, pp 237–258.
6. Merritt J: Advances in orthotics for the patient with rheumatoid arthritis. *J Rheumatol* 14(suppl 15):62–67, 1987.

7. Fess EE, Philips CA: *Hand Splinting: Principals and Methods,* ed 2. St Louis, CV Mosby, 1987, pp 309–324.

8. Stern EB, Ytterberg SR, Krug HE et al: Commercial wrist extensor orthosis: a descriptive study of subject use and preference. *Arthritis Care Res* 10:27–35, 1997.

9. Swigart C, Eaton R, Glickel S et al: Splinting in the treatment of arthritis of the first CMC joint. *J Hand Surg* (Am) 24:86–91, 1999.

10. Backman C: Functional assessment. In Melvin J, Jensen G (eds): Rheumatologic Rehabilitation series: *Assessment and Management,* vol 1. Bethesda, MD, American Occupational Therapy Association, 1998, pp 157–194.

11. Law M, Baptiste S, Carswell A et al: *Canadian Occupational Performance Measure,* ed 2. Toronto, Ontario, Canadian Association of Occupational Therapy, 1994.

12. Backman C, Mackie H: Arthritis hand function test: inter-rater reliability among self-trained raters. *Arthritis Care Res* 8:10–15, 1995.

13. Cailliet R: *Hand Pain and Impairment,* ed 4. Philadelphia, FA Davis, 1994.

14. Jacobs ML, Austin N: *Splinting the Hand and Upper Extremity: Principles and Process.* Philadelphia, Lippincott Williams & Wilkins, 2003.

15. Zoeckler AA, Nicholas JJ: Prenyl hand splint for rheumatoid arthritis. *Phys Ther* 49:377–379, 1969.

16. Biddulph SL: The effect of the Futuro wrist brace in pain conditions of the wrist. *S Afr Med J* 60:389–391, 1981.

17. Eyring EJ, Murray WR: The effect of joint position on the pressure of intra-articular effusion. *J Bone Joint Surg* 46A(6):1235–1241, 1964.

18. Stanley BG, Tribuzi SM: *Concepts in Hand Rehabilitation.* Philadelphia, FA Davis, 1992.

19. Neuberger GB, Smith KV, Black SO et al: Promoting self-care in clients with arthritis. *Arthritis Care Res* 6:141–148, 1993.

20. Backman CL, Deitz JC: Static wrist splint: its effect on hand function in three women with rheumatoid arthritis. *Arthritis Care Res* 1:151–160, 1988.

21. Stern EB, Ytterberg SR, Krug HE et al: Immediate and short-term effects of three commercial wrist orthoses on grip strength and function in patients with rheumatoid arthritis. *Arthritis Care Res* 9:42–50, 1996.

22. Stirrat C: Metacarpophalangeal joints in rheumatoid arthritis of the hand. *Hand Clin* 12:515–529, 1996.

23. Nordenskiold U: Elastic wrist orthosis: reduction of pain and increase in grip force for females with rheumatoid arthritis. *Arthritis Care Res* 3:158–162, 1990.

24. Pagnotta A, Baron M, Korner-Bitensky N: The effect of a static wrist orthosis on hand function in individuals with rheumatoid arthritis. *J Rheumatol* 25:879–885, 1998.

25. Weiss S, LaStayo P, Mills A et al: Prospective analysis of splinting the first carpometacarpophalangeal joint: an objective, subjective, and radiographic assessment. *J Hand Ther* 13:218–227, 2000.

26. Colditz JC: The biomechanics of a thumb carpometacarpophalangeal immobilization splint: design and fitting. *J Hand Ther* 13:228–235, 2000.

27. Melvin JL: Orthotic treatment of the hand: what's new? *Bull Rheum Dis* 44:5–8, 1995.

28. Falconer J: Hand splinting in rheumatoid arthritis: a perspective on current knowledge and directions for research. *Arthritis Care Res* 4:81–86, 1991.

29. Swanson AB: *Flexible Implant Resection Arthroplasty in the Hand and Extremities.* St Louis, CV Mosby, 1973, pp 171–183.

30. Feinberg J: Effect of the arthritis health professional on compliance with use of resting splints by patients with rheumatoid arthritis. *Arthritis Care Res* 5:17–23, 1992.

31. Groth GN, Wilder DM: The impact of compliance of rehabilitation of patients with mallet finger injuries. *J Hand Ther* 7:21–24, 1994.

32. Groth GN, Wulf MB: Compliance with hand rehabilitation: health beliefs and strategies. *J Hand Ther* 8:18–22, 1995.

33. Belcon MC, Haynes RB, Tugwell P: A critical review of compliance studies in rheumatoid arthritis. *Arthritis Rheum* 27:1227–1233, 1984.

34. Moon M, Moon B, Black W: Compliance in splint-wearing behavior of patients with rheumatoid arthritis. *NZ Med J* 83:360–365, 1976.

35. Feinberg J, Brandt KD: Use of resting splints by patients with rheumatoid arthritis. *Am J Occup Ther* 35:173–178, 1981.

36. Nicholas JJ, Gruen H, Weiner G et al: Splinting in rheumatoid arthritis. I. Factors affecting patient compliance. *Arch Phys Med Rehabil* 63:92–94, 1982.

37. Riegger-Krugh C, Keysor JJ: Skeletal malalignments of the lower quarter: correlated and compensatory motions and postures. *J Orthop Sports Phys Ther* 23:164–170, 1996.

38. Loke M: New concepts in lower limb orthotics. *Phys Med Rehab Clinics North Am* 11:477–496, 2000.

39. Keenan MA, Peabody TD, Gronley JK et al: Valgus deformities of the feet and characteristics of gait in patients who have rheumatoid arthritis. *J Bone Joint Surg* 73A:237–247, 1991.

40. Spiegel TM, Spiegel JS: Rheumatoid arthritis in the foot and ankle—diagnosis, pathology and treatment. The relationship between foot and ankle deformity and disease duration in 50 patients. *Foot Ankle* 2:318–324, 1982.

41. Jahss MH: The subtalar complex. In Jahss MH (ed): *Disorders of the Foot.* Philadelphia, WB Saunders, vol 1, 1982, pp 727–763.

42. Deland JT, Wood B: Foot pain. In Kelley WM, Harris ED, Ruddy S, et al (eds): *Textbook of Rheumatology,* vol 1, ed 4. Philadelphia, WB Saunders, 1993, pp 457–469.

43. Billock JN: Clinical evaluation and assessment principles in orthotics and prosthetics. *J Prosthet Orthot* 8:41–44, 1996.

44. Green DR, Carol A: Planal dominance. *J Am Podiatry Assoc* 74:98–103, 1984.

45. Lundberg A, Goldie I, Kalin B, Selvik G: Kinematics of the ankle/foot complex: plantar flexion and dorsiflexion. *Foot Ankle* 9:194–200, 1989.

46. Mann RA: Biomechanics. In Jahss MH (ed): *Disorders of the Foot.* Philadelphia, WB Saunders, vol 1, 1982, pp 37–67.

47. Giannestras N: *Foot Disorders: Medical and Surgical Management,* ed 3. Philadelphia, Lea & Febiger, 1980.
48. Inman VT: Hallux valgus: a review of etiologic factors. *Orthop Clin North Am* 5:59–63, 1974.
49. Thomas WH: Reconstructive surgery and rehabilitation of the ankle and foot. In Kelley WM, et al (eds): *Textbook of Rheumatology.* Philadelphia, WB Saunders, vol 2, 1981, pp 1999–2013.
50. Bouysset M, Tebib J, Noel E et al: Rheumatoid metatarsus: the original evolution of the first metatarsal. *Clin Rheumatol* 10:408–412, 1991.
51. Lorig K, Fries JF (eds): *The Arthritis Helpbook: A Tested Self-Management Program for Coping with Arthritis and Fibromyalgia,* ed 4. Don Mills, Ontario, Addison-Wesley, 1995.
52. Alliare SH, Anderson JJ, Meenan, RF: Reducing work disability associated with rheumatoid arthritis: identification of additional risk factors and persons likely to benefit from intervention. *Arthritis Care Res* 9:349–357, 1996.
53. Katz P: What is the impact of RA on life activities? Modifications and losses of valued activities attributable to rheumatoid arthritis. *Arthritis Care Res* 7:S10, 1994.
54. Mann WC, Hurren D, Tomita, M: Assistive devices used by home-base elderly persons with arthritis. *Am J Occup Ther* 49:810–820, 1995.
55. Helewa A, Goldsmith CH, Lee P et al: Effects of occupational therapy home service on patients with rheumatoid arthritis. *Lancet* 337:1453–1456, 1991.
56. Furst G, Gerber L, Smith C et al: A program for improving energy conservation behaviors in adults with rheumatoid arthritis. *Am J Occup Ther* 41:102–111, 1987.
57. Cordery J, Rocchi M: Joint protection and fatigue management. In Melvin J, Jensen G (eds): Rheumatologic Rehabilitation series, *Assessment and Management.* Bethesda, MD, American Occupational Therapy Association, vol 1, 1998, pp 279–321.
58. Barry MA, Purser J, Hazelman R et al: Effect of energy conservation and joint protection education in rheumatoid arthritis. *Br J Rheumatol* 33:1171–1174, 1994.
59. Yasuda YL: Rheumatoid arthritis and osteoarthritis. In Trombly, CA, Radomski, MV (eds): *Occupational Therapy for Physical Dysfunction,* ed 5. Philadelphia, Lippincott Williams & Wilkins, 2002, pp 1001–1024.
60. Rogers JC, Holm MB: Assistive technology device use in patients with rheumatic disease: a literature review. *Am J Occup Ther* 46:120–127, 1992.
61. Wolfe T: Community resources and assistive devices for people with arthritis. *J Hand Ther* 13:184–192, 2000.
62. Mann WC: Assistive technology for persons with arthritis. In: Melvin J, Jensen G (eds): Rheumatologic Rehabilitation series, vol 1, *Assessment and Management.* Bethesda, MD, American Occupational Therapy Association, 1998, pp 369–392.
63. Nordenskiold U, Grimby G, Hedberg M et al: The structure of an instrument for assessing the effects of assistive devices and altered working methods in women with rheumatoid arthritis. *Arthritis Care Res* 9:358–367, 1996.
64. Hammond A, Lincoln N: Development of the joint protection behavior assessment. *Arthritis Care Res* 12:200–207, 1999.

Additional Readings

1. Alderson M, Starr L, Gow S, Moreland J: The program for rheumatic independent self-management: a pilot evaluation. *Clin Rheumatol* 18:283–292, 1999.
2. Bowker P: *Biomechanical Basis of Orthotic Management.* Boston, MA, Butterworth-Heinemann, 1993.
3. Clark BM: Clinical Basics—Rheumatology: 9. Physical and occupational therapy in the management of arthritis. *Can Med Assoc J* 163:999–1005, 2000.
4. Coppard BM, Lohman H: *Introduction to Splinting: A Critical-Thinking and Problem-Solving Approach.* St Louis, 1996, Mosby-Year Book, 1996.
5. Hammond A, Lincoln N: The effect of a joint protection education programme for people with rheumatoid arthritis. *Clin Rehabil* 13:392–400, 1999.
6. Leonard JB: Joint protection for inflammatory disorders. In Hunter, JM, Mackin, EJ, Callahan, AD (eds): *Rehabilitation of the Hand,* ed 4. St Louis, Mosby-Year Book, 1995, pp 1377–1384.
7. Rogers JC, Holm MB, Perkins L: Trajectory of assistive device usage and user and non-user characteristics: Long-handled bath sponge. *Arthritis Care Res* 6:645–650, 2002.
8. Steultjens EM, Dekker J, Bouter LM et al: Occupational therapy for rheumatoid arthritis: a systematic overview. *Arthritis Care Res* 6:672–685, 2002.
9. Yasuda YL (in collaboration with the AOTA Commission on Practice): *Guidelines for Adults with Rheumatoid Arthritis.* Bethesda, MD, American Occupational Therapy Association, 2000.

Appendix

THE ARTHRITIS SOCIETY
ONTARIO DIVISION
CONSULTATION AND THERAPY SERVICE

FOOT ASSESSMENT

Client Name: _____   Date: _____

Therapist: _____   Duration of foot involvement: _____ years

Reason for assessment: _____

_____

_____

The pain in my _____ over the past _____ is best described as:

_____

No pain   severe pain

PREVIOUS MANAGEMENT:
    Conservative - Shoes: _____
                Orthotics: _____
                Other: _____

    Surgical - _____

FUNCTIONAL MOBILITY REQUIRED: _____

_____

Assessment continues on reverse . . .

CLIENT/THERAPIST GOALS:
    (Pain): _____
    (Gait): _____
    (Footwear:) _____
    (Hygiene/cosmesis) _____
    (Education) _____
    (Other) _____

TREATMENT PLAN:

Education: ☐ Hygiene   ☐ Range of Motion X's
                       ☐ Footwear   ☐ Calf Stretches
                       ☐ Use of mobility aids   ☐ Gait Training
                       ☐ Related disease process   ☐ Modalities _____

Shoe Modifications: ☐ Spot Stretching   ☐ Tongue Pads   ☐ Heel Counter   ☐ Other _____
                        ☐ Insole   ☐ ¾   ☐ Full   Material Used: _____

☐ Components   ☐ long arch   ☐ met. splay   ☐ met. cookie   ☐ met. bar   Material used: _____
                 ☐ lat. wedge   ☐ med. wedge   ☐ heel pad   ☐ heel cup

Referred for: ☐ lift _____ cms. R/L   ☐ rocker   ☐ med./lat. wedge R/L   ☐ med./lat. flare R/L
               ☐ Other _____

Review Date: _____   Change (+) (−) _____mm.

The pain in my _____ over the past _____ is best described as:

├──┤

No pain   severe

OBSERVATIONS AND ASSESSMENT

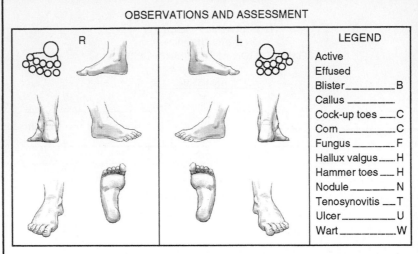

R	L	
	LEGEND	

Active
Effused
Blister _____ B
Callus _____
Cock-up toes ____ C
Corn _____ C
Fungus _____ F
Hallux valgus ____ H
Hammer toes ____ H
Nodule _____ N
Tenosynovitis ___ T
Ulcer _____ U
Wart _____ W

R		L
Toe in / Toe out / Normal	Stance	Toe in / Toe out / Normal
↓ / Normal	One foot balance	↓ / Normal
Invert / Evert / Normal	Hindfoot	Invert / Evert / Normal
↑ / ↓ / Normal Mobile / Rigid	Longitudinal	↑ / ↓ / Normal Mobile / Rigid
↓ / Normal Mobile / Rigid	Metatarsal	↓ / Normal Mobile / Rigid
Mobile / Rigid	Forefoot	Mobile / Rigid
↑ / ↓ / Normal	Toe Off	↑ / ↓ / Normal
Mobile / Rigid	1st MTP	Mobile / Rigid

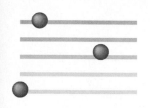

CHAPTER 15

Psychosocial Factors in Arthritis

Donna J. Hawley, RN, EdD

Psychological Distress and Clinical Outcomes

Clinical Outcomes

The impact of any chronic disease for the individual is evaluated by examining the short- and long-term effects of the disease on general health status, often referred to as *health-related quality of life* (HRQOL). HRQOL is a combination of functional ability, symptoms of disease (pain, sleep, fatigue, etc.), social roles and activities including work and school, and emotions and mood.[1] Thus, it represents a perception of well-being that encompasses not only the physiological components of disease but also the consequences that are important to the individual on a daily basis.

More than a decade ago, Fries and Spitz[2] published a hierarchical framework for describing HRQOL (which they called global outcome) that is still relevant and useful today. They listed five broad dimensions: disability, discomfort, financial costs, iatrogenic effects (e.g., drug side effects), and the ultimate outcome, mortality (Figure 15–1). Under each dimension, they described more specific areas. All outcomes and thus HRQOL are interrelated with one area affecting and interconnecting with the other. For example, the financial costs of arthritis and drug side effects interact with pain and psychological distress. Pain management cannot be isolated from managing depression. Adapting to functional loss is inherently interconnected with pain and emotional distress. The relationships among

PHYSICAL REHABILITATION IN ARTHRITIS, Joan M. Walker, PhD, PT, and Antoine Helewa, MSc(Clin Epid), PT, Elsevier Inc. © 2004.

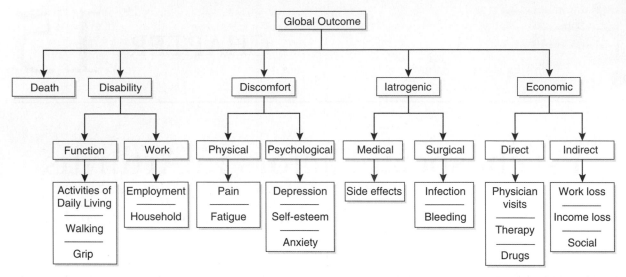

Figure 15-1. The outcomes of rheumatic disorders are shown as a hierarchy with global outcome at the top and becoming more specific under each of the subcategories. (Adapted from Fries JF, Spitz PW: The hierarchy of patient outcomes. In Spilker B (ed): *Quality of Life: Assessments in Clinical Trials.* New York, Raven Press, 1990, pp 25–35.)

disability, chronic pain, and psychological distress are complex and difficult to separate. Nonetheless, current research indicates that the psychological dimension is independent, although related to other outcomes of chronic disease. In this chapter, the psychological aspects of arthritis are explored. These factors are examined both as independent components of disease and as they relate to other disease outcomes, particularly pain and disability.

Although there are more than 100 different types of arthritis and related rheumatic disorders, the majority of the research on psychological aspects remains centered on rheumatoid arthritis (RA). Other types of rheumatic disorders, particularly soft tissues disorders such as fibromyalgia,[3–7] osteoarthritis (OA),[8–10] and systemic lupus erythematosus also have been studied.[11–14] Nonetheless, RA, as the most prevalent of the systemic rheumatic disorders, remains the disease most studied both in individuals and in comparison groups. Information from RA may be used as a model for examining other types of arthritis, as well as a model for studying a variety of painful, systemic chronic disorders.

Early Studies of Psychological Distress

Very early studies of the psychological characteristics of people with RA found evidence of a "rheumatoid

personality" and suggested that certain psychological traits (e.g., self-sacrificing, masochistic, rigid, moralistic, shy, inhibited, and perfectionistic) were present before disease onset or were even causative.[15,16] Most of the studies that led to these conclusions had flaws in study design, evaluation instruments, and statistical procedures. The idea of a rheumatoid personality is no longer considered valid or useful in explaining disease onset or outcome.[17–19]

During the last 25 years well-designed studies using valid and reliable psychological instruments and sophisticated statistical methods have considered the multivariate relationships of social factors, demographic characteristics, and disease severity as elements of observed psychological abnormalities. In recent years, investigators have examined abnormalities of emotional or mental status in arthritis, both cross-sectionally and longitudinally, using depression or depressive symptoms as the psychological factor studied. Depression or depressive symptoms may be considered surrogates for a general state of emotional health. Creed[18] indicated that "anxiety neurosis and depressive illness overlap" and suggested use of the term *depression* for a state of emotional distress that he described as a mixture of anxiety and depression. This convention will be used throughout this chapter. The term depression will be used in this broad context and not as a specific psychiatric diagnosis.

> **A rheumatoid personality is not a valid explanation of disease onset or outcome.**

Prevalence of Depression

Depression has long been accepted as a major problem for people with RA with a prevalence of two to three times that of the general population.[19] For clients with RA, prevalence estimates for actual major depressive disorder are 13% to 17%,[19] and the prevalence of important depressive symptoms in clinical populations is at least 20%.[5,17,18,20] The occurrence of depression in RA is similar to that in other chronic diseases, such as pulmonary disease, diabetes, cancer, chronic cardiovascular disease, and hypertension[18,21] and somewhat less than that found in clients with chronic pain.[18,21,22]

Hawley and Wolfe[5] compared depressive symptoms among more than 6000 clients with various rheumatic disorders seen in a rheumatology clinic (Table 15–1). People with RA reported levels of depressive symptoms similar to those of persons with OA of the knee, hip, or axial skeleton, low back pain, neck pain, and other chronic musculoskeletal problems commonly seen in a rheumatology referral practice. Only clients with OA of the hand had consistently lower depression scores than clients with RA. Clients with fibromyalgia had consistently higher depression levels with almost 30% reporting serious depressive symptoms. The finding that clients with fibromyalgia have high depression scores is consistent with results of other studies.[7,23–25]

In summary, the majority (80%) of people with RA do not have serious depressive symptoms and seem to be managing their lives and their disease. They adapt and develop strategies that enable them to cope with the pain and disability of RA. However, a very significant minority experience depressive symptoms, and many with arthritis have periods in their disease course in which depressive symptoms are problematic.

> **Most people with RA do not present with serious depressive symptoms; they manage their lives and their disease well.**

The challenge for all health professionals is to assist individuals who are experiencing psychological distress. To meet this challenge an understanding of relationships between psychological distress and arthritis is necessary. Three areas are essential to such an understanding. These areas are (1) depressive symptoms and psychological distress demonstrated by people with arthritis; (2) the relationships between disease severity and depressive symptoms; and (3) appropriate interventions and strategies that may improve depression. These three areas are discussed next.

Recognition of Depression and Psychological Distress: Assessment

Characteristics of Depression and Depressive Symptoms

The definitive diagnosis of psychological disturbance or clinical depression requires the use of compre-

Table 15-1. Percentage of Clients with a Rheumatic Disease Who Are at Risk for Serious Depressive Symptoms

Diagnostic Category	N	Percentage of Clients with Probable Depression
Rheumatoid arthritis	1,152	20.4
Fibromyalgia	543	29.3
Osteoarthritis: knee or hip	463	16.8
Osteoarthritis: hand	379	14.2
Neck pain	160	23.1
Low back pain	547	22.7
Osteoarthritis/Axial Overlap*	464	19.6
Other diagnoses*	2,445	18.4

*The osteoarthritis/axial pain overlap group included clients with more than one diagnosis of osteoarthritis, neck pain, or low back pain. The last clinic group, "Other diagnoses" included clients with all other rheumatic disease diagnoses.[5]

hensive interviews using standard diagnostic classification systems.[26] Such diagnosis is beyond the purview of this chapter and is done only by health care professionals with special preparation. However, recognition of psychological distress and depressive symptoms is a part of routine, daily rheumatological practice. Every health care professional working with an individual with arthritis can learn to recognize signs and symptoms of depression and psychological distress and intervene as needed.

Determining the presence of depression in clients requires alertness to the symptoms of depression. Typical symptoms of depression are feelings of sadness, loss of interest in surroundings and in the family, difficulty concentrating, and sluggish thinking. People may withdraw from family and friends, lose interest in work or daily activities, and have feelings of guilt or loss of self-esteem. Certain somatic complaints also are part of depression. Changes in appetite, most often but not always a decrease in appetite, fatigue or lethargy, and problems with sleep including excessive somnolence, insomnia, or early morning awakening are common symptoms. Many of the somatic symptoms typical of depression are an inherent part of a systemic inflammatory process. Sleep disturbances, loss of appetite, weight loss, and fatigue may be part of the disease and may not necessarily be indicative of depression[27,28] (Table 15–2). Separating, for example, the fatigue caused by the disease and fatigue as a symptom of depression can be challenging for the health care professional. Evaluating these common symptoms and complaints of psychological distress (e.g., sadness, sluggish thinking, anorexia, lethargy) in combination with the physical measures common to inflammatory rheumatic disease (e.g., erythrocyte sedimentation rate [ESR], swollen joint count) are necessary for the identification of psychological distress in clients.

Table 15-2. Common Characteristics of Depression*

General Characteristics	Somatic Complaints	Common Signs and Symptoms in Systematic Rheumatic Disorders†
Feelings of sadness; feeling "blue"	Fatigue	Fatigue
Inability to "shake off" feelings of sadness; cannot be "cheered up" by others	Appetite change Anorexia Overeating	Anorexia
Cognitive problems: sluggish thinking; inability to concentrate; memory problems	Sleep problems Hypersomnia Insomnia Early awakening Waking up fatigued	Sleep problems resulting in fatigue
Discouraged about the future	Weight loss or gain	Weight loss
Frequent crying	Psychomotor agitation or retardation	
Loneliness Feelings of being disliked Finding little enjoyment in life Loss of interest in surroundings Suicide		

*Adapted from Depression Subscale, Arthritis Impact Measurement Scales,[29] Beck Depression Inventory,[30] Center for Epidemiological Studies Depression Scale,[31] and Short Geriatric Depression Scale.[32]
†Adapted from Pincus et al,[28] Callahan et al,[27] and Blalock et al.[34]

Self-Report Measures for Depressive Symptoms: Written and Verbal

In addition to being cognizant of depressive symptoms, various self-report written instruments are available and may be used as part of the routine practice of health care professionals. The Center for Epidemiological Studies-Depression Scale (CES-D),[31] the Beck Depression Inventory,[30] and the depression subscale of the Arthritis Impact Measurement Scales (AIMS), original or the mood subscale of AIMS2[29,34] have been used extensively in studies of clients with arthritis. The original AIMS Depression Scale is short, (i.e., six items) and can be easily administered in a busy clinic setting. The six items relate to mood (i.e., enjoyment of activities, low spirits, etc.) during the past month. Somatic items, such as fatigue, appetite, or weight loss or gain, are not part of the scale. The AIMS scale is strongly correlated with the CES-D scale ($r = .81$).[33] The Beck Depression Inventory and the CES-D are both longer than the AIMS Depression Scale with 21 and 20 items, respectively; however, the length is certainly not prohibitive for use in practice and research settings. In addition to these formal scales, the clinician may ask a simple question such as "On a scale of 1 to 10 with 1 being none to 10 being very depressed, rate your feelings of depression or sadness during the last week." Such an inquiry may allow the client to share her or his concerns with the health care professional.

Recognition and Referral

Regardless of the assessment methods used, clinicians need to recognize depressive symptoms and other types of psychological distress in their clients. Interventions as those described in the rest of this chapter may be useful for a majority of clients; however, referrals to other health care professionals should be considered and are appropriate for clients with serious depression. Of course, clients expressing suicidal thoughts require an immediate referral to an appropriate health care professional.

Relationship between Clinical Factors and Psychosocial Factors

Overview

The relationship between disease severity and psychological distress is complex. Anecdotally every clinician knows that certain people with severe disability and pain are not depressed and seem to manage despite their disease. Likewise, some people with apparent mild disease complain of considerable pain, are depressed, and complain of distress that appears to be excessive considering only the disease process. Specifically, chronic long-term pain that is characteristic of arthritis may lead to depression, or chronic pain may be, as stated by Magni and associates,[35] the expression of "an underlying depressive disturbance which is made manifest through the symptom of pain." Similarly, frustrations with the inability to perform usual activities of daily living or inability to complete required work may heighten depressed moods. The corollary that general psychological health may exacerbate pain and disability also is true. Researchers have attempted to sort out these apparent incongruities using a variety of research designs and statistical analyses.

> For clients with serious depression or suicidal thoughts, referral to an appropriate health care professional is essential.

Cross-Sectional Studies

People with depressive symptoms also report higher levels of pain than do those who are not depressed.[19,36-38] The relationship is only moderate and both pain and depression are related to a variety of other demographic, clinical, and social factors. For example, Newman and colleagues[39] reported that demographic variables (especially being female but also education, marital status, age, and social class), functional ability, social isolation, and lower socioeconomic status contributed significantly in explaining depression scores but pain, disease duration, and ESR did not. Several authors also have reported that depression is not related to disease severity measures such as grip strength, morning stiffness, number of painful joints, and ESR.[36,40,41]

Generally higher functional disability also is related to depressive symptoms and to pain. The interrelationship between these three factors is well documented in the literature in both established[42,43] and early disease.[5,44,45] Functional disability is measured in clinical trials, in observational studies, and in regular clinical practice using a variety of self-report questionnaires. When functional ability is measured by self-report questionnaires, separating the degree of functional impairment attributable to disease severity and to depressed mood is difficult.[46,47]

Longitudinal Studies

Longitudinal studies have provided additional clues concerning the relationship between disease characteristics, pain, depression, and demographic and social factors. The three cases studies described in Figure 15–2 illustrate different patterns for adapting to a chronic disease. Depressive symptoms may be a constant in people's lives, a response to disease severity, or a minor part of one's life. Katz and Yelin[20] have followed clients with RA in northern California for more than 10 years using structured telephone interviews. Over a 4-year period, about 4% of the clients were depressed each year and more than 29% experienced depressive symptoms in one or more years. Individuals reporting depressive symptoms in one year were much more likely to report depression in subsequent years. These same authors[48] also found that losing the ability to participate in "valued" activities, specifically "recreational activities" and "social interactions," increased the risk for depression.

There is growing evidence that depressive symptoms may fluctuate in the short term but over several years, they remain essentially stable. Several authors have found that changes in depressive mood were more related to educational level, marital status, age, and lower family income but not to clinical variables such as pain, disability, or joint count in studies of 3 years or more. Over short periods of time (i.e., time between routine outpatient clinic visits or during the first year of disease) depressive symptoms may fluctuate with disease severity measures such as pain, functional disability, and grip strength.[44,49]

Emerging from these cross-sectional and longitudinal studies are two important points. First, although there are relationships between depression, pain, functional ability, and some severity measures, the relationships are moderate. Functional disability, pain, and psychological status are separate concepts and operate to a considerable degree independently of disease severity, disease duration, and even long-term outcome. Second, the characteristics and causes of depression and psychological distress among people with RA are multifactorial and are related more to individual personality, family, and social circumstances than to disease severity. Social factors, such as age, education, gender, marital status, economics, social isolation, and social support are important to our understanding of psychological distress in arthritis. In the next section, we will look at some of these social factors and at interventions addressing these factors.

Management and Interventions

Social Support

Social support is important to the successful management of any chronic disease. Lanza and Revenson[50] define social support as the "...process by which interpersonal relationships promote well-being and protect people from health declines, particularly when they are facing stressful life circumstances." Using this broad definition, social support includes family and friends, health care professionals, community groups, such as church organizations or clubs, self-help educational programs, and formal support groups.

Individuals with RA reporting support from family, particularly spouses, and friends have an advantage over those reporting less support. They indicate higher levels of self-esteem and psychological well-being,[51] adjustment to illness,[52] and depression.[53,54] Support from family and friends may buffer or enhance the coping skills of individuals. Brown and associates,[55] studying the possible buffering effects of social support in the management of arthritis pain, found that individuals with higher satisfaction for emotional support (from a variety of sources) were less depressed at all levels of pain severity.

In examining the support from family and friends, Revenson and colleagues[56] warn that support can be both helpful and nonhelpful or a "double-edged sword." In their study of 101 individuals with newly diagnosed RA (82% women), they found that positive or helpful support was related to lower depression scores and problematic or nonhelpful support was related to higher scores.[56] Affleck and associates[52] asked people with arthritis to describe helpful and unhelpful types of support. In order of frequency, participants mentioned opportunities to express feelings and concerns, encouragement of hope and optimism, and being offered useful information as most helpful. Unhelpful approaches included minimizing the severity of an illness, expressions of pity, pessimistic statements about the future, and unnecessarily solicitous behavior.[52]

In the context of social support, studies most often have concentrated on the support from family, friends, and various social and self-help groups. The importance of support from health professionals is an additional component of social support and is an area for which additional research would be useful. Revenson and colleagues[57] reported that health care professionals were rated as the "source of most helpful support" by 33% to 45% of respondents. Prescribing medications

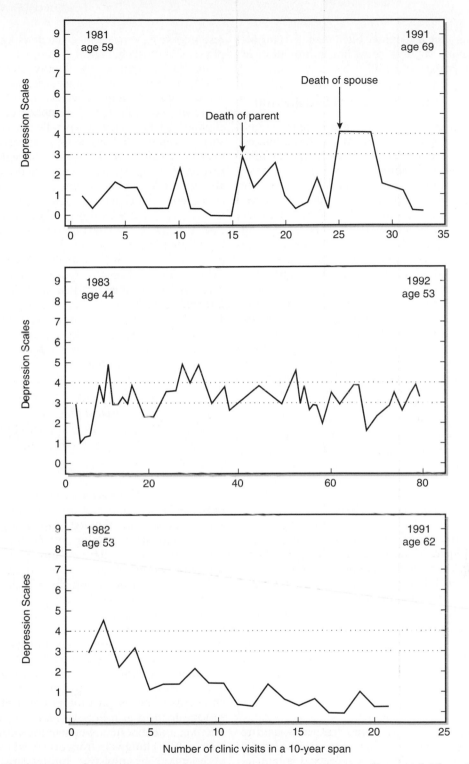

Figure 15-2. Three patterns for the changes in depressive symptoms over time are illustrated. The *y* (vertical)-axis represents the scores on the AIMS Depression Scale with scores ranging from 0 to 10. The *x* (horizontal)-axis represents visits to a specialty rheumatological clinic over about a 10-year period. The *horizontal lines* at 3 and 4 on the *y*-axis are the levels at which depressive symptoms are possibly and probably, respectively, indicative of depression on this particular depression scale.

and treatments were listed more often than less tangible areas of support, such as providing information or emotional support.[57]

Sexual Functioning and Sexual Satisfaction

Studies of the sexual functioning and sexual satisfaction in the chronic rheumatic disorders are limited in number and scope. Perhaps issues of pain, functional status, work disability, psychological distress, or new pharmacologic treatments take precedence over sexual concerns, at least for the researcher. Clients may not wish to discuss their sexual activities with a health professional and consider pain relief and daily functioning as the priority. Pain, functional disability, fatigue, and joint symptoms have been shown to be related to greater sexual dissatisfaction.[58–61] Two authors report that sexual dissatisfaction seems to increase over time for both clients, spouses, and control subjects.[58,60] In an interesting study comparing people with end-stage renal disease (ESRD) to those with RA, lack of desire for sexual activity was more common in men with ESRD, including those with a transplant, compared to men with RA. The same was true for women; however, in all groups the percentage of women reporting lack of desire was much higher (i.e., 20% to 65% higher).[62] The message for the clinician is to remember to ask about sexual satisfaction and to pursue appropriate treatments if the person so desires.

Strategies and Interventions

In addition to support from family, friends, and professionals, specific strategies have been tested and have been shown to relieve depression and improve psychological well-being for clients with arthritis. These strategies including various coping mechanisms, exercise, cognitive-behavioral interventions, and psychoeducational interventions. Each of these strategies except exercise will be discussed. The beneficial effects of exercise are described in Chapters 8 to 13.

Coping Strategies

Coping strategies are the processes, learned skills, and techniques used by an individual to manage a chronic disease, such as RA. These strategies may attenuate the effects of stresses such as pain, or the opposite, and actually exacerbate problems. In addition, the effectiveness of coping strategies may be independent of pain severity or the degree of disability.[63,64] Internal

resources (e.g., personality characteristics, intelligence, physical and psychological energy, education) as well as external resources (e.g., family, income, access to health care services/professionals) are major determiners of the types of coping strategies used.[65]

Brown and colleagues[63] demonstrated that passive coping behaviors, such as depending on others, limiting social activities, and suppressing anger, are positively related to depression. Evers and colleagues[49] reported that passive coping strategies predicted increased disability even 1 year after diagnosis. On the other hand, active coping behaviors, such as staying busy and ignoring or using activities to distract from one's pain, may have a positive effect on depression. In fact, they found that passive coping behaviors may actually intensify the relationship between pain and depression. Felton and associates[64] reported similar descriptive evidence when they studied a variety of chronic diseases including RA. They reported that positive affect is related to two major active coping strategies, i.e., cognitive restructuring and information seeking, whereas negative affect was related to emotional expressions, fantasy, and self-blame. These findings support clinical observations and make intuitive sense.

> Active coping strategies tend to be more effective than passive approaches, but the situation and the individual at a given time play a role.

Table 15–3 lists various coping strategies used by individuals with chronic disease and chronic pain. The strategies are divided into groups labeled as passive and active coping strategies. Although the studies described in the previous paragraph indicate that active coping strategies are more effective in the self-management of chronic disease, the effectiveness of any coping strategy depends on the situation. For example, after initial diagnosis, denial may be a very logical and useful defense mechanism or coping strategy. When a person hears a diagnosis that has a very uncertain and potentially serious outcome, denial is both protective and useful for a short period of time. However, continuing to deny a diagnosis for an extended period of time is not useful. Although seeking help from others is listed as passive coping activity, under some circumstances it is an active approach. Seeking help from others when such help is necessitated by physical limitations is essential, appropriate, and an active strategy. It is only when one depends unnecessarily on others that this strategy becomes a passive activity and ineffective. As stated before, generally speaking, active coping

Table 15-3. Commonly Used Coping Strategies*: A Comparison of Passive and Active Strategies

Passive Coping Strategies	Active Coping Strategies
Denial	
Focusing on the pain or problem	Distraction; selectively ignoring the pain
	Physical activity or exercise
	Imagery
	Avoidance
Isolation from family, friends, social activities	Participation in activities
	Being physically active
	Leisure activities
Seeking comfort from others	Seeking information from knowledgeable others
Telling others about the pain	Professionals
Praying	Read materials about the disease
	Attend self-management classes
Fantasizing/wishing	Cognitive restructuring: reappraise situation
For better medications from the physician	Find positive aspects to life
Dreaming the problem will disappear	Make illness less important in one's life
Daydreaming	Adapt new approaches to managing disease
Blaming others or self	
Dependence on others	Independence
Calling for professional help	Get appropriate help for major tasks
	Maintain as much independence as possible

*Adapted from the work of Brown and Nicassio,[65] Felton et al,[64] and Brown et al.[63]

strategies are more effective than passive approaches, but the effectiveness of any strategy depends on the situation and the individual at a given time.

Interventions

The goal for the clinician is to determine how to use the information about effective and noneffective coping strategies in practice. Assisting people to adapt strategies such as distraction or information seeking rather than ineffective strategies, such as fantasizing or blaming oneself, is well recognized as a vital component of clinical practice. The challenge then for all health care professionals is how to achieve this goal.

Descriptive studies as summarized in the preceding section have provided very useful information about the characteristics of psychological distress and the effectiveness of coping strategies and of social support. Although they are useful diagnostically for the clinician, the next logical step is to move from cross-sectional and longitudinal descriptive studies of social support and coping strategies to studies that test interventions. The typical psychological interventions used in studies of people with RA have been collectively labeled as cognitive-behavioral therapies

or self-management therapies.[46] These types of treatments feature activities such as relaxation techniques, imagery, coping strategies, problem-solving techniques, pain management techniques (e.g., diversion, biofeedback), and communication. Specific details differ from study to study but generally interventions focus on teaching clients techniques that will enable them to manage their own disease. The overall goal is to increase confidence that pain and other symptoms to a large degree are under the individual's control. This confidence or belief that one can master or control a situation is called *self-efficacy*.

Cognitive-Behavioral Therapy

Cognitive-behavioral therapy (CBT) is a psychoeducational approach that emphasizes control of distress/pain or mood by understanding the interaction of emotions and cognition with the physical and behavioral aspects of pain, by learning new skills (e.g., relaxation, diversion, cognitive restructuring), and, finally, by transferring these new skills to everyday life.[67] Leaders of these programs are usually specially trained professionals.

Studies have shown that CBT is an effective treatment for the management of pain and psychological distress for clients with RA and OA,[8] although effects have been only moderate. Studies have shown reductions in self-reported pain and pain behaviors,[68–70] increased use of coping strategies behavior,[71] improvement in feelings of helplessness and self-efficacy.[70,71] In a program emphasizing stress management, Parker and colleagues[72] reported significant improvements in psychological status and pain, but beneficial effects were quite weakened at 15 months after the intervention.

Studies have generally focused on people with long-standing disease. Consistent with recommendations for early treatment of RA with disease-modifying drugs,[73] psychologists have recommended interventions with CBT early in disease.[71,74,75] Recent studies have begun to examine the effectiveness of cognitive-behavioral therapies in early disease and have shown improvements in pain and psychological distress.[72,75] The studies are limited in number and the sample sizes have been small; thus, more studies are needed to determine the effectiveness of CBT in early disease.

Self-Management Interventions

Self-management programs combine presentation of information and problem-solving techniques with group interaction. Emphasis is placed on learning skills, such as flexibility and strengthening exercises, techniques for dealing with depression, using guided imagery for pain control, relaxation techniques, pacing, exercise, and communication with health professionals as well as family members. The Arthritis Self-Management Course (ASMC), developed by Kate Lorig and colleagues in 1979,[76] exemplifies these types of interventions and has been the model for more than 20 years.[76] The program has been fine-tuned with changes to content and methodology,[77] expanded to include all types of chronic disease,[78] and translated into Spanish.[79] Adaptations have been made by others.[80–83] Self-management programs have become widely popular and are now used throughout the world in areas that include Canada, New Zealand, Australia, European countries, and parts of Asia and South America. Programs are often presented by lay leaders.

Several investigators have evaluated the effectiveness of self-management and CBT programs using critical reviews and meta-analyses.[84–89] Improvements in a variety of areas, such as self-efficacy, coping, psychological distress, and pain, as well as reductions in the use of health care services have been modest but clinically important. Several factors must be considered when the short- and long-term outcomes of psychoeducational interventions are examined. First, educational interventions are offered concurrently with medical treatments (e.g., drugs, surgery) that have the more powerful effect on outcomes. It must be recognized *that the medical treatment and education may be synergistic and isolating the unique contribution provided by education is difficult.* Secondly, controlled clinical studies have examined outcomes for groups and not for individuals. Group results guide treatment but are not the only consideration in determining benefit for the individual. Anecdotally, researchers, clinicians, and clients alike testify to the usefulness of educational activities. Lastly, RA is a painful chronic disease with progressive disability and uncertainty over many years; thus, improvement and beneficial effects of therapy are often "very subtle".[90] In summary, studies of psychoeducational interventions have been shown to offer modest, but important, benefits for groups of clients, especially in conjunction with various medical treatments, such as medications and surgery for people with RA.

Complementary Treatments

The term *complementary treatments* has been used for a cadre of interventions known as nontraditional treatments, unconventional treatments, alternative medicine, non-Western medicine, and unorthodox therapies. Boisset and Fitzcharles[91] define such therapies as interventions not "…widely taught in North American medical schools or generally available in North American hospitals."[91] These treatments range from harmless folk treatments (e.g., copper bracelets) to a few expensive and potentially harmful therapies. Recent reports describe usage of complementary treatments among people with arthritis to be 69% to 94%.[92] Estimated usage of these treatments by the general population in the United States is 42%.[92]

Complementary therapy is popular throughout the general population with usage being common regardless of educational background, income level, and health status. The presence of a rheumatic disease may increase the probability of use of such treatments. Two main reasons are advanced to explain why clients with a chronic rheumatic disease find complementary treatments appealing. First, current therapy for arthritis is still not curative. Despite advances in treatments, many of the inflammatory rheumatic diseases are progressive, painful, and disabling. Second, the course of the rheumatic diseases is variable. There may be periods of remission that last a few days to, in rare cases, years. These positive changes occur in response to therapy or may occur spontaneously. Individuals may equate improvement to a visit to the uranium mine, to a change in diet, to a new medication, or to physical therapy, all of which were completed recently. Thus, the two factors of ineffective treatment and variable disease course coupled with a large market (36 million people in the United States alone) have provided a fertile environment for the advent of unconventional treatments.

Examples of complementary treatments include glucosamine, acupuncture, massage, reflexology, homeopathic medications, herbs, vitamins, minerals, special diets of various kinds, fish oil, dimethyl sulfoxide (DMSO), WD-40, urine injections, folk remedies (e.g., copper bracelets, vinegar, honey), venom from various animals, and even sitting in uranium mines. Although usage of these treatments is high among persons with arthritis, studies indicate that people generally continue regular therapy, do not spend large sums of money on such treatments, and do not choose harmful remedies.[91] In fact, the National Institutes of Health, the American College of Rheumatology (ACR), and the Arthritis Foundation have recognized the importance of complementary therapies for clients and have funded studies investigating complementary therapies. The ACR states as part of its position statement:

> The ACR appreciates the current interest in "complementary" and "alternative" therapies and medicines and understands those frustrations and motivations leading to patients' interest in them. The ACR is concerned that simplistic labels for therapies (or hypotheses or publications) may mislead. The ACR welcomes rigorous scientific evaluation of all hypotheses that might improve our understanding and treatments of rheumatic diseases.[93]

Physical therapists and other health care professionals need to be aware of the types of complementary therapies, their costs, and their potential for benefit and harm. Providing information that allows clients to make informed decision about what treatments to use and not use is an important aspect of the role for all health care professionals.

> Establish an environment that encourages the client to share information about the various types of treatments that she or he is using.

Summary

Although the majority of people with all forms of arthritis manage their disease reasonably well, depressive symptoms and psychological distress are common. Relationships between disease characteristics and psychological distress are complex. Strategies for managing the symptoms, the long term outcomes, and the psychological distress of chronic rheumatic diseases are issues important for health care professionals, clients, and their families.

Case Studies

Three case studies of clients with RA illustrate how depression scores change over time and may offer clues for understanding individual differences among people who happen to have a chronic disabling disease. These cases illustrate three characteristic patterns of psychological distress as seen in people with RA over the course of the disease. Similar patterns can probably be found when the clinical course of other chronic disorders is examined. Three graphs, shown in Figure 15–2, depict these three courses. All three women have RA that does not remit for any extended period of time. They each experience progressive disease with gradually increasing disability despite treatment with second-line medications available at the time and intermittent physical therapy as needed during increased disease activity. AIMS Depression scores are shown for each visit to a specialty clinic over about a 10-year period. AIMS Depression scores range from 0 to 10 with scores above 3.00 indicating the presence of possible depressive symptoms and scores above 4.00 indicating probable depression.

Case Study 1

A woman was first seen in the clinic at age 59; she was married with three grown children. She worked full time as college professor at a small private college before her retirement at age 65. She was active in civic groups and, after her retirement, began to participate in water exercise at the local health club. She exhibited little depression at the time of her diagnosis, and her depression scores remained stable and low during the entire 10-year period. Two peaks in her depression scores were noted at the time her mother and husband died. Except during times of stress or family crisis unrelated to her disease, this woman is managing her disease quite effectively, at least from a psychological point of view.

Case Study 2

This case illustrates a second pattern. This client is a woman in whom arthritis was first diagnosed at age 44. She was divorced and had two children in their early twenties who were having some difficulties finding and keeping employment. She worked at a local insurance office as a receptionist but left the position shortly after her diagnosis because of pain. She became eligible for disability payments at age 53. Her depression scores were high at the time of diagnosis and remained high throughout the disease course. She struggled with depression throughout the 10-year period for a variety of reasons. Her scores were relatively stable but consistently high. Her depressive symptoms probably were not related to any great extent to her disease.

Case Study 3

This case illustrates a pattern of high depression early in the disease with a decline soon after diagnosis. This woman was single and traveled extensively as a computer software salesperson for a large company. She was highly productive and enjoyed a very good income. As her disease developed, she found that she could not tolerate the difficulties of air travel, i.e., carrying luggage, hurrying to catch connecting flights, and changing hotels daily. Her productivity began to decline and she was worried about her future income. After the diagnosis, she discussed her situation with her employer. The company made arrangements for a territory that required less travel, reduced her sales responsibilities by 50%, and made her responsible for training of new sales personnel. With these modifications, she was able to continue to work and did not experience a serious decline in her income. This woman experienced high depression scores at the time of her diagnosis. The diagnosis caused her distress as reflected in her initial depression score. Her scores decreased quickly after diagnosis and remained low during the remaining time that she was followed. She has adapted with time to her disease and has learned to cope with her disorder.

In summary, these cases illustrate that the interaction between psychosocial factors and disease are complex and include much more than the severity or the characteristics of the disease. They also demonstrate that many people do manage their disease using various coping strategies. Clients gain support from family, friends, and health care professionals. They attend formal support groups and participate in educational programs, such as the Arthritis Self-Management program. Many people manage very well whereas others do not. The role for all health professionals is to provide assistance to those who are having difficulties managing their disease and to support the independence of those who are managing.

References

1. Gill TM, Feinstein AR: A critical appraisal of the quality of quality-of-life measurements. *JAMA* 272:619–626, 1994.

2. Fries JF, Spitz PW: The hierarchy of patient outcomes. In Spilker B (ed): *Quality of Life: Assessments in Clinical Trials.* New York, Raven Press, 1990, pp 25–35.

3. Buckelew SP, Huyser B, Hewett JE et al: Self-efficacy predicting outcome among fibromyalgia subjects. *Arthritis Care Res* 9:97–104, 1996.

4. Hassett AL, Cone JD, Patella SJ et al: The role of catastrophizing in the pain and depression of women with fibromyalgia syndrome. *Arthritis Rheum* 43:2493–2500, 2000.

5. Hawley DJ, Wolfe F: Depression is not more common in rheumatoid arthritis: a 10 year longitudinal study of 6,608 rheumatic disease patients. *J Rheumatol* 20:2025–2031, 1993.

6. Van Houdenhove B, Neerinckx E, Lysens R et al: Victimization in chronic fatigue syndrome and fibromyalgia in tertiary care: a controlled study on prevalence and characteristics. *Psychosomatics* 42:21–28, 2001.

7. Walker EA, Keegan D, Gardner G et al: Psychosocial factors in fibromyalgia compared with rheumatoid arthritis: I. Psychiatric diagnoses and functional disability. *Psychosom Med* 59:565–571, 1997.

8. Bradley LA, Alberts KR: Psychological and behavioral approaches to pain management for patients with rheumatic disease. *Rheum Dis Clin North Am* 25:215–232, viii, 1999.

9. Hopman-Rock M, Kraaimaat FW, Bijlsma JW: Quality of life in elderly subjects with pain in the hip or knee. *Qual Life Res* 6:67–76, 1997.

10. Rene J, Weinberger M, Mazzuca SA et al: Reduction of joint pain in patients with knee osteoarthritis who have received monthly telephone calls from lay personnel and whose medical treatment regimens have remained stable. *Arthritis Rheum* 35:511–515, 1992.

11. Burckhardt CS, Bjelle A: Perceived control: a comparison of women with fibromyalgia, rheumatoid arthritis, and systemic lupus erythematosus using a Swedish version of the Rheumatology Attitudes Index. *Scand J Rheumatol* 25:300–306, 1996.

12. Cornwell CJ, Schmitt MH: Perceived health status, self-esteem and body image in women with rheumatoid arthritis or systemic lupus erythematosus. *Res Nurs Health* 13:99–107, 1990.

13. Kozora E, Thompson LL, West SG et al: Analysis of cognitive and psychological deficits in systemic lupus erythematosus patients without overt central nervous system disease. *Arthritis Rheum* 39:2035–2045, 1996.

14. Dexter P, Brandt K: Distribution and predictors of depressive symptoms in osteoarthritis. *J Rheumatol* 21:279–286, 1994.

15. Hoffman AL: Psychological factors associated with rheumatoid arthritis: review of the literature. *Nurs Res* 23:218–234, 1974.

16. Moos RH: Personality factors associated with rheumatoid arthritis: a review. *J Chronic Dis* 17:41–55, 1964.

17. Anderson KO, Bradley LA, Young LD et al: Rheumatoid arthritis: review of psychological factors related to etiology, effects, and treatment. *Psychol Bull* 98:358–387, 1985.

18. Creed F: Psychological disorders in rheumatoid arthritis: a growing consensus? *Ann Rheum Dis* 49:808–812, 1990.

19. Dickens C, McGowan L, Clark-Carter D et al: Depression in rheumatoid arthritis: a systematic review of the literature with meta-analysis. *Psychosom Med* 64:52–60, 2002.

20. Katz PP, Yelin EH: Prevalence and correlates of depressive symptoms among persons with rheumatoid arthritis. *J Rheumatol* 20:790–796, 1993.

21. Cassileth BR, Lusk EJ, Strouse TB, et al: Psychosocial status in chronic illness: a comparative analysis of six diagnostic groups. *N Engl J Med* 311:506–511, 1984.

22. Benjamin, S, Morris, S, McBeth, J et al: The association between chronic widespread pain and mental disorder— a population-based study. *Arthritis Rheum* 43:561–567, 2000.

23. Ahles TA, Yunus MB, Riley SD et al: Psychological factors associated with primary fibromyalgia syndrome. *Arthritis Rheum* 27:1101–1106, 1984.

24. Alfici S, Sigal M, Landau M: Primary fibromyalgia syndrome—a variant of depressive disorder? *Psychother Psychosom* 51:156–161, 1989.

25. Yunus MB, Ahles TA, Aldag JC et al: Relationship of clinical features with psychological status in primary fibromyalgia. *Arthritis Rheum* 34:15–21, 1991.

26. American Psychiatric Association: *Diagnostic and Statistical Manual of Mental Disorders (DSM-IV)*, ed 4. Washington, American Psychiatric Association, 1994, p 886.

27. Callahan LF, Kaplan MR, Pincus T: The Beck Depression Inventory, Center for Epidemiological Studies-Depression Scale (CES-D), and General Well-Being Schedule Depression Subscale in rheumatoid arthritis: criterion contamination of responses. *Arthritis Care Res* 4:1–11, 1991.

28. Pincus T, Callahan LF, Bradley LA et al: Elevated MMPI scores for hypochondriasis, depression, and hysteria in patients with rheumatoid arthritis reflect disease rather than psychological status. *Arthritis Rheum* 29:1456–1466, 1986.

29. Meenan RF, Gertman PM, Mason JH et al: The arthritis impact measurement scales. *Arthritis Rheum* 25:1048–1053, 1982.

30. Beck AT, Steer RA, Gabin MG: Psychometric properties of the Beck Depression Inventory: twenty-five years of evaluation. *Clin Psychol Rev* 8:77–100, 1988.

31. Radloff L: The CES-D scale: a self-report depression scale for research in the general population. *Appl Psychol Measure* 1:385–401, 1977.

32. Sheikh JI, Yesavage JA: Geriatric depression scale (GDS): Recent evidence and development of a shorter version. *Clin Gerontol* 51:165–173, 1986.

33. Meenan RF, Mason JH, Anderson JJ et al: AIMS2: the content and properties of a revised and expanded Arthritis Impact Measurement Scales Health Status Questionnaire. *Arthritis Rheum* 35:1–10, 1992.

34. Blalock SJ, DeVellis RF, Brown GK et al: Validity of the Center for Epidemiological Studies depression scale in arthritis populations. *Arthritis Rheum* 32:991–997, 1989.

35. Magni G, Calidieron C, Rigati-Luchini S et al: Chronic musculoskeletal pain and depressive symptoms in the general population: an analysis of the 1st National Health and Nutrition Examination Survey data. *Pain* 43:299–307, 1990.

36. Frank RG, Beck NC, Parker JC et al: Depression in rheumatoid arthritis. *J Rheumatol* 15:920–925, 1988.

37. Hawley DJ, Wolfe F: Anxiety and depression in patients with rheumatoid arthritis: a prospective study of 400 patients. *J Rheumatol* 15:932–941, 1988.

38. McFarlane AC, Brooks PM: An analysis of the relationship between psychological morbidity and disease activity in rheumatoid arthritis. *J Rheumatol* 15:926–931, 1988.

39. Newman SP, Fitzpatrick R, Lamb R et al: The origins of depressed mood in rheumatoid arthritis. *J Rheumatol* 16:740–744, 1989.

40. Bishop D, Green A, Cantor S et al: Depression, anxiety and rheumatoid arthritis activity. *Clin Exp Rheumatol* 5:147–150, 1987.

41. Murphy S, Creed F, Jayson MIV: Psychiatric disorder and illness behaviour in rheumatoid arthritis. *Br J Rheumatol* 27:357–363, 1988.

42. Hagglund KJ, Haley WE, Reveille JD et al: Predicting individual differences in pain and functional impairment among patients with rheumatoid arthritis. *Arthritis Rheum* 32:851–858, 1989.

43. Hawley DJ, Wolfe F: Pain, disability, and pain/disability relationships in seven rheumatic disorders: a study of 1522 patients. *J Rheumatol* 18:1552–1557, 1991.

44. Evers AW, Kraaimaat FW, Geenen R et al: Determinants of psychological distress and its course in the first year after diagnosis in rheumatoid arthritis patients. *J Behav Med* 20:489–504, 1997.

45. Van der Heide A, Jacobs JWG, Vanalbadakuipers GA et al: Physical disability and psychological well being in recent onset rheumatoid arthritis. *J Rheumatol* 21:28–32, 1994.

46. Newman S, Mulligan K: The psychology of rheumatic diseases. *Baillieres Best Pract Res Clin Rheumatol* 14:773–786, 2000.

47. Wolfe F: A reappraisal of HAQ disability in rheumatoid arthritis. *Arthritis Rheum* 43:2751–2761, 2000.

48. Katz PP, Yelin EH: Activity loss and the onset of depressive symptoms: do some activities matter more than others? *Arthritis Rheum* 44:1194–1202, 2001.

49. Evers AW, Kraaimaat FW, Geenen R et al: Psychosocial predictors of functional change in recently diagnosed rheumatoid arthritis patients. *Behav Res Ther* 36:179–193, 1998.

50. Lanza AF, Revenson TA: Social support interventions for rheumatoid arthritis patients: the cart before the horse? *Health Educ Q* 20:97–117, 1993.

51. Fitzpatrick R, Newman S, Lamb R et al: Social relationships and psychological well-being in rheumatoid arthritis. *Soc Sci Med* 27:399–403, 1988.

52. Affleck G, Pfeiffer C, Tennen H et al: Social support and psychological well-being in rheumatoid arthritis. *Arthritis Care Res* 1:71–77, 1988.

53. Fitzpatrick R, Newman S, Archer R et al: Social support, disability and depression: a longitudinal study of rheumatoid arthritis. *Soc Sci Med* 33:605–611, 1991.

54. Goodenow C, Reisine ST, Grady KE: Quality of social support and associated social and psychological functioning in women with rheumatoid arthritis. *Health Psychol* 9:266–284, 1990.

55. Brown GK, Wallston KA, Nicassio PM: Social support and depression in rheumatoid arthritis: a one year prospective study. *J Appl Soc Psychol* 19:1164–1181, 1989.

56. Revenson TA, Schiaffino KM, Majerovitz SD et al: Social support as a double-edged sword: the relation of positive and problematic support to depression among rheumatoid arthritis patients. *Soc Sci Med* 33:807–813, 1991.

57. Revenson TA, Cameron AE, Lanza AF: Perceived help-fulness of patient-provider support transactions: findings from two studies. *Arthritis Care Res* 4:S19, 1991.

58. Blake DJ, Maisiak R, Alarcon GS et al: Sexual quality-of-life of patients with arthritis compared to arthritis-free controls. *J Rheumatol* 14:570–576, 1987.

59. Elst P, Sybesma T, van der Stadt RJ et al: Sexual problems in rheumatoid arthritis and ankylosing spondylitis. *Arthritis Rheum* 27:217–220, 1984.

60. Majerovitz SD, Revenson TA: Sexuality and rheumatic disease: the significance of gender. *Arthritis Care Res* 7:29–34, 1994.

61. Kraaimaat FW, Bakker AH, Janssen E et al: Intrusiveness of rheumatoid arthritis on sexuality in male and female patients living with a spouse. *Arthritis Care Res* 9:120–125, 1996.

62. Toorians AW, Janssen E, Laan E et al: Chronic renal failure and sexual functioning: clinical status versus objectively assessed sexual response. *Nephrol Dial Transplant* 12:2654–2663, 1997.

63. Brown GK, Nicassio PM, Wallston KA: Pain coping strategies and depression in rheumatoid arthritis. *J Consult Clin Psychol* 57:652–657, 1989.

64. Felton BJ, Revenson TA, Hinrichsen GA: Stress and coping in the explanation of psychological adjustment among chronically ill adults. *Soc Sci Med* 18:889–898, 1984.

65. Brown GK, Nicassio PM: Development of a question-naire for the assessment of active and passive coping strategies in chronic pain patients. *Pain* 31:53–64, 1987.

66. Maes S, Leventhal D, DeRidder DTD: Coping and chronic disease. In Zeidner M, Engler N (eds): *Handbook of Coping: Theory, Research, Applications*. New York, Wiley, 1996, pp 221–251.

67. Parker JC, Iverson GI, Smarr KL et al: Cognitive-behavioral approaches to pain management in rheumatoid arthritis. *Arthritis Care Res* 6:207–212, 1993.

68. Applebaum KA, Blanchard EB, Hickling EJ et al: Cognitive behavioral treatment of a veteran population with moderate to severe rheumatoid arthritis. *Behav Ther* 19:489–502, 1988.

69. Bradley LA, Young LD, Anderson KO et al: Effects of psychological therapy on pain behavior of rheumatoid arthritis patients. Treatment outcome and six-month follow-up. *Arthritis Rheum* 30:1105–1114, 1987.

70. O'Leary A, Shoor S, Lorig K et al: A cognitive-behavioral treatment for rheumatoid arthritis. *Health Psychol* 7:527–544, 1988.

71. Parker JC, Frank RG, Beck NC et al: Pain management in rheumatoid arthritis patients: a cognitive-behavioral approach. *Arthritis Rheum* 31:593–601, 1988.

72. Parker JC, Smarr KL, Buckelew SP et al: Effects of stress management on clinical outcomes in rheumatoid arthritis. *Arthritis Rheum* 38:1807–1818, 1995.

73. Emery P, Salmon M: Early rheumatoid arthritis: time to aim for remission? *Ann Rheum Dis* 54: 944–947, 1995.

74. Kraaimaat FW, Brons MR, Geenen R et al: The effect of cognitive behavior therapy in patients with rheumatoid arthritis. *Behav Res Ther* 33:487–495, 1995.

75. Sharpe L, Sensky T, Timberlake N et al: A blind, randomized, controlled trial of cognitive-behavioral intervention for patients with recent onset rheumatoid arthritis: preventing psychological and physical morbidity. *Pain* 89:275–283, 2001.

76. Lorig K, Laurin J, Gines GE: Arthritis self-management: a five-year history of a patient education program. *Nurs Clin North Am* 19:637–645, 1984.

77. Lorig K, Gonzalez V: The integration of theory with practice: a 12-year case study. *Health Educ Q* 19:355–368, 1992.

78. Lorig KR, Ritter P, Stewart AL et al: Chronic disease self-management program: 2-year health status and health care utilization outcomes. *Med Care* 39:1217–1223, 2001.

79. Lorig K, Gonzalez VM, Ritter P: Community-based Spanish language arthritis education program: a randomized trial. *Med Care* 37:957–963, 1999.

80. Barlow JH, Turner AP, Wright CC: A randomized controlled study of the Arthritis Self-Management Programme in the UK. *Health Educ Res* 15:665–680, 2000.

81. Davis P, Busch AJ, Lowe JC et al: Evaluation of a rheumatoid arthritis patient education program: impact on knowledge and self-efficacy. *Patient Educ Couns* 24:55–61, 1994.

82. Lindroth Y, Bauman A, Brooks PM et al: A 5-year follow-up of a controlled trial of an arthritis education program. *Britt's Rheumatol* 34:647–652, 1995.

83. Tail E, Ranker JJ, Sidle ER et al: Health status, adherence with health recommendations, self-efficacy and social support in patients with rheumatoid arthritis. *Patient Educ Couns* 20:63–76, 1993.

84. Satin JA, Buckner W, Seen K et al: Psychological interventions for rheumatoid arthritis: a meta-analysis of randomized controlled trials. *Arthritis Rheum* 47:291–302, 2002.

85. Riesman RP, Koran JR, Tail E et al: Patient education for adults with rheumatoid arthritis (Cochrane Review). *Cochrane Database Syst Rev* CD003688, 2002.

86. Hawley DJ: Psycho-educational interventions in the treatment of arthritis. *Baillieres Clin Rheumatol* 9:803–823, 1995.

87. Hirano PC, Laurent DD, Lorig K: Arthritis patient education studies, 1987–1991: a review of the literature. *Patient Ed Couns* 24:9–54, 1994.

88. Mullen PD, Laville EA, Biddle AK et al: Efficacy of psychoeducational interventions on pain, depression, and disability in people with arthritis: a meta-analysis. *J Rheumatol* 14:33–39, 1987.

89. Mazzuca SA: Does patient education in chronic disease have therapeutic value? *J Chron Dis* 25:521–529, 1982.

90. Fitzpatrick R, Ziebland S, Jenkinson C et al: A comparison of the sensitivity to change of several health status instruments in rheumatoid arthritis. *J Rheumatol* 20:429–436, 1993.

91. Boisset M, Fitzcharles MA: Alternative medicine use by rheumatology patients in a universal health care setting. *J Rheumatol* 21:148–152, 1994.

92. Panush RS: Preface: complementary and alternative therapies for rheumatic disease. II, *Rheum Dis Clin North Am* 26:xv–xx, 2000.

93. American College of Rheumatology: Position statement: "Complementary" and "alternative" therapies for rheumatic disease, Atlanta, American College of Rheumatology, July 11, 1998.

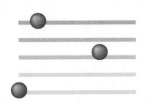

CHAPTER 16

Community-Based Physical Rehabilitation

Barbara Stokes, DIP, PT

Background and Philosophy

Current trends in the provision of health services are focused on more community-based programs. The emphasis is on a "wellness" model with the client assuming responsibility for disease self-management.

A diagnosis of arthritis may carry with it an uncertain prognosis. The onset may vary from slow and insidious to sudden and severe. The course of the disease may be characterized by periods of exacerbation and remission or may be slowly progressive over many years. The implications for the individual's

ability to function may be significant and will vary with age, occupation, and lifestyle. Most often, it is within the community that clients will experience the impact of the disease on their lifestyle. It is, therefore, important that all therapists (occupational and physical therapists and social workers) offer more community-based care in the overall management of clients with arthritis.

What would be an ideal community delivery system for people with arthritis? The service that approximates the ideal may be the community-based program in Ontario, Canada. For more than 50 years, The Arthritis Society in Ontario, Canada, using specially trained personnel, has provided physical therapy (PT), occupational therapy (OT), and social

PHYSICAL REHABILITATION IN ARTHRITIS, Joan M. Walker, PhD, PT, and Antoine Helewa, MSc(Clin Epid), PT, Elsevier Inc. © 2004.

work services to clients with complex forms of arthritis in the home, school, and workplace. The program is funded mainly by a special grant from the provincial Ministry of Health and Long Term Care. All residents of Ontario are eligible for this service under the provincial health insurance scheme. The program is available to about 95% of Ontario residents.

In contrast, the United States has a mostly private health insurance model with health care provision by private facilities and clinicians. Eligibility for rehabilitation services varies and clinicians with special training in arthritis are mainly affiliated with large academic facilities. Additionally, in the managed care model of service delivery the payer may restrict the number of sessions for rehabilitation services. Hospitalization in a rheumatic diseases unit has, for many clients, been shown to control arthritis.[1-3] However, in both Canada and the United States, these units, which traditionally provided a multidisciplinary and specialized approach to disease education and management, have been faced with cost constraints. Thus, numbers of beds and staffing levels have been reduced and designated rehabilitation services have been eliminated. In Canadian hospitals, outpatient rehabilitation services have been reduced or eliminated resulting in excessively long waiting lists. Early intervention, disease education, and self-management are critical to arthritis control. Delays in the provision of disease education and self-management strategies may have a negative impact on outcomes.[2,4] These service delivery constraints have increased the demand for community-based services and focused attention on the importance and relevance of this form of management. In a randomized, controlled trial of OT, the experimental group reported better function at 6 weeks.[5] A randomized, controlled trial of home PT over 6 weeks showed that clients had improved morning stiffness, knowledge of self-management strategies, and self-efficacy. In long-term follow-up, improvements were maintained at 1 year.[6,7] The therapist in the community is uniquely positioned to reinforce, adapt, or expand a disease management program that may have been initiated in a physician's office, in a clinic, or by the client. In many cases, the community-based therapist is the primary contact professional who monitors disease activity, response to drug therapy, and changes resulting from the natural history of the disease or its treatment.

The use of a multidisciplinary approach to disease management in any setting is important. This is especially relevant within the community to minimize the numbers of health care providers going to the client's home, to lend consistency to the management plan, and to reduce costs. The conclusion of an economic evaluation comparing the costs of ambulatory or home-based physiotherapy was that ambulatory care is less expensive.[8] Further, in a study to determine suitability of home- or community-based therapy services, 60% to 75% of clients seen in the home by The Arthritis Society therapists were deemed potential candidates for services in an ambulatory setting.[9] Faced with budgetary constraints and an evident need to improve efficiency while reaching more people with arthritis, The Arthritis Society, in the 1990's broadened it's mandate and expanded services in several ways. First, it developed a primary therapist model of care, in which the first therapist available, regardless of service requested, became the primary therapist or service coordinator.

All Arthritis Society occupational therapists and physical therapists receive the same specialized training in assessment of polyarthritis as part of their orientation.[10] Enhancing the skills of therapists by peer support and consultation supported the shift to this model of service delivery.[11]

Partnerships were established with community facilities, such as small hospitals and community health centers for the provision of clinics and educational/therapeutic groups and physical and occupational therapists provided consultation to other health care providers on management of arthritis. As a result of these changes, between 1995 and 2000, with no increase in budgeted dollars or staff the numbers of people served increased by more than 200%.

Team members may be the family physician, the rheumatologist, physical therapist, occupational therapist, social worker, nurse, and pharmacist. All can contribute importantly either as primary contacts or consultants at any point in the continuum of care. Other support services within the community may include homemaking services, meals on wheels, transport services, pool programs, and various self-help groups. Community-based therapists must be familiar with the support services available to a particular client and must encourage their appropriate use.

Home Assessment

The total assessment of the client with arthritis, with its major components—the history, physical assessment, and functional assessment—has been well detailed in Chapter 5 and the principles apply whatever the setting. However, the importance of a detailed health history cannot be overestimated in the community setting. The client may be referred with simply a diagnosis of "arthritis," and on that basis, with no other relevant information, the therapist enters the client's home. The conventional history contained in a hospital chart is often inaccessible. It therefore is the responsibility of the therapist to obtain, from the client, sufficient information about the disease, its course, and its effects to begin to formulate and establish with the client, realistic management goals. Supplementary information (laboratory or radiographic findings) may be available later, but the health history sets the stage for whatever interventions may be initiated. An algorithm for community-based management of persons with arthritis is shown in Figure 16-1.

The advantages of home assessments are the following:

- Observe the client in his or her own environment.
- Interact with the family.
- Determine the impact of the disease on the client's lifestyle.
- Observe performance of activities of daily living (ADL).
- Provide comfort and convenience for client and family.

Often, it is easier for clients to recall significant clinical events and to divulge sensitive or personal information when they are within the privacy of their own home. Family members may assist in recalling relevant events or changes in the client's functional status. The home is the ideal place to inquire about medication use, including over-the-counter medication, and monitor adherence and side effects. The community-based physical therapist must become familiar with the drugs used in the management of arthritis, their dosages, and expected response time and be alert to possible side effects or interactions (see Chapter 6).

Therapists trained in the standardized assessment techniques, described in Chapter 5, can be as effective as rheumatology fellows in quantifying the effects of joint inflammation and damage in clients with inflammatory arthritis.[10] The active joint count, combined with the duration of morning stiffness, grip strength, and extra-articular features, provides the therapist with invaluable information in planning treatment interventions, monitoring progress, and modifying treatment plans. This information can be conveyed to other treatment team members in a standardized, easily communicated manner (Figure 16-2).

Training in these techniques has been provided by the Ontario Division of The Arthritis Society, Canada, annually since 1976 to more than 450 physical and occupational therapists. An unpublished survey by the Arthritis Community Research and Evaluation Unit in 1992 of 212 physical and occupational therapists who completed the program showed that of the 61% who responded, all reported that they used these skills regularly.[12] Most found the course to be very valuable. Therapists reported that it produced significant changes in their assessment and management of arthritis. This training also enhanced their ability to communicate and interact with other health professionals.

Assessment Equipment

The equipment used in assessing clients with arthritis is minimal. It usually consists of small easily portable items, such as a goniometer, a tape measure, and the modified sphygmomanometer to measure grip strength and strength in affected muscle groups.

> **Equipment used in home assessments should be travel-hardy, simple, and reliable.**

The physical assessment can be easily conducted within the home setting. It is important to be cognizant of the client's tolerance and schedule. Sometimes it is necessary to conduct the total assessment over two or three visits. If this is the case, the client should be provided with some kind of intervention at the first visit, whether it be demonstration of the use of ice packs for an inflamed joint or the provision of educational materials. In this way, the client may be reassured that her or his concerns are being addressed.

The active joint count and damaged joint count can usually be determined quickly with the client on the bed or couch (see Chapter 5). Privacy may be a problem in a household with several small children, dogs, cats, well-meaning neighbors, and ringing telephones! When the clinician makes appointments, it is helpful to explain how long the visit will be, what the client should wear, what activities will take place, and where in the home the assessment will take place. Education about the disease and its treatment begins while the therapist is carrying out the assessment by explaining the purpose of the techniques. Physical findings should be explained in terms that the client can understand.

Another distinct advantage to assessing clients in the home or work environment is the ability to observe how they perform ADL, a difficult if not impossible task in the clinical setting. In the home, the therapist can gather a tremendous amount of information about physical barriers to the performance of many activities, observing everything from the weight and storage of pots and pans to the height of seating, numbers of stairs, and the terrain within and outside the home. The actual functional assessment may be as simple as administering a standardized questionnaire with the

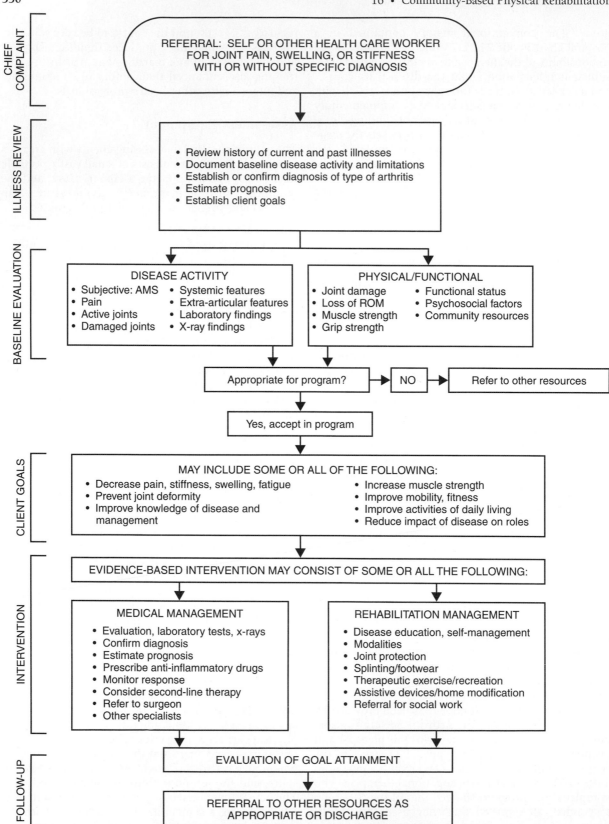

Figure 16-1. Management algorithm in a community-based program for clients with arthritis. *AMS*, morning stiffness; *ROM*, range of motion.

PHYSICAL ASSESSMENT

Patient's Name: _____

Observations:

Gait:

A.M. Stiffness _____ _____
Hrs.   Mins.

Grip Strength: R _____ /20   L _____ /20

Active Joints and Extra-articular Features	**Damaged Joints and Limitations of ROM**
(Definite localized tenderness, stress pain, effusions, not just pain during arc of movement)	(Including lax collaterals, subluxation, bone-on-bone crepitus, malalignment, loss of more than 20% passive ROM. Excluding Heberden's nodes)

No. of active joints _____

Ⓔ Effusion

Ⓧ Tenderness or stress pain

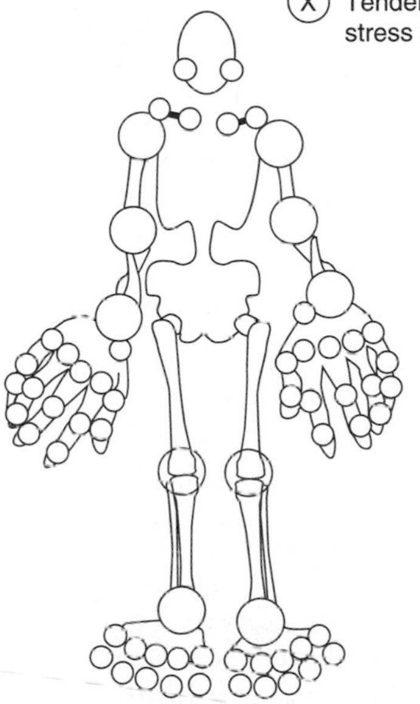

No. of damaged joints _____

● Damage

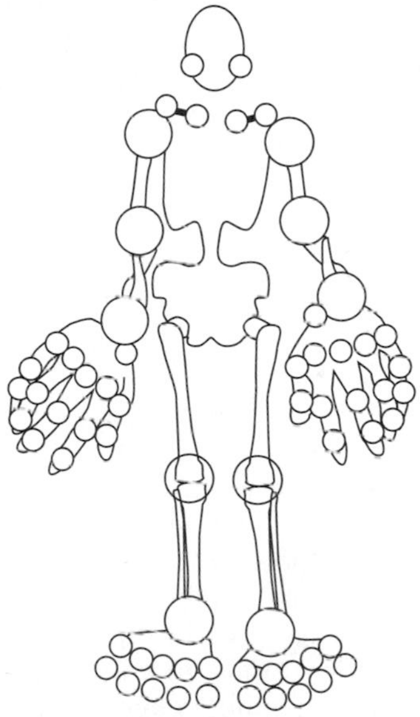

Indicate adjacent to respective fingers the composite range of flexion in centimeters.

WEAK MUSCLE GROUPS													RANGE OF MOVEMENT (SPINE)	
Ms.	Flex		Ext		Abd		Add		E.R.		I.R.		Cervical Spine	Th. Lumbar Spine
Region	R	L	R	L	R	L	R	L	R	L	R			
Should.													LSF FLEX RSF	Fingertip to Floor
Elbow *														_____ cms.
Wrist														Side Flexion: Fingertip to Fib: R cm. L cms.
Hip													LL EXT RR	10 cm. Segments:
Knee														Upper — _____ cms.
Ankle **														Middle — _____ cms. Lower — _____ cms.

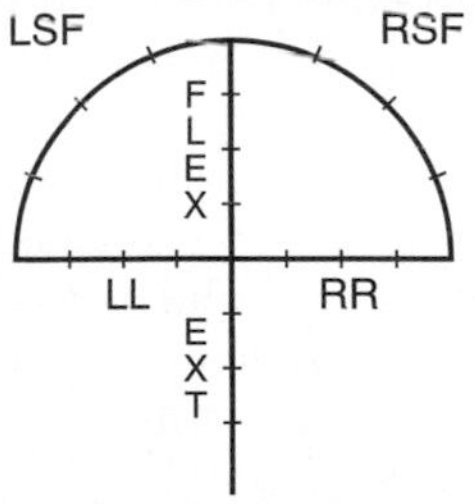

*   Forearm supination and pronation should be recorded under elbow region E.R. and I.R., respectively.
** Foot inversion and eversion should be recorded under ankle E.R. and I.R., respectively.

OF-52A

Figure 16-2. Example of a physical assessment form for use in the community. (From The Arthritis Society, Ottawa, ON, Canada.)

Table 16-1. Examples of Activities Clients May Have Difficulty Performing and Possible Causes and Solutions

Functional Difficulty	Possible Causes	Possible Solutions
Rising from chair	↓ ROM	↑ ROM
	Muscle weakness	Raised cushion
	Joint instability	Strengthen quadriceps
		Surgery
Brushing hair	Limited grasp	Pad handle
	Muscle weakness	Strengthening exercises
	↓ ROM, wrist, elbow, shoulder	Lower head, ↑ ROM
		Long handle
Lifting pots	Weakness, hand, wrist	Strengthening exercises
	Instability, wrist, elbow	Splint wrist
	Pain	Lighter pots
		Slide pots
Carrying files	Pain, wrists	Work splint
	Weakness, fingers, wrists	Strengthening exercises
	↓ ROM, elbow, wrist	Joint protection
		Wheeled cart
		Fewer files

client identifying activities that pose difficulties. Certain impairments such as muscle weakness, loss of range of motion (ROM), or joint instability may be the underlying reason for the difficulty; each of these will require different interventions (Table 16-1). A determination also can be made about the safety or efficiency of particular activities, such as stair climbing and use of a bathtub, and appropriate arrangement of furniture.

The psychosocial effects of the disease upon clients are more easily observed in the home setting. The therapist has the opportunity to watch family interactions, to ask family members about the impact of the illness upon the family, and to determine the roles and expectations of each member in the household. The therapist also has the opportunity to identify the level of understanding about the disease and its management within the family unit and to determine what level of involvement of family members may be appropriate for education.

The four components of the assessment—detailed history, physical assessment, functional assessment, and psychosocial factors—assist in the identification and the setting of realistic treatment goals, specific to that client and her or his own environment.

Identification of Management Goals

It is vitally important in this age of consumer awareness and escalating health care costs to determine at the outset what the client wishes or expects from the care provider, what her or his treatment goals are, and whether these goals are realistic or achievable. The client needs sufficient information about the disease, implications, and management to make an informed decision about which interventions are realistic and acceptable. Therapy in the home is an expensive service. Although most of the management of the disease must be the client's responsibility, regular monitoring of disease activity and treatment response by the caregivers will be required.

The Rheumatoid Arthritis Management Protocol was developed by The Arthritis Society in 1998 and is based on evidence in the literature where available and in its absence on the consensus of The Arthritis Society therapists and other experts in rheumatology (available from The Arthritis Society, Ontario Division). A retrospective chart review for 1993 to 1994 of Arthritis Society clients with rheumatoid arthritis (RA) identified the most common goals of treatment.[13] Goals were grouped according to the International Classification of Impairments, Activities and Participation (ICIDH-2) developed by the World Health Organization[14] to ensure a holistic approach to management. Each goal stands alone and includes a suggested management plan and references, assuming that a systematic and comprehensive assessment has been conducted.

Modification or progression of the treatment goals should be based on periodic reassessments. The client and the physical or occupational therapist can negotiate a mutually agreeable "contract" based on a list of mutually agreed goals, management strategies, and, wherever possible, outcome measures to determine if these goals have been met. Planning for discharge from active treatment must start on the first visit with the client actively participating in this process (see Figure 16-1).

Family members and other caregivers can take part in the goal-setting process and must become aware of the proposed management plan. They may assist with the application of various modalities, taking on some household tasks or learning about the level of emotional support the client may need. At this point, referral to other support services such as homemaking or social work may be necessary.

Management Plan

Only when the total assessment (history, physical and functional assessment) is completed, psychosocial issues are addressed, and the client goals are identified can the treatment program be established. It is particularly important in the home setting to develop a treatment program that is simple, that responds to the client's goals, and that is relevant to the individual (see Figure 16-1). A program that requires a great deal of equipment can be complicated and time consuming and may be cast aside as other family or household demands take precedence. Inappropriate equipment also can increase pain and the level of discomfort.

The disease itself may be very active at the time of referral. The client may be exhausted, experiencing significant pain, and be unable to actively participate in a full exercise program. Physical and occupational therapists have limited but important roles to play at this point. Service provision in the home setting allows the client to conserve energy by eliminating the need to dress for going out, arrange transport, and travel to and from an outpatient setting. It is critical that the first steps of medical management are underway, but response to medications may not yet have occurred. During this interval, the therapist must provide emotional support and educate the client and the caregivers about the nature of the disease and its management. The importance of rest, the value of joint protection, and energy conservation techniques can be introduced at this time. There are a number of useful booklets detailing these principles that can be left with the client to provide reinforcement and to inform other household members (see Appendix I).

Disease Education

One of the primary treatment goals is disease education, in relation to the natural history, prognosis, medical and rehabilitation management, and the range of therapeutic interventions that may be available. This includes information about the role of PT modalities, exercise, and use of assistive devices. Clients will have varied needs for information. It is important to recognize the readiness of the recipient to comprehend the vast amount of information that may be required to adjust to the demands of the disease and to accept the diagnosis of a chronic and progressive illness. Some individuals may be able to assimilate only very basic information because of anxiety or depression; others may demand very technical and sophisticated reading materials. Others may be vulnerable to well-meaning but possibly misguided friends and family who will bombard them with materials on alternative therapies or "quack" remedies.

A great deal of client educational material pertaining to specific conditions and to treatment methods has been published by The Arthritis Society in Canada, the Arthritis Foundation in the United States, and similar organizations in the United Kingdom, Australia, New Zealand, and other countries. Appendix I contains information on obtaining these materials. This information is usually in the form of easily understood pamphlets or brochures. A number of audiocassettes and videotapes have been produced that can be loaned to or purchased by the client.

Web Sites

In recent years a number of web sites have been developed, which provide information not only about the disease and its treatment options but also about sources to inform and assist clients in accessing resources and in managing their condition. Therapists should be familiar with reliable web sites and should caution clients that much health information on the Internet is not peer reviewed and that they should check information with their health care provider.

There also are many books published and widely distributed about arthritis and its management. These have variable content and quality. Clients may require some guidance in selecting reading materials or web sites. Two companion books, *Arthritis: A Comprehensive Guide to Understanding Your Arthritis* and *The Arthritis Helpbook,* are recommended by the Arthritis Foundation and The Arthritis Society for use in an arthritis self-management program (see Appendix I). These books provide an excellent resource for all therapists who should be thoroughly familiar with the content of any material provided. They can be left with the client to read and discussed at a subsequent visit. This material is not a substitute for one-on-one or even group education sessions but is used to reinforce the information provided by the community-based therapist.

It is generally helpful to educate the client about the disease process in terms that she or he can understand. Using the illustrations in the pamphlets may be helpful in explaining the effects of the inflammatory process on the joints and on other body systems. Explaining the processes that can cause joint damage and limit motion, as well as the meaning of certain symptoms enhances the client's ability to self-monitor her or his disease and to understand the rationale behind the proposed treatment strategies. Disease-specific educational groups may be an efficient means of providing education and allowing clients to discuss the information and share experiences.

Rest, both general and local, has been shown to reduce joint inflammation.[3,15] In the early stages of the disease, the importance of rest should be emphasized as an item over which the client can take direct control and a means by which she or he can participate in the overall management of the disease. In the home setting, the therapist can assist in teaching the client to break up daily activities into manageable components and to schedule rest in the daily timetable.

Often, when the community-based therapist sees clients in the workplace, it is useful to meet with the employer or the occupational health nurse; education about arthritis can be provided and their cooperation gained in accommodating the special needs of the employee. For example, modification of the workspace or scheduled rest periods may be required.

Incorporated into the education package and useful in the early stages of the intervention is the teaching of joint protection and energy conservation techniques. These principles, which are addressed in Chapter 14, can be introduced early to a client whose disease activity is still very limiting. These principles can be reinforced and reviewed throughout the treatment process.

> Being able to observe how the client functions at home is a clear advantage for the community-based therapist.

In summary, excellent printed materials, as well as audiocassettes and videotapes, are available to reinforce one-on-one client education.

Medication Usage

Working in the community places additional responsibility on community-based therapists, because they are often the only health care professional with regular, ongoing contact with the client. Physician appointments may be several months apart, and when they do occur, the client's anxiety or the physician's schedule may not provide opportunity to clarify issues or address concerns about medication dosage, side effects, or response. Many clients do not understand the difference between analgesics and anti-inflammatory drugs. This is particularly true of nonsteroidal anti-inflammatory drugs (NSAIDs) in their many forms. Clients often will not take their NSAID in the therapeutic range because, "I don't like to take a lot of pills." A client also may not understand the use of the slower-acting disease-remitting agents (DMARDs) and may be extremely disappointed, for example, when they notice no change in their status after 2 weeks of taking methotrexate.

The community-based therapist must be aware of the actions and interactions of the various drugs prescribed, must be alert to the potential side effects, and must educate the client in this regard. Alternative therapies have become popular in recent years and clients may inquire about their use. Because many of these products have not been studied in the long term, are not regulated, and can be expensive, clients should be advised to consult with their physician or pharmacist about potential interactions with prescription medication. It is important to encourage adherence to the medication scheme and to report, to the physician, any changes, adverse or beneficial, that may be occurring as a result of medication use.

Modalities in the Home

For most clients, the presence of active synovitis makes it difficult to achieve analgesia through the use of thermal modalities or electrical stimulation. Pain relief is usually the result of adequate response to anti-inflammatory therapy; however, the application of pain-relieving physical agents may provide some short-term relief, and these agents are particularly useful before or after clients engage in therapeutic exercise or ADL.

The choice of thermal modalities is influenced by client preference. Clients often are reluctant to apply ice to painful joints, but with adequate explanation resistance to the idea can be overcome. The use of ice applications to acutely inflamed joints can be beneficial by reducing pain sensation and decreasing muscle spasm,[16] in addition to having an anti-inflammatory effect.[17] In addition, brief strokes with ice over the bellies of atrophied muscles will facilitate movement (see Chapter 9).

Applications of heat can be local or general and are usually preferred, both to relieve stiffness and to prepare for exercise. Often, clients report that a warm shower assists with relief of morning stiffness and that they can move more easily to do their exercises after the application of heat.

Safety

The use of modalities in the home setting must be governed by practical considerations, with a particular emphasis on safety issues. Careful explanation must be given to the client about the indications for the use of any of the range of modalities available for home use and potential risks that can result from overuse or misuse. It is not unusual when first visiting clients in the home to discover that they already are inappropriately applying various forms of heat, such as electric heating pads. For example, some elderly clients may wrap a heating pad around a knee and sleep with it on at low heat; this practice causes tissue damage. Other misuses that are potentially hazardous are the use of analgesic rubs in conjunction with heating pads or hot water bottles, insufficient layers of toweling between the source of heat and the client's skin, and the application of heat or cold to areas that may have impaired circulation or sensation. It is therefore critical that clients are well educated about use of these modalities, particularly since they are generally applying them without supervision.

Alternative to Wax Baths

One popular form of treatment in the home setting for many years was the use of wax baths for the relief of stiffness and pain in the hands. Short-term benefits have been reported after wax application and active exercise.[18] Wax application, although still used in the clinical setting, is potentially hazardous because of the risk of fire from improper heating procedures and the risk of burns if the temperature is not well controlled. It also is time consuming and cumbersome to the client.[19] An alternative that is safer and easier is the use of *rubber gloves and oil*. A generous application of mineral oil or baby oil to the hands followed by putting on ordinary rubber gloves and then immersing the hands in hot tap water for 5 to 10 minutes is a more practical solution. Clients report that it eases morning stiffness.

Pain-Relieving Modalities

These are widely available commercially and can be costly. Clients should be advised of the availability of these items. Some may be loaned for evaluation, but generally it is preferable to use simple, inexpensive items found in most households.

A 1-lb package of frozen peas or corn makes an effective and reusable *ice pack* when wrapped in a damp towel, molding well to the joint and being light and easy to handle. Clients should be advised against applying ice directly to the skin, because they may sustain a burn, particularly if they rest the weight of the body part on top of the ice.

The use of *moist heat* is advisable, because it allows more even distribution of heat over the affected area and reduces the risk of burns and moist applications cool down gradually. A hot water bottle wrapped in a damp towel molds well to the affected joint, as does a wet facecloth placed in a microwave safe plastic bag and heated for 1 minute in a microwave oven and then wrapped in a damp towel.

> **Warn clients with Raynaud's phenomenon against the use of either heat or ice for their hands or feet because of the risk of tissue damage.**

The Use of Electrical Modalities

The use of modalities such as ultrasound or interferential currents is impractical in the home setting. Ultrasound (US) units tend to lose their calibration when carried in cars and in and out of homes. Furthermore, the frequency with which US can be used is problematic, and evidence of its efficacy in treating inflammatory polyarthritis is lacking.[20] Effects of interferential current on clients with arthritis has not been studied and the equipment is simply not available for home use.

Many studies on the effects of transcutaneous electrical nerve stimulation (TENS) have been carried out; however, those that were conducted on clients with RA were flawed.[21-23] The portability and relatively low cost of the units make TENS suitable for home use. In many cases, however, clients with limited hand function find TENS difficult to apply. Also, with the multiple sites involved in inflammatory arthritis, TENS becomes impractical. Some community-based programs stock a few TENS units to lend to clients to evaluate, and in some situations, such as refractory shoulder or neck pain, clients report relief with use of these units. Purchase or rental for home use may be possible.

In summary, many thermal modalities can be applied simply and inexpensively in the home. In some situations, if one or two joints remain problematic, a trial of some therapy in an outpatient setting or referral to another facility may be appropriate in the short term.

Rest

Local Rest

Relief of pain may be achieved through the use of support to affected joints and training in proper rest positions. Devices such as resting splints for the hands, wrists, and knees may reduce inflammation through local rest of affected joints and relieve associated muscle spasm (see Chapter 14 for details on orthotics).

Hand Splints

Morning stiffness lasting more than 1 hour is considered to be an indication for hand resting splints, as is persistent wrist and metacarpophalangeal (MCP) joint effusion or tenosynovitis. Pain and swelling may be relieved by immobilization and support.[24] Many clients, however, find a full hand splint too restrictive for independent use at home. The community-based therapist must be aware of the limitations that such splints impose and recognize the importance of maintaining a client's independence in applying the splints, turning light switches on and off, pulling up bedclothes, or even scratching her or his nose! Because of its considerable limitations, the full hand splint, particularly with the thumb incorporated, is usually unsatisfactory for home use. A more acceptable alternative is a splint that leaves the thumb and web space between the thumb and index finger free, but supports the MCPs and allows opposition of the thumb and little finger for minimal light hand function. Motion sensor lighting may be useful for hand splint wearers. Some clients are advised to wear the right hand splint during one night and the left during the next night, until they get used to the splints and are able to rest undisturbed by these appliances.

Knee Splints

Support for inflamed knees with associated spasm of the hamstrings and lack of extension may be provided by means of commercially available knee splints or by molded thermoplastic splints. These are easily applied by the client and fastened with Velcro. They should maintain the knee in as much extension as possible, without exerting an uncomfortable force.

Home Manufacture of Splints

There are many thermoplastic materials available that are suitable for fabrication of splints in the client's home. The materials can be precut and easily heated in a standard oven or an electric frying pan. A simple portable kit containing scissors, splinting materials, Velcro, stockinette, and a heat gun for spot molding is all that is needed for home use. Printed instructions on the use and care of splints should be provided. Clients should be cautioned against applying analgesic rubs before wearing splints, because this can produce skin rash or even burns. At every visit, the therapist should check splints for fit and pressure points and modify the splints if necessary.

Neck Care

The neck needs special attention for relief of pain and maintenance of correct postural alignment. Use of too many pillows under the head should be avoided. Often neck and shoulder pain can be attributed to inadequate neck support during rest. Therefore, the client should be taught to support the cervical spine by means of specially shaped pillows, neck rolls, or cervical ruffs. These can be fabricated from stockinette stuffed with dressing roll or fiberfill batting. Usually two small ruffs fit better and are more comfortable than one large ruff. The advantage of using ruffs is that they stay in place during sleep and also can be helpful when the client is in the upright position. The client should be advised to be alert to the presence of neurologic signs, such as dizziness, blurred vision, or numbness and tingling in the extremities, which could develop from atlantoaxial subluxation. Although such occurrences are rare and the therapist should avoid alarming the client unduly, these symptoms should be promptly reported and investigated. Working with the client in her or his own setting provides the opportunity to identify postures or habits that help or hinder, to solve problems, to demonstrate the use of appropriate support, and to demonstrate alternative positioning using the client's own furnishings.

General Rest

For general rest, client education materials often describe proper resting positions. Illustrations show the client resting supine, with one small, flat pillow under the neck, arms at the sides, and knees out absolutely straight. These instructions are totally unrealistic, because few, if any, clients can relax or are able to sleep in this posture. To relax, *the joints must be adequately supported*. The presence of effusion in the knees or hamstring spasm will render a client unable to straighten the knees completely in the supine position. Traditionally clients are told not to use pillows under the knees unless there is some support, because relaxation will be impossible and pain may increase. If splinting is not possible or practical, the client can be instructed to use a towel folded several times to support the knees *in as much extension as possible*. Resting of the forearm on a pillow laid lengthwise beside the client may assist in alleviating pain in shoulders and elbows. A small pillow or folded towel in the axilla can provide relief for painful shoulders by holding the arm in slight abduction. Bedclothes should be lightweight and should not restrict movement of the feet and ankles. If needed, a cardboard carton can be used to lift the bedclothes from the feet, and sheepskin elbow or heel protectors are sometimes helpful.

General Relaxation

Relaxation techniques may be helpful for clients with intractable pain that cannot be controlled with analgesics and other modalities. These techniques may be used in combination with modalities and medication to maximize their effectiveness. Clients also may choose from the array of available relaxation audiocassettes, selected music, or guided imagery to assist in managing their pain. The client's emotions and behaviors and those of the family can influence the experience of pain. Education about pain and pain management options should be communicated to the client and family. Whatever the client chooses as the most beneficial form of pain control, she or he needs to be assured that the pain is real. Each client needs to recognize which types of pain respond to which interventions such as heat, ice, and splinting and when to seek assistance from health professionals for treatment modifications or further medical intervention.

Therapeutic Exercise

Perhaps the most challenging aspect of providing home PT and rehabilitation is delivering therapeutic exercise, which is, after all, the very essence of what is unique to the practice of PT. (See Chapter 9 for principles of exercise therapy in inflammatory conditions, and Chapter 13 for cardiovascular fitness in clients with arthritis.) This section deals with exercise prescription within the community setting.

In the acute stage of the condition clients are often fatigued and depressed and in pain, with an understandable apprehension about moving the affected joints. They may be deconditioned owing to the effects of the disease, or they may be following a program of rest and have been told to avoid exercise. Clients require considerable education about the purpose and different types of therapeutic exercise and encouragement to participate in designing an acceptable, custom-tailored exercise program.

Adherence to an Exercise Program

To enhance adherence, the exercise program must be relevant, pain free, and short in duration. Poor adherence is likely if the program is time consuming, complicated, or causes increased pain. Careful explanation should be given about the purpose of the three types of exercises prescribed: mobilizing, strengthening, and conditioning. The time of day at which the exercise program is carried out will depend on many factors. Ideally, exercise should be done at a time when the client has the least pain and is not fatigued. However, this may not be possible because of other competing lifestyle factors. The physical therapist should work with the client to identify the means by which the exercises can be incorporated into everyday activity.

The physical therapist should design a short, simple exercise program for certain target areas, especially if the client has identified a specific functional problem, such as inability to rise unassisted from a chair. If this problem is due to muscle weakness, the exercise program can be focused on quadriceps strengthening. Difficulty reaching objects on shelves may be addressed by increasing shoulder ROM. Pointing out the improvements in function that result from the exercise can provide the client with an incentive to continue.

Morning stiffness affecting the hands may interfere with dressing activities. A few minutes of gentle hand exercises in warm water may relieve the stiffness and make dressing easier. Mid morning may be the least painful period of the day and therefore a good time to perform other ROM and strengthening exercise. Some clients take their morning medication and return to bed until it takes effect and then perform their exercises.

> Enhance exercise adherence by using a short program with a clear purpose that considers the client's comfort, ease of performance, and functional gains.

Mobilizing Exercises

Mobilizing exercises are indicated to increase ROM in affected joints, increase flexibility, and relieve stiffness. Actively inflamed joints should be moved gently through the available range, once or twice daily for no more than three repetitions. This may require assistance from a family member or other caregiver if the client is weak or has difficulty moving a shoulder, for example. The assistant should merely support the weight of the affected limb and allow the client to carry out the actual movement. As the inflammation decreases, the client can be taught to move through the available range and then attempt to go a little farther to begin to stretch tight joint structures. For example, with forward flexion of the shoulder, the client can be taught to use a doorway, slide the hand up the door frame as far as possible, hold for a few seconds, and then attempt to reach up a little farther. Pulleys can be useful for regaining ROM in the shoulders and are easily mounted in a doorway, for example, using a single pulley, sash cord, and pipe insulation for handles, all inexpensive and available in hardware stores.

Hold-relax techniques can be of great value in regaining lost ROM and relieving stiffness in periarticular structures. These techniques can be taught to the client or to an assistant and modified in the home setting very easily. Clients should be warned that it is inadvisable to apply a force across more than one affected joint. An example of the self-applied hold-relax technique is for the client to use the side of the bed or front of an upholstered chair to provide isometric resistance to the hamstrings followed by voluntary relaxation of these muscles and then active extension of the knee.

The pain and limitation of movement caused by inflammatory arthritis often results in reflex inhibition and disuse atrophy. Muscle weakness, combined with ROM and endurance losses, can result in difficulties with ADL.

> **Disease management should include daily exercise to improve ROM, build strength and control, and increase endurance.**

Strengthening Exercises

When joints are actively inflamed, the client should be advised not to perform many repetitions, not to exercise to the point of fatigue, and to avoid resisted movements. The muscles acting on inflamed joints should be exercised isometrically to maintain and increase strength and endurance. These exercises are easily performed in the home setting and require only minimal equipment. For example, the knee can be positioned over a large juice can wrapped in a towel and the heel supported to perform isometric quadriceps exercises in mid range.

When joint inflammation has subsided and muscle strength has improved, the exercise program can be increased to include movement, beginning gradually and using low resistance. Strengthening exercises should be performed once daily.

Although clients can be taught to self-resist various muscle groups, clients with hand/wrist involvement may find this difficult. The community-based therapist then can instruct other household members to apply resistance, or teach the client to use belts, resistive rubber bands, tubing, or other elastic materials. Because clients will be expected to carry out the exercise program unsupervised, it is important to remind them to monitor the number of repetitions and that the strengthening exercises should be pain free. Exercises that cause increased joint pain or swelling should be discontinued until the community-based therapist can reassess and modify the program.

It is important to tailor the program to the specific needs of the individual client, bearing in mind the need to incorporate this aspect of disease management into the client's lifestyle. The community-based therapist should determine, with the client, how the program can fit into her or his daily schedule and should emphasize that ADL are an adjunct but not a substitute for therapeutic exercise.

Conditioning Exercise

In recent years, the importance of maintaining physical fitness has replaced the emphasis previously placed on rest and avoidance of strenuous activity. People with arthritis experiencing pain, fatigue, or disability may abandon activities enjoyed previously such as gardening, skiing, or cycling. They may have a sense of loss, depression, and further deconditioning as a result of inactivity.

Exercise/Recreation in the Community

The community-based therapist can encourage the client to resume conditioning exercise by exploring alternatives or adapting activities. In many communities, recreational programs designed for people with physical limitations, such as low-impact aerobic classes, walking groups, and pool exercise programs, are available. These activities may be appropriate for clients, but because of fear of pain, lack of self-confidence, and depression, some clients may be reluctant to participate. The community-based therapist can be of great assistance in providing reassurance and encouragement to clients to use appropriate resources.

Pool exercise programs for people with arthritis are becoming increasingly popular and available. Frequently, water fitness instructors consult physical therapists about exercises that are suitable for people with arthritis. It is preferable that the pool be accessible by graduated steps or ramp and that the temperature be warm, ideally about 85° F (29° C). Pool exercise can provide benefits for clients, because the warmth of the water promotes relaxation and the buoyancy of the water assists with ROM. Water also offers controlled resistance for strengthening activities. A pool program can be recreational and may enhance social interaction among participants.

The community-based therapist may accompany the client to a designated pool program or exercise group to determine whether the program offered is suitable or the facility is safe and accessible. The community-based therapist may consult with the instructor and provide reassurance to the client about the potentially new experience of a pool/exercise program.

Other clients may wish to pursue more self-directed activities, such as cycling or cross-country skiing. Advice should be provided to the client about suitable types of activities and to the equipment used. Ski pole handles can be padded and bicycle seats and handlebars adjusted to allow the client to perform the activity in a safe and pain-free manner. Again, clients must learn to pace themselves by starting slowly and building up their tolerance levels and watching for signs of increased joint pain or swelling.

The management of arthritis demands a great deal of the client both physically and emotionally. To improve the client's overall sense of well-being, attention must be paid to pursuits the client finds pleasurable and rewarding. If the activity can be suitably adapted and increases the client's strength, tolerance, and sense of well-being, it is well worth the therapist's effort.

Audiovisual Aids to Exercise

Because the client will not be receiving direct supervision at home, the exercises must be carefully taught, and the provision of written exercise materials can be helpful. The language should be very clear and specific. Sometimes it is helpful to develop an exercise chart so that clients can check off which exercises they have performed on a daily basis. Clients also can record which exercises they have found difficult in a diary that can be reviewed by the community-based therapist on subsequent visits. There are many pamphlets and exercise sheets available, some of which are produced by pharmaceutical companies and others by hospital departments. Some of these have excellent and very clear illustrations that can serve as good reminders for starting positions and desired movements. Clients may adhere better to a personalized exercise prescription that they wrote out using their own terms.

Many audiocassettes and videotapes for exercising are available; these vary in content and quality. Some of them can be useful as a resource for clients, but the exercises should be reviewed with the community-based therapist and customized for the individual client. Otherwise, there is a risk of harm if the client performs an exercise incorrectly or does too many repetitions, resulting in unnecessary or inappropriate exercise. Therefore, although these materials are a useful adjunct to treatment, they must be accompanied by specific instructions about the purpose, frequency, number of repetitions, and progression or modification of the exercises.

With the increasing availability of computer-based exercise programs that enable individual item selection and instruction, exercise pamphlets can be tailor made for individual clients.

Ambulation

The importance of supportive and comfortable footwear cannot be overestimated (see Chapter 14). In the home, the community-based therapist can examine the footwear habitually worn around the house by the client, look at the shoes the client may have tried or prefers, and encourage adaptation or replacement of footwear. Basic footwear modifications are easy to perform in the home. Insoles can be fabricated with thermoplastics, or metatarsal and longitudinal arch supports can be put in existing shoes. The community-based therapist should have available a list of recommended brands of shoes and the sources for shoes and other modifications, such as names of suppliers of orthotics or retail outlets. It also is helpful to provide a handout on the recommended features of shoes.

On occasion the community-based therapist may accompany the client to the shoe store or orthotist to ensure that proper fit and adaptation are obtained. It may be difficult to convince the client of the value of good, supportive, and often expensive footwear. By pointing out the number of uncomfortable shoes the client may have tried and discarded and the associated expense of continually purchasing unsuitable shoes, the community-based therapist may convince the client to accept the recommended footwear and to absorb the cost. When the client has properly fitted and comfortable footwear, she or he frequently adheres to the suggestions and finds it easier to tolerate walking and standing.

In some communities, there are special footwear outlets, occasionally with orthotists who have special knowledge of foot pathological conditions and who can work with the client and the community-based therapist to find acceptable solutions for foot problems. Mobile, visiting suppliers who will see a client at home to provide fitting and adaptation services may be available in some regions. Referral to an occupational therapist is appropriate in many circumstances when the client's foot problems are complex and require specialized modification. Similarly, referral to chiropodists or special outpatient foot clinics for management of problem nails, calluses, bunions, or skin breakdown may be indicated.

Clients should be carefully taught about foot care and instructed in the importance of monitoring skin conditions and care of areas of pressure that may occur. Clients with limited mobility may have difficulty reaching and seeing these areas. The use of a hand-held mirror may help, as well as having family members check on foot conditions.

> **Improper foot care can lead to infection.**

Ambulatory Aids

Ambulatory aids can be of great value whether a client has a single knee or hip involvement, as in osteoarthritis, or multiple inflamed joints, such as in RA. Properly used, they afford joint protection and an element of pain relief, allowing a client more mobility in the home and in the community. Used inappropriately, they can put a client at risk of falls and may reinforce poor posture.

Canes and Crutches

Some clients "borrow" canes from relatives or friends that are too long or too short. Many misguidedly use the cane in the wrong hand. It is, therefore, important to assess clients carefully for the prescription of canes, crutches, or walkers. Clients should be educated about the dangers inherent in holding on to

furniture or leaning against walls to get around their home. Caution should be given about the risks of loose carpets or slippery floors.

Adjustable canes are easily available and can be lent to a client for a trial. Some clients may have difficulty with the conventional rounded handle of a cane. There are some types of canes on the market with specially molded hand grips. The community-based therapist may modify a cane handle with wide rubber bands or some other material to make it easier for the client to grasp. Instruction in measurement for the correct length of a walking aid may be required.

Clients with arthritis of the upper limbs usually have great difficulty managing conventional axillary crutches because of the need to transfer weight through the elbows and wrists. If crutches are necessary, either postsurgically or when joints are painful or unstable, then forearm support crutches are recommended. These permit the weight to be distributed over the forearm and therefore avoid pressure on inflamed joints of the hands and wrists. They can be cumbersome for some clients and a nuisance for indoor use or use on stairs, and the Velcro straps securing the forearm can be problematic. Forearm crutches, however, are helpful outdoors or in shopping malls.

> **Clients using walking aids should regularly check the tips for wear, use ice pick tips when appropriate, and be able to manage steps/stairs.**

Walkers

Many types of walkers are available; some are very simple and lightweight, some have features such as a carrying basket that converts to a seat, and some have various types of wheels. When a walker is prescribed, it is helpful to assess the specific needs of the client, particularly within the home, because many factors must be taken into consideration. These include the ability of the client to lift and move the walker safely, the layout of the rooms and furniture, and the requirement to use stairs.

Often a walker supplied in an outpatient or rehabilitation center appears suitable but may be unsafe or unsuitable at home. This is exemplified by the case of an elderly, frail lady with advanced RA who, after total knee arthroplasty, moved well in the corridors and gymnasium of the rehabilitation center using a high delta walker. She was discharged to her small bungalow with this walker, which proved to be too cumbersome and unwieldy. In attempting to move the walker through a doorway and around a corner, the client fell, pulling the walker down on top of herself and sustaining a fractured femur. For this client, a home assessment by a community therapist immediately after discharge may have prevented this unfortunate occurrence.

Scooters

Motorized scooters have become popular and are in widespread use, but should be prescribed only when the physically challenged client is likely to become homebound without such assistance. These vehicles can be cumbersome in the ordinary home and are very expensive, although some insurance schemes will partially cover the cost. The client may require assistance to be able to transfer safely. Scooters may, nevertheless, permit freedom of movement for very mobility-limited clients who otherwise might not be able to get out in the community. These vehicles are sometimes very helpful to clients who can use them at work. In some instances, the scooters permit clients to continue their employment.

> In selection of ambulatory aids, the client's physical ability to use the aid and the environment the aid must be used in should be considered.

Activities of Daily Living

The common goal for most clients with arthritis is to maintain their independence within their home and community. This goal is achieved in a variety of ways. The provision of aids and adaptations may, for many clients, provide the solution to problems with ADL. Aids and adaptations, however, should be provided judiciously.

They should be used in the acute phase of the disease to protect inflamed joints or to allow the performance of an activity that would otherwise not be possible because of pain and weakness. For example, the use of a raised toilet seat for a client with painful, effused knees and weak quadriceps would be appropriate but is not a substitute for the exercise program necessary to preserve or increase ROM and strengthen the quadriceps. With proper management and disease control, the client will not require this aid. Similarly, the provision of a reaching device may be indicated for a client who cannot bend because of limitation of joint movement. Again, an exercise program may restore joint mobility and eliminate the need for the device. If the disease progresses and joint damage

occurs precluding improvement of ROM or joint stability, such devices become necessary.

Facilitating a client's ability to carry out ADL is a very tangible means of gaining a client's confidence because she or he can immediately perceive the impact of using a tap turner or a raised cushion. It is important, however, not to provide clients with equipment that is neither needed nor wanted and will not therefore be used. It is often more appropriate to lend a piece of equipment for clients to evaluate over a period of time than it is to ask them to purchase an expensive item they may not use.

When working in the home setting, it is easy to determine whether a client is not using the cane or the raised cushion, because these items may not be visible or may be hidden deep in a closet. Working with the client to achieve maximum function and independence can be greatly enhanced by first-hand observation, and use of concrete examples can reinforce the principles of joint protection and energy conservation.

Safety Concerns

One of the primary considerations when therapists work with a client to achieve increased function and independence is the issue of safety. Many times, clients will adapt to altered functional status by using poor body mechanics, leaning on unstable pieces of furniture, or grabbing at towel bars or the sink. The community-based therapist should carefully observe activities such as transfers from the bed, chairs, and the bathtub or shower, movement about the kitchen, and use of stairs and educate the client about the inherent hazards within the home setting. Any piece of equipment that is supplied should be checked for safe installation and use. The community-based therapist should identify for the client, potentially unsafe activities, such as lifting and reaching, and hazards, such as loose scatter mats, stairs without rails, and slippery surfaces. Fall prevention programs are available in many communities and booklets for distribution to clients are available as a resource (see Appendix I).

> The client should be alerted to safety concerns, both within and outside the home.

Within the household, many simple adjustments can be made with little expense or effort, such as raising the height of chairs, changing faucet handles to levers, reorganizing kitchen shelves, and teaching the client easier ways to perform certain tasks. Simply by watching a client move about the home or carry out a few kitchen activities, the community-based therapist can be of great assistance in identifying and helping to correct poor body mechanics or work habits. An OT referral is appropriate if extensive modification to the household appears indicated. The occupational therapist has skills and resources that will enhance the client's function and independence.

> **Assist clients to investigate financial support or tax deductions for home modifications.**

Visiting the Workplace

Visiting a client in the workplace provides the opportunity for the community-based therapist to directly observe work habits, posture, tools involved, and organization of the workspace and to demonstrate alternatives or modify existing equipment or furnishings. The community-based therapist has an important role to play in determining the client's level of disease activity and physical capability of carrying out their job responsibilities.

The occupational therapist should assist in making modifications for a specific client in the workplace. In many communities, occupational therapists with rheumatology experience are actively working in this capacity. Businesses are becoming more aware of the importance of ergonomics. Modifications and updating of furnishings and equipment are being made, not only to prevent injury in the workplace but also to facilitate employment for people with physical limitations. Often, with appropriate information and explanation, employers are able to provide rest breaks or adapted equipment to facilitate the individual's return to work. In large organizations, there may be facilities available to allow the client to lie down for a break or to perform the prescribed exercise routine. There may be nursing staff available to assist in monitoring the client's condition and, in some instances, the provision of educational presentations or printed materials is welcomed by the organization. A meeting with the client, employer, fellow workers, and other treatment team members, as appropriate, can result in a satisfactory return to the workplace and exemplifies the concept of a team approach within the community.

Perioperative Management

Ideally, consideration of surgical intervention should take place before the development of contractures, severe deformity, and loss of function. Early consultation for orthopaedic surgery may be encouraged by the community-based therapist for preventive or prophylactic procedures, such as synovectomy or arthroscopic débridement because the success rates are greater earlier in the disease process. Pain is the primary indication for surgery and can lead to weakness and deconditioning along with loss of function. The community-based therapist can assist the client in considering the risks and benefits of surgery in a realistic manner, taking into account the client's expectations, lifestyle, home situation, and available resources for support. Education can be provided about the surgical procedure itself and pre- and postoperative care using illustrated materials available from the Arthritis Foundation, The Arthritis Society, or individual orthopaedic surgeons (see also Chapter 7 and 11).

Preoperatively many clients are unable to exercise adequately because of pain. In Canada, there are long waiting periods before hip and knee arthroplasty, leaving clients discouraged and anxious. The role for the community-based therapist at this time is to work with the client to achieve pain relief and to exercise the supporting muscle groups safely and effectively. The therapist should encourage the client to continue with as much exercise as is tolerable to maintain cardiovascular fitness. Clients often find that exercising in a warm pool can relieve pain and provide a comfortable means of maintaining fitness levels. The provision of assistive devices such as raised toilet seats, grab bars, and walking aids can be of great benefit in helping the client maintain independence. Pamphlets, illustrations, and information about the procedure itself can be provided to the client and to the family. Discussing the postoperative program is helpful in assisting the client to determine what resources will be necessary and available after surgery. Ensuring that the necessary support is in place can be very reassuring to the client and to the family.

Other Resources

In the institutional setting, the roles of various team members may be strictly defined, but in the community, a multiskilled approach is essential to provide more efficient and cost-effective service. For example, in Ontario, Arthritis Society social workers operating from regional offices are well poised to provide consultation services to the Society's physical therapists, occupational therapists, and clients.

> **Social workers are excellent client advocates in dealing with government bureaucracy and employers.**

The client may require an advocate to assist with the formalities of benefits, disability pensions, financial assistance for the purchase of special equipment, or returning to work on a part-time basis. Family or personal counseling may be needed to help clients and families cope with the impact of arthritis. Emotional support groups facilitated by a social worker have been shown to influence coping skills and lessen depression in clients with RA.[25] At various stages throughout the course of the disease, the client may require modification of the drug regimen; consultation with a pharmacist, chiropodist, or orthopedic surgeon; or referral to vocational rehabilitation services. The therapist providing care in the community should ensure that appropriate communication takes place between the service providers and that the client can recognize when to seek advice or services.

Discharge Planning

Discharge planning ideally begins at the time of the first visit of the community-based therapist to the client. This is the time when the relationship between the physical or occupational therapist and the client begins. It should be clear, especially with a client who has a long-term, chronic disease, that resources are available to assist her or him in achieving realistic goals. The major responsibility, however, rests with the client, who must assume an active role in the selection and implementation of treatment strategies. It is easy for clients seen at home to establish a dependence either on the service or on the care provider. Although this may be gratifying to the provider, the therapist must remember that the purpose of the intervention is to allow the client to remain active and independent within the community. The ultimate aim of the therapist is to provide disease education and self-management methods with information on resources.

Because the course of the disease is unpredictable and the severity is variable, the needs of individual clients will differ. Coping strategies unique to each person often will determine how much is required. Other treatment team members should be involved in discharge planning, so that the client is not left feeling abandoned. It is useful to communicate to the client,

on reassessment, what progress has been made, what outcomes are expected from the treatment program, and what indicators are being used to recognize achievement of the goals related to treatment (see Figure 16-1). When discharge is planned, it is sometimes helpful to taper off the frequency of visits, spacing them out from weekly, for example, to every 2 weeks or once monthly, so that the therapist may help the client confirm her or his ability to manage independently. Another strategy is to arrange a monthly telephone check. On discharge, clients are advised to call the community-based therapist if new problems arise or when they have specific concerns.

Research Questions

1. Does disease education by the physical therapist/occupational therapist/social worker in a group setting enhance treatment adherence and self-efficacy?
2. Is rehabilitation in the ambulatory setting as effective as rehabilitation delivered individually in the home setting.
3. Are the short-term gains from dynamic exercise (heart rate exceeds 60% of age-related maximum heart rate) maintained over 12 months?

Summary

The advantages of service provision in the home are obvious for clients with a chronic condition that results in energy depletion and can cause significant functional and psychological problems. Bridging the gap between the hospital or outpatient department, the community-based therapist can assist the client in applying the principles of self-management and treatment strategies that may have been initiated in a clinical setting but must be incorporated into an individual's lifestyle. As part of a team that may have few or many members, the community based therapist has the opportunity and obligation to mobilize community resources, to advocate on behalf of the client, and to work in a variety of settings, creatively employing multidisciplinary skills to enable the client to adapt and to maintain function and independence within her or his own community.

Case Studies

The following two case studies provide examples of the value of community-based care to individuals with arthritis.

Case Study 1

Mrs. K., a 39-year-old married woman with three sons, worked as a retail buyer and had an active life style until she developed progressive, symmetrical, seropositive RA. Her family physician had prescribed naproxen, which was only partially effective. No longer able to work after 18 months, she was referred to a rheumatologist who prescribed methotrexate and chloroquine. She was referred to The Arthritis Society for physical and occupational therapy.

At the first home visit, Mrs. K.'s own treatment goals were relief of both pain and motion restriction, which would allow her to return to work, manage her household activities, and resume cross-country skiing and tennis.

Physical Assessment.

- Morning stiffness of 2 hours
- Grip strength: 84/20 right (R); 92/20 left (L)
- 18 active joints (6 with effusions)
- 12 damaged joints
- Decreased ROM in L knee, both wrists, both shoulders, and in proximal interphalangeal joints of both hands
- Decreased muscle strength affecting shoulder girdle, quadriceps, and both wrists
- *Functional assessment* showed the following:
- Walking difficulties due to foot and knee pain
- Difficulty climbing stairs and rising from sitting
- Problems in self-care and household chores due to hand, wrist, and shoulder pain and weakness
- Inability to work caused by fatigue, lack of endurance, and upper extremity involvement
- Decreased social and recreational activities

Additionally, Mrs. K. was experiencing depression and family difficulties.

Treatment Plan.

Mrs. K.'s goals were to learn more about the disease, how to manage the pain and stiffness, and to regain ROM and strength to return to her previous active lifestyle and return to work. A treatment plan was negotiated between the community-based therapist and the client to include the following:

- Reinforcement of disease education provided by the rheumatologist and pharmacist with additional reading materials provided for client and family
- Instruction in the application of heat for shoulders and hands and the application of ice to swollen joints
- Exercise to maintain and increase ROM in affected joints and isometric exercise for major muscle groups
- Provision of a raised toilet seat, tap turners, and jar opener
- Fabrication of polyethylene work splints
- Referral to an occupational therapist for footwear modifications and reinforcement of joint protection and energy conservation techniques
- A meeting between the physical therapist, husband, and sons to answer questions and suggest redistribution of household chores to reduce stress on the client

Progress.

The physical therapist visited weekly over the next 6 weeks to monitor progress and adjust therapy as required. On assessment at 6 weeks, Mrs. K. reported reduction of morning stiffness to 1 hour, an increase in her energy, and increased ability to carry out ADL. The active joint count was 12 with 2 effusions, ROM had improved in shoulders and wrists, but the left knee remained hot and swollen and lacked 10 degrees of extension. Grip strength had improved to 130/20 (R) and 142/20 (L).

Mrs. K. felt that her arthritis was beginning to respond to therapy and that she was making good use of the joint protection and energy conservation techniques she had been shown. Work splints were made in The Arthritis Society splint clinic that enabled her to carry out light kitchen duties, and the footwear modifications had reduced her foot pain. She also reported that her husband was becoming angry and frustrated because of her inability to go to work, the cost of medications, and the increased work-load on family members. The client was considering returning to work and discontinuing her medication because of cost.

The physical therapist reported the client's status to the rheumatologist who injected the left knee with good result. Referral was made to a homemaking service. At that point, both the therapist and client felt that the exercise program could be increased moderately in scope and intensity and that a referral to social work was indicated because of the increased financial and family stresses.

The social worker was able to secure financial assistance to pay for the medications and to work with the client and her husband toward resolving the family problems.

Over the next 4 months, the community-based therapist decreased the frequency of her visits, because Mrs. K. was able to carry out the treatment program independently and was learning to monitor her disease activity. In consultation with the occupational therapist and the social worker, it was felt that although Mrs. K. was responding well to the overall treatment program, she was becoming socially isolated and withdrawn. Physically, she was ready to begin a more active exercise program and could benefit from a recreational activity. She agreed to attend weekly hydrotherapy sessions at a warm pool, which she enjoyed and which allowed her to interact socially with others. At this point, the community-based therapist discontinued regular visits and referred Mrs. K. to an emotional support group conducted in The Arthritis Society facilities by the social worker.

Nine months after referral, a visit to Mrs. K.'s workplace by the community-based therapist to provide consultation on the need for modifications enabled the client to return to work on a part-time basis. The community-based therapist visited Mrs. K. at home, once more, to reassess her situation and determine whether the treatment goals had been achieved. Mrs. K. had 20 minutes of morning stiffness, six active joints, grip strength of 192/20 (R) and 212/20 (L); ROM was full in both shoulders and the left knee and 75% in both wrists; and she was largely independent in performing ADL but still required assistance with cleaning and laundry. Although unable to play tennis, she was able to resume cross-country skiing on gentle terrain, limiting herself to brief periods. On discharge the client felt she had, at least partially, fulfilled her treatment goals. Although some of the family stresses remained, the treatment program had resulted in Mrs. K. becoming an informed and active participant in the management of her disease. She was able to integrate the treatment strategies into her lifestyle, appropriately utilizing professional services and community resources.

Case Study 2

Mrs. H. was a 76-year-old widow with widespread osteoarthritis (OA) affecting both hands, knees, and hips. She relocated from another city to share a small apartment with her son. Because of increasing functional limitations, she was referred to The Arthritis Society by her family physician for physical therapy. The physical therapist met with Mrs. H. and her son in their home. Both were concerned with Mrs. H.'s increasing difficulty with ambulation, transfers, and bathing, as well as her social isolation and depression.

Physical Assessment.

- Bony enlargement, limitation of motion of distal and proximal interphalangeal joints bilaterally, carpometacarpal joint involvement of both thumbs, muscle wasting, loss of dexterity
- Pain, crepitus on movement of right knee, 20-degree flexion contracture, 75 degrees of flexion, quadriceps wasting and weakness
- Left knee, which had undergone an arthroplasty, pain free with ROM of 0 to 95 degrees
- Hips, limited to 50% of full ROM, pain on lateral rotation and flexion

Functional Assessment.

- Ambulation limited to 20 feet and slow and painful, holding on to furniture for support
- Difficulty with transfers
- Difficulty with self-care due to decreased dexterity and difficulty with meal preparation due to limited mobility and strength

Treatment Plan.   Mrs. H.'s goals were relief of pain and increased independence in ambulation, self-care, and meal preparation. She also wanted to be able to go shopping and to socialize. Her son was anxious about her depression and her physical condition. The treatment plan included the following:

- Discussion with family physician, prescription of analgesics, and referral to a rheumatologist for potential surgical intervention
- Application of oil and rubber glove routine for hands
- Instruction of Mrs. H.'s son in application of moist heat to hips and right knee and positioning at rest; instruction in ROM exercises for knees and hips within tolerance and isometric exercises for quadriceps, hamstrings, and hip extensors

Care was transferred to the occupational therapist for the following:

- Provision of tap turners, jar opener, and padded handles of utensils
- Fabrication of working splints
- Addressing of safety issues (chair height, use of raised toilet seat, bath bench, and bars; instruction in use of walker; removal of loose carpets)
- Referral to Friendly Visitors

Mrs. H. was referred by the rheumatologist to an orthopedic surgeon who recommended a total R. knee arthroplasty. Before surgery she required reassurance and encouragement to strengthen her lower extremities. She was able to move about the apartment using a walker, but her tolerance was low and she was unable to go outdoors independently.

After surgery and a brief period in a rehabilitation center, she was discharged to her son's home. The Arthritis Society physical therapist visited again to assess Mrs. H.'s safety and to follow up on her exercise program. Mrs. H. was able to carry out her exercise program unsupervised, was ambulating well with a walker within the apartment, but was afraid to go outdoors or even to go to the mailroom alone. The treatment program was to do the following:

- Increase the scope and intensity of exercises
- Progress to ambulation indoors with one cane
- Commence hydrotherapy to increase strength, endurance, and social contacts

Mrs. H. was reluctant to attempt ambulation outside of the apartment, even with her son. With the physical therapist accompanying her, she gradually increased her confidence and was able to walk to the nearest street corner within a few weeks. She was fearful of attending hydrotherapy sessions on her own, so the physical therapist arranged for her son to accompany her for the first few sessions, after which she met another participant who offered to drive her to and from the pool.

Three months after her hospitalization, Mrs. H. was able, with the use of aids, to prepare meals independently, perform self-care, and ambulate. She was planning a move into her own apartment and had arranged for a homemaker to assist with housework. The occupational therapist from The Arthritis Society visited the new apartment with Mrs. H. and made suggestions for modifications to the bathroom and kitchen to enhance her independence.

At the time of discharge, Mrs. H. was attending a seniors' group as well as the hydrotherapy program. The community-based team was effective in assisting Mrs. H. to achieve independence within the community.

Skeleton Case History

Age: 33
Gender: Male
Occupation: Hospital orderly
Onset: 4 years
Stage: Acute
Severity: Moderate
Adherence: Medium
Issues: Efficacy of medication, difficulty performing job

References

1. Helewa A, Bombardier C, Goldsmith CH et al: Cost effectiveness of inpatient and intensive outpatient treatment of rheumatoid arthritis. *Arthritis Rheum* 32:1505–1514, 1989.
2. Anderson RB, Needleman RD, Gatter RH et al: Patient outcome following inpatient vs outpatient treatment of rheumatoid arthritis. *J Rheumatol* 15:556–560, 1988.
3. Swezey RL: Rheumatoid arthritis: the role of the kinder and gentler therapies. *J Rheumatol* 17(suppl 25):8-13, 1990.
4. Katz S, Vignos PJ, Moskowitz W et al: Comprehensive outpatient care in rheumatoid arthritis: a controlled study. *JAMA* 206:1249–1254, 1968.
5. Helewa A, Goldsmith CH, Lee P et al: Effects of occupational therapy home service on patients with rheumatoid arthritis. *Lancet* 337:1453–1456, 1991.
6. Bell MJ, Lineker SC, Wulkins AL et al: A randomized controlled trial to evaluate the efficacy of community based physical therapy in the treatment of people with rheumatoid arthritis. *J Rheumatol* 25:231–237, 1998.
7. Lineker SC, Bell MJ, Wilkins A et al: Improvements following short term home based physical therapy are maintained at one year in people with moderate to severe rheumatoid arthritis. *J Rheumatol* 28:165–168, 2001.
8. Li LC, Coyte PC, Lineker SC, et al: Ambulatory care of home based treatment? An economic evaluation of two physiotherapy delivery options for people with rheumatoid arthritis. *Arthritis Care Res* 13:183–190, 2000.
9. Badley EM, Rothman LM: Determining suitability for home versus community based ambulatory therapy services for adults with arthritis. *Arthritis Care Res* 1:27–34, 1996.
10. Helewa A, Smyth HA, Goldsmith CH et al: The total assessment of rheumatoid polyarthritis—evaluation of a training program for physiotherapists and occupational therapists. *J Rheumatol* 14:87–92, 1987.
11. Lineker SC, Wood H, Badley EM et al: Evaluation of the primary therapist model of service delivery as implemented by The Arthritis Society, Consultation and Rehabilitation Service: phase I: therapist survey. Working Paper 98-5, Toronto, ON, Arthritis Community Research and Evaluation Unit, 1998.
12. The Arthritis Society: Internal report to The Arthritis Society. Ontario Division 1993, rev. 1996, unpublished.
13. Lineker SC, Wilkins A: A retrospective chart review of the CTS goal oriented recording system. Working Paper 95-5, Toronto, ON, Arthritis Community Research and Evaluation Unit, 1995.
14. *ICIDH-2: International Classification of Impairments, Activities and Participation. A Manual of Dimensions of Disablement and Health.* Beta-1 draft for field trials, Geneva, World Health Organization, 1997.
15. Minor MA, Westby MD: Rest and exercise. In Robbins L, Burckhardt CS, Hannan MT et al (eds): *Clinical Care in the Rheumatic Diseases,* ed 2. Atlanta, American College of Rheumatology, 2001.
16. Kirk JA, Kersley GC: Heat and cold in the physical treatment of rheumatoid arthritis of the knee: a controlled trial. *Ann Phys Med* 9:270–274, 1968.
17. Williams J, Harvey J, Tannenbaum H: Use of superficial heat versus ice for the rheumatoid arthritis shoulder: a pilot study. *Physiother Can* 38:8–13, 1986.
18. Oosterveld FGJ, Rasker JJ, Jacobs JWG et al: The effect of local heat and cold therapy on intraarticular and skin surface temperature of the knee. *Arthritis Rheum* 35:146–151, 1992.
19. Dellhag B, Wollersjo I, Bjelle A: Effect of active hand exercise and wax bath treatment in rheumatoid arthritis patients. *Arthritis Care Res* 5: 87–92, 1992.
20. Falconer J, Hayes KW, Chang RW: Therapeutic ultrasound in the treatment of musculoskeletal conditions. *Arthritis Care Res* 3:85–91, 1990.
21. Simmonds MJ, Kumar S: Pain and the placebo in rehabilitation using TENS and laser. *Disabil Rehabil* 16: 13–20, 1994.
22. Kumar VN, Redford JB: Transcutaneous nerve stimulation in rheumatoid arthritis. *Arch Phys Med Rehabil* 63:595–596, 1982.
23. Langley GB, Sheppeard H, Johnson M et al: The analgesic effects of transcutaneous electrical nerve stimulation and placebo in chronic pain patients: a double blind non-crossover comparison. *Rheumatol Int* 4:119–123, 1984.
24. Feinberg J, Brandt KD: Use of resting splints by patients with rheumatoid arthritis. *Am J Occup Ther* 35:555–561. 1981.
25. Gignac MAM: An evaluation of a psychotherapeutic group intervention for persons having difficulty coping with musculoskeletal disorders. *Social Work Health Care* 32:57–75, 2000.

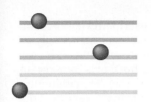

CHAPTER 17

Special Topics in Clinical Research and Health Status Instruments

Antoine Helewa, MSc(Clin Epid), PT

Overview

In this chapter special topics in arthritis research will be reviewed and some of the problems encountered in the design architecture and methodology in rehabilitation trials, systematic reviews, or meta-analyses will be exposed. Compared with research in the field of medicine, physical rehabilitation research in arthritis is still in its infancy, despite important advances made in the past decade. This is evident in the small number of well-designed scientific articles reported in print or electronic journals; the lack of rigor in design architecture of reported trials; and the methodological deficiencies revealed in systematic reviews and meta-analyses. These three issues are interrelated and can

only be resolved by massive investment in scientific manpower and research grants by governments at all levels as well as disease-specific not-for-profit organizations, such as the Arthritis Foundation in the United States, The Arthritis Society in Canada, The British Rheumatism Council in the United Kingdom, and similar organizations worldwide. Also, there is a need for greater commitment to science on the part of rehabilitation professional associations who continue to be preoccupied largely by professional issues to the detriment of the rehabilitation sciences.

Massive investment in the research and advertising of drugs by the pharmaceutical industry has created a critical imbalance in the minds of interested investigators who are attracted by easy access to research funds, contrary to the public's perceptions of clinical priorities. Tallon and associates,[1] in a recent article, showed a mismatch between the amount of published work on

PHYSICAL REHABILITATION IN ARTHRITIS, Joan M. Walker, PhD, PT, and Antoine Helewa, MSc(Clin Epid), PT, Elsevier Inc. © 2004.

different interventions and the degree of interest of consumers. A review of published and unpublished studies showed that the evidence base in osteoarthritis research is dominated by studies of pharmaceutical agents and surgical interventions by 59% and 26%, respectively. Only 6% of 930 studies related to physical therapy and exercise and a mere 3% to client education. Of the studies of pharmaceutical interventions, 89% were commercially funded compared with 2% of physical rehabilitation interventions. On the other hand, consumers chose first knee replacements (36%), followed by education and advice at 21%, as issues that are important to their well being.[1] Only 4% of consumers rated pharmaceutical agents as their first choice; 3% rated physical therapy first. The low rating of physical therapy, the only rehabilitation profession reviewed, may reflect consumers' poor understanding of the benefits of its interventions.

The second half of this chapter contains a review and critical appraisal of important health status instruments that are currently used in evaluating arthritis-related rehabilitation interventions. These must be distinguished from instruments used in clinical practice, where the thrust is to evaluate individual clients rather than group outcomes or patterns of disease. However, some clinical measures can be used to evaluate research strategies, but most of these have been addressed in Chapter 5, as well as in the management chapters of this text, and will not be included here.

Special Topics in Physical Rehabilitation Research

Senior clinicians and administrators often repeat a litany of criticisms when asked to participate or support research related to physical rehabilitation. Included among these are the following: interventions require long periods of observation to show any effects, which makes the research costly; the clinical effects tend to be borderline even when they show statistical significance; the interventions are difficult to mask; and outcome measures used in these trials have little relevance to clinical questions and are therefore difficult to interpret. Similar views were held in the past by surgeons, namely that surgical procedures are impossible to evaluate in randomized, clinical trials (RCTs). Fortunately, these criticisms are decreasing as researchers in the area have been able to address some of these difficulties in numerous clinical trials published in the past two decades. Nonetheless, some methodological problems remain, which will require greater attention by investigators when designing trials,

and by grant reviewers, manuscript reviewers, and those engaged in systematic reviews or meta-analyses when asked to approve such works.

To illustrate this point, authors of seven recent systematic reviews related to physical rehabilitation interventions in rheumatoid arthritis[2-8] reported the following inadequacies in research design and methods in some of the trials reviewed:

- Incomplete literature review
- Poor design architecture; few RCTs on specific interventions
- Poor description of baseline characteristics
- Inadequate masking of control or experimental interventions
- Inadequate descriptions of trial maneuvers
- Improper allocation of clients to treatment groups
- Absence of sample size estimates and small sample sizes
- Outcome measures that lacked accuracy and precision
- Lack of standardization in outcome measures and measurement periods
- Short duration of interventions
- Concurrent therapy resulting in confounding of variables
- Lack of accounting for dropouts and clients who entered and completed the trial
- Large number of missing values
- Lack of standardization of reported data
- Lack of intent-to-treat (effectiveness) analysis

These inadequacies, similar to those found in fields other than arthritis, often will lead to serious biases that can compromise the validity of study results and undermine the theoretical foundations of professional practice. The following topics address some of the concerns listed above that may be of assistance to investigators in the field:

- The research question
- Statement of hypotheses
- Rigor of research design
- Validity of the research
- Importance of study results
- Impact of results on clinical management

The Research Question

Early in the research enterprise the research question must be asked. It should have clinical relevance, be answerable, and be feasible. It should have the potential to have an impact on practice or contribute to theoretical foundations of practice. Because the research question is the focus of the research problem it should identify the sample of clients to be studied and the intervention that will be applied.[9] The variable that will measure the effects of the intervention on clients can be mentioned or left open-ended. In controlled trials, the control intervention, be it a placebo an active treatment or no treatment, need not be mentioned at this early stage. An example of a research question asked in a study may read as follows: "Are the outcomes of clients with ankylosing spondylitis improved at 4 months after they received 4 weeks of home physical therapy?"

Statement of Hypotheses

Two hypotheses are advanced. The first is the *null hypothesis* (H^0), or hypothesis of no difference. By referring to the research question above and using the Bath Ankylosing Spondylitis Functional Index (BASFI) as the primary outcome measure, H^0 can be stated as follows: "There will be no change in the BASFI at 4 months between the groups receiving home physical therapy and those not." The second is the *alternate hypothesis* (H^A). Using the example above H^A will read as follows: "There will be a change." H^0 is stated first to demonstrate no bias on the part of the investigator. If H^0 cannot be proven, then the investigator will accept H^A because evidence demonstrated that a change occurred. Unlike the above example an H^0 value can be unidirectional, whereby the word *'change'* is substituted for improvement or deterioration. These statements bind investigators to a predetermined path from which they may not deviate. Quite often statements of hypotheses are omitted from research protocols or in reporting results, making it difficult to determine where investigator bias lies.

Rigor of Research Design

There is a hierarchy of research design which places *randomized, clinical trials* at the top of a certainty scale (Table 17-1).[10] Because RCTs are more complex in design, cost more to carry out, and take longer to execute, they have been avoided by a majority of investigators who may be working on tight timelines, with ticking tenure clocks or considerations for promotion. Further, because investigators in physical rehabilitation do not have the same clout as their colleagues in medicine, they have not been as successful in garnering research grants large enough to carry out RCTs.

However, RCTs continue to be favored by research funding agencies, editors of high-impact journals, and reviewers of meta-analyses. Therefore, investigators who work on RCTs are better rewarded in the end than those who want to make an impression with high productivity and shorter timelines. In recent decades investigators in the rehabilitation sciences generally and especially those working industriously in arthritis research have increasingly shifted their sights to RCTs. This trend is more evident in research protocols and in scientific publications, and the consequence is enhancement of the credibility of rehabilitation research in arthritis. In the next decade, meta-analytic research will be reaping a more abundant harvest of RCTs, from which firmer conclusions may be drawn about evidence in the physical rehabilitation of clients with arthritis.

In the past, concern about inherent bias in *quasi-experimental and observational studies* has limited their use in comparing treatments. When results of observational studies were compared with results of

Table 17-1. The Certainty Scale, Levels of Evidence in Clinical Trials

Evidence	Level	Certainty Scale
Large randomized trials with low false-positive and low false-negative errors	I	↓
Small randomized trials with high false-positive and/or high false-negative errors	II	
Nonrandomized, concurrent cohort comparisons between contemporaneous subjects who did and did not receive the intervention	III	
Nonrandomized, historical cohort comparisons between current subjects who did receive the intervention and former subjects who did not	IV	
Case series without control subjects	V	

Adapted from Sackett D, Haynes RB, Tugwell P: *Clinical Epidemiology: A Basic Science for Clinical Medicine.* Boston, Little Brown, 1989 p2S. With permission.

RCTs using similar outcome measures and interventions, observational studies showed better treatment effects than RCTs. This difference was attributed to poor design, less intensive control of study methods, and a variety of other biases. Despite of their lower cost, longer timelines, and broader range of patients, the Cochrane Collaboration and other reviewers of meta-analyses have shunned observational studies.

Two recent systematic reviews of medical therapies challenged the current consensus about a hierarchy of research design in clinical research that places RCTs at the top of the certainty scale (Table 17-1).[11,12] Using similar methodologies, one study reviewed the results of observational studies with the results of RCTs on the same interventions and using similar outcome measures[11]; the other compared the results of meta-analyses of RCTs with those of meta-analyses of observational studies of the same interventions since 1984.[12] Both reviews reported that observational studies did not systematically overestimate the magnitude of the effects of treatment, compared with those in RCTs on the same topic. These results were attributed to improved design and research methods and better control of biases in observational studies since 1984. Unfortunately, these results do not yet apply to the field of physical rehabilitation, reported in current meta-analyses, in which observational studies continue to overestimate treatment effects compared to RCTs. Improvements in research methods of observational studies in this field may in the future yield results similar to those found recently in medical research.

Validity of the Research

A study is considered valid if the treatment effect reported represents the true direction and magnitude of the treatment effect. In other words, the results must represent an unbiased estimate of the treatment effect and not be affected by systematic errors that could lead to false conclusions.[13] In certain conditions, factors such as age, sex, and disease severity may confound study results, if these characteristics are not equally represented among clients in study or control groups. The following approaches may help reduce systematic errors and enhance the validity of study results.

Random Allocation

The true benefit of random allocation is derived from the assumption that both known and unknown client characteristics are evenly distributed between treatment or control groups. This creates groups of clients who at the start of the study have identical risks for the events that investigators are trying to prevent. The allocation method must be described in detail, such as tossing a coin or using a standard text listing of random numbers.[14] Allocation must be concealed from clinicians administering the experimental or control therapy, as well as from those who will be independently assessing study outcomes, a process often referred to as double masking or double blinding. Masking is critical because it will prevent clinicians or assessors from either consciously or unconsciously distorting the balance between the groups being compared.

Accounting for Clients

Ideally, the number of clients admitted to a study must match the number who completed the study, because lost clients could have events that may change study conclusions. Acceptable losses should be in the 5% to 10% range and should be included in the analysis by assigning worst-case scenario values to losses in the group that improved and best-case scenario values to losses in the group that deteriorated.[14] After random allocation, clients should be analyzed in the group to which they have been assigned, even if they accidentally received the wrong treatment or did not fully adhere to the prescribed intervention. This form of analysis is referred to as an *intent-to-treat* or *effectiveness analysis*. Excluding clients who did not complete the trial from the analysis (often referred to as *efficacy analysis*) may result in an imbalance in numbers between treatment groups and no consideration of clients who potentially have favorable outcomes. This reduces the benefit of randomization and will distort study results.

Similarity of Groups at Baseline

Clients admitted to a trial should have similar known characteristics that are measurable at baseline. These usually include age, gender, disease severity, height, weight, laboratory findings, and so on. A table displaying baseline characteristics, accompanied by an analysis comparing these characteristics, is usually shown at the start of the results section of an article. Random allocation provides a measure of reassurance that known and unknown characteristics are well balanced 1 time out of 20, provided the sample size is adequate. Large differences in baseline characteristics could compromise the validity of a study. An additional strategy to ensure comparability of groups is to stratify clients before randomization into prognostic factors that may influence results.[13] These prognostic factors could be one or more characteristic, such as disease severity, age, or sex. After stratification, clients then are allocated to different groups within strata, thus ensuring that at the very least, certain important characteristics are in balance among the groups. For example, in rheumatoid arthritis (RA), the prognosis of clients with severe disease is worse than that of those with mild disease, and men tend to have more severe disease than women. Therefore, stratification before randomization for severity levels and gender will ensure that those characteristics are in balance between the groups.

Equal Assignment to Therapy

Aside from the experimental therapy, clients within treatment groups should be treated equally. It is tempting to provide more time and attention to clients in the experimental group, if clinicians providing the interventions are not masked to treatment groups, as in single-masked trials. This is especially critical in rehabilitation research when the application of placebo therapy is sometimes impossible. In addition, clinicians administering the therapy may be tempted to provide additional interventions consciously or unconsciously to one group or another depending on the direction of their bias. Thus, equal time and attention should be assigned to treatment groups. Additionally, if other therapy is required, such as anti-inflammatory therapy for clients receiving different rehabilitation interventions, these must be applied in the same manner to the different treatment groups.

> There are few ways to do a study properly and a thousand ways to do a study badly!

Importance of Study Results

In reviewing or reporting on an article on therapy, first determine how large the treatment effect was, then if large enough, how important it is to your practice. These effects are measured in terms of their statistical significance, clinical importance, or relative risk reduction.[14]

Statistical significance merely tells whether a difference is likely to be real not whether it is important or large. It is a statement of the likelihood that this difference may or may not be due to chance alone. An arbitrary level of probability of less than 5% (usually expressed as $P < .05$) is often used, indicating that the probability of this difference being real (or due to chance alone) is less than 5%.

Clinical importance refers to the importance of a difference in clinical outcomes between experimental and control groups and usually is described in terms of the magnitude of the results. In other words, is the

difference important to clinicians and would it lead to clinicians abandoning an old treatment for a new one? If study results are shown to be statistically significant and clinically important, then the results are important enough to incorporate the new treatment in one's practice.

Relative risk reduction (RRR) refers to the risk of occurrence of unwanted events among subjects receiving the experimental treatment relative to control subjects. It is commonly expressed in percentages. An RRR of 60% means that the prevention strategy reduced the risk of unwanted events in experimental subjects by 60%, relative to control subjects. RRR is not a precise estimate of true treatment effects; rather it is a point estimate. This means that the true value lies in the neighborhood usually expressed as a confidence interval (CI).

The preceding paragraphs give a cursory description of statistical methods that help in determining the magnitude of treatment effects. The reader should consult statistical or research methodology texts to obtain a good grasp of these issues.

Impact of Results on Client Management

Study inclusion and exclusion criteria define the population studied. If a client meets the criteria of a particular study, then the results would apply to him or her. If a client does not meet the criteria, a clinician must find a compelling reason why the results should or could apply.[13]

Also, a clinician must be satisfied about the following:

- The experimental therapy is described in sufficient detail to allow replication with precision.
- The therapy was clinically and biologically sensible.
- The therapy is available.
- The investigators were aware of the possibility of co-intervention (providing other therapies that could distort the results) or contamination of the maneuver (whether control clients consciously or unconsciously received the experimental therapy).

For example, in a study of occupational therapy (OT) management of clients with RA, if all the clients received OT as well as physical therapy (PT), it would be difficult to attribute the benefits to OT alone.

Also, if some of the clients in one group received PT or if some of the clients were randomly assigned to the wrong group, this could lead to contamination of the experimental maneuver, because PT in RA could provide benefits similar to those of OT.

The primary outcome measure used in a study must be specific to the diagnosis or condition studied, the research question asked, and the experimental intervention under investigation. For example, a depression scale will not measure the impact of joint protection techniques, measures of inflammation will not measure the impact of therapeutic exercise, and an erythrocyte sedimentation rate will not measure the severity of fibromyalgia.

Lastly, the treatment benefits shown must be worth the potential harm due to side effects of the therapy, and the costs must be reasonable and within the ability of the client or third-party coverage to bear.

In summary, there are few ways to do a study properly and thousands of ways to do it wrong. In physical rehabilitation of clients with arthritis more studies are needed that address the concerns reviewed above, so that accumulating evidence can be reviewed systematically and metanalytic statistical techniques can be used.

Health Status Instruments

Chronic rheumatic diseases can affect several aspects of a client's life. Functional disability may exist, psychological stress may increase, and socio-economic losses may result.[15] As mentioned in the management chapters of this text, these effects can be assessed by using measures that focus on a specific clinical aspect of a client's status, such as muscle strength or active joint counts, or focus on multidimensional measures that may assess a number of aspects simultaneously.[15] The focus of this section will be on health status instruments (HSI). These instruments have certain properties: they target a client's functional, psychological or socio-economic status, and generally have taken the form of self-administered or interviewer-administered questionnaires. Therefore, they rely on clients' impressions, rather than on professional observations.[15]

HSIs have the following characteristics and differ from one another in some aspects of client status:

- They all address items related to functional ability.
- Most contain items related to work and social status.
- The rest cover dimensions related to sleep, satisfaction with care received, health costs, or side effects of therapy.

Some of their *advantages* include the following: (1) they provide a broad and fairly comprehensive assessment of client status using one instrument;

(2) they are easy and inexpensive to use because they do not consume a health professional's time; and (3) they can be as precise and accurate as traditional clinical measures.[13] They also can be disease specific, intervention specific and research question specific. Some of their *disadvantages* are the following: (1) they provide breadth at the cost of depth, e.g., not enough detail on hand function to assess the effects of hand rehabilitation; (2) they cannot be used to generate a single composite measure of client status, because the components are dissimilar and valued differently by different clients; and (3) their scoring and content are not generally familiar to practicing clinicians and, therefore, their current usefulness to clinicians can be limited.

Factors to Consider in Choosing an Instrument

Before reviewing some of the instruments commonly used in rheumatology, we should ask, "What factors should be considered to help us determine whether an instrument is *precise* and *accurate*?"

Precision

A measurement is said to be precise when it has the same value each time it is measured. Precision and its related concepts of reliability and consistency are affected by random error. The greater the error, the less precise is the instrument. There are four interacting sources of random error: observer variability, subject variability, instrument variability, and variability due to the test environment.[9] Precision of an instrument has a very important influence on the power of a study; the more precise the instrument is, the greater is its statistical power at a given sample size to estimate mean values and to test hypotheses.[16]

Factors that contribute to instrument precision are (1) standardization of measurement methods, (2) training and certification of observers, (3) refinement of the instrument, and (4) accounting for variability due to order of measurement.

Accuracy

A measurement is said to be accurate if it actually represents what it is intended to represent and when its inherent systematic error is minimal. As with precision, the same sources of systematic error apply here, namely, contribution of bias due to observer, subject, instrument, and the environment.[9] Factors that contribute to instrument accuracy are (1) prediction of an outcome of interest (*predictive validity*), (2) agreement with other approaches for measuring the same characteristic (*convergent validity*), and (3) intuitive sense of the instrument (*face validity*).

As well as precision and accuracy, other factors to consider in choosing an instrument are the following:

- Sensitivity to different characteristics of the object being measured: In other words, does it pick up differences where differences are known to exist?
- Responsiveness: Does it measure change in health status when real change has occurred?
- Specificity for the characteristic being measured
- Safety or causing no harm to the subject under observation
- Reasonable cost of application
- Minimal time to apply: Inordinately lengthy measurements can affect cost, fatigue of the subject, and safety of application.

Three types of health status instruments will be reviewed below: a health related quality of life instrument, general arthritis instruments, and condition-specific instruments. All these instruments have been tested extensively for accuracy and precision; they are also sensitive, responsive, specific to the characteristic measured, safe, and cost little to apply. (Appendix II provides a sample of each of these instruments.)

Health-Related Quality-of-Life Instruments

Health-related quality-of-life instruments (HRQOLs) are multidimensional instruments that probe quality of life in broad terms and allow comparative analyses between very diverse conditions, such as arthritis and cardiovascular disease.[17] HRQOL instruments are, in general, less responsive than arthritis-specific instruments, but capture elements of health beyond the scope of the latter. For this reason they are often used with arthritis-specific instruments in research studies as secondary outcome measures.[17]

The SF-36

This HRQOL instrument is the one most commonly used in arthritis-related research. The acronym stands for the Medical Outcomes Study (MOS) 36-Item Short Form Health Survey.[18] The SF-36 is a 36-question multidimensional instrument that measures general quality of life over the last month or week and has been tested extensively for precision and accuracy in a variety of populations and disease groups. Normative data are available for the United States and several European countries.[18,19] It takes 5 to 10 minutes to complete, is scored quickly, and has been paired with disease-specific instruments in clinical investigations. It measures three major health attributes (functional status, well-being, and overall health status), and eight health concepts:

- Limitations of physical activities because of health problems
- Limitations in social activities because of emotional or physical problems
- Limitations in usual role activities because of physical health problems
- Bodily pain
- General mental health
- Limitations in usual role activities because of emotional problems
- Vitality
- General health problems.

It can be administered by a trained interviewer in person, by telephone or computer.

General Arthritis Instruments

Two instruments will be reviewed: the Arthritis Impact Measurement Scale (AIMS)[20] and the Health Assessment Questionnaire (HAQ).[21] These two instruments were originally designed to probe general issues encountered by clients with arthritis; however, they also have been used extensively in specific conditions.

The AIMS

This widely used instrument has been extensively validated in different clinical settings and translated into several languages. The instrument was revised and expanded by Meenan and colleagues in 1992[20] as AIMS 2, the version in current use. It is a self-administered, multidimensional index using 42 items to probe 9 separate dimensions: mobility, physical activity, dexterity, social role, social activity, activities of daily living (ADL), pain, depression, and anxiety. It includes three subscales related to arm function, ability to work, and support from family and friends (see Appendix II). Clients also are asked about satisfaction with current level of function, impact of arthritis on health status, and prioritization of three areas in which clients would like to see improvement. The dimensions are arranged in a Guttman scale order, so that clients who fail for an item also tend to fail for all lower items in that dimension. Items are scored on a 5-point adjectival scale that varies from item to item. The instrument takes more than 20 minutes to complete, limiting its use to research studies.

The Health Assessment Questionnaire

This instrument in its original form is 20 pages long and deals with costs, side effects of medications, utilization of services, and functional capacity. The version that is in common use and that has been extensively tested, is the *short, 2-page functional disability scale.* This scale is extracted from the long version and consists of 24 questions. Eight dimensions of function are assessed, all related to ADL: dressing and grooming, arising, eating, walking, hygiene, reach, grip, and mobility and work in the home and outside. It also includes questions related to use of aids and help from others, as well as a visual analogue pain scale. Items are scored on a 4-point adjectival scale: performing an activity "without any difficulty" scored as 0 to "unable to do" scored as 3 (see Appendix II). Several condition-specific versions, such as the RA-HAQ, a new short, modified version, the MHAQ, and a difficult 8-item DHAQ version, have been developed and were recently reviewed by Wolfe.[22] He concluded that the original functional disability scale, the HAQ, performed better than the other versions for detecting treatment change (responsiveness) and for identifying the extent of the functional disability.

Condition-Specific Instruments

There are four condition-specific instruments in common use: the Bath Ankylosing Spondylitis Functional Index (BASFI),[23] the Fibromyalgia Impact Questionnaire (FIQ),[24] the McMaster Toronto Arthritis Patient Preference Disability Questionnaire (MACTAR),[25] and the Western Ontario and McMaster Universities Osteoarthritis Index (WOMAC).[26] All four instruments have been tested in numerous studies for their precision, accuracy, and responsiveness.

The Bath Ankylosing Spondylitis Functional Index

This unidimensional instrument is 1 page long and comprises 10 questions to which the response is marked on a 10-cm visual analogue scale (VAS) from "easy" to "impossible." The VAS enhances responsiveness in that each item has a potential 101 responses (i.e., one response to each millimeter of the 0- to 100-mm scale). Respondents are asked to indicate their level of ability within the last week. The categories are specific to functional problems encountered by clients with spondyloarthropathies and include activities such as putting on socks, picking up objects, reaching above the head, getting up from sitting, and so on (see Appendix II). A recent review of 27 clinical trials using the BASFI and the Dougados Functional Index (DFI)[27] (another spondyloarthropathy-specific instrument) showed that both are valid and reliable measures of functional ability in clients with ankylosing spondylitis; however, in physical therapy trials responsiveness was better with the BASFI than with the DFI.[28]

The Fibromyalgia Impact Questionnaire

This is a short, 1-page, 10-item instrument designed specifically to assess the impact of fibromyalgia on clients.[24] The first item is subdivided into 10 subitems dealing with functional abilities; the remaining items probe several dimensions, which include general well-being, ability to work, pain, fatigue, sleep, stiffness, and anxiety and depression. Scoring of dimensions varies considerably. For functional abilities a 4-point adjectival scale is used: "always" is scored as 0 and "never" is scored as 4. For items 2 and 3, a numeric scale is used. For the remainder a VAS is used, with each line describing a different state, e.g., "no problem" at one end of item 4 to "great difficulty" at the other end and "no tiredness" at one end of item 6 to "very tired" at the other end and so on (see Appendix II). Subjects are able to choose not to answer questions that do not apply to them and to leave unanswered certain dimensions that do apply or are most difficult. This approach leads to underestimation in scoring certain functional abilities, thereby distorting comparisons among groups.[29]

The McMaster Toronto Arthritis Patient Preference Disability Questionnaire

This measurement used chiefly in RA is administered by a trained interviewer and employs an approach based on the selection of disability signals by individual clients.[25] The index quantifies the specific functional priorities of each client, which are identified by open-ended questioning at the time of the initial assessment. Specifically, clients are asked to describe limitations in functional abilities, work, leisure, social roles, and sexuality and then to rank the importance of performing these activities without pain (see Appendix II). Using a detailed protocol, the interviewer probes for answers. As may be expected the cost of administration is high compared with that for other instruments. However, this innovative approach to measurement continues to attract attention and has been shown to be valid and responsive in clinical trials.[30]

The Western Ontario and McMaster Universities Osteoarthritis Index

This instrument is self-administered and is specially designed to measure dimensions particularly relevant to osteoarthritis of the hip or knee joints.[26] It is tridimensional, measuring pain, stiffness, and physical disability using either the Likert scale or the VAS (see Appendix II). The clinometric (clinical measurement) properties of the WOMAC have been shown to be accurate, precise, and responsive.[31] It is used worldwide and has been translated into more than 10 languages. Its brevity (about 10 minutes) and simple scoring make it attractive for use in a clinical setting.

Other Condition-Specific Instruments

A number of other condition-specific instruments have been developed for systemic lupus erythematosus,[32] fatigue,[33] coping,[34] and helplessness[35]; however, they tend to be too exotic and complex and are rarely used in the field of physical rehabilitation. Several juvenile idiopathic arthritis instruments have been developed but have not been well tested for accuracy and precision. These are well reviewed in Chapter 8 for interested readers.

Discussion

Over the past three decades, research activities and the development of health status instruments in physical rehabilitation have expanded. Although many obstacles encountered in early studies recently have been overcome, much remains to be achieved. Three areas deserve special attention: acceleration and enhancement of well-designed clinical trials, multicenter collaboration in research, and further refinement in health assessment instruments and quantitative clinical measures.

> Quality research demands enhancement of collaboration between clinicians and academic-based clinical scientists.

Early in this chapter, I showed that the state of the art in rehabilitation research was deficient. Well-designed clinical trials appear to be the exception rather than the rule, funding is scarce, and competition for limited funds is fierce. This bleak assessment is improving as more clinical scientists, individuals who are competitive and well trained, are coming into the field. This new generation of clinical scientists will be able to carry the torch further than has been possible to date. To accelerate this process, national and international collaboration in clinical trials is needed. A multicenter trial approach as proposed here will increase the number of well-designed trials required to answer important clinical questions and help globalize research in physical rehabilitation. One of the critical problems in clinical research is finding clients who meet study criteria and none of the exclusions. A multicenter trial approach is sometimes the only route to overcome this problem, especially in research related to rare conditions. Not all studies have to be an RCT in design. In fact, some research questions cannot be addressed in an RCT design. Further, it has been shown earlier in this chapter that well-designed observational studies can be as valid as RCTs.[11,12]

In the past decade, the practice environment in physical rehabilitation has shifted from hospital-based services to private clinics and other community-based services. These services in many instances have been privatized, and billing is made to third-party payers. Although privatization creates its own incentives for efficiency and cost containment, there is a risk that services become volume driven. The impact of these trends on research activities in this field has not been determined. Cooperation between clinicians and university-based clinical scientists must be enhanced, or the whole research enterprise may flounder. The former should be asking the research questions and applying the treatment maneuvers on clients in their practices, and the latter should be seeking funding, designing the study and its methods, and evaluating its results. Both groups should not shy away from the effort because the cost of the whole enterprise can be supported by successful research applications, including the cost of research assistants, statisticians, and clinical personnel. Clinicians, clients, and scientists only can be enriched by these collaborations.

As research results on the efficacy of therapy are published in scientific journals, transfer of this new knowledge to clients and clinicians is imperative. Mechanisms should be established for this knowledge transfer, which can be disseminated by professional journals, associations, or other forums, such as focus groups or as treatment guidelines, thereby setting new standards of evidence-based practice.

The field of rehabilitation desperately needs one or two electronic journals to disseminate information expeditiously. It takes a minimum of 6 months for existing print journals to publish an article. On the other hand, electronic journals can have a turnaround time of 2 to 4 weeks, and editors of these journals are not as concerned about costs and, therefore, are not hounding authors to reduce the amount of material submitted (in itself, this may demand a higher standard of critical reading by clinicians!). Electronic publishing will finally yield a rich harvest of clinical trials and will help feed data to systematic reviews and meta-analyses. Whereas some reviews to date have shown no beneficial treatment effects for certain interventions or only borderline results, as more trials addressing similar questions are added to these reviews, thereby expanding the sample size, clinically important effects might emerge.

Although a number of health assessment instruments are available for use in clinical trials, most have not been designed with physical rehabilitation in mind. There is an urgent need to develop more condition-specific and intervention-specific measures that could demonstrate the efficacy of rehabilitation interventions. The same mantra could be repeated for quantitative clinical outcome measures. Although the availability of clinical measures has improved, unfortunately their reception and usage by the majority of clinicians remain lukewarm.

Summary

In this chapter, I reviewed and discussed special topics in arthritis research as they pertain to the field of physical rehabilitation and reviewed and described health assessment instruments in common use. The selected research topics were derived from critiques embedded in published systemic reviews of research studies reviewed by these authors.[2-8] It is interesting to note that these systematic reviews did not include any meta-analytic statistics, because each review contained only a small number of studies that met the review criteria, and the research questions, primary outcomes used, treatment methods investigated, and treatment dosages were not homogeneous. This observation is a clear indication that more and better research must be done using outcomes that are compatible with the research question asked and that are precise and accurate.

The outcome measures, in the form of health assessment instruments, reviewed can be recommended for use in future trials because their precision, accuracy, and responsiveness have been established. However, more work is needed on these instruments, and others need be developed that are more specific to the field of physical rehabilitation.

References

1. Tallon D, Chard J, Dieppe P: Relation between agendas of the research community and the research consumer. *Lancet* 355:2037–2040, 2000.
2. Robinson V, Brosseau L, Casimiro L et al: Thermotherapy for treating rheumatoid arthritis (Cochrane Review). The Cochrane Library, Issue 3, Oxford, Update Software, 2002.
3. Steultjens EMJ, Dekker J, Bouter LM et al: Occupational therapy for rheumatoid arthritis: a systematic review. *Arthritis Care Res* 47:672–685, 2002.
4. Casimiro L, Brosseau L, Robinson V et al: Therapeutic ultrasound for the treatment of rheumatoid arthritis (Cochrane Review). The Cochrane Library, Issue 3, Oxford, Update Software, 2002.
5. Casimiro L, Brosseau L, Milne S et al: Acupuncture and electroacupuncture for the treatment of RA (Cochrane Review). The Cochrane Library, Issue 3, Oxford, Update Software, 2002.
6. Pelland L, Brosseau L, Casimiro L et al: Electrical stimulation for the treatment of rheumatoid arthritis (Cochrane Review). The Cochrane Library, Issue 3, Oxford, Update Software, 2002.
7. Brosseau L, Welch V, Wells G et al: Low level laser therapy (classes I, II and III) for treating rheumatoid arthritis (Cochrane Review). The Cochrane Library, Issue 3, Oxford, Update Software, 2002.
8. Verhagen AP, de Vet HCW, de Bie RA et al: Balneotherapy for rheumatoid arthritis and osteoarthritis (Cochrane Review). The Cochrane Library, Issue 3, Oxford, Update Software, 2002.
9. Helewa A, Walker JM: *Critical Evaluation of Research in Physical Rehabilitation*. Philadelphia, WB Saunders, 2000.
10. Sackett DL, Haynes RB, Tugwell P: *Clinical Epidemiology: A Basic Science for Clinical Medicine*. Boston, Little, Brown, 1989.
11. Kjell B, Hartz AJ: A comparison of observational studies and randomized controlled trials. *N Engl J Med* 342:1878–1886, 2000.
12. Concato J, Nirav S, Horwitz RI: Randomized, controlled trials, observational studies, and the hierarchy of research designs. *N Engl J Med* 342:1887–1892, 2000.
13. Guyatt GH, Sackett DL, Cook DJ: Users guide to the medical literature. II. How to use an article about therapy and prevention. Are the results of the study valid? *JAMA* 270:2598–2601, 1993.
14. Sackett DL, Richardson WS, Rosenberg W, Haynes RB: *Evidence-Based Medicine: How to Practice and Teach EBM*. New York, Churchill Livingstone, 1997.
15. *Dictionary of the Rheumatic Diseases*, vol III. *Health Status Measurements*, Atlanta, American College of Rheumatology, Contact Associates International, 1998.
16. Hulley SB, Cummings SR: *Designing Clinical Research. An Epidemiologic Approach*. Baltimore, Williams & Wilkins, 1988.
17. Bellamy N: Evaluation of the Patient: B. Health Assessment Questionnaires. In Klippel JH (ed): *Primer on the Rheumatic Diseases*, ed 12. Atlanta, Arthritis Foundation, 2001.
18. Ware JE, Sherbourne CD: The MOS 36-Item Short Form Health Survey (SF-36). I. Conceptual frame-work and item selection. *Med Care* 30:473–483, 1992.
19. Scott A, Garrod T: Quality of life measures: use and abuse. *Baillieres Best Pract Res Clin Rheumatol* 14:663–687, 2000.
20. Meenan RF, Mason JH, Anderson JJ et al: AIMS 2: the content and properties of a revised and expanded Arthritis Impact Measurement Scales health status questionnaire. *Arthritis Rheum* 35:1–10, 1992.

21. Fries JF, Spitz P, Kraines RG et al: Measurement of patient outcome in arthritis. *Arthritis Rheum* 23:137–145, 1980.

22. Wolfe F: Which HAQ is best? A comparison of the HAQ, MHAQ and RA-HAQ, a difficult 8-item HAQ (DHAQ), and a rescored 20 item HAQ (HAQ 20): analyses in 2491 rheumatoid arthritis patients following leflunomide initiation. *J Rheumatol* 28:982–989, 2001.

23. Calin A, Garrett S, Whitelock H et al: A new approach to defining functional ability in ankylosing spondylitis: the development of the Bath Ankylosing Spondylitis Functional Index. *J Rheumatol* 21:2181–2185, 1994.

24. Burckhardt CS, Clark SR, Bennett RM: The Fibromyalgia Impact Questionnaire: development and validation. *J Rheumatol* 18:728–733, 1991.

25. Tugwell P, Bombardier C, Buchanan WW et al: The MACTAR Patient Preference Disability Questionnaire—an individualized functional priority approach for assessing improvement in physical disability in clinical trials in rheumatoid arthritis. *J Rheumatol* 14:446–451, 1987.

26. Bellamy N, Buchanan WW, Goldsmith CH et al: Validation study of WOMAC: a health status instrument for measuring clinically important patient relevant outcomes to anti-rheumatic drug therapy in patients with osteoarthritis of the hip or knee. *J Rheumatol* 15:1833–1840, 1988.

27. Dougados M, Gueguen A, Nakache JP et al: Evaluation of a functional index and an articular index in ankylosing spondylitis. *J Rheumatol* 15:302–307, 1988.

28. Ruof G, Stucki G: Comparison of the Dougados Functional Index and the Bath Ankylosing Spondylitis Functional Index: a literature review. *J Rheumatol* 26:955–960, 1999.

29. Wolfe F, Hawley DJ, Goldenberg DL et al: The assessment of functional impairment in fibromyalgia (FM): Rasche analysis of 5 functional scales and the development of the FM Health Assessment Questionnaire. *J Rheumatol* 27:1989–1999, 2000.

30. Verhoeven AC, Boers M, van der Linden S: Validity of the MACTAR questionnaire as a functional index in a rheumatoid arthritis clinical trial. *J Rheumatol* 27:2801–2809, 2000.

31. Bellamy N: WOMAC: a 20 year experiential review of a patient-centered self-reported health status questionnaire. *J Rheumatol* 29:2473–2476, 2002.

32. Bombardier C, Gladman DD, Urowitz MB et al: Derivation of the SLEDAI: a disease activity index for lupus patients. The Committee on Prognosis Studies in SLE. *Arthritis Rheum* 35:630–640, 1992.

33. Belza BL, Henke CJ, Yelin EH et al: Correlates of fatigue in older adults with rheumatoid arthritis. *Nurs Res* 42:93–99, 1993.

34. van Lankveld W, van't Pad Bosch P, van de Putte L et al: Disease-specific stressors in rheumatoid arthritis: coping and well-being. *Br J Rheumatol* 33:1067–1073, 1994.

35. Stein MJ, Wallston KA, Nicassio PM: Factor structure of the Arthritis Helplessness Index. *J Rheumatol* 15:427–432, 1988.

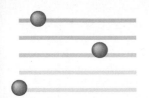

APPENDIX I

Resources

Educational Materials

A. For Children

The following fun workbooks can help children understand.

1. Falco JL, Block DV, Vostrejs MD et al: *JRA and Me—A Fun Workbook*. Atlanta, Rocky Mountain Juvenile Arthritis Center, Arthritis Foundation, 1987. Approximately $7.00 US.
   For school-aged children, this workbook contains puzzles, games, worksheets
2. *Coloring Books and Interactive Games*. Houston, Texas Children's Hospital; www2.texaschildrens hospital.org.
3. Kids on the Block, Inc.; www.kotb.com/kob2.htg/ arth.htm. Programs in the United States, Canada, Hong Kong, and New Zealand. In the United States >30 topics are in 700 communities; sites have children's pages.
   Educational puppet programs are designed to inform children about experiences of having a medical illness or disability, as well as, programs on social-safety issues.
4. The Arthritis Foundation: *Decision Making for Teenagers with Arthritis*. Free; available through the www.arthritis.org store web site.
5. Arthritis Insight/JRA World. PO Box 441571, Indianapolis, IN 46244.; http://jraworld.arthritis insight.com/about/contact.html.
   Nonmedical web site that allows children with arthritis to write in and share stories and ideas about their disease; also includes the monthly Junior Warrior Award for a child with JRA.

PHYSICAL REHABILITATION IN ARTHRITIS, Joan M. Walker, PhD, PT, and Antoine Helewa, MSc(Clin Epid), PT, Elsevier Inc. © 2004.

6. Ability OnLine Support Network. 104 1120 Finch Avenue West, Toronto, ON, Canada M3J 3H7; www.abilityonline.org.
   A computer friendship organization that connects kids with special needs, providing friendship and support.

B. For Parents and Teachers

1. Aldape VT: *Nicole's Story: A Book about a Girl with Juvenile Rheumatoid Arthritis*. Lerner Publications Company, Minneapolis, 1996. $21.27 US. Available through Amazon.com.
2. Barrett Singer AT: *Coping with Your Child's Chronic Illness*. San Francisco, Robert D. Reed Publishers, 1999. Available through http://www.arthritis.ca/ programs%20and%20resources/book%20store/ju venile%20arthritis/.
3. Bloorview MacMillan Children's Centre: *Kids Get Arthritis Too!* Toronto, ON, Bloorview MacMillan Children's Centre (416-425-6220, ask for the Arthritis Program), 1996.
4. Huegel K: *Young People and Chronic Illness*. Minneapolis, Free Spirit Publishing, 1998.
5. Parson N. *Working with Your School and Educational Rights*. Presented at the 1997 American Juvenile Arthritis Organization Regional Conference, Pennsylvania, Mount Laurel Resort, August 27, 1997; www.arthritis.org/resources/ classroom.asp.
6. The Arthritis Foundation: *Raising a Child with Arthritis: A Parent's Guide*. Atlanta, Arthritis Foundation, 2000. $14.95 US. Available through the www.arthritis.org store web site.
7. The Arthritis Foundation: *Arthritis in Children*. Atlanta, Arthritis Foundation, 2000. Free. Available through the www.arthritis.org store web site.
8. The Arthritis Foundation: *When Your Student Has Arthritis*. Atlanta, Arthritis Foundation, 2000,

28 pages. Free. Available through the www.arthritis.orgstore web site.

9. The Arthritis Foundation: *Decision Making for Teenagers with Arthritis*. Atlanta, Arthritis Foundation, 2000. Free. Available through the www.arthritis.org store web site.

10. Tucker L, DeNardo B, Stebulis J et al: *Your Child with Arthritis: A Family Guide For Caregiving*. Baltimore, John Hopkins University Press, 1996. $15.00 US. Available through Amazon.com.

C. For Health Professionals on Juvenile Arthritis

1. Exercise videotape for young children: *Shake, Rattle and Roar*. $12 plus shipping and handling. Available through the www.arthritis.org store web site.

2. Exercise videotape for school-aged children: *Where Are the Indians?* A videotape by the Physical Therapy Department of Texas Scottish Rite Hospital. $7 US. Available by writing to Deanna Carman, Physical Therapy Department, Texas Scottish Rite Hospital for Children, 2222 Welborn, Dallas, TX 75219.

D. For Adults

1. Aladjem H: *Understanding Lupus*. New York, Macmillan Publishing, 1985.
   "Extremely comprehensive and authoritative; some information only relevant to Americans… possibly of more interest to health professionals."—Arthritis Foundation.

2. Arthritis Foundation: *Change Your Life! Simple Strategies to Lose Weight, Get Fit and Improve Your Outlook*. Atlanta, Arthritis Foundation, 2002.

3. Arthritis Foundation: The Arthritis Foundation's Tips for Good Living with Arthritis. Atlanta, Arthritis Foundation, 2001.

4. Blau S, Schultz D: *Lupus: The Body Against Itself*. New York, Doubleday, 1984.
   "Well written and informed."—Arthritis Foundation.

5. Ediger B: *Coping with Fibromyalgia*. Toronto, ON, FM Facts, 1991.
   Generally clear and useful.

6. Eriendssonit J: *Car Driving with Ankylosing Spondylitis*. East Sussex, UK, The Ankylosing Spondylitis International Federation & National Ankylosing Spondylitis Society, 1998.

7. Fries JF: *Arthritis: A Comprehensive Guide to Understanding Your Arthritis*. Don Mills, ON, Addison-Wesley, 1986.

Factual information for readers with average education.

8. Horstman J: The supplement guide: Get smart about the herbs, vitamins and other remedies you take. *Arthritis Today* July/August:33-49, 2001.

9. Klippel JH (ed): *Primer on Rheumatic Diseases*, Appendix 4, *Supplementary Guide*, ed 12. Atlanta, Arthritis Foundation, 2001.
   Lists dietary supplements commonly used by people with arthritis, with review of their safety and efficacy.

10. Lorig K, Fries JF: *The Arthritis Helpbook*. Don Mills, ON, Addison-Wesley, 1990.
    Text used in arthritis self-management programs offered in the United States, Australia, New Zealand, and Canada. Six-week program with sessions 2 hours a week, taught in classes of 10 to 14 people. Sessions are led by trained volunteers. This text teaches individuals to become arthritis self-managers.

11. Missouri Arthritis Rehabilitation Research & Training Center, Information Dissemination Project: Series of brochures on gardening, ergonomics, workplace accommodation, etc., for persons with arthritis. Available from MARRTC, 13 Walkter Williams, Columbia, MO 65211; fax: 573-884-3437; MARRTC@missouri.edu.

12. Phillips RH: *Coping with Rheumatoid Arthritis*. New York, Avery Publishing Group, 1988.
    General reading, comprehensive.

13. Pitzele SK: *We Are Not Alone: Learning to Live with Chronic Illness*. New York, Workman Publishing, 1986.
    "Written by a lupus sufferer…comprehensive and inspirational."—Arthritis Foundation.

14. Sobel D: *Arthritis: What Works*. New York, St. Martin's Press, 1991.
    Based on a survey not true research.

Exercise

1. ARRTC: *Good Moves for Everybody* ($30 US ppd); *Good Moves II* (for beginners, $25 US), exercise videotapes, Missouri Arthritis Rehabilitation Research & Training Center, Columbia, University of Missouri. Order from The Health Connection, 601 Business Loop 70W, Ste. 219 Parkade Center, Columbia, MO 65201.

2. Arthritis Foundation: *PACE I and PACE II*, exercise videotapes, Atlanta, Arthritis Foundation.

3. Arthritis Foundation: *Walk with Ease*, 2002 (text); *Walk with Ease*, 2003 (audiotape). Atlanta, Arthritis Foundation.

4. Arthritis Foundation: *Pool Exercise Program (PEP)*, exercise video, $33.95 US ppd. Order from Cox Entertainment, PO Box 23451, Pleasant Hill, CA 94523.

5. Arthritis Foundation: *Arthritis Self-Management Course.*
   Contact your local Arthritis Foundation or Society Chapter office for local programs and training opportunities.

6. Arthritis Society/Foundation: Recreational exercise programs and aquatics programs (AFYAP/AFAP and Plus).

7. Ellert G: *Arthritis and Exercise: A User's Guide to Fitness and Independence.* Vancouver, BC, 1985, Trelle Enterprises.

8. Erson T: *Courageous Pacers—The Complete Guide to Running, Walking and Fitness for Kids.* Corpus Christi, TX, Pro-Activ Publications, 1993.

9. Francis L, Francis P: *A Pre-Aerobic Exercise Program.* San Diego State University, supported by Reebok International, Avon, MA.

10. Francis PR, Francis L: *If it Hurts Don't Do It: Tune Up Your Body for Pain-Free, Injury Free Life Long Fitness.* Rocklin, CA, Prima Publishing and Communications, 1988, 161 pp.

11. Gairdner J: *Fitness for People with Rheumatoid Arthritis.* Markham, ON, Fitzhenry & Whiteside, 1986.
    Not in depth but generally "information is accurate and advice appropriate"—Arthritis Foundation.

12. Jetter J, Kadlec N: *The Arthritis Book of Water Exercise.* London, Granada, 1985.

13. Krasevec JA, Grimes DC: *HydroRobics™: A Water Exercise Program for Individuals of All Ages and Fitness Levels,* ed 2. West Point, NY, Leisure Press, 1985, 224 pp.

14. Lorig K, Fries JF: *The Arthritis Helpbook,* ed 5. Don Mills, ON, Addison-Wesley, 2001.

15. Rockport Walking Institute: *The Rockport Fitness Walking Test.* Available from Rockport Walking Institute, PO Box 480, Marlboro, MA 01752 (include stamped, self-addressed envelope).

16. ROM Institute: *ROM Dance: A Range of Motion Exercise and Relaxation Program.* Instructional materials and training available from ROM Institute, New Ventures of Wisconsin Inc, 3601 Memorial Drive, Madison, WI 53704.

17. Sayce V, Fraser I: *Exercise Beats Arthritis, An Easy-to-Follow Programme of Exercises,* ed 3. Boulder, CO, Bull Publishing, 1998.

18. Sobel D, Klein AC: *What Exercises Work.* New York, St. Martin's Press, 1993.

Intimacy

1. Foltz-Gray D: Rekindling intimacy. *Arthritis Today* March/April, 16–65, 2003.
   Offers tips on how to return to the loving closeness previously experienced.

2. Houtchens CJ: *A Guide to Intimacy with Arthritis.* Atlanta, Arthritis Foundation, 1998. Free copy available from the Arthritis Foundation, 1300 West Peachtree Street, Atlanta, GA 30309 or through www.arthritis.org.
   Offers tips on recreating intimacy as well as seven pain-free positions for people with arthritis.

3. Sandowski CL: *Sexual Concerns When Illness or Disability Strikes.* Springfield, IL, Charles C Thomas, 1990.

4. Sipski ML: *Sexual Function in People with Disabilities and Chronic Illness: A Health Professional's Guide.* Rockville, MD, Aspen Publishers, 1997.

5. www.sexualhealth.com, a web site offering advice to those with disability and chronic conditions.

Periodicals

1. *Arthritis Today.* Bimonthly magazine available from the Arthritis Foundation and its chapters with $20 US or more membership donation.

2. *AS NEWS.* Quarterly publication of the Ankylosing Spondylitis Association (US). Ankylosing Spondylitis Association, 511 North La Cienega #216, Los Angeles, CA 90048.

3. *Living with Arthritis.* Monthly newsletter published by the Association for People with Arthritis, PO Box 954, 6 Commercial Street, Hicksville, NY 11802. Phone: 1-800-323-2243.

4. *Arthritis News,* a publication of The Arthritis Society of Canada ceased publication in Spring 2003.

Peer-Reviewed Journals

Journals are listed by ISI journal citation reports of Rheumatology Impact Factors 2002:

Arthritis and Rheumatism (American College of Rheumatology)
Annals of Rheumatic Diseases
Seminars in Arthritis and Rheumatism
Rheumatology (formerly *British Journal of Rheumatology*)
The Journal of Rheumatology
Osteoarthritis and Cartilage (Osteoarthritis Research Society [OARS])
Rheumatic Diseases Clinics of North America

Lupus
Clincal and Experimental Rheumatology
Scandinavian Journal of Rheumatology (Sweden)
Arthritis Care and Research (Arthritis Health Professions Association [AHPA], American College of Rheumatology)
Bulletin on Rheumatic Diseases (Arthritis Foundation [ARF], Atlanta)
Rheumatology International
Clinical Rheumatology (Brussels)
Balliere's Best Practice & Research. Clinical Rheumatology (London)
Zeitschrift fur Rheumatologie
Journal of Musculoskeletal Pain
Joint, Bone, Spine (formerly Revue du Rhematisme, France)

Additional Peer Reviewed Journals

Experimental Rheumatology
Reports on Rheumatic Diseases. Topical Reviews "Series 2" (Arthritis & Rheumatism Council for Research [ARC] for Research, Great Britain);
Reports on Rheumatic Diseases. Practical Problems "Series 2" (ARC for Research, Great Britain)
Rheumatic Diseases/Reports on Rheumatic Diseases (ARF, London)

Organizations

1. **The Arthritis Foundation**
   1314 Spring Street NW, Atlanta, GA 30309
   Phone: 404-872-7100; fax: 404-872-0457
   For publications: PO Box 7669, Atlanta, GA 30357-0669
   Phone: 1-800-283-7800 (US only)
   www.arthritis.org
   Offers a rich variety of resources of general information, advocacy, children, services, treatments, and types of arthritis. Single copies of publications available from state chapters, bulk orders from the Foundation, some items at lower cost to members, some materials in other languages.
2. **American Juvenile Arthritis Organization**
   1330 West Peachtree Street NW, Atlanta, GA 30309
   Phone: 404-872-7100
   www.arthritis.org/resources/kidpower.asp
   Advocacy group for all interested in juvenile rheumatoid arthritis.
3. **Arthritis Health Professions Association (AHPA)**
   AHPA (USA) was replaced by the ARHP (see later)
   AHPA (Canada), The Arthritis Society, 393

University Avenue, Ste 1700, Toronto, ON, Canada M5G 1E6
E-mail: ahpa@arthritis.ca
Multidisciplinary professional organization concerned with all issues related to arthritis.
4. **The Arthritis Society of Canada**
   National Office, 393 University Avenue, Ste 1700, Toronto, ON, Canada M5G 1E6
   Phone: 1-800-321-1433; fax: 416-979-8366
   Phone, Ontario Division: 416-979-7228
   www.arthritis.ca
   Addresses of provincial offices may be obtained from the National Office.
5. **Arthritis Foundation of Australia**
   National Office, PO Box 121, Sydney, NSW 2001, Australia
   Phone: 02-221-2456
6. **Arthritis Foundation of New Zealand**
   National Office, PO Box 10-020, Wellington, New Zealand
   Phone: 04-721-427
7. **Association of Rheumatology Health Professionals (ARHP)**
   Division of the American College of Rheumatology, 1800 Century Plaza, Suite 250, Atlanta, GA 30345-4300
   www.rheumatology.org
8. **Leagues against Rheumatism** (check ILAR home page, or World Health Organization [WHO]) for currency of addresses listed below)
   A. AFLAR (African): Professor G.M. Mody (President), Private Bag 7, Congella 4013, Durban, South Africa
   Phone: 27-31-2604284; fax: 27-31-2604482
   E-mail: modva@med.und.ac.za
   B. APLAR (Asia Pacific): Chen Shun-Le, MD (President), Rheumatology & Immunology Unit, Ren Ji Hospital, Shanghai No 2 Medical University, 145 Shan Dong Zong Road, China
   Phone: 86 21 832 50477; fax: 91 21 632 60930
   E-mail: slchen@online.sh.cr
   C. EULAR (European): Prof. Dr. J.R. Kaiden (President), Medizinische Klinik III, Universitat Erlangen-Numberg, Krankenhausstrasse 12, C-91054 Erlangen, Germany
   Phone: 49 9131 853 3363; fax: 49 9131 853 4770
   E-mail: kaiden@med3.med.unierlangen.de
   D. ILAR (International): Prof. T. El-Hadidi, 38 Kambiz Str., 12311 Dokki, Cairo, Egypt
   Phone: 20-2-760 9344; fax: 202 340 0362
   E-mail: thadidi@ilarportal.org
   E. Allied Health Professionals (Section of ILAR): Prof. J.J. Rasker, University of Twente, Department of Rheumatology & Communication

Studies, PO Box 217, 7500 AE Enschede, The Netherlands
Phone: 31-53-4894048; fax: 31-53-4894259
E-mail: j.j.rasker@wmw.utwente.ni

F. **PANLAR (Pan America):** A.J. Reginato, MD (President), Department of Medicine, Cooper Hospital/UMC, 401 Haadon Evenne, Camden, NJ 06103
Phone: 1-609-757-4818; fax: 1-609-757-7803
E-mail: ajreginato@aol.com

9. **Lupus Canada**
040-635 6th Avenue SW, Calgary, AL, Canada T2P 0T5
Phone: 1-800-265-4613
Branches in 10 provinces providing information and support.

10. **Lupus Foundation of America Inc.**
1300 Piccard Drive, Suite 200, Rockville MD 20850
www.lupus.org

11. **National Fibromyalgia Syndrome Association**
6380 East Tanque Verde, Suite D, Tucson, AZ 85715
Phone: 520-733-1570
www.afsafund.org

12. **National Institute of Arthritis and Musculoskeletal and Skin Diseases (NIAMS)**
National Institutes of Health, 1 AMS Circle, Bethesda, MD 20892-3675
Phone: 301-565-2966
www.niams.nih.gov/hi/topics/juvenile_arthritis/juvarthr.htm

13. **National Osteoporosis Association**
1231 22nd Street, Washington, DC 20037
Phone: 202-223-2226
www.nof.org

14. **Osteoporosis Society of Canada**
Box 280, Station Q, Toronto, ON, Canada M4T 2M1

15. **National Center for Complementary & Alternative Medicine**
NCCAM Clearinghouse, PO Box 8218, Silver Spring, MD 20807-8218
http://nccam.nih.gov

Spondylitis Associations

Canada: Ontario Spondylitis Association (five chapters), Ankylosing Spondylitis Association of British Columbia, Manitoba Ankylosing Spondylitis Association.

For addresses contact The Arthritis Society (see earlier).

United States of America: Ankylosing Spondylitis Association, 511 N La Cienega #216, Los Angeles, CA 90048. Phone: 310-652-0609

Contact for addresses of state support groups (29 states). Supplies educational materials, patient guidebook and videos and publishes a quarterly: AS NEWS.

United Kingdom: The Ankylosing Spondylitis International Federation & National Ankylosing Spondylitis Society, PO Box 179, Mayfield, East Sussex, UK TN20 6ZL

United Kingdom Offices of Arthritis & Rheumatism Council for Research (ARC):

ARC, Copeman House, St. Mary's Gate, Chesterfield, Derbys, England S41 7TD. Phone: 44 011 246-558033

ARC, 17 Cleland Park South, Bangor, County Down, N Ireland BT20 3EW ARC, PO Box 304, Swansea, Wales SA1 1W2 ARC, 140 High Street, Lochee, Dundee, Scotland DD2 3BZ

Audiovisual Materials

1. *ARHP Teaching Slide Collection CD-ROM for Clinicians and Educators, Assessment and Management of Rheumatic Diseases,* 3rd ed. 328 slides. Appropriate for professionals and lay-client audiences. ($29 US ARHP members, $59 nonmembers). Available from American College of Rheumatology (ARC), Atlanta, GA; www.rheumatology.org/products (also from ARC 800 slide set *ACR Clinical Slide Collection on the Rheumatic Diseases.* 1999, $750 members, $790 nonmembers; vol II, 1998 CD-ROM for both PC and MAC [$79 members, $99 nonmembers]).

2. ARRTC: *Good Moves for Everybody.* Exercise videotape. Arthritis Rehabilitation Research & Training Center, Columbia, University of Missouri (see Exercise section).

3. Arthritis Foundation: *Pool Exercise Program (PEP).* (See Exercise section.)

4. Arthritis Foundation: *PACE: People with Arthritis Can Exercise.* Two videocassettes, Parts I and II. Available from the Arthritis Foundation (Phone: 1-800-207-8633) or at www.arthritis.org; Tapes are $19.50 each.

5. NASA: *The Water Workout-Exercise Video.* $1/2$ hour VHS, National Ankylosing Spondylitis Association, Los Angeles, CA.

6. NASA: *Fight Back Exercise.* Videotape, 35 min VHS, National Ankylosing Spondylitis Association, Los Angeles, CA.

7. Vostrejs, MD: *Aquonastics.* Denver, CO, National Jewish Center for Immunology and Respiratory Medicine, 1986.

Assistive Devices

1. ABLE DATA, 8630 Fenton Street, Suite 930, Silver Spring, MD 20910
   An on-line repository of assistive technology products and devices
   Phone: 1-800-227-0216
   www.abledata.com
2. American Occupational Therapy Association (AOTA), AOTA Arthritis Resource Guide, Product Department, 1383 Piccard Drive, PO Box 1726, Rockville, MD 20849-1725
   Phone: 1-800-729-9626
   www.aota.org
3. Canadian Association of Occupational Therapists (CAOT), OT Resources and Links - OT Works, CTTC Building, 3400-1125 Colonel By Drive, Ottawa, ON, Canada K1S 5R1
   Phone: 1-800-434-2268
   www.caot.ca
4. AliMed, Inc., 297 High Street, Dedham, MA 02026
   Phone: 1-800-225-2610; fax: 1-800-437-2966
   www.alimed.com
5. E.R.P. Group Professional Products Ltd., 3232 Autoroute Laval West, Laval, QU, Canada H7T 2H6; phone: 1-800-361-3537; fax: 450-687-8035
   www.erp.ca
6. Independent Needs Centre, 100 Amber Street, Unit 1, Markham, ON, Canada L3R 3A2
7. North Coast Medical, 18305 Sutter Boulevard, Morgan Hill, CA 95037-2845
   Phone: 1-800-821-9319; fax: 1-877-213-9300
   www.ncmedical.com
8. Sammons Preston Rolyan, 4 Sammons Court, Bolingbrook, IL 60440
   Phone: 1-800-323-5547; fax: 1-800-547-4333
   United States: www.sammonspreston.com; Canada: www.sammonspreston.ca
9. Silver Ring Splint Company, PO Box 2856, Charlottesville, VA 22902

Phone: 804-971-4052; fax: 804-971-8828
Contact local occupational therapists who may have the measuring kit.
10. Smith & Nephew Inc., 185-A Courtneypark Drive, Mississauga, ON, Canada L5T 2T6
    Phone: 905-670-1131; fax: 905-670-1135
    www.smith-nephew.com
11. W. Kearns, 435 Dwyer Road, Saint John, NB, Canada E2M 4T6
    Phone: 506-672-908 (evening)
    E-mail: billk@nbnet.nb.ca
    Canadian supplier of silver ring splints; contact local occupational therapists for measurement

Web Sites

Note: As web users recognize, web addresses may change at any time, the Internet is a dynamic environment.
American Academy of Orthopaedic Surgeons (AAOS); www.orthoinfo.aaos.org; a general information site for both health professionals and for individuals with arthritis
American Academy of Sleep Medicine; www.aasmnet.org
American College of Rheumatology and ARHP; www.rheumatology.org
American Chronic Pain Association; www.theacpa.org
American Pain Society; www.ampainsoc.org
Arthritis Foundation; www.arthritis.org/resources; resources for both health professionals and individuals with arthritis
International Myopain Society; www.theacpa.org
Joint and Bone; www.jointandbone.org; news on rheumatology and its drug therapy
Missouri Arthritis Rehabilitation Research & Training Center (MARRTC); www.muhealth.org
Physician's Desk Reference; www.pdr.net/getting well/ arthritis/consumers.html

Health Status Assessment Instruments in Common Use

1. **Arthritis Impact Measurement Scales 2 (AIMS2).** From Meenan RF, Mason JH, Anderson JJ, et al: AIMS2. The content and properties of a revised and expanded arthritis impact measurement scales health status questionnaire. *Arthritis Rheum* 35:1–10, 1992. With permission.
2. **Bath Ankylosing Spondylitis Functional Index (BASFI).** From Calin A, Garrett S, Whitelock H, et al: A new approach to defining functional ability in ankylosing spondylitis: the development of the Bath Ankylosing Spondylitis Functional Index. *J Rheumatol* 21:2281–2285, 1994. With permission.
3. **Fibromyalgia Impact Questionnaire (FIQ).** From Burckhardt CS, Clark SR, Bennett RM: The Fibromyalgia Impact Questionnaire: development and validation. *J Rheumatol* 18:728–733, 1991. With permission.
4. **Health Assessment Questionnaire (HAQ) Disability and Discomfort Scales (revision 1994; Short Form).** From Fries JF, Spitz P, Kraines RG, Holman HR: Measurement of patient outcome in arthritis. *Arthritis Rheum* 23:137–145, 1980. With permission.
5. **McMaster Toronto Arthritis Patient Preference Disability Questionnaire (MACTAR).** From Tugwell P, Bombardier C, Buchanan WW, et al: The MACTAR Patient Preference Disability Questionnaire—an individualized functional priority approach for assessing improvement in physical disability in clinical trials in rheumatoid arthritis. *J Rheumatol* 14:446–451, 1987. With permission.
6. **Short-Form Health Survey (SF-36).** From Ware JE Jr, Sherbourne CD: The MOS 36-item short-form health survey (SF-36). I. Conceptual framework and item selection. *Med Care* 30(6):473–483, 1992. With permission.
7. **Western Ontario and McMaster Universities Osteoarthritis Index (WOMAC)—VA3.0.** From Bellamy N, Buchanan WW, Goldsmith CH, et al: Validation study of WOMAC: a health status instrument for measuring clinically important patient relevant outcomes to anti-rheumatic drug therapy in patients with osteoarthritis of the hip or knee. *J Rheumatol* 15:1833–1840, 1988. With permission.

ARTHRITIS IMPACT MEASUREMENT SCALES 2 (AIMS2)

Courtesy of the originator

Source: *Arthritis Rheum* 35:1–10, 1992.

Contact Address: Robert F. Meenan MD, MPH
                     The Arthritis Center
                     Boston University School of Medicine
                     Conte Building
                     80 East Concord Street
                     Boston, MA
                     USA 02118-2394

Telephone: 617-638-4310
Fax: 617-638-5226

Please check (X) the most appropriate answer for each question.

These questions refer to MOBILITY LEVEL.

DURING THE PAST MONTH . . .	All Days (1)	Most Days (2)	Some Days (3)	Few Days (4)	No Days (5)	
1. How often were you physically able to drive a car or use public transportation?	____	____	____	____	____	8/
2. How often were you out of the house for at least part of the day?	____	____	____	____	____	9/
3. How often were you able to do errands in the neighborhood?	____	____	____	____	____	10/
4. How often did someone have to assist you to get around outside your home?	____	____	____	____	____	11/
5. How often were you in a bed or chair for most or all of the day?	____	____	____	____	____	12/

AIMS

These questions refer to WALKING AND BENDING.

DURING THE PAST MONTH . . .	All Days (1)	Most Days (2)	Some Days (3)	Few Days (4)	No Days (5)	
6. Did you have trouble doing vigorous activities such as running, lifting heavy objects, or participating in strenuous sports?	____	____	____	____	____	13/
7. Did you have trouble either walking several blocks or climbing a few flights of stairs?	____	____	____	____	____	14/
8. Did you have trouble bending, lifting, or stooping?	____	____	____	____	____	15/
9. Did you have trouble either walking one block or climbing one flight of stairs?	____	____	____	____	____	16/
10. Were you unable to walk unless assisted by another person or by a cane, crutches, or walker?	____	____	____	____	____	17/

AIMS2 Continued

Please check (X) the most appropriate answer for each question.

These questions refer to HAND AND FINGER FUNCTION.

DURING THE PAST MONTH . . .	All Days (1)	Most Days (2)	Some Days (3)	Few Days (4)	No Days (5)	
11. Could you easily write with a pen or pencil?	____	____	____	____	____	18/
12. Could you easily button a shirt or blouse?	____	____	____	____	____	19/
13. Could you easily turn a key in a lock?	____	____	____	____	____	20/
14. Could you easily tie a knot or a bow?	____	____	____	____	____	21/
15. Could you easily open a new jar of food?	____	____	____	____	____	22/

AIMS

These questions refer to ARM FUNCTION.

DURING THE PAST MONTH . . .	All Days (1)	Most Days (2)	Some Days (3)	Few Days (4)	No Days (5)	
16. Could you easily wipe your mouth with a napkin?	____	____	____	____	____	23/
17. Could you easily put on a pullover sweater?	____	____	____	____	____	24/
18. Could you easily comb or brush your hair?	____	____	____	____	____	25/
19. Could you easily scratch your low back with your hand?	____	____	____	____	____	26/
20. Could you easily reach shelves that were above your head?	____	____	____	____	____	27/

AIMS

These questions refer to SELF-CARE TASKS.

DURING THE PAST MONTH . . .	Always (1)	Very Often (2)	Sometimes (3)	Almost Never (4)	Never (5)	
21. Did you need help to take a bath or shower?	____	____	____	____	____	28/
22. Did you need help to get dressed?	____	____	____	____	____	29/
23. Did you need help to use the toilet?	____	____	____	____	____	30/
24. Did you need help to get in or out of bed?	____	____	____	____	____	31/

AIMS

These questions refer to HOUSEHOLD TASKS.

DURING THE PAST MONTH . . .	Always (1)	Very Often (2)	Sometimes (3)	Almost Never (4)	Never (5)	
25. If you had the necessary transportation, could you go shopping for groceries without help?	____	____	____	____	____	32/

AIMS2 Continued

Please check (X) the most appropriate answer for each question.

26. If you had kitchen facilities, could you prepare your own meals without help?   ____ ____ ____ ____ ____   33/

27. If you had household tools and appliances, could you do your own housework without help?   ____ ____ ____ ____ ____   34/

28. If you had laundry facilities, could you do your own laundry without help?   ____ ____ ____ ____ ____   35/

AIMS

These questions refer to SOCIAL ACTIVITY.

DURING THE PAST MONTH . . .	All Days (1)	Most Days (2)	Some Days (3)	Few Days (4)	No Days (5)	
29. How often did you get together with friends or relatives?						36/
30. How often did you have friends or relatives over to your home?						37/
31. How often did you visit friends or relatives at their homes?						38/
32. How often were you on the telephone with close friends or relatives?						39/
33. How often did you go to a meeting of a church, club, team, or other group?						40/

AIMS

These questions refer to SUPPORT FROM FAMILY AND FRIENDS.

DURING THE PAST MONTH . . .	Always (1)	Very Often (2)	Sometimes (3)	Almost Never (4)	Never (5)	
34. Did you feel that your family or friends would be around if you needed assistance?						41/
35. Did you feel that your family or friends were sensitive to your personal needs?						42/
36. Did you feel that your family or friends were interested in helping you solve problems?						43/
37. Did you feel that your family or friends understood the effects of your arthritis?						44/

AIMS

These questions refer to ARTHRITIS PAIN.

DURING THE PAST MONTH . . .	Severe (1)	Moderate (2)	Mild (3)	Very Mild (4)	None (5)	
38. How would you describe the arthritis pain you usually had?						45/

AIMS2 Continued

Please check (X) the most appropriate answer for each question.

	All Days (1)	Most Days (2)	Some Days (3)	Few Days (4)	No Days (5)	
39. How often did you have severe pain from your arthritis?	___	___	___	___	___	46/
40. How often did you have pain in two or more joints at the same time?	___	___	___	___	___	47/
41. How often did your morning stiffness last more than 1 hour from the time you woke up?	___	___	___	___	___	48/
42. How often did your pain make it difficult for you to sleep?	___	___	___	___	___	49/

AIMS

These questions refer to WORK.

DURING THE PAST MONTH . . .	Paid work (1)	House work (2)	School work (3)	Unemployed (4)	Disabled (5)	Retired (6)	
43. What has been your main form of work?	___	___	___	___	___	___	50/

If you answered unemployed, disabled, or retired, please skip the next four questions and go to the next page.

DURING THE PAST MONTH . . .	All Days (1)	Most Days (2)	Some Days (3)	Few Days (4)	No Days (5)	
44. How often were you unable to do any paid work, house work, or school work?	___	___	___	___	___	51/
45. On the days that you did work, how often did you have to work a shorter day?	___	___	___	___	___	52/
46. On the days that you did work, how often were you unable to do your work as carefully and accurately as you would like?	___	___	___	___	___	53/
47. On the days that you did work, how often did you have to change the way your paid work, housework, or school work is usually done?	___	___	___	___	___	54/

AIMS

These questions refer to LEVEL OF TENSION.

DURING THE PAST MONTH . . .	Always (1)	Very Often (2)	Sometimes (3)	Almost Never (4)	Never (5)	
48. How often have you felt tense or high strung?	___	___	___	___	___	55/
49. How often have you been bothered by nervousness or your nerves?	___	___	___	___	___	56/

AIMS2 Continued

Please check (X) the most appropriate answer for each question.

50. How often were you able to relax without difficulty?   _____ _____ _____ _____ _____   57/

51. How often have you felt relaxed and free of tension?   _____ _____ _____ _____ _____   58/

52. How often have you felt calm and peaceful?   _____ _____ _____ _____ _____   59/

AIMS

These questions refer to MOOD.

DURING THE PAST MONTH . . .	Always (1)	Very Often (2)	Sometimes (3)	Almost Never (4)	Never (5)	
53. How often have you enjoyed the things you do?	_____	_____	_____	_____	_____	60/
54. How often have you been in low or very low spirits?	_____	_____	_____	_____	_____	61/
55. How often did you feel that nothing turned out the way you wanted it to?	_____	_____	_____	_____	_____	62/
56. How often did you feel that others would be better off if you were dead?	_____	_____	_____	_____	_____	63/
57. How often did you feel so down in the dumps that nothing would cheer you up?	_____	_____	_____	_____	_____	64/

AIMS

These questions refer to satisfaction with each health area.

DURING THE PAST MONTH . . .	Very Satisfied (1)	Somewhat Satisfied (2)	Neither Satisfied Nor Dissatisfied (3)	Somewhat Dissatisfied (4)	Very Dissatisfied (5)	
58. How satisfied have you been with each of these areas of your health?						
MOBILITY LEVEL (example: do errands)	_____	_____	_____	_____	_____	65/
WALKING AND BENDING (example: climb stairs)	_____	_____	_____	_____	_____	66/
HAND AND FINGER FUNCTION (example: tie a bow)	_____	_____	_____	_____	_____	67/
ARM FUNCTION (example: comb hair)	_____	_____	_____	_____	_____	68/
SELF-CARE (example: take bath)	_____	_____	_____	_____	_____	69/

AIMS2 Continued

Please check (X) the most appropriate answer for each question.

HOUSEHOLD TASKS
(example: housework)   ____   ____   ____   ____   ____   70/

SOCIAL ACTIVITY
(example: visit friends)   ____   ____   ____   ____   ____   71/

SUPPORT FROM FAMILY
(example: help with problems)   ____   ____   ____   ____   ____   72/

ARTHRITIS PAIN
(example: joint pain)   ____   ____   ____   ____   ____   73/

WORK
(example: reduce hours)   ____   ____   ____   ____   ____   74/

LEVEL OF TENSION
(example: felt tense)   ____   ____   ____   ____   ____   75/

MOOD
(example: down in dumps)   ____   ____   ____   ____   ____   76/

AIMS

These questions refer to arthritis impact on each area of health.

DURING THE PAST MONTH . . .	Not a Problem for Me (0)	Due Entirely to Other Causes (1)	Due Largely to Other Causes (2)	Due Partly to Arthritis and Partly to Other Causes (3)	Due Largely to My Arthritis (4)	Due Entirely to My Arthritis (5)	
59. How much of your problem in each area of health was due to your arthritis?							
MOBILITY LEVEL (example: do errands)	____	____	____	____	____	____	8/
WALKING AND BENDING (example: climb stairs)	____	____	____	____	____	____	9/
HAND AND FINGER FUNCTION (example: tie a bow)	____	____	____	____	____	____	10/
ARM FUNCTION (example: comb hair)	____	____	____	____	____	____	11/
SELF-CARE (example: take bath)	____	____	____	____	____	____	12/
HOUSEHOLD TASKS (example: housework)	____	____	____	____	____	____	13/
SOCIAL ACTIVITY (example: visit friends)	____	____	____	____	____	____	14/
SUPPORT FROM FAMILY (example: help with problems)	____	____	____	____	____	____	15/

AIMS2 Continued

Please check (X) the most appropriate answer for each question.

ARTHRITIS PAIN
(example: joint pain)   _____ _____ _____ _____ _____ _____   16/

WORK
(example: reduce hours)   _____ _____ _____ _____ _____ _____   17/

LEVEL OF TENSION
(example: felt tense)   _____ _____ _____ _____ _____ _____   18/

MOOD
(example: down in dumps)   _____ _____ _____ _____ _____ _____   19/

You have now answered questions about different AREAS OF YOUR HEALTH. These areas are listed below. Please check (X) up to THREE AREAS in which you would MOST LIKE TO SEE IMPROVEMENT. Please read all 12 areas of health choices before making your decision:

check = 1
blank = 0

60. AREAS OF HEALTH   THREE AREAS FOR IMPROVEMENT

MOBILITY LEVEL
(example: do errands)   _____   20/

WALKING AND BENDING
(example: climb stairs)   _____   21/

HAND AND FINGER FUNCTION
(example: tie a bow)   _____   22/

ARM FUNCTION
(example: comb hair)   _____   23/

SELF-CARE
(example: take bath)   _____   24/

HOUSEHOLD TASKS
(example: housework)   _____   25/

SOCIAL ACTIVITY
(example: visit friends)   _____   26/

SUPPORT FROM FAMILY
(example: help with problems)   _____   27/

ARTHRITIS PAIN
(example: joint pain)   _____   28/

WORK
(example: reduce hours)   _____   29/

LEVEL OF TENSION
(example: felt tense)   _____   30/

MOOD
(example: down in dumps)   _____   31/

Please make sure that you have checked no more than THREE AREAS for improvement.

AIMS2 Continued

BATH ANKYLOSING SPONDYLITIS FUNCTIONAL INDEX (BASFI)

Courtesy of the authors and the Editor, *J Rheumatol* 21:2281–2285, 1994.

Contact Address: Dr. Andrei Calin, MD, FRCP, RNHRD
                   Upper Borough Walls
                   Bath BA1 7RL
                   England
Email: <calinandrei@hotmail.com>
Telephone: 44-1225-421760
Fax: 44-1225-473437

PLEASE DRAW A MARK ON EACH LINE BELOW TO INDICATE YOUR LEVEL OF ABILITY WITH EACH OF THE FOLLOWING ACTIVITIES DURING THE LAST WEEK:

N.B. An aid is a piece of equipment which helps you to perform an action or movement

EXAMPLE:

EASY_____IMPOSSIBLE

1) Putting on your socks or tights without help or aids (e.g., sock aid)

EASY_____IMPOSSIBLE

2) Bending forward from the waist to pick up a pen from the floor without an aid

EASY_____IMPOSSIBLE

3) Reaching up to a high shelf without help or aids (e.g., helping hand)

EASY_____IMPOSSIBLE

4) Getting up out of an armless dining room chair without using your hands or any other help

EASY_____IMPOSSIBLE

5) Getting up off the floor without help from lying on your back

EASY_____IMPOSSIBLE

6) Standing unsupported for 10 minutes without discomfort

EASY_____IMPOSSIBLE

7) Climbing 12–15 steps without using a handrail or walking aid. One foot on each step

EASY_____IMPOSSIBLE

8) Looking over your shoulder without turning your body

EASY_____IMPOSSIBLE

9) Doing physically demanding activities (e.g., physiotherapy exercises, gardening, or sports)

EASY_____IMPOSSIBLE

10) Doing a full day's activities whether it be at home or at work

EASY_____IMPOSSIBLE

FIBROMYALGIA IMPACT QUESTIONNAIRE (FIQ)

Courtesy of the authors and the Editor, *J Rheumatol* 18:728–733 1991.

Contact Address: Dr. R.M. Bennett
Division of Arthritis and Rheumatic Diseases
Department of Medicine-L329A
Oregon Health Sciences University
3181 SW Sam Jackson Park Road
Portland, OR
USA 97201-3098
Telephone: 503-494-8963
Fax: 503-494-4348

	Always	Most times	Occasionally	Never
1. Were you able to:				
a. Do shopping	0	1	2	3
b. Do laundry with a washer and dryer	0	1	2	3
c. Prepare meals	0	1	2	3
d. Wash dishes/cooking utensils by hand	0	1	2	3
e. Vacuum a rug	0	1	2	3
f. Make beds	0	1	2	3
g. Walk several blocks	0	1	2	3
h. Visit friends/relatives	0	1	2	3
i. Do yard work	0	1	2	3
j. Drive a car	0	1	2	3

2. Of the 7 days in the past week, how many days did you feel good?

    1   2   3   4   5   6   7

3. How many days in the past week did you miss work because of your fibromyalgia? (If you don't have a job outside the home leave this item blank.)   1   2   3   4   5

4. When you did go to work, how much did pain or other symptoms of your fibromyalgia interfere with your ability to do your job?

    No problem   Great difficulty

5. How bad has your pain been?

    No pain   Very severe pain

6. How tired have you been?

    No tiredness   Very tired

7. How have you felt when you got up in the morning?

    Awoke well rested   Awoke very tired

8. How bad has your stiffness been?

    No stiffness   Very stiff

9. How tense, nervous, or anxious have you felt?

    Not tense   Very tense

10. How depressed or blue have you felt?

    Not depressed   Very depressed

HEALTH ASSESSMENT QUESTIONNAIRE (HAQ-SF)

Health Assessment Questionnaire (HAQ) Disability and Discomfort Scales (revision 1994; Short Form). From Fries JF, Spitz P, Kraines RG, Holman HR: Measurement of patient outcome in arthritis. *Arthritis Rheum* 23:137–145, 1980. With permission.

Contact Address: James F. Fries
  Division of Immunology and Rheumatology
  Department of Medicine
  Stanford University School of Medicine
  1000 Welsh Road, Suite 203
  Palo Alto, Ca, USA 94304
Telephone: 415-723-6003
Fax: 415-723-9656

Name_____ Date_____

In this section we are interested in learning how your illness affects your ability to function in daily life. Please feel free to add any comments on the back of this page.

Please check the response which best describes your usual abilities OVER THE PAST WEEK:

	Without ANY Difficulty	With SOME Difficulty	With MUCH Difficulty	UNABLE To Do	
DRESSING & GROOMING Are you able to:					
Dress yourself, including tying shoelaces and doing buttons?	_____	_____	_____	_____	
Shampoo your hair?	_____	_____	_____	_____	**DRESSNEW**
ARISING Are you able to:					
Stand up from a straight chair?	_____	_____	_____	_____	
Get in and out of bed?	_____	_____	_____	_____	**RISENEW**
EATING Are you able to:					
Cut your meat?	_____	_____	_____	_____	
Lift a full cup or glass to your mouth?	_____	_____	_____	_____	
Open a new milk carton?	_____	_____	_____	_____	**EATNEW**_____
WALKING Are you able to:					
Walk outdoors on flat ground?	_____	_____	_____	_____	
Climb up five steps?	_____	_____	_____	_____	**WALKNEW**_____

PATKEY#_____

QUESTDAT_____

HAQADMIN_____

QUESTYPE____2____

PMSVIS____1____

RASTUDY_____

QUESTNUM_____

HAQ-SF Continued

Please check any **AIDS OR DEVICES** that you usually use for any of these activities:

_____ Cane
_____ Walker
_____ Crutches
_____ Wheelchair

_____ Devices used for dressing (button hook, zipper pull, long-handled shoe horn, etc.)
_____ Built-up or special utensils
_____ Special or built-up chair
_____ Other (Specify: _____)

Please check any categories for which you usually need **HELP FROM ANOTHER PERSON**:

_____ Dressing and Grooming
_____ Arising

_____ Eating
_____ Walking

Please check the response which best describes your usual abilities **OVER THE PAST WEEK**:

	Without ANY Difficulty	With SOME Difficulty	With MUCH Difficulty	UNABLE To Do
HYGIENE Are you able to:				
Wash and dry your body?	_____	_____	_____	_____
Take a tub bath?	_____	_____	_____	_____
Get on and off the toilet?	_____	_____	_____	_____
REACH Are you able to:				
Reach and get down a 5-lb object (such as a bag of sugar) from just above your head?	_____	_____	_____	_____
Bend down to pick up clothing from the floor?	_____	_____	_____	_____
GRIP Are you able to:				
Open car doors?	_____	_____	_____	_____
Open jars which have been previously opened?	_____	_____	_____	_____
Turn faucets on and off?	_____	_____	_____	_____
ACTIVITIES Are you able to:				
Run errands and shop?	_____	_____	_____	_____
Get in and out of a car?	_____	_____	_____	_____
Do chores such as vacuuming or yardwork?	_____	_____	_____	_____

Please check any **AIDS OR DEVICES** that you usually use for any of these activities:

_____ Raised toilet seat
_____ Bathtub seat
_____ Jar opener (for jars previously opened)

_____ Bathtub bar
_____ Long-handled appliances for reach
_____ Long-handled appliances in bathroom
_____ Other (Specify: _____)

DRSGASST_____
RISEASST_____
EATASST_____
WALKASST_____

HYGNNEW_____

REACHNEW_____

GRIPNEW_____

ACTIVNEW

HAQ-SF Continued

Please check any categories for which you usually need HELP FROM ANOTHER PERSON:

_____Hygiene   _____Gripping and opening things

_____Reach   _____Errands and chores

We are also interested in learning whether or not you are affected by pain because of your illness. **How much pain have you had because of your illness IN THE PAST WEEK:**

PLACE A <u>VERTICAL</u> (|) MARK ON THE LINE TO INDICATE THE SEVERITY OF THE PAIN

NO   SEVERE
PAIN   PAIN

0   100

HYGNASST_____
RCHASST_____
GRIPASST_____
ACTVASST_____

PAINSCAL_____

HAQ-SF

McMASTER TORONTO ARTHRITIS PATIENT PREFERENCE DISABILITY QUESTIONNAIRE (MACTAR)

Courtesy of Dr. Peter Tugwell and the Editor, *J Rheumatol* 14:446–451, 1987.

Contact Address: Dr. Peter Tugwell
                   Department of Medicine
                   Ottawa General Hospital
                   501 Smyth Road
                   Ottawa, Ontario
                   Canada
Telephone: 613-737-8900
Fax: 613-737-8851

Baseline

1. Do you think your arthritis limits your ability to carry out any of your activities? i.e., Are there activities that you used to have no problems with before you had arthritis that you now find painful or have difficulty with because of arthritis?

   (Interviewer lists disabilities)

2. Does your arthritis limit:
   (a) Any (other) activities around the house such as getting around, cooking, housework, dressing, etc.

   (b) Any (other) activities at your work/outside the home/driving, etc.

   (c) Any (other) activities such as athletic (e.g., bowling, swimming, golf), or nonathletic (e.g., needlework, wood work, etc.)

   (d) Any (other) social activities such as visiting, playing cards, going to church, etc.

3. Which of these activities would you most like to be able to do without the pain or discomfort of your arthritis?

4. Which of these activities would you *next* most like to be able to do without the pain or discomfort of your arthritis?

   (The rest of the activities are rank ordered in the same way.)

Follow-up

Each of the disabilities identified at baseline is reviewed as follows:

Since the first interview 8 weeks ago have you noticed any change in your ability to (Name of Disability)   ☐ No   ☐ Yes

If yes, has your ability to _____ Improved ☐ or become Worse ☐

In the past 2 weeks, were you able to do the following tasks without the use of splints and/or mechanical aids?

	Yes, Without Difficulty	Yes, With Some Difficulty	No, Too Difficult To Do
(a) Turn your head from side to side?	____	____	____
(b) Comb your hair (at back of head)?	____	____	____
(c) Close your drawers (with arms only)?	____	____	____
(d) Open drawers?	____	____	____
(e) Lift a full teapot?	____	____	____
(f) Lift a cup with one hand to drink from it?	____	____	____
(g) Turn a key in a lock?	____	____	____
(h) Cut meat with a knife?	____	____	____
(i) Butter bread?	____	____	____
(j) Wind a watch?	____	____	____

MACTAR Continued

(k)	Walk?	___		___
(l)	Walk without:			
	1. Someone's help	___	___	___
	2. Crutches	___	___	___
	3. A walking stick	___	___	___
(m)	Stand up with your knees straight?	___	___	___
(n)	Stand up on your toes?	___	___	___
(o)	Bend down to pick something off the floor?	___	___	___
(p)	Walk up a flight of stairs?	___	___	___
(q)	Walk down a flight of stairs?	___	___	___
(r)	Wash your face and hands?	___	___	___
(s)	Prepare meals?	___	___	___
(t)	Dress/undress yourself?	___	___	___
(u)	Stand up from a chair?	___	___	___
(v)	Do light housework?	___	___	___
(w)	Get on or off the toilet?	___	___	___
(x)	Shave yourself?	___	___	___
(y)	Go shopping?	___	___	___

MACTAR

SHORT FORM HEART SURVEY (SF-36)

Courtesy of the authors and the Editor, *Med Care* 30:473–483, 1992.

Contact Address: John E. Ware Jr., Ph.D.
CEO and Chief Science Officer
Quality Metric Incorporated
640 George Washington Highway, Suite 201
Lincoln, RI 02865
Telephone: 401-334-8800 ext: 242
Fax: 401-334-8801

Your Health and Well-Being

This survey asks for your views about your health. This information will help keep track of how you feel and how well you are able to do your usual activities. *Thank you for completing this survey!*

For each of the following questions, please mark an ☒ **in the one box that best describes your answer.**

1. **In general, would you say your health is:**

Excellent	Very good	Good	Fair	Poor
▼	▼	▼	▼	▼
☐1	☐2	☐3	☐4	☐5

2. **Compared to one week ago, how would you rate your health in general now?**

Much better now than one week ago	Somewhat better now than one week ago	About the same as one week ago	Somewhat worse now than one week ago	Much worse now than one week ago
▼	▼	▼	▼	▼
☐1	☐2	☐3	☐4	☐5

3. The following questions are about activities you might do during a typical day. Does <u>your health now limit you</u> in these activities? If so, how much?

	Yes, limited a lot ▼	Yes, limited a little ▼	No, not limited at all ▼
a <u>Vigorous activities</u>, such as running, lifting heavy objects, participating in strenuous sports	☐₁	☐₂	☐₃
b <u>Moderate activities</u>, such as moving a table, pushing a vacuum cleaner, bowling, or playing golf	☐₁	☐₂	☐₃
c Lifting or carrying groceries	☐₁	☐₂	☐₃
d Climbing <u>several</u> flights of stairs	☐₁	☐₂	☐₃
e Climbing <u>one</u> flight of stairs	☐₁	☐₂	☐₃
f Bending, kneeling, or stooping	☐₁	☐₂	☐₃
g Walking <u>more than a mile</u>	☐₁	☐₂	☐₃
h Walking <u>several hundred yards</u>	☐₁	☐₂	☐₃
i Walking <u>one hundred</u> yards	☐₁	☐₂	☐₃
j Bathing or dressing yourself	☐₁	☐₂	☐₃

4. During the <u>past week</u>, how much of the time have you had any of the following problems with your work or other regular daily activities <u>as a result of your physical health</u>?

	All of the time ▼	Most of the time ▼	Some of the time ▼	A little of the time ▼	None of the time ▼
a Cut down on the <u>amount of time</u> you spent on work or other activities	☐₁	☐₂	☐₃	☐₄	☐₅
b <u>Accomplished less</u> than you would like	☐₁	☐₂	☐₃	☐₄	☐₅

c Were limited in the <u>kind</u> of work or other
activities .... ☐₁ .... ☐₂ .... ☐₃ .... ☐₄ .... ☐₅

d Had <u>difficulty</u> performing the work or other
activities (for example, it took extra effort) .... ☐₁ .... ☐₂ .... ☐₃ .... ☐₄ .... ☐₅

5. **During the <u>past week</u>, how much of the time have you had any of the following problems with your work or other regular daily activities <u>as a result of any emotional problems</u> (such as feeling depressed or anxious)?**

	All of the time	Most of the time	Some of the time	A little of the time	None of the time
	▼	▼	▼	▼	▼

a Cut down on the <u>amount of time</u> you spent
on work or other activities .... ☐₁ .... ☐₂ .... ☐₃ .... ☐₄ .... ☐₅

b <u>Accomplished less</u> than you would like .... ☐₁ .... ☐₂ .... ☐₃ .... ☐₄ .... ☐₅

c Did work or other activities <u>less carefully</u>
than usual .... ☐₁ .... ☐₂ .... ☐₃ .... ☐₄ .... ☐₅

6. **During the <u>past week</u>, to what extent has your physical health or emotional problems interfered with your normal social activities with family, friends, neighbors, or groups?**

Not at all	Slightly	Moderately	Quite a bit	Extremely
▼	▼	▼	▼	▼
☐₁	☐₂	☐₃	☐₄	☐₅

7. **How much <u>bodily</u> pain have you had during the <u>past week</u>?**

None	Very mild	Mild	Moderate	Severe	Very severe
▼	▼	▼	▼	▼	▼
☐₁	☐₂	☐₃	☐₄	☐₅	☐₆

8. During the <u>past week</u>, how much did <u>pain</u> interfere with your normal work (including both work outside the home and housework)?

Not at all	A little bit	Moderately	Quite a bit	Extremely
▼	▼	▼	▼	▼
☐₁	☐₂	☐₃	☐₄	☐₅

9. These questions are about how you feel and how things have been with you <u>during the past week</u>. For each question, please give the one answer that comes closest to the way you have been feeling. How much of the time during the <u>past week</u>...

	All of the time	Most of the time	Some of the time	A little of the time	None of the time
	▼	▼	▼	▼	▼
a Did you feel full of life?	☐₁	☐₂	☐₃	☐₄	☐₅
b Have you been very nervous?	☐₁	☐₂	☐₃	☐₄	☐₅
c Have you felt so down in the dumps that nothing could cheer you up?	☐₁	☐₂	☐₃	☐₄	☐₅
d Have you felt calm and peaceful?	☐₁	☐₂	☐₃	☐₄	☐₅
e Did you have a lot of energy?	☐₁	☐₂	☐₃	☐₄	☐₅
f Have you felt downhearted and depressed?	☐₁	☐₂	☐₃	☐₄	☐₅
g Did you feel worn out?	☐₁	☐₂	☐₃	☐₄	☐₅
h Have you been happy?	☐₁	☐₂	☐₃	☐₄	☐₅
i Did you feel tired?	☐₁	☐₂	☐₃	☐₄	☐₅

10. During the <u>past week</u>, how much of the time has your <u>physical health or emotional problems</u> interfered with your social activities (like visiting friends, relatives, etc.)?

All of the time	Most of the time	Some of the time	A little of the time	None of the time
▼	▼	▼	▼	▼
☐₁	☐₂	☐₃	☐₄	☐₅

11. How TRUE or FALSE is <u>each</u> of the following statements for you?

	Definitely true	Mostly true	Don't know	Mostly false	Definitely false
a. I seem to get sick a little easier than other people	$\square_1$	$\square_2$	$\square_3$	$\square_4$	$\square_5$
b. I am as healthy as anybody I know	$\square_1$	$\square_2$	$\square_3$	$\square_4$	$\square_5$
c. I expect my health to get worse	$\square_1$	$\square_2$	$\square_3$	$\square_4$	$\square_5$
d. My health is excellent	$\square_1$	$\square_2$	$\square_3$	$\square_4$	$\square_5$

THANK YOU FOR COMPLETING THESE QUESTIONS!

WESTERN ONTARIO AND McMASTER UNIVERSITIES OSTEOARTHRITIS INDEX (WOMAC)-VA3.0

Courtesy of the originator.

Source: J Rheumatol 15:1833–1840, 1988.

Contact Address: Dr. Nicholas Bellamy
                    Division of Rheumatology
                    Victoria Hospital
                    P.O. Box 5375
                    London, Ontario
                    Canada N6A 4G5
Telephone: 519-667-6815
Fax: 519-667-6687

INSTRUCTIONS TO PATIENTS

In Sections A, B, and C questions will be asked in the following format and you should give your answers by putting an "X" on the horizontal line.

NOTE:

1. If you put your "X" at the left-hand end of the line, i.e.,

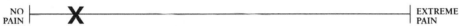

    then you are indicating that you have no pain.

2. If you place your "X" at the right-hand end of the line, i.e.,

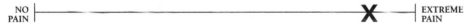

    then you are indicating that your pain is extreme.

3. Please Note:

    a) that the further to the right-hand end you place your "X" the **more** pain you are experiencing.

    b) that the further to the left-hand end you place your "X" the **less** pain you are experiencing.

    c) **Please do not** place your "X" outside the end markers.

You will be asked to indicate on this type of scale the amount of pain, stiffness, or disability you are experiencing. Please remember the further you place your "X" to the right, the more pain, stiffness, or disability you are indicating that you experience.

WOMAC Continued

Section A

INSTRUCTIONS TO PATIENTS

The following questions concern the amount of pain you are currently experiencing due to arthritis in your hips and/or knees. For each situation please enter the amount of pain recently experienced (please mark your answers with an "X").

QUESTION: How much pain do you have?

1. Walking on a flat surface.

    NO |—————————————————————————| EXTREME
    PAIN | | PAIN

2. Going up or down stairs.

    NO |—————————————————————————| EXTREME
    PAIN | | PAIN

3. At night while in bed.

    NO |—————————————————————————| EXTREME
    PAIN | | PAIN

4. Sitting or lying.

    NO |—————————————————————————| EXTREME
    PAIN | | PAIN

5. Standing upright.

    NO |—————————————————————————| EXTREME
    PAIN | | PAIN

Section B

INSTRUCTIONS TO PATIENTS

The following questions concern the amount of joint stiffness (not pain) you are currently experiencing in your hips and/or knees. Stiffness is a sensation of restriction or slowness in the ease with which you move your joints (please mark your answers with an "X").

1. How **severe** is your stiffness **after first wakening** in the morning?

    NO |—————————————————————————| EXTREME
    STIFFNESS | | STIFFNESS

2. How **severe** is your stiffness after sitting, lying or resting **later in the day**?

    NO |—————————————————————————| EXTREME
    STIFFNESS | | STIFFNESS

WOMAC Continued

Section C

INSTRUCTIONS TO PATIENTS

The following questions concern your physical function. By this we mean your ability to move around and to look after yourself. For each of the following activities, please indicate the degree of difficulty you are currently experiencing due to arthritis in your hips and/or knees (please mark your answers with an "X").

QUESTION: What degree of difficulty do you have with:

1. Descending stairs.

NO DIFFICULTY |————————————————————————| EXTREME DIFFICULTY

2. Ascending stairs.

NO DIFFICULTY |————————————————————————| EXTREME DIFFICULTY

3. Rising from sitting.

NO DIFFICULTY |————————————————————————| EXTREME DIFFICULTY

4. Standing.

NO DIFFICULTY |————————————————————————| EXTREME DIFFICULTY

5. Bending to floor.

NO DIFFICULTY |————————————————————————| EXTREME DIFFICULTY

6. Walking on flat.

NO DIFFICULTY |————————————————————————| EXTREME DIFFICULTY

7. Getting in/out of car.

NO DIFFICULTY |————————————————————————| EXTREME DIFFICULTY

8. Going shopping.

NO DIFFICULTY |————————————————————————| EXTREME DIFFICULTY

9. Putting on socks/stockings.

NO DIFFICULTY |————————————————————————| EXTREME DIFFICULTY

10. Rising from bed.

NO DIFFICULTY |————————————————————————| EXTREME DIFFICULTY

11. Taking off socks/stockings.

NO DIFFICULTY |————————————————————————| EXTREME DIFFICULTY

12. Lying in bed.

NO DIFFICULTY |————————————————————————| EXTREME DIFFICULTY

WOMAC Continued

13. Getting in/out of bath.

NO |————————————————————————————————————| EXTREME
DIFFICULTY   DIFFICULTY

14. Sitting.

NO |————————————————————————————————————| EXTREME
DIFFICULTY   DIFFICULTY

15. Getting on/off toilet.

NO |————————————————————————————————————| EXTREME
DIFFICULTY   DIFFICULTY

16. Heavy domestic duties.

NO |————————————————————————————————————| EXTREME
DIFFICULTY   DIFFICULTY

17. Light domestic duties.

NO |————————————————————————————————————| EXTREME
DIFFICULTY   DIFFICULTY

WOMAC

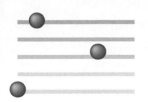

APPENDIX III

Bibliography

ACSM's Guidelines for Exercise Testing and Prescription, ed 6. Philadelphia, Lippincott Williams & Wilkins, 2002.

Akeson WH, Amiel D, Abel MF et al: Effects of immobilization on joints. *Clin Orthop* 219:28–37, 1987.

American Physical Therapy Association: Guide to physical therapy practice, 2nd edition. *Phys Ther* 81:9–744, 2001.

Ansell BM, Rudge S, Schaller JG: *Color Atlas of Pediatric Rheumatology.* London, Wolfe Publishing, 1992.

Badley EM, Ibanez D: Socioeconomic risk factors and musculoskeletal disability. *J Rheumatol* 21:515–522, 1994.

Badley EM, Rasooly I, Webster GK: Relative importance of musculoskeletal disorders as a cause of chronic health problems, disability and health care utilization: Findings from the 1990 Ontario Health Survey. *J Rheumatol* 21:505–514, 1994.

Banwell BF: Physical therapy in arthritis management. In Ehrlich GE (ed): *Rehabilitation Management of Rheumatic Conditions,* ed 2. Baltimore, Williams & Wilkins, 1986, pp 264–284.

Cassidy JT (ed): *Textbook of Rheumatology.* New York, Churchill Livingstone, 1990.

Cole B, Finch E, Gowland C et al: In Basmajian J (ed): *Physical Rehabilitation Outcome Measures,* ed 2. Toronto, ON, Canadian Physiotherapy Association, 2002.

Conference on outcome measures in rheumatoid arthritis clinical trials. Maastrich, the Netherlands April 29–May 3, 1992. *J Rheumatol* 20:525–603, 1993.

Connor EP (product manager): *Physicians' Desk Reference.* Montvale, Medical Economics Data Production Company, 2002.

Felson DT, Anderson JJ, Boers M et al: The American College of Rheumatology preliminary core set of disease activity measures for rheumatoid arthritis trials. *Arthritis Rheum* 36:729–740, 1993.

Frank RG, Hagglund KJ, Schopp LH et al: Disease and family contributors to adaptation in juvenile rheumatoid arthritis and juvenile diabetes. *Arthritis Care Res* 11:166–176, 1988.

Gallin JI, Goldstein IM, Snyderman R (eds): *Inflammation: Basic Principles and Clinical Correlates,* ed 2. New York, Raven Press, 1992.

Guyatt G, Rennie D (eds): *User's Guide to the Medical Literature. A Manual for Evidence-based Clinical Practice.* Chicago, Ill AMA Press, 2002.

Hawley DJ, Wolfe F: Depression is not more common in rheumatoid arthritis: a 10 year longitudinal study of 6,608 rheumatic disease patients. *J Rheumatol* 20:2025–2031, 1993.

Helewa A, Bombardier C, Goldsmith CH et al: Cost-effectiveness of inpatient and intensive outpatient treatment of rheumatoid arthritis. A randomized, controlled trial. *Arthritis Rheum* 32:1505–1514, 1989.

Helewa H, Goldsmith CH, Lee P et al: Effects of occupational therapy home service on patients with rheumatoid arthritis. *Lancet* 337:1453–1456, 1991.

Helewa H, Goldsmith CH, Smythe HA: Patient, observer and instrument variation in the measurement of strength of shoulder abductor muscles in patients with rheumatoid arthritis using a modified sphygmomanometer. *J Rheumatol* 13:1044–1049, 1986.

Helewa A, Smythe HA, Goldsmith CH: Can specially trained physiotherapists improve the care of patients with rheumatoid arthritis? A randomized health care trial. *J Rheumatol* 21:70–79, 1994.

Helewa A, Smythe HA, Goldsmith CH et al: The total assessment of rheumatoid polyarthritis-evaluation of a training program for physiotherapists and occupational therapists. *J Rheumatol* 14:87–92, 1987.

Helewa A, Walker JM: *Critical Evaluation of Research in Physical Rehabilitation.* Philadelphia, WB Saunders, 2002.

Jamison L, Ogden D: *Aquatic therapy using PNF Patterns.* Tucson, AZ, Therapy Skill Builders, 1994.

Klippel JH (chief ed): *Primer on the Rheumatic Diseases,* ed 12. Atlanta, Arthritis Foundation, 2001.

Klippel JH, Dieppe PA (eds): *Rheumatology.* St Louis, Mosby Yearbook, 1994.

Kovar PA, Allegrante JP, Mackenzie CR et al: Supervised fitness walking in patients with osteoarthritis of the knee: A randomized, controlled trial. *Ann Intern Med* 116:529–534, 1992.

PHYSICAL REHABILITATION IN ARTHRITIS, Joan M. Walker, PhD, PT, and Antoine Helewa, MSc(Clin Epid), PT, Elsevier Inc. © 2004.

Kraag G, Stokes B, Groh J et al: The effects of comprehensive home physiotherapy and supervision on patients with ankylosing spondylitis-an 8-month follow up. *J Rheumatol* 21:261–263, 1994.

Kuettner K et al (eds): *Articular Cartilage and Osteoarthritis.* New York, Raven Press, 1992.

Levy AS, Marmar E: The role of cold compression dressings in the postoperative treatment of total knee arthroplasty. *Clin Orthop* 297:174–178, 1993.

Lorig KR, Ritter P, Stewart AL et al: Chronic disease self-management program: 2-year health status and health care utilization outcomes. *Med Care* 39:1217–1223, 2001.

Lundon K: *Orthopedic Rehabilitation Science. Principles for Clinical Management of Nonmineralized Connective Tissue.* New York, Butterworth Heinemann, 2003.

McCain GA, Bell DA, Mai FM et al: A controlled study of the effects of a supervised cardiovascular fitness training program on the manifestations of primary fibromyalgia. *Arthritis Rheum* 31:1135–1141, 1988.

Melvin J, Jensen G (eds): *Rheumatologic Rehabilitation Series,* vols 1–5. Bethesda, MD, American Occupational Therapy Association, 1998–2000. (vol 1: *Assessment and Management,* 1998).

Melvin J, Wright V (eds): *Pediatric Rheumatic Diseases.* Bethesda, MD, American Occupational Therapy Association, 2002.

Minor MA, Kay DR. Arthritis. In Durstine JL, Moore GE (eds): *ACSM's Exercise Management for Persons with Chronic Diseases and Disabilities,* ed 2. Champaign, IL, Human Kinetics, 2003.

Moncur C: Physical therapy competencies in rheumatology. *Phys Ther* 65:1365–1372, 1985.

Mow VC, Radcliffe A: *Basic Orthopaedic Biomechanics,* ed 2. Philadelphia, Lippincott-Raven, 1997.

National Arthritis Data Workgroup: Arthritis prevalence and activity limitations. *Morb Mortal Weekly Rep* 4:433–438, 1994.

Newman S, Mulligan K: The psychology of rheumatic diseases. *Baillieres Best Pract Res Clin Rheumatol* 14:773–786, 2000.

Panush RS (ed): Complementary and alternative therapies for rheumatic disease. *Rheum Dis Clin,* Part I, 25:XIII-XVIII, November 1999; Part II, 21:XV-XX, February 2000.

Price LG, Hewett JE, Kay DR et al: Five-minute walking test of aerobic fitness for people with arthritis. *Arthritis Care Res* 1:33–37, 1988.

Rapoff MA: Evaluating and enhancing adherence to regimens for pediatric rheumatic diseases. In Melvin J, Wright V (eds): *Pediatric Rheumatic Diseases.* Bethesda, MD, American Occupational Therapy Association, 2002, pp 127–140.

Repchinsky C (ed): *CPS,* ed 37. Ottawa, ON, Canadian Pharmaceutical Association, 2002.

Riesman RP, Koran JR, Tail E, Ranker JJ: Patient education for adults with rheumatoid arthritis (Cochrane Review). *Cochrane Database Syst Rev* CD003688, 2002.

Robbins L et al (eds): *Clinical Care in the Rheumatic Diseases,* ed 2. Atlanta, Association of Rheumatology Health Professionals, American College of Rheumatology, 2001.

Ruddy S, Harris ED, Sledge CB et al (eds): *Kelley's Textbook of Rheumatology,* ed 6, vols 1 and 2. Philadelphia, WB Saunders, 2001.

Salter RB: *Continuous Passive Motion (CPM): A Biological Concept for the Healing and the Generation of Articular Cartilage, Ligaments, and Tendons: From its Origination to Research to Clinical Applications.* Baltimore, Williams & Wilkins, 1993.

Schlapbach P, Gerber NJ (eds): *Physiotherapy: Controlled Trials and Facts,* vol 14. Rheumatology, Basel, Karger, 1991.

Semble EL, Loeser RF, Wise CM: Therapeutic exercise for rheumatoid arthritis and osteoarthritis. *Semin Arthritis Rheum* 20:32–40, 1990.

Seymour R: *Prosthetics and Orthotics: Lower Limb and Spinal.* Philadelphia, Lippincott Williams & Wilkins, 2003.

Sheon RP, Moskowitz RW, Goldberg VM (eds): *Soft Tissue Rheumatic Pain: Recognition, Management, Prevention,* ed 3, vols I and II. Baltimore, Williams & Wilkins, 1996.

Smythe HA, Buskila D, Gladman DD: Performance of scored palpation, a point count, and dolorimetry in assessing unsuspected nonarticular tenderness. *J Rheumatol* 20:352–357, 1993.

Spilker B (ed): *Quality of Life: Assessments in Clinical Trials.* New York, Raven Press, 1990.

Stenstrom CH, Minor MA: Evidence for the benefit of strengthening and aerobic exercise in rheumatoid arthritis. *Arthritis Care Res* 49:428–434, 2003.

Stokes BA, Helewa A, Goldsmith CH et al: Reliability of spinal mobility measurements in ankylosing spondylitis patients. *Physiother Can* 40:338–344, 1988.

Trombly CA, Radomski MV (eds): *Occupational Therapy for Physical Dysfunction,* ed 5. Philadelphia, Lippincott Williams & Wilkins, 2002.

van Baar ME, Assendelft Wjj, Dekker J et al: Effectiveness of exercise therapy in patients with osteoarthritis of the hip or knee: A systematic review of randomized clinical trials. *Arthritis Rheum* 43:1361–1369, 1993.

Wolfe F, Pincus T (eds): *Rheumatoid Arthritis, Pathogenesis, Assessment, Outcome and Treatment.* New York, Marcel Dekker, 1994.

World Health Organization: 715. Osteoarthrosis and allied disorders. In *International Classification of Diseases,* rev 9, Clinical Modification (ICD-9-CM 2001), vols 1 and 3. Chicago, American Medical Association, 2002.

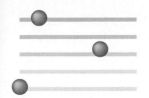

Glossary

accuracy A measurement that actually represents what it is intended to represent

active joint A joint considered to have active inflammation when any of three conditions are present: effusion, tenderness, or stress pain

ACR American College of Rheumatology, previously American Rheumatism Association

adherence Extent to which a person's behavior (e.g., follow diet, activity, splint use) corresponds to health advice; preferred term to *compliance*

aggrecan Grouping of collagen protein monomers in articular cartilage

AIMS Arthritis Impact Measurement Scales (not to be confused with Piper's AIMS for infants)

angiogenesis Formation of new blood vessels (neovascularization)

antalgic gait Person leans over painful hip when weight bearing to reduce contraction of painful hip abductors

ARA American Rheumatism Association, *former* name of the American College of Rheumatology

arteritis Inflammation of arteries

arthrodesis Surgical fusion of a joint

arthroplasty The operative procedure of reconstruction of a diseased joint

ASA Acetylsalicylic acid or aspirin

ARHP Association of Rheumatology Health Professionals (part of ACR, formerly ARA)

ASMC The Arthritis Self-Management Course (Arthritis Foundation, US)

avascular necrosis Cell/tissue death due to loss of blood supply

Baker's cyst Leakage of joint synovial fluid into an adjacent bursa, commonly seen at the knee due to increased intra-articular pressure, also popliteal cyst

bamboo spine Ossification of periphery of intervertebral discs, and spinal ligaments, seen on radiographs

BASFI Bath Ankylosing Spondylitis Functional Index

BASDAI Bath Ankylosing Spondylitis Disease Activity Index

Biologics Biological response modifiers, drugs with chemical messengers that coordinate the autoimmune process

Bouchard's nodes Osteophytes on the proximal interphalangeal (PIP) joints

boutonnière "Button hole" deformity of digit due to erosion of the central extensor mechanism over the proximal interphalangeal joint (PIP), flexion contractures of PIP with hyperextension of distal phalangeal (DIP) joint

Bunnell's sign Test to distinguish between synovitis of proximal interphalangeal joint (PIP) and spasm of intrinsic muscles

case control design A study that identifies persons with the disease of interest and a suitable control group of persons without the disease

CES-D The Center for Epidemiological Studies-Depression Scale

Chondroadherin Leucine-rich repeat protein

Clubbing Enlargement of distal digit pads with increased convexity of the nail and loss of normal angle between nail and cuticle; in fingers or toes

cock up deformity Dorsal subluxation of metatarsal phalangeal (MTP) joint(s)

COF Coefficient of friction, the shear force needed to make one surface slide on another divided by the normal force pressing them together

cohort study Prospective (forward in-time) study with two groups, one with the risk factor(s) and a matched control group without the risk factor(s); used to compare rates of disease occurrence or incidence between the two groups

complement system A group of 20 plasma proteins involved in the body's defense and immune systems

CPPD Calcium pyrophosphate dihydrate-crystal deposition disease

CRP C-reactive protein, a nonspecific indicator of the presence of inflammation

CPT Community physical therapy

crepitus Palpable or audible grating sensation produced by roughened surfaces rubbing against one another; articular or extra-articular, as in tendon sheaths

PHYSICAL REHABILITATION IN ARTHRITIS, Joan M. Walker, PhD, PT, and Antoine Helewa, MSc(Clin Epid), PT, Elsevier Inc. © 2004.

CTAP-III   A connective tissue activating protein

cytokines   Extracellular messenger proteins, peptide growth factors secreted by a variety of inflammatory cells with multiple biological activities (examples are transforming growth factor [TGF], platelet-derived growth factor [PDGF])

cytotoxic   Adverse effects on cells, associated with drug therapy

Damage-Duration Index   Index of rate of destruction; number of "damaged" joints divided by disease duration, in years

De Quervain's tenosynovitis   Inflammation and stenosis of tendon sheaths at base of thumb

débridement   Surgical cleaning of debris in a joint

decordin   Interstial proteoglycan-associated molecule that can bind to collagen

DMARDs   Disease-modifying antirheumatic drugs (also slow-acting antirheumatic drugs [SAARDs])

Dupuytren's contracture   Thickening and contractures of palmar aponeurosis causing severe flexion of the fourth and fifth fingers

enthesis   Ligament-bone junction

epidemiology   The study of the distribution and determinants of health-related states and events in populations and the application of this study to the control of health problems

ESR   Erythrocyte sedimentation rate, a nonspecific indicator of the presence of inflammation

fibromyalgia tender points   Characteristic "active" sites that are tender and can be distinguished from equally characteristic "control" points that are nontender

fibromodulin   Collagen-binding protein

fibromyalgia (FM)   Widespread pain and tenderness at 11 or more of 18 defined sites

FSI   Functional Status Index

genu recurvatum   Hyperextension of the knee (*genu*); the upper thigh (femur) and lower leg (tibia, fibula) are angled forward of the knee joint

genu valgus   Knock knees, lateral angulation of the leg in relation to the thigh and knee

genu varum   Bow legs, medial angulation of the leg in relation to the thigh and knee

hallax valgus   Lateral deviation of the phalanges at the first metatarsophalangeal (MTP) joint

hammer toes   Hyperextension of MTP joints with flexion or hyperextension of the distal interphalangeal (DIP) joints

HAQ   Health Assessment Questionnaire

hemarthrosis   Joint effusion containing blood products, forms rapidly

Heberden's nodes   Excessive bone formation (osteophytes) at joint margins, seen in digits (especially distal interphalangeal [DIP] joints) of clients with osteoarthritis

hemosiderin   An iron blood corpuscle pigment

HLA-B27   Histocompatibility antigen found in clients with ankylosing spondylitis, indicator of relative risk when present (positive)

hydroxyapatites   Crystals of calcium salts

hyperplasia   Increase in cell number

hypertrophy   Increase in size

hyperuricemia   Supersaturation of urate in serum, seen in gout

IAP   Intra-articular pressure within intact joint cavity, normally negative

IGF-I, IGF-II   Insulin-like growth factors

IL-1   Interleukin-1, a pro-inflammatory mediator

incidence   Rate of occurrence of new cases of a disease during a given period, in a defined population at risk

inflammatory arthritis   Damage to a joint characterized by a process of inflammation

intra-articular therapy   Injection of drugs directly into a joint

iontophoresis   Topical administration of active drug ions that can be driven through the skin by a continuous direct current

JA   Juvenile arthritis, also known as juvenile rheumatoid arthritis, juvenile idiopathic arthritis

JAFAR   Juvenile Arthritis Functional Assessment Report

JAQQ   Juvenile Arthritis Quality of Life Questionnaire

JASI   Juvenile Arthritis Functional Status Index

JIA   Juvenile idiopathic arthritis

JRA   Juvenile rheumatoid arthritis, also known as juvenile arthritis, juvenile idiopathic arthritis

keratocan   Nonproteoglycan protein that can bind to collagen

keratoconjunctivitis   Impaired secretion of tears, dry eyes, part of Sjögren's syndrome

lubricin   Glycoprotein found in synovial fluid

lumican   Proteoglycan collagen associated molecule

mallet deformity   Deformity of DIP joint, results from attenuation or rupture of distal extensor attachment

microklutziness   Type of incoordination and proposed mechanism for damage by repetitive impulse loading

N of 1 study   Entire experiment within a single patient including randomization of intervention(s)

NSAIDs   Nonsteroidal anti-inflammatory drugs

Onycholysis   Pitting of nails and dystrophic changes in psoriatic arthritis

Opera-glass hand (la main en lorgnette)   Shortening (telescoping) of digits produced by destruction and resorption of the ends of the phalanges

orthotic (splints)   Externally applied devices that support/protect/stabilize a joint or enhance its function

osteoarthritis (degenerative joint disease, osteoarthrosis)   Process characterized by thinning and destruction of articular cartilage, remodeling of bony surfaces

osteopenia   Radiological term for thinning or deficiency of bone (not synonymous with osteoporosis)

osteophyte   Formation of new bone at joint margins (bony spur)

osteoporosis   Decreased bone density, increased bone fragility and fractures

paleopathology   The study of disease and trauma in extinct societies

pannus   Inflammatory fibrinous exudate, highly vascular, contains several cell types, spreads over joint surfaces, and destroys articular cartilage; characteristic of rheumatoid arthritis

PAR-Q Physical Activity Readiness Questionnaire

pauciarticular Arthritis involving four or fewer joints

photophobia Intolerance of light

pencil and cup deformity Results from joint erosion, tapering of proximal phalanx, and bony proliferation of distal phalanx; seen on radiographs of clients with psoriatic arthritis

Phalen's sign Numbness or paraesthesias in distribution of the median nerve

polyarticular Arthritis involving five or more joints

precision A measurement that has nearly the same value each time it is measured; related concepts are reliability and consistency

PRELP Basic leucine-rich repeat nonproteoglycan protein found in connective tissues

prevalence The proportion of cases identified in a population at a given point in *time (point prevalence)* or during a specified interval *(period prevalence),* or at any time *(lifetime prevalence)*

PT Physical therapy, physiotherapy, physical therapist, physiotherapist

randomized clinical trial (RCT) An experiment in which subjects are allocated at random to two or more groups to receive different interventions or a placebo

reactive arthritis Nonsuppurative inflammatory process due to an infectious process at a distance from the primary process

reliability (consistency) The degree of stability in a measurement, when repeated under identical conditions; the degree to which a measure is free of random error

reproducibility Ability to achieve the same response/outcome in repeated trials (test-retest reliability or stability over time)

responsiveness Ability of a measures to detect *clinically important change,* after application of a treatment maneuver

rheumatoid factor Antibody (usually of IgM isotype) that reacts with antigenic determinants on the immunoglobulin molecule, an anti-antibody

rheumatoid nodules Cutaneous signs of subcutaneous nodules in tendons or ligaments; rarely on deep structures (e.g., vocal cords, heart valves)

RIL Repetitive impulsive loading, excessive mechanical loading

Romanus lesions Bone erosions at anterior margin vertebral bodies

Schöber test In the erect position a mark is made at S1 and another mark 10 cm above; subject flexes the spine and the change in distance between the two marks is recorded

Sclerodactyly Tight shiny atrophic appearance of digits in scleroderma

scleroderma (systemic sclerosis) Generalized disorder of collagen

sclerosis Thickening

sensitivity Ability to detect true positives in diagnostic tests

septic arthritis Due to a bacterial infection

seronegative arthritis Inflammatory arthritic conditions in which results of the serological test for rheumatoid factor are characteristically negative

SLE Systemic lupus erythematosus, an inflammatory disease affecting many organs

specificity Ability to detect true negatives in diagnostic tests; having a defined and limited effect/outcome (i.e., drug therapy, exercise)

spondylitis Arthritis of the vertebral column

spondylolisthesis Slippage of one vertebra on the vertebra below

spondylolysis Separation of pars interarticularis that allows vertebra slippage on the one below

Still's disease JRA with a systemic onset

Swan-neck deformity Deformity of digit due to "bowstringing" of the collateral ligaments causing combined hyperextension of proximal interphalangeal (PIP) joints and flexion of distal interphalangeal (DIP) joints

syndesmophytes Bony bridges between vertebral bodies due to calcification then ossification of outer fibers of the annulus

synovectomy Removal of synovial tissues by surgery

synovial lining tissue (SLT) Term that has replaced the former inappropriate "synovial membrane"; covers most intra-articular structures

tidemark Junction between the uncalcified and calcified layers of articular cartilage

Tinel's sign Tingling in median nerve distribution, often seen with carpal tunnel syndrome

TNF Tumor necrosis factor, a pro-inflammatory mediator

tophi Deposits of monosodium urate crystals in and around joints in gouty arthritis

validity Degree to which a test measures what it purports to measure, concept related to accuracy

VAS Visual Analogue Scale, a line of known length on which clients score their symptoms

vasculitis Inflammation of blood vessels

WOMAC Western Ontario and McMaster Universities Osteoarthritis Index

xerophthalmia Dry eyes (keratoconjunctivitis) due to chronic inflammation of lacrimal and salivary glands

xerostomia Dry mouth due to impaired secretions of salivary glands

"zigzag" deformity In hand, radial deviation of carpus at wrist with radial angulation of metacarpals and ulnar deviation at metacarpophalangeal (MCP) joints

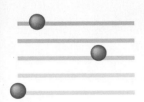

Index

Page numbers followed by "f" indicates figures, "t" indicates tables.